AF905276

Atlas of Diagnostic Imaging in Dermatology

Clarissa Canella Moraes do Carmo
Editor

Ana Luisa Sampaio • Robertha Nakamura
André da Silva Cartell • Bruna Duque-Estrada
Associate Editors

Atlas of Diagnostic Imaging in Dermatology

A Practical Approach

Springer

Editor
Clarissa Canella Moraes do Carmo, MD, MS, PhD, Post-doc
Radiology
Universidade Federal Fluminense – UFF and Clínica CDPI and ALTA
Rio de Janeiro, Brazil

Associate Editors
Ana Luisa Sampaio, MD, MS
Dermatologist in Private Practice
Rio de Janeiro, Brazil

Dermatologist at State University of Rio de Janeiro (UERJ)
Pedro Ernesto Hospital (HUPE)
Rio de Janeiro, Brazil

André da Silva Cartell, MD, MS, PhD
Adjunct Professor at Faculdade de Medicina da Universidade Federal do Rio Grande do Sul
Rio de Janeiro, Brazil

Dermatologist and Dermatopathologist in Private Practice
Rio de Janeiro, Brazil

Robertha Nakamura, MD, MS
Coordinator of the Center for Nail Studies at the Institute of Dermatology Professor Rubem David Azulay
Rio de Janeiro, Brazil

Bruna Duque-Estrada, MD, MS
Universidade Federal de São Paulo
Rio de Janeiro, Brazil

Professor in the Hair Disorders Department at the Instituto de Dermatologia Professor Rubem David Azulay
Rio de Janeiro, Brazil

ISBN 978-3-031-77986-2 ISBN 978-3-031-77987-9 (eBook)
https://doi.org/10.1007/978-3-031-77987-9

© The Editor(s) (if applicable) and The Author(s), under exclusive license to Springer Nature Switzerland AG 2025

This work is subject to copyright. All rights are solely and exclusively licensed by the Publisher, whether the whole or part of the material is concerned, specifically the rights of translation, reprinting, reuse of illustrations, recitation, broadcasting, reproduction on microfilms or in any other physical way, and transmission or information storage and retrieval, electronic adaptation, computer software, or by similar or dissimilar methodology now known or hereafter developed.
The use of general descriptive names, registered names, trademarks, service marks, etc. in this publication does not imply, even in the absence of a specific statement, that such names are exempt from the relevant protective laws and regulations and therefore free for general use.
The publisher, the authors and the editors are safe to assume that the advice and information in this book are believed to be true and accurate at the date of publication. Neither the publisher nor the authors or the editors give a warranty, expressed or implied, with respect to the material contained herein or for any errors or omissions that may have been made. The publisher remains neutral with regard to jurisdictional claims in published maps and institutional affiliations.

This Springer imprint is published by the registered company Springer Nature Switzerland AG
The registered company address is: Gewerbestrasse 11, 6330 Cham, Switzerland

If disposing of this product, please recycle the paper.

Clarissa Canella Moraes do Carmo
To my father, Marco Antonio (in memoriam), always awaiting the day of our reunion.
To my mother, Ellyete, for being my example and love.
To my husband, Guilherme, for the complicity, love, and unconditional support.
To my children, Maria Clara, Beatriz, and Felipe, for being my world, my life, and the reason for everything.

Ana Luisa Sampaio
To Thiago Jeunon, who supports me in every moment and shares his life with me.
To my family, for their constant support.
To Luna Azulay and Alexandre Gripp, my inspiring teachers.
To Vivi, Maria, Haizza, Paulinha, Camila, and Dani, who were exceptional partners in the development of the chapters.

André da Silva Cartell
To my parents, Oscar Cartell (in memoriam) and Edir Valente (in memoriam).

Bruna Duque-Estrada
To God for the wisdom, strength, and inspiration.

To my parents who taught me that study, ethics, and constant hard work always prevail.
To my wonderful family, Leandro, Arthur, and Antonia, who support me unconditionally and understand the many hours dedicated to study and work.
To my great and inspiring mentors, Celso Sodré, Antonella Tosti, and Sergio Hirata.
To all the colleagues who contributed by sharing cases that enriched our work, especially Dr. Clarissa Canella, and to my collaborators Maria Carolina Zafra, Lara Franceschetto, Bruna Barroso, and Ana Letícia Boff for their dedication to the sections on hair diseases.

Robertha Nakamura
To my parents, Marlly de Carvalho and Hugo Nakamura, for teaching me that dreams are achieved through dedication and continuous learning.
To my mentor, Professor Robert Baran, whose example continues to inspire me.
To my dear friends and fellow explorers in the world of nails, Andreia Leverone, Nathália Matos, and Renata Villa Verde, whose support and camaraderie have been invaluable throughout this journey.

Preface

Dermatologic imaging is a growing field worldwide, encompassing everything from dermatologic lesions to aesthetic alterations. Advances in technology have enabled the use of high and ultra-high frequency ultrasonography probes, making it possible to visualize and analyze complex, millimeter-scale skin structures. It is important to remember that dermatologic imaging is not limited to ultrasonography. Magnetic resonance imaging is a powerful tool, allowing for the accurate analysis of structures through dynamic and functional sequences. Moreover, this imaging method now enables the generation of 3D images, biomodel printing, and the analysis of cases in virtual and augmented reality, utilizing all available technology to provide our patients the best possible treatment, with quality, precision, and accuracy.

I emphasize that clinical evaluation is paramount, and to correctly assess the image of a dermatologic lesion, it is essential to access clinical data, analyze the lesion, and have a basic understanding of dermatology. This atlas was designed with the intention of making the reader's routine easier and more practical, enabling quick consultation of the clinical, histopathological, and radiological aspects of the main dermatologic lesions, including conventional radiography, computed tomography, high-frequency ultrasonography, magnetic resonance imaging with surface coil, and 3D virtual images. With the help of the best team I could ask for, we created overlay indications on more than 600 images to make the consultation more educational, eliminating the need for long and complex captions. The division of chapters by body region were conceived with practical radiologic reasoning in mind, as applied in real-life clinical scenarios – the same approach I strive to teach my residents every day.

Love, dedication, persistence, and resilience sum up this atlas. I hope you enjoy reading it and that it inspires you to share in my passion I for diagnostic imaging of dermatologic lesions.

Rio de Janeiro, Brazil — Clarissa Canella Moraes do Carmo

Acknowledgments

To my children, Maria Clara (Aiaia), Beatriz (Naná), and Felipe (Badiba), for all the moments we weren't together, with the certainty that I will be a source of great pride for you one day. You are the reason for everything.

To my husband, Guilherme, for the patience and encouragement during the most difficult times. Thank you for being by my side in joy and sorrow, in health and in sickness, every day of my life.

I thank my mother, Ellyete, for being my greatest professional example and for providing me with the opportunity to acquire all the knowledge I have today, always standing by my side.

To my father, Marco Antônio (in memoriam), for the values he taught me, the greatest of which was resilience, following his premature and unexpected passing.

To my dear stepmother, Maria Cláudia, for always being an excellent second mother and for giving me a wonderful brother, Rafael, a life partner.

To my grandmothers, Elly (in memoriam) and Terezinha (in memoriam), wherever they may be, awaiting our reunion.

To my eternal residents, who made this dream possible, Carolina, Jessica, Ludmila, Priscila, Philippe, Weydler, and Tatiana.

To the friends and co-editors of this atlas, Ana Luisa, Andre, Bruna, and Robertha, who accepted this challenge and embarked on this crazy, exhausting, and rewarding journey with me.

To the friends I admire so much personally and professionally, Silvana Mendonça, Flavia Costa, Marcelo Bordalo, and Rodrigo Aguiar, gratitude for your support, encouragement, and generosity.

To all the teachers who have been a part of my life, each leaving their mark and teaching, contributing to my education, especially Professor Erica Braga Jorge, for the time we spent together in middle school.

To my great mentors, Professors Anne Cotten, Donald Resnick, and Edson Marchiori, for embracing me with total dedication, competence, attention, and kindness. I will be eternally grateful for teaching me and inspiring my love for scientific work and academic life.

To the professional colleagues, friends and family who make life light, fun, and at the same time are a support during turbulent moments.

To my patients, who teach me much more than medicine every day.

Contents

Part II Scalp

Part III Face, Ears and Nose

Editors and Contributors

About the Editors

Clarissa Canella Moraes do Carmo, MD, MS, PhD, Post-doc Adjunct Professor of Radiology at the Fluminense Federal University – UFF

Invited Professor in the Postgraduate Program in Radiology at the Federal University of Rio de Janeiro – UFRJ

Radiologist specializing in Dermatology and Musculoskeletal Imaging at DASA – RJ

Coordinator of the Medical Residency and Specialization Program in Radiology at DASA – Rio de Janeiro

Master's degree in Radiology from the Federal University of Rio de Janeiro – UFRJ

PhD's degree in Radiology from the Federal University of Rio de Janeiro – UFRJ

Postdoctoral degree in Radiology from the Federal University of São Paulo – UNIFESP

Scientific Researcher at the Biodesign Laboratory from DASA-PUC

Coordinator of the Outreach Program of the International Skeletal Society – ISS

Bruna Duque-Estrada, MD, MS Dermatologist in Private Practice – Clinica BCM Dermatologia Especializada

Professor of the Hair Diseases Department at Instituto de Dermatologia Prof. Rubem David Azulay – SCMRJ

Post-graduate in Dermatology at Instituto de Dermatologia Prof. Rubem David Azulay – SCMRJ

Master in Medicine (recognized equivalence) at University of Porto, Portugal

Master's degree in Internal Medicine and Dermatology from the Federal University of Rio de Janeiro – UFRJ

PhD fellow at Universidade Federal de São Paulo, Brazil

Board certified Dermatologist by the Brazilian Society of Dermatology – SBD

Member of the International Trichoscopy Society

Ana Luisa Bittencourt Sampaio Jeunon Vargas, MD, MS Dermatologist in Private Practice

Medical Residency in Internal Medicine at Universidade Federal do Rio de Janeiro – UFRJ

Medical Residency in Dermatology at State University of Rio de Janeiro – UERJ

Master's degree in Internal Medicine and Dermatology from the Federal University of Rio de Janeiro – UFRJ

PhD student at the Faculty of Medical Sciences – State University of Rio de Janeiro – UERJ

Board-certified in Dermatology by Sociedade Brasileira de Dermatologia – SBD

Robertha Carvaho Nakamura, MD, MS Dermatologist in Private Practice

Professor of the Centro de Estudos das Unhas – CEU at Instituto de Dermatologia Prof. Rubem David Azulay – SCMRJ

Medical Residency in Internal Medicine at Santa Casa da Midericórdia do Rio de Janeiro – SCMRJ

Medical Residency in Dermatology at Instituto de Dermatologia Prof. Rubem David Azulay – SCMRJ

Master's degree in Internal Medicine and Dermatology from the Federal University of Rio de Janeiro – UFRJ

Board certified Dermatologist by the Brazilian Society of Dermatology – SBD

André da Silva Cartell, MD, MS, PhD Dermatolophatologist in Private Practice

Preceptor of the Medical Residency Program in Pathology at the Hospital de Clínicas de Porto Alegre

Professor at the Federal University of Rio Grande do Sul – UFRS

Board certified Dermatologist by the Brazilian Society of Dermatology – SBD

Contributors

André da Silva Cartell, MD, MS, PhD Adjunct Professor at Faculdade de Medicina da Universidade Federal do Rio Grande do Sul, Rio de Janeiro, Brazil
Dermatologist and Dermatopathologist in Private Practice, Rio de Janeiro, Brazil

Ana Luisa Sampaio, MD, MS Department of Dermatology, Hospital Universitario Pedro Ernesto, Universidade Estadual do Rio de Janeiro—UERJ, Rio de Janeiro, Brazil

Felipe Aguinaga, MD Instituto de Dermatologia Professor Rubem David Azulay, Santa Casa da Misericórdia do Rio de Janeiro, Rio de Janeiro, RJ, Brazil
Department of Dermatology, Hospital Universitario Pedro Ernesto, Universidade Estadual do Rio de Janeiro—UERJ, Rio de Janeiro, Brazil

Alessandro Aita, MD, MS Musculoskeletal and Dermatological Imaging, Universidade Federal do Piaui—UFPI Ininga, Teresina, Brazil

Vinicius Arcoverde, MS Biodesign Lab DASA—PUC—Rio de Janeiro, Rio de Janeiro, RJ, Brazil

Luna Azulay, MD, MS, PhD Professor Rubem David Azulay Institute of Dermatology—Santa Casa RJ, Rio de Janeiro, RJ, Brazil
State University of Rio de Janeiro—UERJ, Pedro Ernesto Hospital—HUPE, Rio de Janeiro, RJ, Brazil

Thaís Emanuelle Freire Barbosa, MD Marcilio Dias Naval Hospital and National Cancer Institute—INCA, Rio de Janeiro, RJ, Brazil

Ana Leticia Boff, MD Santa Casa Hospital, Porto Alegre, RS, Brazil
Dermathopathologist Private Practice, Clinica Dermapat, Porto Alegre, RS, Porto Alegre, RS, Brazil

Caroline Brandão, MD, MS Oncological Dermatology Gávea, Rio de Janeiro, Brazil

Leonardo Rodrigues Campos, MD, MS Department of Pediatric Rheumatology, Antônio Pedro University Hospital—UFF, Niterói, RJ, Brazil

Ana Paula Kunning Casqueiro, MD Clinica Multi-Imagem Ipanema—RJ, Rio de Janeiro, RJ, Brazil
Musculoskeletal Imaging at DASA—RJ, Rio de Janeiro, RJ, Brazil

Miguel Angel Ceccarelli, MD Nail Diseases Outpatient Clinic at Dermatology Department, Hospital Universitário Pedro Ernesto—Universidade Estadual do Rio de Janeiro—UERJ, Maracanã, Rio de Janeiro, Brazil

Mario Chaves, MD Department of Dermatology, Hospital Universitario Pedro Ernesto, Universidade Estadual do Rio de Janeiro—UERJ, Rio de Janeiro, Brazil
Dermatologic Surgery Outpatient Clinic at HCAP, Carlos Chagas Foundation, Rio de Janeiro, Brazil

Ana Maria Doffemond Costa, MD Clinica Ana Doffemond, Belo Horizonte, Brazil

Flavia Martins Costa, MD, MS, PhD Universidade Federal do Rio de Janeiro—UFRJ, Rio de Janeiro, Brazil
Department of Radiology, Diagnóstico das Americas—DASA—Rio de Janeiro, Rio de Janeiro, Brazil

Marina Ramos Costa, MD Instituto de Dermatologia Professor Rubem David Azulay- Santa Casa da Misericórdia do Rio de Janeiro, Rio de Janeiro, Brazil
State University of Rio de Janeiro—UERJ, Pedro Ernesto Hospital—HUPE, Rio de Janeiro, RJ, Brazil

Romer Braga da Silva, MD Rede Amil, DASA and Prevent—Rio de Janeiro, Centro, Rio de Janeiro, Brazil

Carolina Ávila de Almeida, MD, MS Faculty of Medicine of Valença—UniFaa, Valença, Brazil
Federal University of Rio de Janeiro—UFRJ, Rio de Janeiro, Brazil

Laila Klotz de Almeida Balassiano, MD, MS Sector of Dermatology and Post Graduate Course in Medical Clinics—UFRJ, Federal University of Rio de Janeiro, Rio de Janeiro, RJ, Brazil
Federal University of Rio de Janeiro—UFRJ, Rio de Janeiro, RJ, Brazil

Haizza Cristina de Almeida Cabral Monteiro, MD State University of Rio de Janeiro—UERJ, Pedro Ernesto Hospital—HUPE, Rio de Janeiro, RJ, Brazil
Department of Dermatology, Hospital Rio-Barra and Rede D'Or São Luiz, Rio de Janeiro, RJ, Brazil

Tatiana de Almeida Gonçalves Secco, MD Clinica de Diagnostico por Imagem and Fleury Group—RJ, Barra da Tijuca, Rio de Janeiro, Brazil
Musculoskeletal Imaging at DASA—RJ, Barra da Tijuca, Rio de Janeiro, Brazil

Marcia Castilho Farme de Amoedo, MD Private Dermatology Practice, Rio de Janeiro, Brazil

Daniel Cunha de Araújo, MD Hospital das Clínicas da Universidade de São Paulo—USP, Rio de Janeiro, Brazil
Hospital Universitário Pedro Ernesto, Universidade Estadual do Rio de Janeiro—UERJ, Rio de Janeiro, Brazil

Paula Figueiredo de Marsillac, MD, MS State University of Rio de Janeiro—UERJ, Hospital Universitário Pedro Ernesto, Rio de Janeiro, RJ, Brazil

Elisa de Oliveira Barcaui, MD, MS, PhD Ultrasonography, Clinica Dermatologica de Ipanema—CDI—Rio de Janeiro, Rio de Janeiro, RJ, Brazil

Julia de Oliveira Barcaui Souza Marques Faculty of Medicine, Rio de Janeiro, RJ, Brazil

Maria de Oliveira Buffara, MD State University of Rio de Janeiro—UERJ, Pedro Ernesto Hospital—HUPE, Rio de Janeiro, RJ, Brazil

Ellyete de Oliveira Canella, MD, MS Breast Radiology Center, Hospital Quinta d'Or São Cristóvão, Rio de Janeiro, Brazil

Priscilla Haui de Oliveira Galuzzi Fonseca, MD Clinica CDPI and ALTA—Rio de Janeiro, Barra da Tijuca, Rio de Janeiro, RJ, Brazil

Tadeu de Rezende Vergueiro, MD, MS Centro de Cirurgia da Pele Tijuca, Rio de Janeiro, Brazil

Fernanda Franco de Sá, MD Clinica Franco de Sa—Rio de Janeiro, Rio de Janeiro, RJ, Brazil

Marcos Decnop, MD Department of Radiology, Instituto Nacional De Cancer—INCA, Centro, Rio de Janeiro, Brazil

Gabriella di Giunta, MD, MS, PhD Federal University of Santa Catarina, Florianópolis, SC, Brazil

Marcelo Bragança dos Reis Oliveira Seba, MD, MS, PhD Universidade Federal do Rio de Janeiro—UFRJ, Rio de Janeiro, Brazil
Trauma-Orthopaedics Service, Orthopaedic Oncology, Federal University of Rio de Janeiro—UFRJ, Rio de Janeiro, Brazil

Ana Beatriz Vargas dos Santos, MD, PhD State University of Rio de Janeiro—UERJ, Pedro Ernesto Hospital—HUPE, Rio de Janeiro, RJ, Brazil

Ludmila do Valle Vieira Gusmão, MD Marcilio Dias Naval Hospital, Dermatological Imaging Department of DASA – Rio de Janeiro, Rio de Janeiro, Brazil

Alejandra Galeano España, MD Clinica Dermobarra, Rio de Janeiro, Brazil

Tatiana Fazecas, MD, MS Radiology Department, Hospital Municipal Jesus—HMJ and Diagnósticos da América—DASA, Rio de Janeiro, Brazil

Luiza Feres, MD Clinica Vanessa Metz, Ipanema—Rio de Janeiro, Galeria Fórum de Ipanema, Rio de Janeiro, Brazil

Rodrigo Gaudio, MD, MS Antônio Pedro University Hospital—UFF, Niterói, RJ, Brazil
Autoimmunity Center (NAI)—AMIL, Niterói, RJ, Brazil

André Francisco Gomes, MD Clinica Diagnóstico Avançado por Imagem—DAPI—Curitiba, Curitiba, Brazil

Michelle Azevedo Gomes, MD, MS Head and Neck Oncological Surgery, National Institute of Cancer—INCA, Rio de Janeiro, Brazil

Bruna Barroso Gonçalves, MD Hair Diseases Department, Instituto de Dermatologia Professor Rubem David Azulay - Santa Casa de Misericórdia do Rio de Janeiro, Rio de Janeiro, Brazil

Simone Guarçoni, MD Clinica ALTA—Rio de Janeiro, Botafogo, Brazil

Livia Guidoni, MD DERMUS Specialized Ultrasound, Hospital Universitario Cassiano Antonio Moraes—UFES Santos Dumont, Vitória, Brazil

Manuela Boleira Sieiro Guimarães, MD, MS Dermatology Department, Policlinica Geral do Rio de Janeiro, Centro, Castelo, RJ, Brazil

Weydler Hottz, MD Clinica CDPI—DASA—Rio de Janeiro, Rio de Janeiro, RJ, Brazil

Matilde Iorizzo, MD, MS, PhD Private Dermatology Practice, Bellinzona, Switzerland

Veronica Rodrigues Bogado Leite, MD Hospital Universitario Antonio Pedro, Universidade Federal Fluminense—UFF, Niterói, Brazil

Andreia Pizarro Leverone, MD, MS Nail Study Center—Institute of Dermatology Professor Ruben David Azulay, Santa Casa da Misericórdia do Rio de Janeiro, Centro, Rio de Janeiro, RJ, Brazil

Renata Valente Lisboa, MD, MS Faculty of Medicine of Valença—Rio de Janeiro—UNIFAA, Valença, Brazil

Flávio Barbosa Luz, MD, MS, PhD Department of Dermatology, Universidade Federal Fluminense—UFF, Dermatologic Surgery and Mohs Micrographic Surgery—UFF, Centro de Cirurgia da Pele—Rio de Janeiro, Centro, Niterói, Brazil

Viviane Maria Maiolini, MD Faculty of Medicine, Cancer Institute of the State of São Paulo—ICESP, University of São Paulo—FMUSP, São Paulo, RJ, Brazil

Philippe Alcântara Gonçalves Martins, MD Bronstein DASA—Tijuca, Rio de Janeiro, Brazil
Américas Medical City, Barra da Tijuca, Rio de Janeiro, Brazil

Nathália Matos, MD Dermatology Department of Fundação de Medicina Tropical Doutor Heitor Vieira Dourado, Manaus, Brazil

Silvana Machado Mendonça, MD Clinica de Diagnostico por Imagem, Clinica Cavallieri, Barra da Tijuca, Rio de Janeiro, RJ, Brazil
Dermatology and Musculoskeletal Imaging at Diagnóstico das Américas—DASA—RJ, Rio de Janeiro, RJ, Brazil

Vanessa Metz, MD Clinica Vanessa Metz, Ipanema—Rio de Janeiro, Galeria Fórum de Ipanema, Rio de Janeiro, Brazil

Lara Franceschetto Milleri, MD BCM Dermatologia Especializada - Private Practice, Rio de Janeiro, Brazil

Fernada Miraldi, MD, MS Fonte Imagem Medicina Diagnóstica, Casa de Saúde São José and Fleury Group, Rio de Janeiro, Brazil

Robertha Nakamura, MD, MS Institute of Dermatology Professor Rubem David Azulay, Rio de Janeiro, RJ, Brazil
Dermatology by the Brazilian Society of Dermatology, Rio de Janeiro, RJ, Brazil
Dermatology from the Federal University of Medicine at Rio de Janeiro, Rio de Janeiro, RJ, Brazil
Nail Study Center—Institute of Dermatology Professor Ruben David Azulay, Santa Casa da Misericórdia do Rio de Janeiro, Rio de Janeiro, RJ, Brazil

Tatiana Venâncio Nakamura, MD Instituto Humanizare in Juína, Juína, Brazil

Mary Lane Alves Nemer, MD Clinica DERMUS—Ultrassonografia Especializada, Vitória, Brazil

Camila Silveira Nobre, MD Private Dermatology Practice, Rio de Janeiro, RJ, Brazil
State University of Rio de Janeiro—UERJ, Pedro Ernesto Hospital—HUPE, Rio de Janeiro, RJ, Brazil

Talita Caldas Oliveira, MD Department of Dermatology, Fluminense Federal University—UFF, Hospital Universitario Antonio Pedro—HUAP, Niterói, Brazil

Maria Carolina Zafra Páez, MD Zafra Dermatology Private Clinic, Rio de Janeiro, Brazil
BCM Dermatologia Especializada, Private Practice, Rio de Janeiro, Brazil

Fernanda Philadelpho Arantes Pereira, MD, MS, PhD Alta Excelência Diagnóstica and Clínica de Diagnóstico por Imagem DASA, Barra da Tijuca, Rio de Janeiro, Brazil

Izabela Machado Flores Pereira, MD Felício Rocho Hospital—FELUMA, Belo Horizonte, Brazil

Davi Berardo Porciuncula, MD Pathologist in Private Practice – Diagnósticos da América – DASA, Rio de Janeiro, Brazil

Jéssica Gonçalves Povill, MD Clinica de Diagnostico por Imagem, Dermatological Imaging at DASA, Barra da Tijuca, Rio de Janeiro, Brazil

Carolina Andrea Fernández Quiroga, MD, MS, PhD Internal Medicine Radiology and Dermatological Imaging, Cutaneous Ultrasound Unit, Dermatology Department, Hospital Moisès Broggi, Barcelona, Spain

Gerson Ribeiro, MS Biodesign Lab DASA—PUC—Rio de Janeiro, Rio de Janeiro, Brazil

Leila Riedel, MD Doppler Imaging Diagnostic Clinic—Niterói, Postgraduate Program in Dermatological Ultrasound at Lapidare—São Paulo, General Ultrasound at Unissom—Rio de Janeiro, Niterói, Brazil

Rachel Marina Sá Rosado, MD Dermatologist and Rheumatologist in Private Practice, Rio de Janeiro, RJ, Brazil

State University of Rio de Janeiro—UERJ, Pedro Ernesto Hospital—HUPE, Rio de Janeiro, RJ, Brazil

Felipe Mauricio Soeiro Sampaio, MD, MS Private Dermatology Practice, Rio de Janeiro, Brazil

Mariana Franco Ferraz Santino, MD, MS Dermatology Division, Universidade Federal do Rio de Janeiro—UFRJ, Rio de Janeiro, Brazil
Hospital São Vicente de Paulo and Hospital Copa D'or, Rio de Janeiro, Brazil

Stacy Smith, MD, MS, PhD Division of Musculoskeletal Imaging and Intervention at Brigham and Women's Hospital, Harvard Medical School, Boston, MA, USA

Roberto Souto, MD, MS Hospital Universitario Pedro Ernesto, Universidade Estadual do Rio de Janeiro—UERJ, Rio de Janeiro, Brazil

Ana Paula Stutz, MD Department of Radiology, Universidade Federal Fluminense—UFF, Centro, Niterói, Brazil

Curt Mafra Treu, MD, MS, PhD Department of Dermatologic Surgery and Cutaneous Oncology, Policlinica Geral do Rio de Janeiro—PGRJ and Hospital Federal de Bonsucesso, Castelo, Brazil

Renata Brandão Villa Verde, MD Marcilio Dias Naval Hospital, Lins de Vasconcelos, Rio de Janeiro, RJ, Brazil

Glauber Voltan, MD, MS, PhD Instituto Humanizare in Juína, NervUS Project, Juína, Brazil

Heron Werner, MD, MS, PhD Clinica ALTA—DASA—Rio de Janeiro, Rio de Janeiro, RJ, Brazil
Universidade Federal do Rio de Janeiro—UFRJ, Rio de Janeiro, RJ, Brazil
Biodesign Lab DASA—PUC—Rio de Janeiro, Rio de Janeiro, Brazil

Ximena Wortsman, MD, MS, PhD Faculty of Medicine, Department of Dermatology, Universidad de Chile, Santiago, Chile
Department of Dermatology, School of Medicine, Pontificia Universidad Catolica de Chile, Santiago, Chile
Department of Dermatology and Cutaneous Surgery, Miller School of Medicine, University of Miami, Miami, FL, USA
Institute for Diagnostic Imaging and Research of the Skin and Soft Tissues, Santiago, Chile

Julia Diva Zavariz, MD Radiology Institute of Clinical Hospital, São Paulo University, Cerqueira César, São Paulo, Brazil

Clarissa Canella Moraes do Carmo, MD, MS, PhD, Post-doc Fluminense Federal University—UFF, Rio de Janeiro, Brazil
Federal University of Rio de Janeiro—UFRJ, Rio de Janeiro, Brazil
Diagnóstico das Américas—DASA—RJ, Rio de Janeiro, Brazil
Biodesign Laboratory, DASA-PUC, Rio de Janeiro, Brazil

Bruna Duque-Estrada, MD, MS BCM Dermatologia Especializada, Private Practice, Rio de Janeiro, Brazil
Universidade Federal de São Paulo, São Paulo, Brazil
Hair Diseases Department, Instituto de Dermatologia Professor Rubem David Azulay – Santa Casa da Misericórdia do Rio de Janeiro, Rio de Janeiro, Brazil

Part I
Anatomy

Chapter 1
Anatomy of Skin: Clinical, Imaging, and Histological Aspects

Ana Luisa Sampaio, André da Silva Cartell, Ludmila do Valle Vieira Gusmão, Carolina Ávila de Almeida, Luiza Feres, Vanessa Metz, Fernanda Franco de Sá, and Clarissa Canella Moraes do Carmo

Understanding skin anatomy goes beyond just what we see on the surface. This chapter introduces the basics of skin structure by looking at it in three different ways: histology, ultrasonography, and MRI with surface coil. Histology is like taking a close-up look under a microscope, where we can see the different layers of the

A. L. Sampaio
Department of Dermatology, Hospital Universitario Pedro Ernesto, Universidade Estadual do Rio de Janeiro—UERJ, Rio de Janeiro, Brazil

A. da Silva Cartell
Adjunct Professor at Faculdade de Medicina da Universidade Federal do Rio Grande do Sul, Rio de Janeiro, Brazil

Dermatologist and Dermatopathologist in Private Practice, Rio de Janeiro, Brazil

L. do Valle Vieira Gusmão
Marcilio Dias Naval Hospital, Dermatological Imaging Department of DASA - Rio de Janeiro, Rio de Janeiro, Brazil

C. Á. de Almeida
Faculty of Medicine of Valença—UniFaa, Valença, Brazil

Federal University of Rio de Janeiro—UFRJ, Rio de Janeiro, Brazil

L. Feres · V. Metz
Clinica Vanessa Metz, Ipanema—Rio de Janeiro, Galeria Fórum de Ipanema, Rio de Janeiro, Brazil

F. F. de Sá
Clinica Franco de Sa—Rio de Janeiro, Rio de Janeiro, RJ, Brazil

C. Canella Moraes do Carmo (✉)
Fluminense Federal University—UFF, Rio de Janeiro, Brazil

Federal University of Rio de Janeiro—UFRJ, Rio de Janeiro, Brazil

Diagnóstico das Américas—DASA—RJ, Rio de Janeiro, Brazil

Biodesign Laboratory, DASA-PUC, Rio de Janeiro, Brazil

© The Author(s), under exclusive license to Springer Nature Switzerland AG 2025

C. Canella Moraes do Carmo (ed.), *Atlas of Diagnostic Imaging in Dermatology*,
https://doi.org/10.1007/978-3-031-77987-9_1

skin and how they are made up of tiny cells. Ultrasonography allows us to see inside the skin, showing us the different layers and any changes or issues that might be happening. MRI with surface coil, on the other hand, gives us a very detailed picture of the skin, showing even deeper layers and structures. By combining these three methods, we get a full understanding of how the skin is built and how it works. This chapter is useful for anyone studying or working with skin, as it explains the important details of skin anatomy in a clear and simple way.

1.1 Anatomy [1, 2]

- The skin, the largest organ of the human body, plays essential functions and presents a complex structure composed of different layers and cells.
- The skin consists of three layers:
  - the epidermis
  - the dermis
  - the hypodermis, which is composed of subcutaneous adipose tissue and in some areas, it may contain striated muscle, the dartos, as in the nipple and scrotal sac.
- Significant variation in skin thickness, ranging from less than 1.0 mm on the eyelids to 4.0 mm on the back.
- The skin presents different anatomical features, such as glabrous, non-glabrous (hairy), volar, acral, anogenital, photoexposed, and non-photoexposed skin.

1.1.1 Epidermis (Fig. 1.1)

- The epidermis is a keratinized stratified squamous epithelium.
- It is composed of five layers:
  - Stratum corneum (horny layer): The outermost layer, made up of dead, flattened cells that are filled with keratin. These cells continuously shed and are replaced by new cells from the layers below.
  - Stratum lucidum (clear layer): This thin, clear layer is only present in thick skin, such as the palms of the hands and soles of the feet. It provides an extra layer of protection.
  - Stratum granulosum (granular layer): In this layer, the skin cells begin to flatten and accumulate keratin, a protein that provides a protective barrier. The cells also start to die as they move toward the surface.

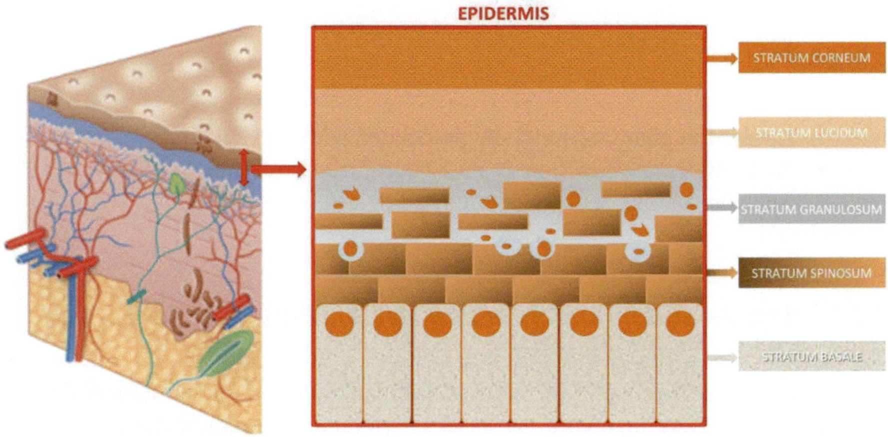

Fig. 1.1 Diagram illustrating the structure of human skin, focusing on the epidermis layer. The left side shows a cross-section of the skin, highlighting layers and blood vessels. The right side zooms into the epidermis, detailing its five layers: stratum corneum, stratum lucidum, stratum granulosum, stratum spinosum, and stratum basale. Each layer is labeled and depicted with distinct colors and textures to represent their unique characteristics

  - Stratum spinosum (spiny layer): Above the basal layer, this layer provides strength and flexibility to the skin. The cells here are connected by desmosomes, which give them a spiny appearance under a microscope.
  - Stratum basale (basal layer): This is the deepest layer, where new skin cells (keratinocytes) are generated. It also contains melanocytes, which produce the pigment melanin, giving skin its color.

- Keratinocytes are the most numerous cells in the epidermis, comprising approximately 80% of the epidermal population. The differentiation process of keratinocytes lasts an average of 28 days:
- There are other different cell types in epidermis, accounting for 20% of epidermal population:

  - Melanocytes:

    - Dendritic cells producing melanin, located in the basal layer.
    - Melanin protects proliferative cells in the skin against ultraviolet radiation and has antioxidant functions.
    - Transfer of melanin to keratinocytes occurs by apocopation.
    - The number of melanocytes varies between 500 and 2000/mm^2, decreasing with age.

  - Langerhans cells:

    - Immunological dendritic cells account for 2–3% of the epidermal population.

    - Located in the upper half of the epidermis and involved in presenting antigens to T lymphocytes.
  - Merkel cells:
    - Located in glabrous areas and associated with nerve fibers.
    - Neuroendocrine function as slow neuroreceptors.
    - Specific staining with cytokeratin 20.

1.1.2 Dermo-Epidermal Junction (DEJ) (Figs. 1.2 and 1.3) [3]

- Also known as the zone of the basal membrane or dermo-epidermal junction.
- Complex structure involving the basal membrane of keratinocytes and dermal collagen.
- The thickness of the basal membrane varies between 60 and 140 nanometers.
- Layers of the dermo-epidermal junction:
  - Basal layer of keratinocyte: Hemidesmosomes and anchoring filaments.
  - Basal membrane
  - Lucid layer: Contains antigens of bullous pemphigoid, laminin, and fibronectin.
  - Dense Layer: Collagen type IV.
  - Sublamina densa

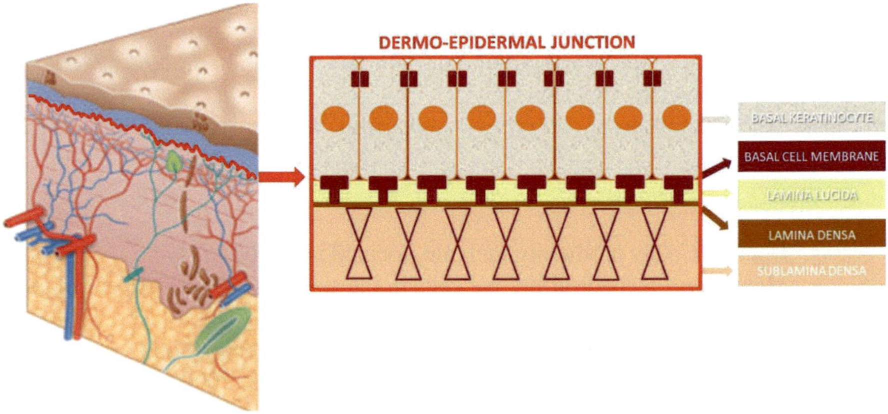

Fig. 1.2 The image illustrates the structure of the skin, focusing on the dermo-epidermal junction. On the left, a cross-section of the skin shows layers including the epidermis, dermis, and subcutaneous tissue, with visible blood vessels and nerve endings. On the right, a detailed diagram highlights the dermo-epidermal junction, labeling components such as basal keratinocyte, basal cell membrane, lamina lucida, lamina densa, and sublamina densa. The diagram emphasizes the connection between the epidermis and dermis

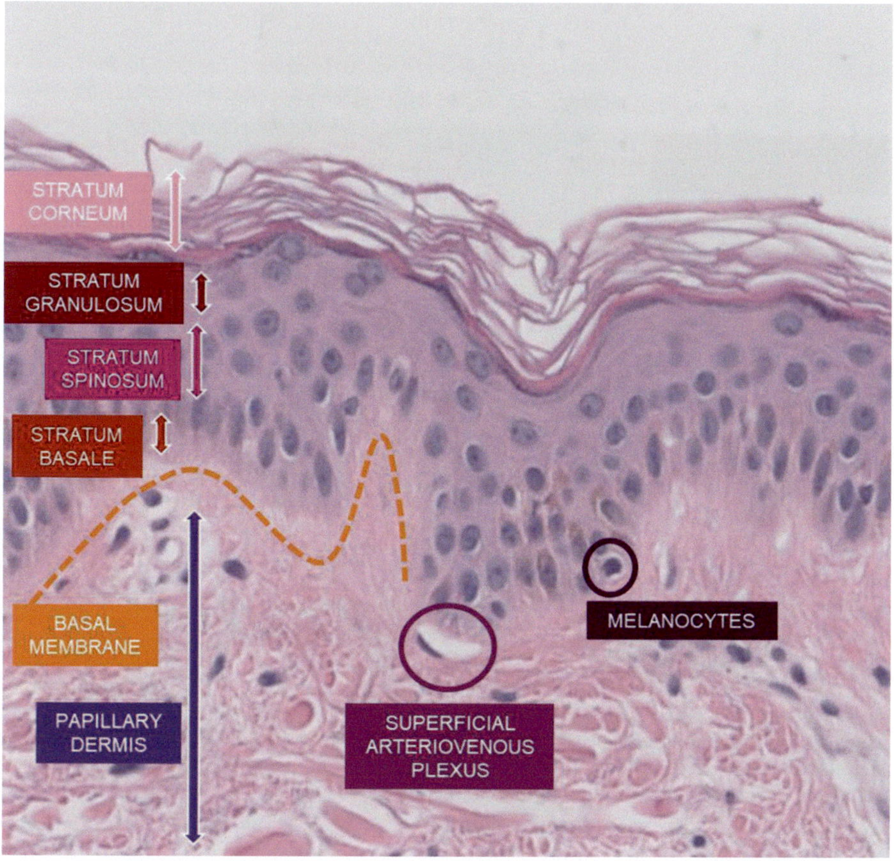

Fig. 1.3 A histological image of human skin layers, labeled with different strata (H&E X10). The outermost layer is the stratum corneum, followed by the stratum granulosum, stratum spinosum, and stratum basale. Below these is the basal membrane and the papillary dermis. The image highlights melanocytes and the superficial arteriovenous plexus. Each layer is color-coded and marked with arrows indicating their position and thickness

1.1.3 Dermis and Subcutaneous Adipose Tissue (Figs. 1.4, 1.5, 1.6, and 1.7) [4]

- Dermis aspects:
  - The dermis is primarily composed of collagen and elastin fibers. The papillary dermis contains Meissner's corpuscles (specialized sensory receptors), while sweat glands are mainly located in the deep reticular dermis and hypodermis.
  - Divided into
    - papillary dermis, that is rich in collagen types I and III, forming dermal ridges or rete ridges.

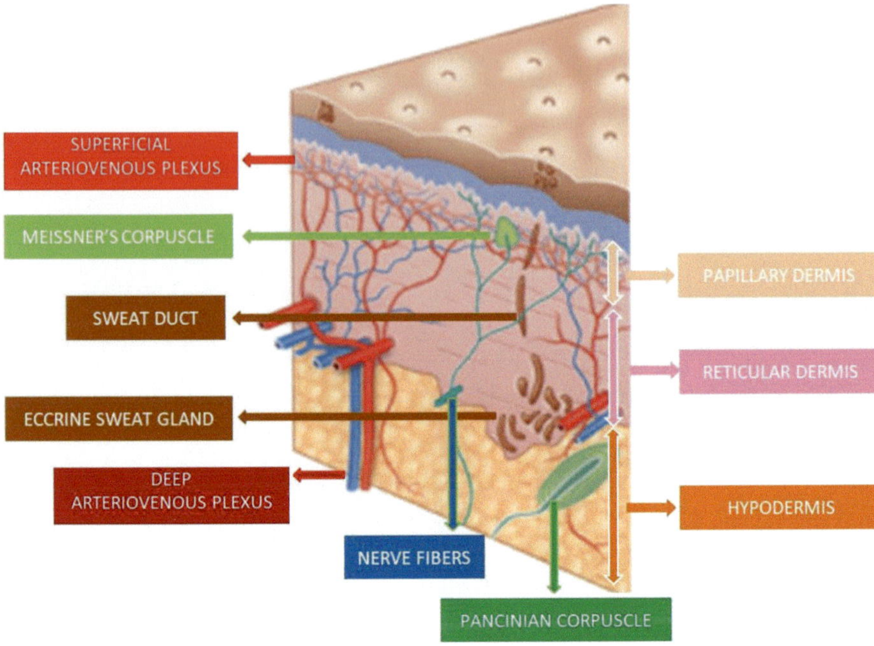

Fig. 1.4 Diagram of a cross-section of human glabrous skin showing labeled layers and structures. The top layer is the epidermis, followed by the papillary dermis and reticular dermis. Key structures include the superficial and deep arteriovenous plexus, Meissner's corpuscle, sweat duct, eccrine sweat gland, nerve fibers, and Pacinian corpuscle. The hypodermis is the bottom layer. Each component is color-coded and labeled for clarity

    - periadnexal (or dermis).
    - reticular dermis, that is composed of dense bands of collagen type I.
  - For hairy (non-glabrous) skin, we can also observe in dermis:
    - hair follicles = tubular structures extend from the epidermis to the dermis.
    - sebaceous glands = associated with hair follicles, produce sebaceous secretion for hair and scalp lubrication.
    - sweat glands.
    - arrector pili muscles = smooth muscles attached to hair follicles.

- Hypodermis aspects:
  - Also called subcutaneous adipose tissue.
  - Contains subcutaneous fat, superficial fascia, perforating blood vessels, and nerves.
  - Divided into lobes of mature adipocytes, separated by connective tissue septa.
  - Divided into
    - lobular
    - septal
    - mixed

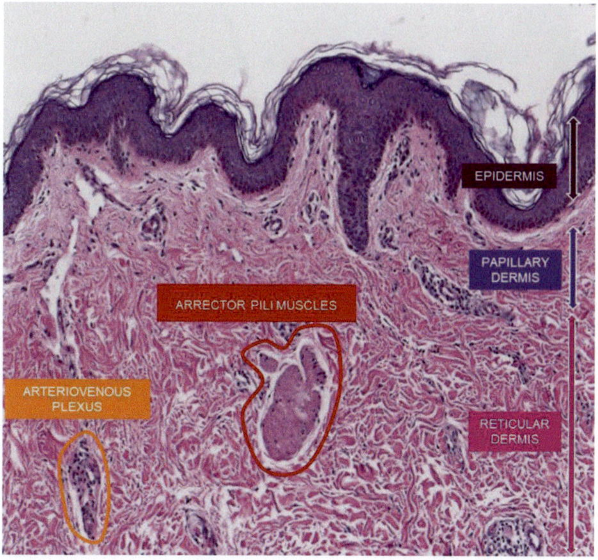

Fig. 1.5 A histological image of human glabrous skin layers stained in hematoxylin and eosin (H&E X10). Labeled structures include the Epidermis at the surface, with the underlying Papillary and Reticular layers of the dermis. Two structures are highlighted the Arrector Pili Muscles and the Arteriovenous Plexus. The image shows the intricate structure and organization of skin tissue

- Vascularization and innervation:
  - Two parallel vascular plexuses: superficial vascular plexus and deep vascular plexus.
  - Presence of lymphatic vessels, nerves, and vascular anastomoses in acral areas.
  - Glomus, glomus bodies, or Sucquet–Hoyer channels are important anastomosed structures for regulating blood flow.
  - Nerves and Meissner and Vater-Pacini corpuscles are common in soles, palms, and acral skin.
- Cutaneous lymphatic network:
  - Variable and complex although little studied.
  - Importance in the excision of malignant neoplasms, such as melanoma.
- Skeletal muscle tissue:
  - Occurs within the dermis in external genitalia (dartos) and the nipple areola.

1.1.4 Functions and Properties of the Skin [5]

- Protection:
  - Protection against physical and chemical trauma.
  - Barrier against the penetration of chemical agents, including drugs and toxins.
  - Prevents unregulated loss or entry of water, electrolytes, ultraviolet radiation, and infections.

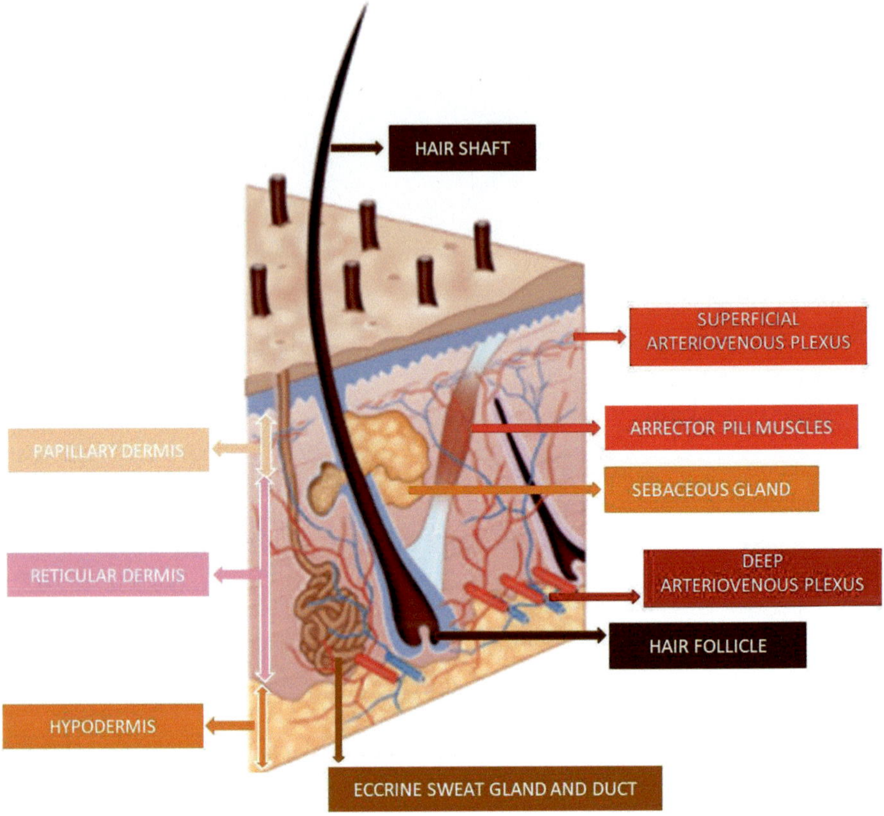

Fig. 1.6 A detailed cross-sectional diagram of human non-glabrous skin layers and structures. The outermost layer shows the hair shaft protruding from the surface. Below, the papillary dermis and reticular dermis are labeled, with the hypodermis at the base. Key structures include the hair follicle, sebaceous gland, and eccrine sweat gland and duct. The diagram also highlights the superficial and deep arteriovenous plexus, and the arrector pili muscles. Each component is color-coded and labeled for clarity

  - Immune barrier through the presence of dendritic cells, resident T lymphocytes and cytokine production.
- Sensory information:
  - Provision of sensory information such as heat, cold, rough, or smooth texture.
- Thermal regulation:
  - Maintains mechanisms for controlling and maintaining body temperature.
  - Involvement in processes such as vasodilation, vasoconstriction, and sweat evaporation.
- Synthesis of vitamin D:
  - In response to sunlight exposure

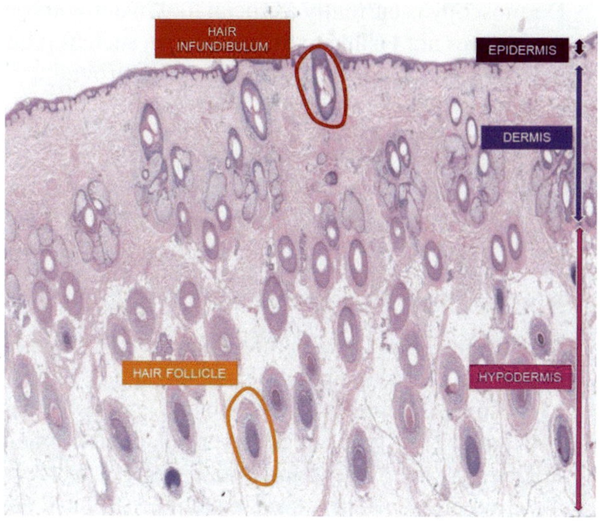

Fig. 1.7 A histological image of human non-glabrous skin showing three distinct layers: epidermis, dermis, and hypodermis, stained in hematoxylin and eosin (H&E X10). The image highlights a hair infundibulum in the epidermis with a red label and circle, and a hair follicle in the dermis with an orange label and circle

- Containment of internal organs:
  - Maintains the integrity of internal organs due to their elasticity.
  - Collaboration with skeletal muscles in containment and protection.
- Expression of physical and sexual identity:
  - Contributes to physical and sexual identity through characteristics such as color, texture, and quantity of hair.
  - Social elements, such as tribal identity, are reflected in scars, piercings, and tattoos.
- Nonverbal communication:
  - Apocrine glands secrete pheromones that play a role in chemical communication.
- Adaptation and regeneration:
  - Adaptation to environmental stimuli
  - Capacity for self-healing and self-regeneration in response to injuries

1.2 Dermoscopy [6–8]

Dermoscopy is also known as dermatoscopy, skin surface microscopy, epiluminescence microscopy, and incident light microscopy. It is a noninvasive diagnostic imaging technique that involves the use of a device with integrated lighting and magnification systems that allow clear visualization of the structures and patterns of the surface and subsurface of the skin [1–3].

Dermoscopy is currently a crucial tool in dermatology and allows dermatologists to see features not visible to the naked eye, such as pigment network patterns, blood vessels, and fine details of skin lesions. By providing a clearer view of these structures, dermoscopy significantly improves the accuracy of diagnosing conditions.

1.2.1 Dermatoscope Components (Fig. 1.8) [9–11]

A dermatoscope typically consists of the following components:

- Magnifying lens: Usually offers 10× to 20× magnification, allowing for detailed examination of skin and nail structures [1, 2, 12].
- Light source: Illuminates the skin and nail, enhancing the visibility of subungual structures. This light can be either polarized or non-polarized [1, 2, 12].
- Polarizing filters: These are used to reduce surface reflections, enabling the visualization of deeper structures within the skin and nail [1, 2, 12].
  - Polarized light reduces surface reflections, allowing for better visualization of deeper structures such as blood vessels, pigmentation, and dermal changes [5, 7, 10, 12].
  - Non-polarized light highlights surface details and is better suited for examining the superficial aspects of the lesion, such as texture, keratin changes, and surface irregularities. Non-polarized light may show details like scaling, surface ridges, or superficial pigmentation more clearly [5, 7, 10, 12].
- Contact plate: A transparent plate that is placed directly on the examination of the nail and skin surface. It helps in stabilizing the dermatoscope and sometimes requires the application of an interface fluid [1, 2, 12]. This fluid, often a gel or

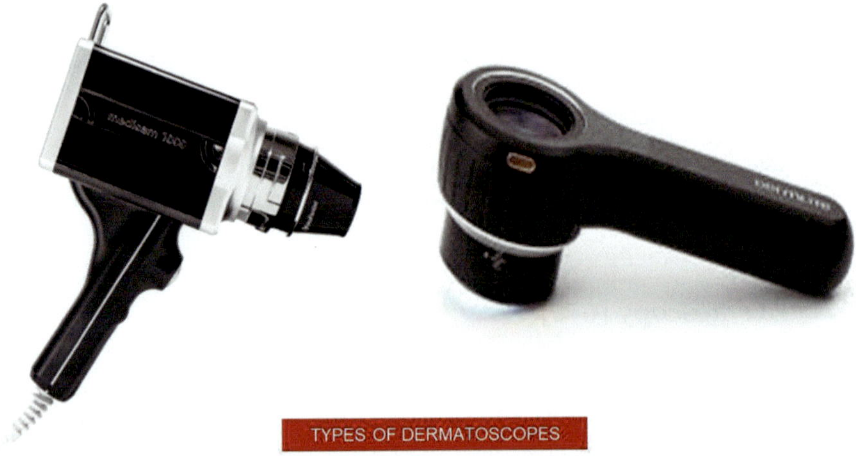

Fig. 1.8 Two types of dermatoscopes are shown. On the left is a handheld dermatoscope labeled photofinder video dermoscope, featuring a black and silver design with a cord. On the right is a black, compact dermatoscope with a lens

alcohol, helps eliminate air bubbles and improves the optical coupling between the nail, the skin and the dermatoscope. This results in clearer images and better visualization of both superficial and deeper structures. The fluid can also minimize reflections when non-polarized light is used, allowing for better assessment of the nail's morphology and any underlying conditions [1, 5, 13].

- Battery or power source: Powers the light source and any other electronic components [1, 2, 12].
- Camera and imaging system: Some dermatoscopes include integrated cameras for capturing images of the lesions for documentation and further analysis [1, 2, 12].

Various instruments can be employed for skin analyses. Handheld dermatoscopes offer greater clarity but provide lower magnification (×10), making them suitable for evaluating some lesions; however, they may not consistently assess vascular architecture. Conversely, video dermatoscopes are versatile tools capable of achieving much higher magnifications (up to ×200) [5, 6].

1.2.2 Dermoscopic Aspects of Normal Non-Glabrous Skin (Fig. 1.9) [6]

Epidermis

- Stratum corneum: The outermost layer, typically seen as a translucent or slightly opaque layer on dermoscopy. It may appear as a shiny surface due to the reflection of light.
- Epidermal ridges: The patterns of ridges and furrows are visible, giving a granular texture to the skin surface.

Dermal-epidermal junction

- Pigment network: This is a characteristic feature in some skin types, showing a mesh-like pattern due to the distribution of melanin within the epidermis.

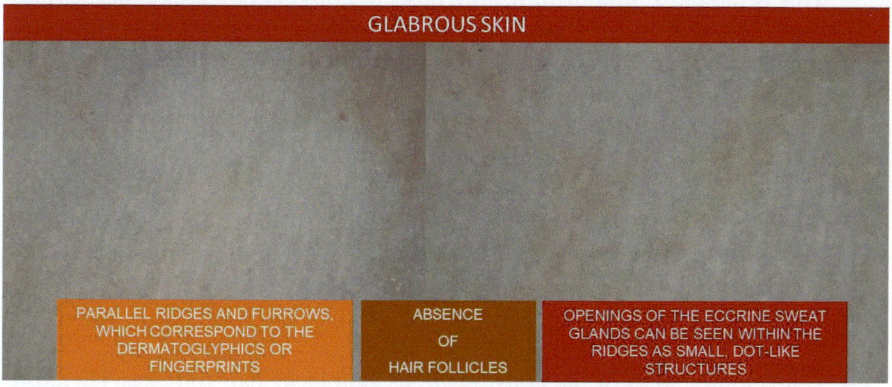

Fig. 1.9 Images showing the dermoscopic aspects of non-glabrous skin (X10)

- Linear and reticular pigmentation: Normal skin often shows a regular, linear, or reticular (net-like) pigmentation pattern, which can be seen in the dermal-epidermal junction.

Dermis

- Papillary dermis: The upper layer of the dermis, which may exhibit fine, looped blood vessels and a delicate texture.
- Vascular structures: Normal dermis contains capillaries and small blood vessels, which can appear as fine reddish or bluish lines or spots under dermoscopy.

Hair follicles

- Follicular openings: Dermoscopy reveals hair follicle openings as small, round structures scattered across the skin surface.
- Follicular patterns: The arrangement and density of hair follicles can vary, appearing as regular or irregular patterns depending on the area of the body.

Sebaceous glands

- Sebaceous ducts: These are less prominent in normal dermoscopy but can be identified as small, round, or oval structures near hair follicles.

Sweat glands

- Sweat pores: Although not always visible, in some cases, sweat pores might be seen as tiny openings on the skin surface.

Skin texture

- Smooth to slightly rugose: Normal skin texture varies from smooth to slightly rough or pebbly, depending on individual skin types and anatomical locations.

1.2.3 Dermoscopic Aspects of Normal Glabrous Skin (Fig. 1.10) [6, 14–16]

- Parallel ridge pattern:
  - This is the most prominent feature observed in glabrous skin under dermoscopy. The skin shows a pattern of parallel ridges and furrows, which correspond to the dermatoglyphics or fingerprints.
  - The ridges appear as slightly darker linear structures, while the furrows between them are lighter.
- Sweat gland openings:
  - Small, dot-like structures can be seen within the ridges. These are the openings of the eccrine sweat glands, which are abundant in glabrous skin. These dots are usually darker than the surrounding skin.
- Absence of hair follicles:
  - Unlike other areas of the body, glabrous skin lacks hair follicles. Therefore, under dermoscopy, no hair shafts, follicular openings, or associated structures (like sebaceous glands) are observed.

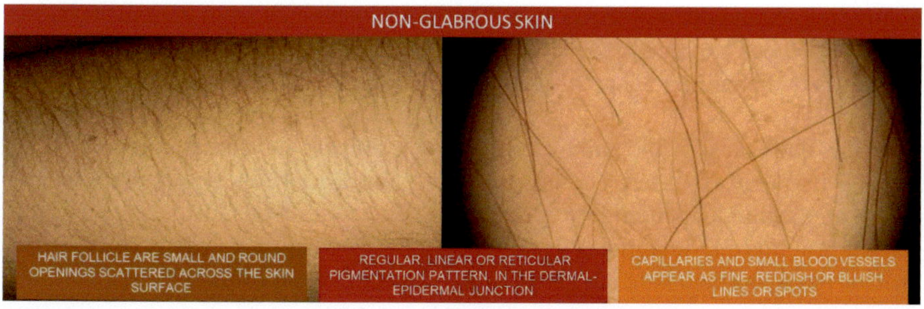

Fig. 1.10 Images showing the dermoscopic aspects of non-glabrous skin (x10 and x20)

- Furrows:
  - The furrows between the ridges are slightly paler and can appear as thin white lines separating the ridges.
- Homogeneous background:
  - The background skin tone under dermoscopy is typically homogeneous, without significant color variation. The color is usually consistent with the individual's skin tone.
- No pigment network:
  - The typical pigment network seen in pigmented lesions of the skin is absent in glabrous skin. This is because the skin on the palms and soles has a different structure, with thicker epidermis and less prominent melanin patterns.

1.3 Imaging Technique [17]

Imaging is crucial for characterizing skin lesions, confirming clinical suspicions, and determining the extent of involvement. High-frequency ultrasonography (HFUS) is increasingly used for the initial assessment of skin lesions. While conventional radiography can detect or confirm underlying bone involvement, HFUS is particularly useful for identifying most skin structures with high-resolution images and detailed anatomy. Different frequency ranges allow for visualization of both superficial and deeper structures.

Computed tomography (CT) offers high-resolution imaging but, similar to radiography, is limited to identifying soft tissue components and bone lesions. Magnetic resonance imaging (MRI) with surface coil is considered an emerging technique for evaluating skin lesions due to its high resolution, excellent inherent contrast, and ability to provide detailed anatomical visualization using surface coils. Proper positioning and stabilization of the coil at the central portion of the lesion are essential for obtaining diagnostic-quality images.

Recent advances in 3D reconstruction of images from 3T MRI with surface coil have further improved the visualization and understanding of lesion extent, even for non-radiologist medical professionals. The images obtained from 3T MRI with isotropic sequences can be imported into 3D Slicer software, allowing for image segmentation and enabling 3D reconstruction for virtual navigation and 3D printing of the model.

In this book on skin and nail lesions, the radiographic and computed tomography findings frequently overlap. Therefore, they will be described together in most cases where applicable, depending on the disease being discussed. Likewise, MRI with surface coil and 3D imaging will only be included when their use is relevant and provides a clear diagnostic advantage for the specific condition.

1.3.1 Radiography and Computed Tomography (Fig. 1.11)

- Radiography is a technique used to visualize the internal structure of the human body, particularly bones. It works by passing X-ray beams through the body. These beams are absorbed at different rates by different tissues, with denser structures like bones absorbing more X-rays. The X-rays that pass through are captured on an X-ray detector, creating an image that shows various densities, allowing for the differentiation between bones and softer tissues.
  - Advantages:
    - Quick and widely available.
    - Excellent method for bone imaging.
    - Cost-effective, being relatively inexpensive compared to other imaging techniques.
  - Disadvantages:
    - Limited soft tissue detail.
    - Radiation exposure.
    - Two-dimensional images, which may not fully capture the complexity of some anatomical structures.

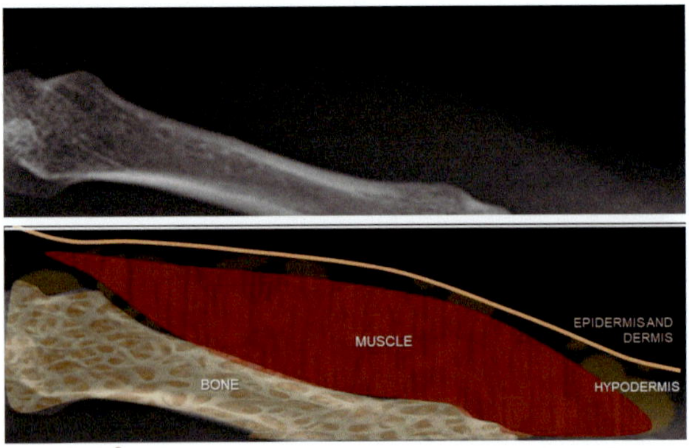

Fig. 1.11 The image is divided into two sections. The top section shows an X-ray of a bone and soft tissues, highlighting its structure. The bottom section is a labeled diagram of a cross-section of the same area, showing layers from bottom to top: bone, muscle, hypodermis, and epidermis and dermis. The labels provide a clear understanding of the anatomical layers (Philips Duo Diagnost R&F Room Digital RF and Tomo System)

- Computed tomography is an imaging method used to create detailed cross-sectional images of the human body. It works by taking multiple X-ray measurements from different angles around the structure and then using computer processing to combine these measurements into a comprehensive image. This technique provides more detailed and precise images compared to traditional X-rays, allowing for better visualization of internal structures.
  - Advantages:
    - Highly detailed images of bones, soft tissues, and blood vessels, allowing for accurate diagnosis.
    - The procedure is quick, making it valuable in emergency situations.
    - 3D reconstruction, offering a comprehensive view of complex structures.
  - Disadvantages:
    - Radiation exposure that involves higher doses of radiation compared to regular X-rays
- Normal skin appears as a thin soft-tissue attenuation layer over the subcutaneous fat, which has variable thickness. The different layers of the skin are otherwise not readily discernible on routine radiography or computed tomography.
- The use of these techniques primarily focuses on analyzing bone lesions or occasionally detecting foreign bodies.

1.3.2 Ultrasonography (Figs. 1.12 and 1.13) [12, 18, 19]

- Ultrasonography is a medical imaging technique that uses high-frequency sound waves to create images of structures inside the human body. A transducer emits high-frequency sound waves, which bounce off tissues and organs, creating echoes. The transducer detects these echoes and sends the data to a computer, which produces real-time images on a monitor.
  - Advantages
    - Noninvasive method.
    - Does not use ionizing radiation, making it safer than X-rays and CT scans.
    - Real-time imaging, providing immediate visual feedback, useful for guiding procedures.
    - Widely accessible.
  - Disadvantages
    - Limited penetration, especially in bone or gas.
    - The quality of the images and the accuracy of the interpretation can vary based on the skill of the radiologist.
    - Resolution, not providing as detailed images as other imaging techniques like MRI with surface coil or CT.

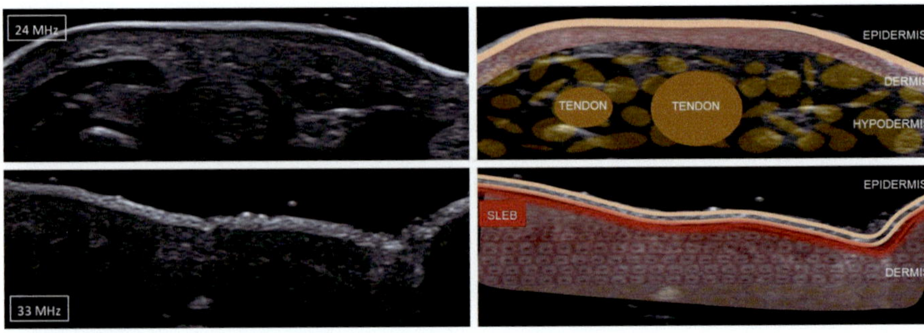

Fig. 1.12 The image is a comparison of ultrasonography scans of the glabrous skin at different frequencies probes. The top left shows a 24 MHz ultrasonography scan, while the top right is a labeled diagram highlighting the epidermis, dermis, hypodermis, and tendons. The bottom left shows a 33 MHz ultrasonography scan, and the bottom right is a labeled diagram showing the epidermis, dermis, and subepidermal low echogenic band (SLEB) (Aplio i800, Canon Medical Systems)

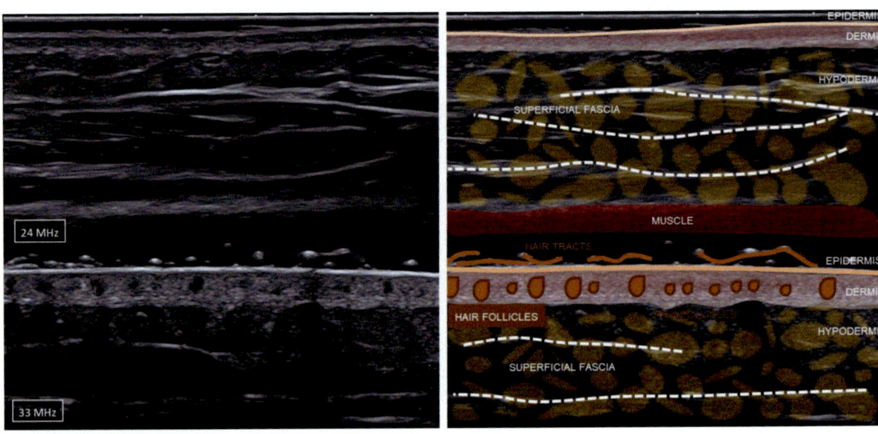

Fig. 1.13 The image shows a side-by-side comparison of an ultrassonography scan and a labeled diagram of human nonglabrous skin layers. The left side displays a grayscale ultrasonography image at frequencies of 24 MHz and 33 MHz, highlighting the skin's internal structure. The right side is a color-coded diagram labeling the epidermis, dermis, hypodermis, superficial fascia, muscle, hair tracts, and hair follicles. The diagram provides a detailed view of the skin's anatomy, with each layer distinctly marked (Aplio i800, Canon Medical Systems)

- Regarding transducer frequencies, we currently have several options available:
  - An 18 MHz transducer is ideal for evaluating lesions approximately 12–15 mm deep.
  - A 24 MHz transducer is suitable for lesions 6–8 mm deep.
  - A 33 MHz transducer is best for lesions with a depth of 4–6 mm.
  - A 15 MHz transducer is sometimes required to complement the evaluation of adjacent structures during a skin examination. This probe is particularly well-suited for assessing muscles, deeper joints, and peripheral nerves, as it allows adequate visualization of deeper tissues without significant loss of image

quality. It is useful for evaluating muscle architecture, joint effusions, synovial hypertrophy, and nerve morphology.

- Nowadays, we have both portable and console ultrasonography machines available.
  - Console machine:
    - Typically have more powerful processors, leading to faster and more accurate imaging.
    - Offer a greater range of features and capabilities compared to portable models.
    - Higher image quality.
    - Console machines are not easily moved, limiting their use to specific locations.
    - Less practical for bedside or emergency use compared to portable models.
    - Tend to be more expensive.
    - Their lack of portability makes them less suitable for point-of-care applications, where immediate imaging is required at the patient's location.
  - Portable machine:
    - Portable machines can be easily transported to different locations, making them highly versatile.
    - Their smaller size allows for use in tight spaces and makes them convenient for bedside examinations.
    - Generally, portable machines are less expensive compared to console ones.
    - They typically have less powerful processors, which may affect the speed and accuracy of imaging.
    - The image quality may not be as high as that of non-portable machines, potentially limiting diagnostic capabilities.
    - Achieving optimal image quality can take more time, which can be a drawback in fast-paced clinical settings.
- Anatomy
  - Epidermis:
    - The echogenicity of the epidermis is a result of the high content of keratin.
    - On ultrasonography, it appears as a bright hyperechoic line in non-glabrous skin and as a bilaminar parallel hyperechoic structure in the palmar and plantar skin.
  - Dermis:
    - The echogenicity of the dermis depends on the collagen content, appearing as hyperechoic band, however, less bright than the epidermis.
    - The dermis thickness is different depending on body region, being thinner on the face and thicker on the back.
    - The UV radiation over time causes a deposit of glycosaminoglycans on the photoaged skin, also called elastosis, which may be shown in the upper dermis, which can be detected on ultrasonography as a subepidermal low-echogenicity band (SLEB).

  - Using ultrahigh-frequency probe (more than 50 MHz), the villous hair located in the body appears as a hyperechoic monolaminar structure.
- Hypodermis:
  - The echogenicity of the hypodermis is a result of the fatty tissue. The hypodermis presents hypoechogenicity, owing to fatty lobules, with hyperechoic fibrous septa in between.
  - On power Doppler, low-flow arterial and venous vessels are commonly detected in the hypodermis. Capillaries in the papillary dermis can also be visualized in certain conditions, such as inflammation or neovascularization.

1.3.3 MRI (Fig. 1.14) [13, 17]

- Medical imaging technique used to produce detailed images of internal structures, with exceptional detail and the capability to differentiate tissue origins.
- The patient lies inside a cylindrical machine that generates a strong magnetic field. Radio waves are transmitted through the body, causing hydrogen atoms in the tissues to align and then return to their original positions. This movement produces signals that the MRI machine detects. A computer processes these signals to create detailed cross-sectional images of the body.
- Advantages
  - High-resolution images
  - Noninvasive
- MRI does not use ionizing radiation, making it safer for repeated use.

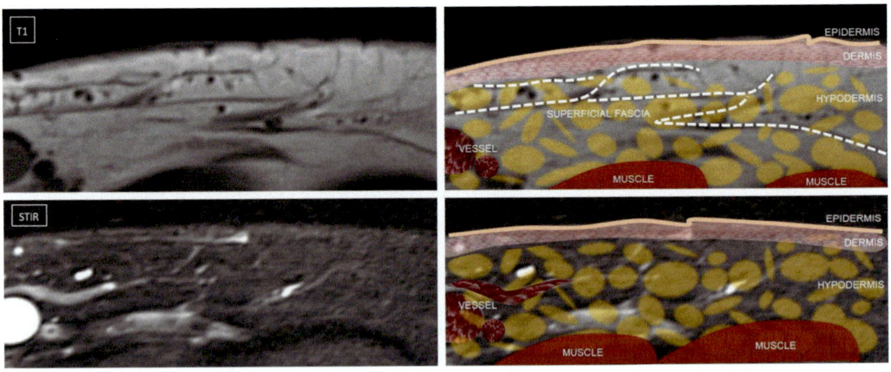

Fig. 1.14 The image consists of two rows, each with two panels. The left panels show MRI with surface coil scans on T1-weighted and STIR images depicting cross-sectional views of human skin. The right panels are labeled illustrations of the same sections, highlighting anatomical layers: epidermis, dermis, hypodermis, superficial fascia, vessels, and muscle. The illustrations use color and labels to differentiate between the layers and structures (Magnetom Prisma 3T MRI, Siemens)

- It can be used to image almost any part of the body. For dermatological conditions, a surface coil must be used. While the epidermis and dermis cannot be differentiated by this technique, dermal and hypodermal lesions are very well-studied, particularly tumoral lesions. These can be reconstructed, segmented, and have 3D images generated.
- Disadvantages
  - MRI machines are expensive to operate and not as widely available as other imaging techniques, especially the surface coil.
  - MRI scans can take 20 min to over an hour, which is longer than other imaging procedures.
  - The enclosed space of the MRI machine can be uncomfortable for some patients.
  - Patients with metal implants, especially pacemakers may not be able to undergo an MRI due to the strong magnetic field.
- Basic MRI sequences:
  - T1-Weighted Sequences (T1)
    - A basic anatomical sequence where fat appears bright (hyperintense) and water appears dark (hypointense).
    - Excellent for assessing anatomical details, such as skin layers, subcutaneous fat, and lesion margins. Helps define fat-containing lesions or detect fat infiltration.
  - T2-Weighted Sequences (T2):
    - A fluid-sensitive sequence where water-containing structures appear bright (hyperintense).
    - Highlights edema, fluid collections, inflammation, cysts, and tumors with high water content.
  - Fat-Suppressed T2-Weighted or STIR (Short Tau Inversion Recovery):
    - A modified T2-weighted sequence that suppresses fat signal.
    - Enhances contrast by making fluid and inflammation bright (hyperintense) while suppressing bright fat signal, being ideal for detecting edema, cellulitis, abscesses, or tumor margins.
  - Proton Density with Fat Saturation (PD FS):
    - A sequence with intermediate contrast between T1 and T2, often combined with fat suppression.
    - Provides high resolution and is good for evaluating small superficial structures, including fine skin layers, tendon insertions, and nerves.
  - Post-Contrast T1-Weighted with Fat Saturation (T1 FS Gd):
    - A T1-weighted sequence performed after injecting a contrast agent (gadolinium), with fat suppression applied.

    - Highlights vascularized lesions, inflammation, and tumor enhancement. Helps distinguish between solid and cystic lesions.

  - 3D T2-Weighted Sequences:

    - A 3D imaging technique with high-spatial resolution.
    - Allows fine anatomical details, multi-planar reconstructions, and precise surgical planning, especially for lesions involving face, scalp, or digits.

- Anatomy [17]

  - On T2-weighted images, normal epidermis appears hyperintense relative to the underlying dermis and shows as a linear line with intermediate signal intensity on T1-weighted spin-echo images.
  - The subcutaneous fat appears bright and is traversed by vessels with flow voids and the superficial fascia on both T1- and T2-weighted images.
  - Define morphologic assessment, such as size and depth, as well as the description of the relationship with underlying critical structures such as periosteum, muscle, and nasal cartilage. The origin of the tissue can be especially determined when multiple sequences are used, such as:

    - DWI (diffusion-weighted imaging): This sequence measures the random movement of water molecules within tissues. It is particularly useful for detecting areas with restricted diffusion within lesions, which often indicates a higher cell content.
    - Chemical-shift imaging: This technique exploits differences in the resonant frequencies of fat and water protons to distinguish between these tissues. It is valuable for identifying fat within tissues.
    - Perfusion imaging: This sequence evaluates the flow of blood through tissues, providing information about tissue vascularity and perfusion.
    - SWI (susceptibility-weighted imaging): This technique enhances the contrast between tissues based on their magnetic properties. It is particularly sensitive to blood, iron, and calcium.

References

1. Lindberg MR, Lamps LW. Diagnostic pathology: normal histology. 2nd ed. Elsevier; 2018.
2. Werner B. Biópsia de pele e seu estudo histológico: Por quê? Para quê? Como? Parte I. An Bras Dermatol. 2009;84:391–5.
3. Barnhill RL, Crowson AN, Magro CM, Piepkorn MW, Kutzner H, Desman GT. Barnhill's dermatopathology. 4th ed. McGraw Hill/Medical; 2019. https://dermatology.mhmedical.com/content.aspx?bookid=2802&sectionid=238125236.
4. Elder DE, Elenitsas R, Murphy GF, Rosenbach M, Rubin AI, Seykora JT, et al. Lever's dermatopathology: histopathology of the Skin. 12th ed. Lippincott Williams & Wilkins; 2022.
5. Patterson JW. Weedon's skin pathology. 6th ed. Elsevier; 2024.
6. Nirmal B. Dermatoscopy: physics and principles. Indian J Dermatopathol Diagn Dermatol. 2017;4:27.

7. Campos-do-Carmo G, Ramos-e-Silva M. Dermoscopy: basic concepts. Int J Dermatol. 2008;47:712–9.
8. Kittler H, Marghoob AA, Argenziano G, Carrera C, Curiel-Lewandrowski C, Hofmann-Wellenhof R, et al. Standardization of terminology in dermoscopy/dermatoscopy: results of the third consensus conference of the International Society of Dermoscopy. J Am Acad Dermatol. 2016;74:1093–106.
9. Lencastre A, Lamas A, Sá D, Tosti A. Onychoscopy. Clin Dermatol. 2013;31:587–93.
10. Sathe NC, Saleh HM. Onychoscopy. StatPearls Publishing; 2024.
11. Pan Y, Gareau DS, Scope A, Rajadhyaksha M, Mullani NA, Marghoob AA. Polarized and nonpolarized dermoscopy. Arch Dermatol. 2008;144:828–9.
12. Wortsman X. Atlas of dermatologic ultrasound. Cham: Springer International Publishing; 2018. https://doi.org/10.1007/978-3-319-89614-4.
13. Kim J, Kim JY, Chun KA, Jee W-H, Sung M-S. MR imaging manifestations of skin tumors. Eur Radiol. 2008;18:2652–61.
14. Hirata SH, Yamada S, Almeida FA, Enokihara MY, Rosa IP, Enokihara MMS, et al. Dermoscopic examination of the nail bed and matrix. Int J Dermatol. 2006;45:28–30.
15. Alessandrini A, Starace M, Piraccini BM. Dermoscopy in the evaluation of nail disorders. Skin Appendage Disord. 2017;3:70–82.
16. Ronger S, Touzet S, Ligeron C, Balme B, Viallard AM, Barrut D, et al. Dermoscopic examination of nail pigmentation. Arch Dermatol. 2002;138:1327–33.
17. Ginat DT, Cipriani NA. Introduction: skin anatomy, imaging approaches, and dermatology terminology. In: Neuroradiological imaging of skin diseases and related conditions. Cham: Springer International Publishing; 2019. p. 1–6.
18. Wortsman X, Jemec GBE, Villani A. Ultrasound and other imaging methods. In: Baran & Dawber's diseases of the nails and their management. Chichester: Wiley; 2018. p. 140–74. https://doi.org/10.1002/9781119323396.ch5.
19. Wortsman X. Common applications of dermatologic sonography. J Ultrasound Med. 2012;31:97–111. https://doi.org/10.7863/jum.2012.31.1.97.

Chapter 2
Anatomy of Scalp: Clinical, Imaging, and Histological Aspects

Maria Carolina Zafra Páez, Ludmila do Valle Vieira Gusmão, André da Silva Cartell, Ximena Wortsman, Carolina Ávila de Almeida, Clarissa Canella Moraes do Carmo, and Bruna Duque-Estrada

The human scalp, a complex structure composed of multiple layers, plays a vital role in protecting the underlying cranial structures. Understanding the anatomy of the scalp is essential for both clinical and surgical practices, as it consists of diverse tissues, including this chapter delves into the intricate architecture of the scalp, providing a detailed exploration of its anatomical features. Additionally, this chapter explores the most recent imaging modalities that have revolutionized the evaluation of these conditions, such as trichoscopy, ultrasonography, and magnetic resonance imaging (MRI) with surface coil, offering insights into their applications in visualizing the scalp's layers and diseases.

M. C. Z. Páez
Zafra Dermatology Private Clinic, Rio de Janeiro, Brazil

BCM Dermatologia Especializada, Private Practice, Rio de Janeiro, Brazil

L. do Valle Vieira Gusmão
Marcilio Dias Naval Hospital, Dermatological Imaging Department of DASA - Rio de Janeiro, Rio de Janeiro, Brazil

A. da Silva Cartell
Adjunct Professor at Faculdade de Medicina da Universidade Federal do Rio Grande do Sul, Rio de Janeiro, Brazil

Dermatologist and Dermatopathologist in Private Practice, Rio de Janeiro, Brazil

X. Wortsman
Faculty of Medicine, Department of Dermatology, Universidad de Chile, Santiago, Chile

Department of Dermatology, School of Medicine, Pontificia Universidad Catolica de Chile, Santiago, Chile

Department of Dermatology and Cutaneous Surgery, Miller School of Medicine, University of Miami, Miami, FL, USA

Institute for Diagnostic Imaging and Research of the Skin and Soft Tissues, Santiago, Chile

© The Author(s), under exclusive license to Springer Nature Switzerland AG 2025
C. Canella Moraes do Carmo (ed.), *Atlas of Diagnostic Imaging in Dermatology*,
https://doi.org/10.1007/978-3-031-77987-9_2

2.1 Anatomy [1]

2.1.1 *Skin Structure of the Scalp (Figs. 2.1, 2.2 and 2.3)*

- The epidermis on the scalp presents the same histological appearance as the epidermis on the rest of the body. The structure of the epidermis consists of the stratum basale, stratum spinosum, stratum granulosum, and stratum corneum.
- The underlying dermis contains hair follicles, sebaceous glands, sweat glands, and arrector pili muscles:
  - Hair follicles
    - Tubular structures that comprise an outer and inner sheath.
    - The outer root sheath provides structural support, extending from the epidermis to the hair bulb.

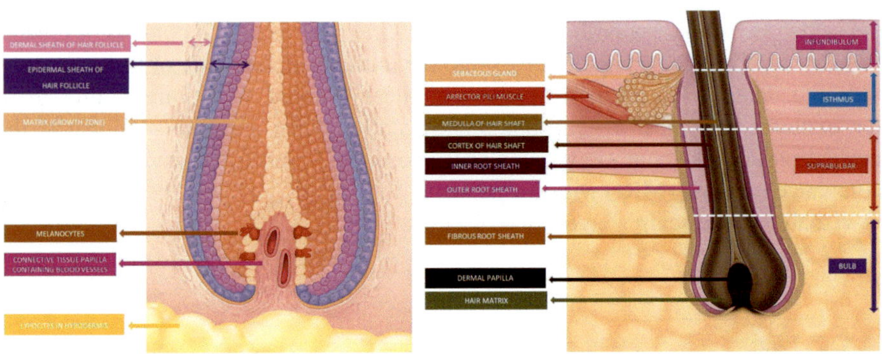

Fig. 2.1 Schematic diagram of the hair follicle of the scalp

C. Á. de Almeida
Faculty of Medicine of Valença—UniFaa, Valença, Brazil

Federal University of Rio de Janeiro—UFRJ, Rio de Janeiro, Brazil

C. Canella Moraes do Carmo (✉)
Fluminense Federal University—UFF, Rio de Janeiro, Brazil

Federal University of Rio de Janeiro—UFRJ, Rio de Janeiro, Brazil

Diagnóstico das Américas—DASA—RJ, Rio de Janeiro, Brazil

Biodesign Laboratory, DASA-PUC, Rio de Janeiro, Brazil

B. Duque-Estrada
BCM Dermatologia Especializada, Private Practice, Rio de Janeiro, Brazil

Universidade Federal de São Paulo, São Paulo, Brazil

Hair Diseases Department, Instituto de Dermatologia Professor Rubem David Azulay – Santa Casa da Misericórdia do Rio de Janeiro, Rio de Janeiro, Brazil

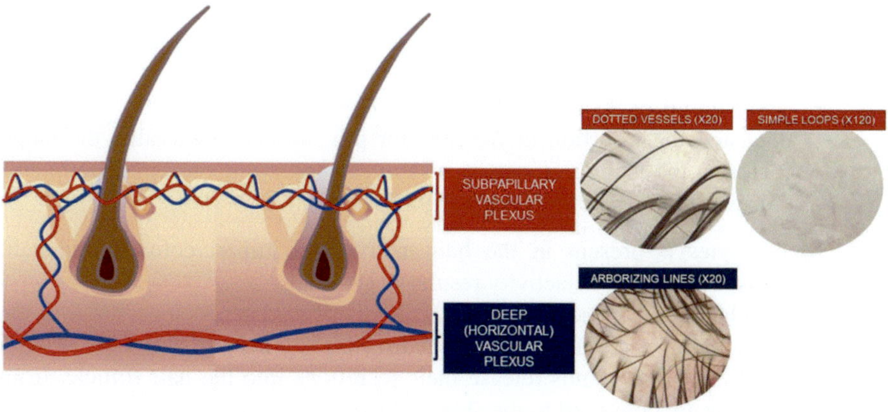

Fig. 2.2 Schematic diagram of the human scalp illustrating the superficial and deep vascular plexus

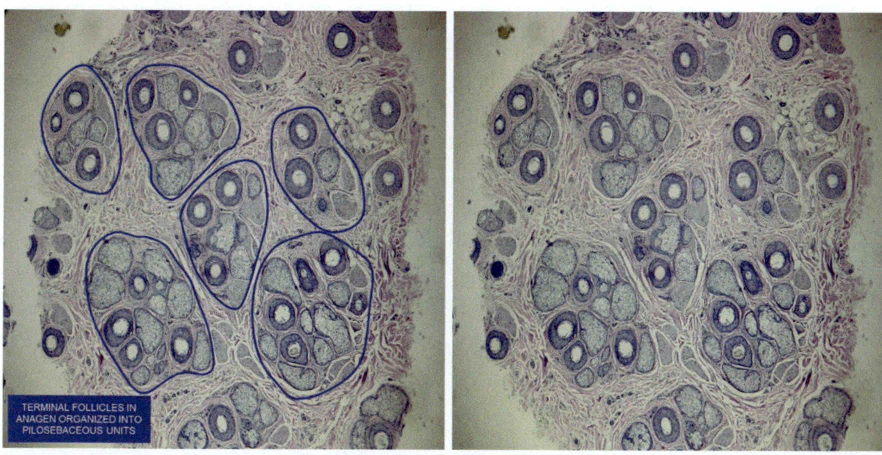

Fig. 2.3 Histological findings of the human scalp (H&E x40)

- The inner root sheath surrounds the growing hair shaft, providing support, maintaining its integrity, and facilitating its passage as it emerges from the follicle.
- The hair bulb, at the follicle base, contains actively germinative cells, responsible for hair growth.
- Mesenchymal dermal papilla, a connective tissue structure, nourishes the hair bulb and influences hair growth. The dermal papilla is a small, finger-like projection at the base of the hair follicle, which play a key role in hair growth by delivering nutrients and signaling molecules to the growing hair.
- Sebaceous glands, linked to the hair follicle, produce sebum for hair and scalp lubrication. The glandular activity may vary among individuals.

- Arrector pili muscle is a smooth muscle attached to hair follicles. They contract during stress or cold responses and in pilocarpine testing, causing hair to stand on end (goosebumps).
- The isthmus of the hair follicle is the region between the sebaceous gland duct and the insertion of the arrector pili muscle Essentially, the bulge region in the isthmus serves as a stem cell reservoir, ensuring continuous hair growth and skin repair throughout life.

– Melanocytes = present in the hair matrix and impart color to the hair. Decreased melanocytic activity results in gray hair.
– Sweat glands = Eccrine sweat glands are distributed across most areas of the body, including the scalp, and secrete directly onto the surface of the skin. In contrast, apocrine glands release their secretions into the hair follicle, from which they are conveyed to the skin surface.
– Blood vessels = supply nutrients and oxygen to follicles and skin and are divided into a superficial and a deep vascular plexus. The superficial vascular plexus is a network of arterioles and venules, interconnected together in the dermis and running just below the epidermis. Capillaries formed here extend more superficially within the papillary dermis. The deep vascular plexus, on the other hand, is found deeper, in the reticular dermis, these capillaries are distributed around the hair follicles and sweat glands.
– Scalp nerves = hair follicles are extensively innervated by nerve endings that function as highly sensitive mechanoreceptors. These nerve fibers, especially those encircling the hair bulb, are activated by hair movement, enabling the perception of tactile stimuli and subtle vibrations.

2.1.2 Scalp Layers (Fig. 2.4) [2]

- Epidermis and Dermis:
  The outermost layer, dermal cells, hair follicles, sebaceous glands, and sweat glands.
- Connective tissue (dense subcutaneous tissue): Dense subcutaneous tissue (connective tissue):
  A dense layer of subcutaneous fat and fibrous tissue. This fibrofatty layer connects the skin to the epicranial aponeurosis.
  Contains blood vessels and nerves that supply the scalp.
- Epicranial Aponeurosis (galea aponeurotica):
  Fibrous sheet of connective tissue that serves as a tendon, connecting the muscles of the scalp. It links the frontalis muscle (in the forehead) to the occipitalis muscle (at the back of the head), forming part of the occipitofrontalis muscle. This structure plays a key role in facial expressions, scalp movement, and maintaining scalp integrity.

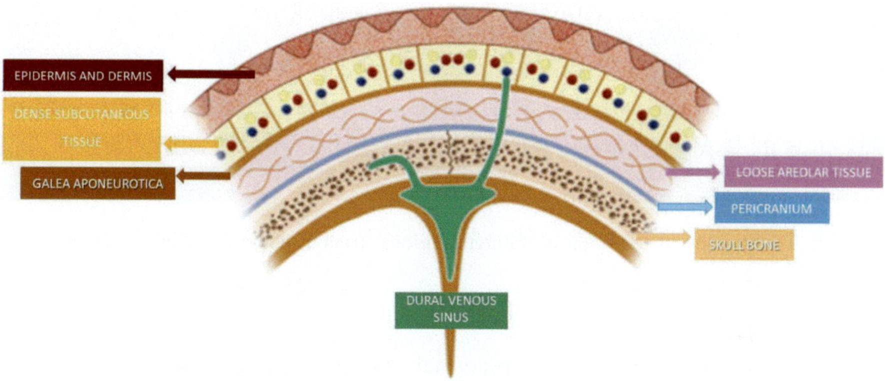

Fig. 2.4 Schematic diagram of the human scalp. Each layer is color-coded and labeled with arrows pointing to the respective sections

- Loose areolar connective tissue:
  Loose connective tissue that provides flexibility and mobility to the scalp. A sponge-like layer that allows the first three layers to move over the pericranium and skull.
  It is also known as the "danger zone" because infections can spread easily in this layer.
- Pericranium:
  The periosteum of the skull bones, a dense layer of connective tissue that adheres tightly to the surface of the skull.

2.2 Trichoscopy Aspects of the Scalp (Fig. 2.5) [3]

Trichoscopy is a noninvasive diagnostic technique used to examine the scalp and hair under magnification, typically with a dermatoscope or a specialized trichoscope. This method allows dermatologists to visualize the hair shafts, scalp skin, hair follicles, and blood vessels in great detail. Below are the anatomical features observed on trichoscopy of the scalp:

Hair follicles

- Follicular openings are the most prominent feature of the normal scalp under dermoscopy. Hair follicle openings are visible as small, round structures filled with hair shafts. In dark skin phototypes, follicular openings are prominent by the contrast of the honeycomb pigmented network. In normal scalp, follicles are distributed in a relatively regular pattern, with varying density depending on the scalp area. The distribution can help in assessing normal hair growth and identifying abnormalities.
- Hair shafts emerge from the center of the follicular ostia, in a parallell pattern. The number of hair shafts per follicular ostia may vary among individuals, age groups, ethnicity, and according to the scalp areas. Hair density and the pattern of scalp emergency can help differentiate various types of scalp conditions.

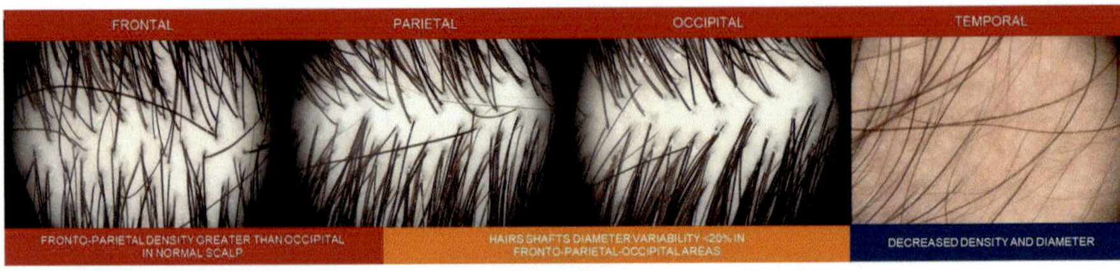

Fig. 2.5 Trichoscopy of the scalp in different regions: frontal, parietal, occipital, and temporal areas (x20)

Sweat glands

- The acrosyringium is the intraepidermal portion of the eccrine sweat duct. It's the final segment of the eccrine sweat gland that spirals through the epidermis and opens at the skin surface. It can be observed as pinpoint white dots, which surround larger follicular ostia under trichoscopy, specially in dark skin phototypes and sun-damaged scalp.

Vascular structures

- The normal scalp has a rich vascular network which may have different trichoscopic patterns: thin arborizing vessels, linear vessels, and dotted vessels. A pale pink background may be observed in Caucasians. Abnormal patterns, as twisted loops, glomerular vessels, or thick arborizing vessels, are observed in many inflammatory scalp conditions.

Pigmentation

- Normal scalp skin typically exhibits a relatively uniform pigmentation. However, the scalp may show slight variations in color depending on skin type and hair color. In dark skinphototypes, the honeycomb pigmentes network may present varying shades of brown.

Scaling or crusting

- Absence of excessive scaling: In healthy scalp, dermoscopy typically does not reveal significant scaling or crusting. Mild interfollicular and perifollicular scaling might be present in senile patients, but it should not be excessive or indicative of pathology.

2.3 Hair Growth Phases (Fig. 2.6) [4]

- Anagen phase:
  - Active growth phase
  - Hair bulb rooted in the subcutaneous tissue
  - Cells in the hair matrix divide rapidly
  - Contributes to continuous hair elongation
  - Can last for several years

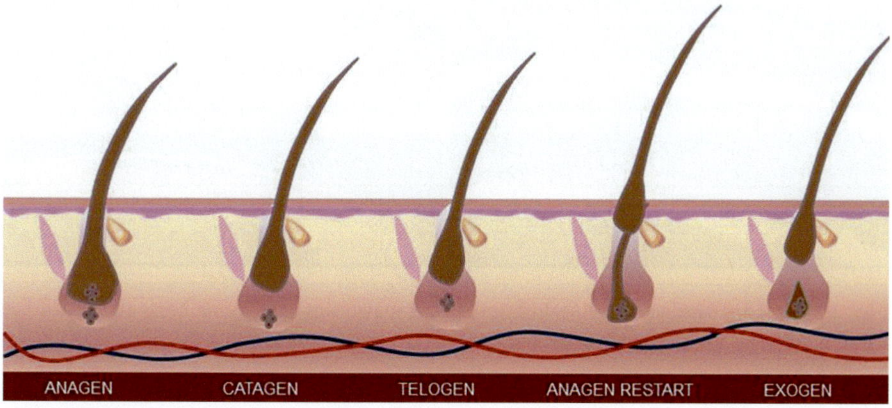

Fig. 2.6 Diagram illustrating the hair growth cycle with four stages: Anagen, Catagen, Telogen, and Exogen

- Catagen phase:
  - Transition phase marking the end of active growth phase
  - Hair follicle shrinks, detaches from the blood supply, and moves upward
  - Short duration, lasting a few weeks.
- Telogen phase:
  - Resting phase with no active growth in the old hair bulb.
  - Old hair bulb remains in the upper dermis, as new hair bulb begins to grow beneath it, in the subcutaneous.
  - Telogen typically lasts 2–3 months. The exogenous phase of the former hair shaft inside the hair follicle occurs while a new hair shaft in the anagen phase emerges inside the follicular ostia.

2.4 Imaging Technique [5]

2.4.1 Radiography and Computed Tomography (Fig. 2.7)

- On radiographic images, the scalp layers may not be distinctly visible due to the limitations of radiography in differentiating soft tissue structures.
- When utilizing advanced imaging techniques such as computed tomography, the following anatomical features of the scalp can be observed:
  - Skin:
    Appears as a thin outermost layer, usually presenting intermediate density.

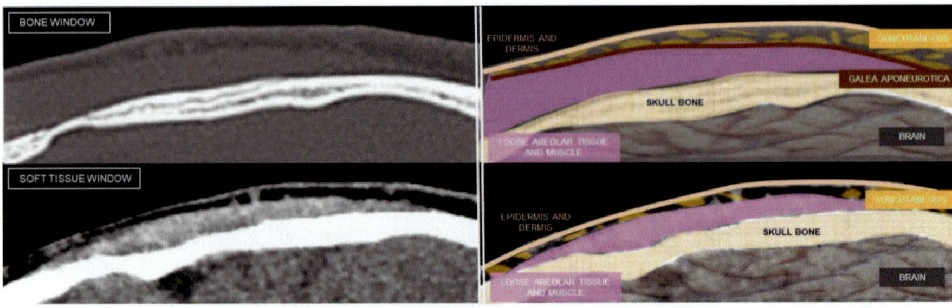

Fig. 2.7 Imaging aspects of the scalp layers in computed tomography on bone and soft tissue window with a labeled diagram on the right, detailing the anatomical structures (Philips Brilliance CT 64-slice)

- Connective tissue:
  The dense subcutaneous connective tissue layer, containing fat, blood vessels, and nerves, can be visualized more clearly, appearing as a slightly less dense layer compared to the skin.
- Aponeurosis and loose areolar connective tissue:
  May be thin and challenging to distinguish, usually these layers are seen together on CT.
- Pericranium:
  This periosteal layer adheres to the outer surface of the skull bones, appreciated on CT scans as the layer immediately adjacent to the skull bones.

2.4.2 *Ultrasonography (Fig. 2.8) [6–9]*

- Skin:
  The outermost layer appears as hyperechoic line due to the reflection of ultrasonography waves at the skin surface. It may be slightly thicker in scalp due to the presence of hair follicles and sebaceous glands.
- Hair follicles:
- The hair follicles show as dermal hypoechoic bands with oblique disposition. Longitudinally, it contains the proximal deep dermal follicle bulb and the distal superficial hair shaft, the relative position of which depends on the growth phase:
  - In the telogen phase the hair bulb is in a superficial subdermal location.
  - In the anagen or active growth phase the hair bulb is in the deep dermis/subcutaneous tissue.
  - In the catagen or transition phase it is found in an intermediate position.

Using ultrahigh-frequency probe (more than 50 MHz), the hair tracts located on the scalp show a trilaminar hyperechoic appearance owing to the keratin content and their disposition. The two outer layers compose the cuticle-cortex complex and the inner layer corresponds to the medulla [2].

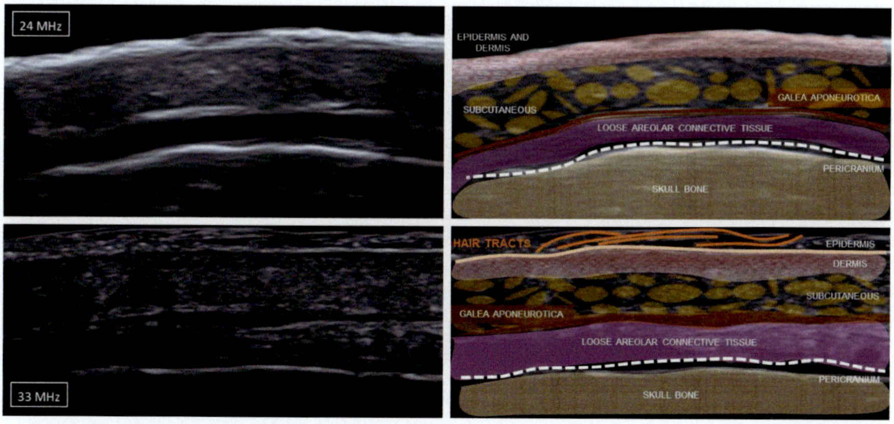

Fig. 2.8 Imaging aspects of the scalp layers in ultrasonography with a 24 and 33 MHz probes, with a labeled diagram on the right, detailing the anatomical structures (Aplio i800, Canon Medical Systems)

- Hair shafts appearance
  - Well-organized, uniformly thick hypoechoic bands with a bottom-heavy or parallel configuration corresponding to hair follicles and shafts.
  - The proximal portions of the hair shafts appeared to blend seamlessly into the hypoechoic subcutaneous tissue, due to the similar echogenicity between these structures and surrounding fat.
  - Uncommon findings can be observed, such as miniaturized hairs (thin, vertically oriented hypoechoic lines confined to the dermis), variation in hair shaft diameter and telogen follicles (small and ovoid follicular structures).
- Dense subcutaneous tissue (Connective tissue):
  Located beneath the skin, this layer appears hypoechoic with scattered hyperechoic strands representing connective tissue and fibrous septa between the fat lobules.
  Contains blood vessels, which can be seen as anechoic tubular structures, and nerves seen as fine echogenic lines.
- Galea aponeurotica:
  This fibrous sheet appears as a thin, hypoechoic band corresponded to the galeal layer (epicraneous muscle and its aponeurosis), separating the subcutaneous tissue from the underlying loose areolar connective tissue.
  Due to its fibrous nature, it provides a distinct echogenic boundary.
- Loose areolar connective tissue:
  Appears hypoechoic compared to the galea aponeurotica and the pericranium.
  This layer is more echolucent, providing a relatively clear space where fluid or infections might spread, known as the "danger zone."
- Pericranium:
  The periosteum of the skull bones appears as a thin, hyperechoic line closely apposed to the outer surface of the skull. Its echogenicity is due to the tight adherence to the skull bones (Fig. 2.9).

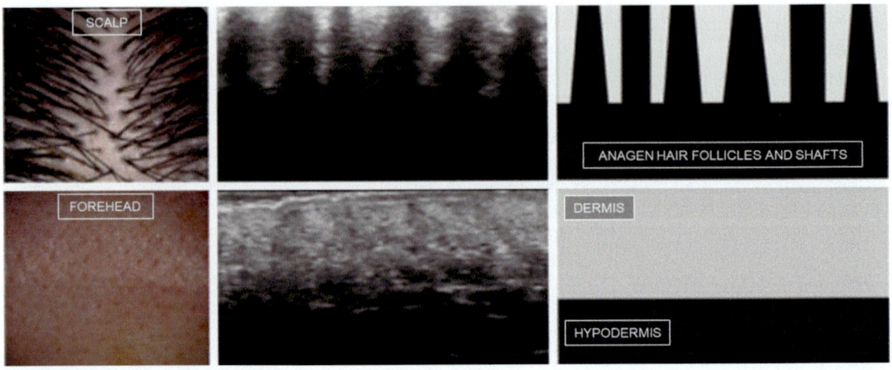

Fig. 2.9 Imaging aspects of the scalp and forehead layers in ultrasonography with a 70 MHz probe. Reprinted from Journal of Dermatological Science, 102 (2021), Kinoshita-Ise M, Ohyama M, Ramjist JM, Foster FS, Yang VXD, Sachdeva M, Sade S, Shear NH, Ultra high-frequency ultrasound with seventy-MHz transducer in hair disorders: Development of a novel noninvasive diagnostic methodology, Pages 167-174, Copyright (2025), with permission from Elsevier

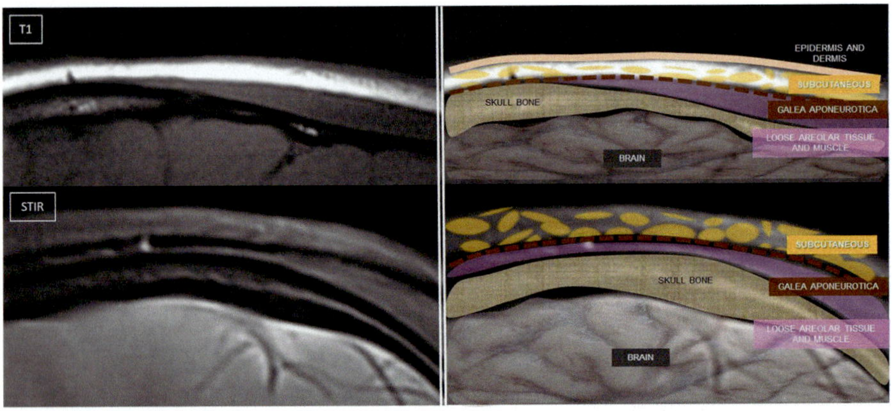

Fig. 2.10 Imaging aspects of the scalp layers in MRI with surface coil, with a labeled diagram on the right, detailing the anatomical structures (Magnetom Prisma 3T MRI, Siemens)

2.4.3 MRI (Fig. 2.10) [10]

On 3T MRI with a surface coil, the following anatomical features of the scalp can be observed:

- Skin:
  Appears as a thin outermost layer, presenting intermediated signal on T1- and T2-weighted images.

- Dense subcutaneous tissue (Connective tissue)
  This layer can be identified due to the signal differences between fat and other soft tissues, showing hypersignal on T1- and T2-weighted images.
- Galea Aponeurotica:
  On MRI, especially T2-weighted images, it may appear as a low-intensity line between the connective tissue and loose areolar connective tissue.
- Loose areolar connective tissue:
  It can be identified as a layer with variable intensity due to the presence of fat and small blood vessels.
- Pericranium:
  It can sometimes be seen as a thin layer of tissue closely apposed to the bone. The external cortical bone presents lack of signal on T1- and T2-weighted images, the medullary bone shows hypersignal on T1- and T2-weighted images and internal cortical bone also presents lack of signal on T1- and T2-weighted images.

References

1. Lindberg MR, Lamps LW. Diagnostic pathology: normal histology. 2nd ed. Elsevier; 2018.
2. Werner B. Biópsia de pele e seu estudo histológico: Por quê? Para quê? Como? Parte I. An Bras Dermatol. 2009;84:391–5.
3. Barnhill RL, Crowson AN, Magro CM, Piepkorn MW, Kutzner H, Desman GT. Barnhill's Dermatopathology. 4th ed. McGraw Hill/Medical; 2019. https://dermatology.mhmedical.com/content.aspx?bookid=2802&sectionid=238125236.
4. Patterson JW. Weedon's skin pathology. 6th ed. Elsevier; 2024.
5. Wortsman X, GBE J, Villani A. Ultrasound and other imaging methods. In: Baran & Dawber's diseases of the nails and their management. Chichester: Wiley; 2018. p. 140–74. https://doi.org/10.1002/9781119323396.ch5.
6. Wortsman X, Wortsman J, Matsuoka L, Saavedra T, Mardones F, Saavedra D, et al. Sonography in pathologies of scalp and hair. Br J Radiol. 2012;85:647–55.
7. Wortsman X. Common applications of dermatologic sonography. J Ultrasound Med. 2012;31:97–111. https://doi.org/10.7863/jum.2012.31.1.97.
8. Seery GE. Surgical anatomy of the scalp. Dermatol Surg. 2002;28:581–7.
9. Al-Nuaimi Y, Baier G, Watson REB, Chuong C-M, Paus R. The cycling hair follicle as an ideal systems biology research model. Exp Dermatol. 2010;19:707–13.
10. Kim J, Kim JY, Chun KA, Jee W-H, Sung M-S. MR imaging manifestations of skin tumors. Eur Radiol. 2008;18:2652–61.

Chapter 3
Anatomy of the Ears, Nose, Lips, and Eyes: Clinical, Imaging, and Histological Aspects

André da Silva Cartell, Ana Luisa Sampaio, Ludmila do Valle Vieira Gusmão, Michele Azevedo Gomes, Luiza Feres, Vanessa Metz, Fernanda Franco de Sá, Carolina Ávila de Almeida, and Clarissa Canella Moraes do Carmo

The intricate structures of the ears, nose, lips, and eyes are essential components of the human face, each serving crucial sensory and functional roles. Understanding the anatomy and histology of these regions is fundamental for medical professionals in fields such as otorhinolaryngology and ophthalmology. Recent advancements in imaging technologies like ultrasound (USG) and magnetic resonance imaging (MRI) with surface coil have significantly enhanced our ability to visualize these complex tissues, allowing for more precise diagnosis and treatment planning. This chapter delves into the detailed anatomy and histology of the ears, nose, lips, and eyes while exploring how modern imaging techniques are utilized to assess and understand these vital structures. Through a comprehensive examination of these elements, we aim to provide a thorough understanding of their normal and pathological states, which is crucial for effective medical intervention.

A. da Silva Cartell
Adjunct Professor at Faculdade de Medicina da Universidade Federal do Rio Grande do Sul, Rio de Janeiro, Brazil

Dermatologist and Dermatopathologist in Private Practice, Rio de Janeiro, Brazil

A. L. Sampaio
Department of Dermatology, Hospital Universitario Pedro Ernesto, Universidade Estadual do Rio de Janeiro—UERJ, Rio de Janeiro, RJ, Brazil

L. do Valle Vieira Gusmão
Marcilio Dias Naval Hospital, Dermatological Imaging Department of DASA - Rio de Janeiro, Rio de Janeiro, Brazil

M. A. Gomes
Head and Neck Oncological Surgery, National Institute of Cancer—INCA, Rio de Janeiro, Brazil

L. Feres · V. Metz
Clinica Vanessa Metz, Ipanema—Rio de Janeiro, Galeria Fórum de Ipanema, Rio de Janeiro, Brazil

© The Author(s), under exclusive license to Springer Nature Switzerland AG 2025

C. Canella Moraes do Carmo (ed.), *Atlas of Diagnostic Imaging in Dermatology*,
https://doi.org/10.1007/978-3-031-77987-9_3

3.1 Ears

3.1.1 Anatomy (Fig. 3.1) [1–5]

- Skin:
  - The epidermis on the ears presents the same histological appearance as on the rest of the body. The structure of the epidermis, consisting of the same layers (stratum basale, stratum spinosum, stratum granulosum, and stratum corneum).

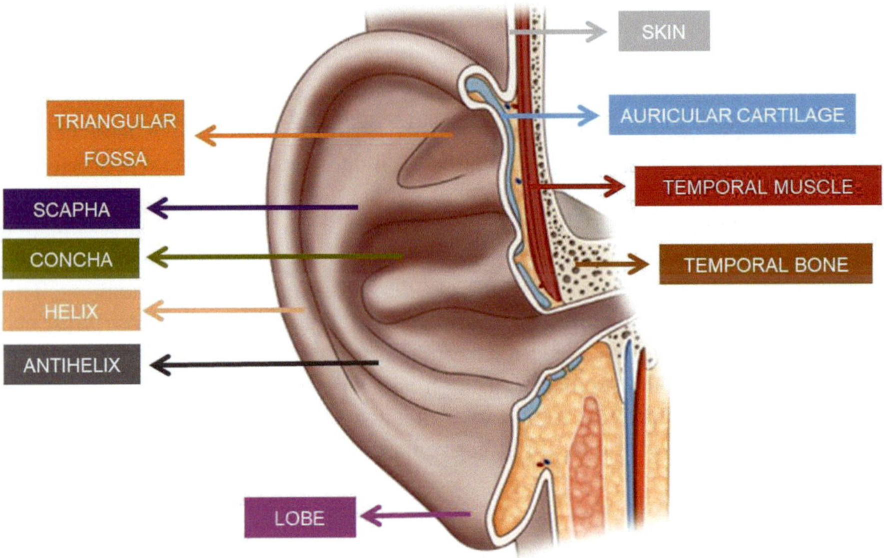

Fig. 3.1 Diagram of the human ear anatomy. Labels point to the triangular fossa, scapha, concha, helix, and antihelix on the outer ear. The lobe is marked at the bottom. Internal structures include the auricular cartilage, temporal muscle, and temporal bone. The skin layer is also indicated. Each part is color-coded for clarity

F. F. de Sá
Clinica Franco de Sa—Rio de Janeiro, Rio de Janeiro, RJ, Brazil

C. Á. de Almeida
Faculty of Medicine of Valença—UniFaa, Valença, Brazil

Federal University of Rio de Janeiro—UFRJ, Rio de Janeiro, Brazil

C. Canella Moraes do Carmo (✉)
Fluminense Federal University—UFF, Rio de Janeiro, Brazil

Federal University of Rio de Janeiro—UFRJ, Rio de Janeiro, Brazil

Diagnóstico das Américas—DASA—RJ, Rio de Janeiro, Brazil

Biodesign Laboratory, DASA-PUC, Rio de Janeiro, Brazil

  - The underlying dermis contains cutaneous appendages, such as sebaceous glands and hair follicles.
- Cartilage:
  - Mainly composed of elastic cartilage, characteristically basophilic in hematoxylin-eosin staining.
  - The peripheral ear contains denser cartilage, while the central part is more flexible.
- Auricular muscle
  - The auricular muscles are a group of three small muscles around the ear. They are involved in the movement of the ear.
  - Auricularis anterior = arises from the galea aponeurotica and inserts into the anterior part of the helix of the ear. Supplied by the temporal branch of the facial nerve.
  - Auricularis superior = arises from the galea aponeurotica and inserts into the upper part of the cranial surface of the auricle (the external part of the ear). Supplied by the temporal branch of the facial nerve.
  - Auricularis posterior = arises from the mastoid part of the temporal bone and inserts into the lower part of the cranial surface of the auricle. Supplied by the posterior auricular branch of the facial nerve.
- External auditory canal:
  - Stratified squamous epithelium lines the external auditory canal.
  - Ceruminous glands in the canal skin produce cerumen.
- Middle and inner ear:
  - Transition from skin to respiratory epithelium in the internal auditory canal, specifically a ciliated pseudostratified columnar epithelium.
  - Presence of sensory structures such as the cochlea and vestibular system in the inner ear.

3.1.2 Radiography and Computed Tomography [6]

- Radiography is not typically used to visualize the soft tissue structures of the ear, including the skin. It primarily shows bony structures such as the ear canal and the bones of the middle ear.
- Computed tomography shows:
  - Skin and subcutaneous tissue: Appears as a thin indistinguishable outer layer of low attenuation compared to the higher attenuation bone structures.
  - Cartilage: Visualized as a structure with intermediate attenuation between the skin and bone.

– Ear canal: Is well-visualized, showing the bony and cartilaginous portions.
– Middle and inner ear: Detailed images of the bony structures of the middle and inner ear, including the ossicles and cochlea, but the skin is only a faint outline.

3.1.3 *Ultrasonography (Fig. 3.2) [6, 7]*

- Epidermis:
  – Appears as a hyperechoic outer layer due to the reflection of ultrasonography waves at the skin surface.
- Dermis:
  – Appears as a hypoechoic layer between epidermis and subcutaneous tissue.
- Subcutaneous tissue:
  – Visible as a hypoechoic layer beneath the dermis, containing fat and connective tissue.

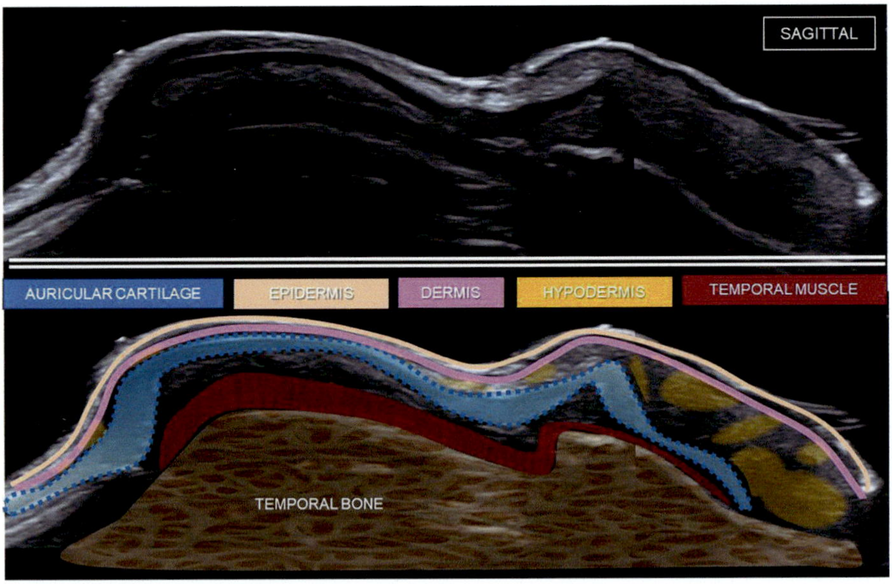

Fig. 3.2 The image shows a sagittal ultrasonographic scan of the ear with 24 MHz probe and a labeled diagram below it. The diagram illustrates the layers of the ear, including auricular cartilage, epidermis, dermis, hypodermis, temporal muscle, and temporal bone. Each layer is color-coded and labeled for clarity (Aplio i800, Canon Medical Systems)

- Cartilage:
  - The auricular cartilage appears as a more hypoechoic structure compared to the subcutaneous tissue but less hypoechoic than the bone.
  - The cartilage is thick at the antihelix border of the auricula. The mean thickness in the normal cartilage at the antihelix border (middle third in the transverse axis) is around 0.8 ± 0.1 mm (range, 0.7–0.9 mm).
- Auricular muscle
  - Hypoechoic layer with fibrillar appearance adjacent the bone
- Ear lobule
  - Which is a one-layer structure and consists of only skin because of the absence of cartilage in this area. It is comparable with the normal sonographic anatomy of skin elsewhere on the body.
  - The mean thickness of the lobule in the healthy individuals is around 6.9 ± 1 mm (range, 5.9–8.1 mm)

3.1.4 MRI (Fig. 3.3) [6, 8]

- Skin:
  - Appears as a thin, hyperintense line on T1-weighted images and a variable intensity on T2-weighted images.
- Subcutaneous tissue:
  - Visible as a layer with intermediate to high signal intensity on T1-weighted images and higher intensity on T2-weighted images due to fat content.

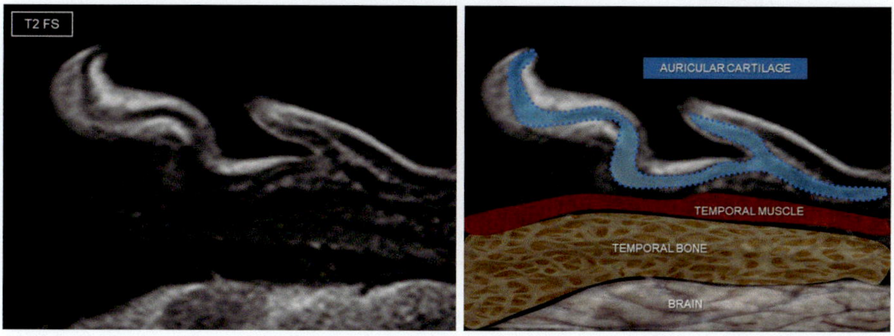

Fig. 3.3 The image consists of two panels. The left panel shows a sagittal T2-weighted MRI of the ear, highlighting the internal structures in grayscale. The right panel is an annotated version of the same scan, with colored labels identifying key anatomical features (Magnetom Prisma 3T MRI, Siemens)

- Cartilage:
  - The auricular cartilage shows intermediate signal intensity on T1- and T2-weighted images.
- Auricular muscle:
  - Shows intermediate signal intensity on T1-weighted images and intermediate to high signal intensity on T2-weighted images. It is well-defined and can be differentiated from surrounding structures due to the high contrast
- Ear canal:
  - Well-visualized with clear differentiation between the bony and cartilaginous portions.
- Middle and inner ear:
  - Excellent soft tissue contrast, allowing detailed visualization of the structures within the middle and inner ear, including the ossicles, cochlea, vestibule, and membranous labyrinth.

3.2 Nose

3.2.1 Anatomy (Fig. 3.4) [2–5]

The nose consists of external structures (such as the nasal bridge, tip, and nostrils) and internal components (including the nasal cavity, septum, conchae, and mucosa).

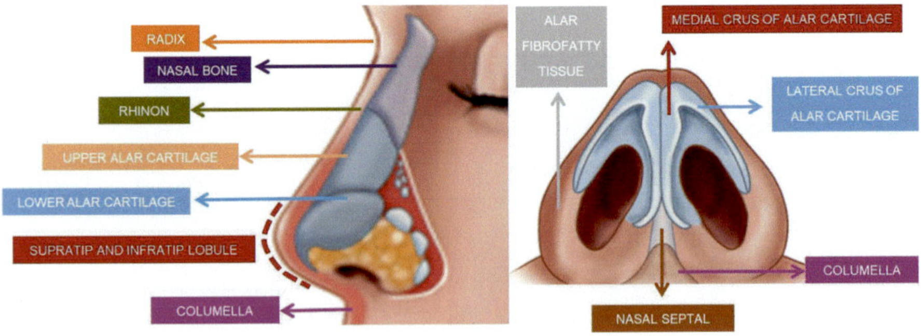

Fig. 3.4 Diagram illustrating the anatomy of the nose. The left side shows a sagittal view with labeled parts: radix, nasal bone, rhinon, upper and lower alar cartilage, supratip and infratip lobule, and columella. The right side displays an axial view highlighting the alar fibro-fatty tissue, medial and lateral crus of alar cartilage, columella, and nasal septal. Each label is color-coded for clarity

- External structures
  - Nasal bridge = the upper, bony part of the nose that forms the bridge between the forehead and the nasal tip. Composed of the nasal bones and the frontal process of the maxilla.
  - Nasal tip (apex) = the rounded end of the nose. Mainly composed of cartilage, including the lower lateral cartilages.
  - Nostrils (nares) = the external openings of the nose. Surrounded by the alar cartilages and bordered by the nasal vestibule.
  - Columella = the tissue that separates the nostrils. Made of cartilage and skin.
  - Ala = the flared, external sides of the nostrils. Comprised of the alar cartilages and surrounding skin.
- Internal components
  - Nasal cavity = The hollow space behind the nose that is divided into two halves. Lined with mucous membranes and divided by the nasal septum.
  - Nasal septum = the partition that divides the nasal cavity into left and right sides. Composed of bone (the perpendicular plate of the ethmoid bone and the vomer) and cartilage (the septal cartilage).
  - Nasal conchae (turbinate bones) = Bony structures within the nasal cavity that help warm and humidify the air. Nasal cartilage contributes to external shape and supports the nostrils.
  - Nasal mucosa = The lining of the nasal cavity that is rich in blood vessels and mucus-secreting glands. Helps trap particles and pathogens, and humidify the air.
  - Olfactory region = The area at the roof of the nasal cavity responsible for the sense of smell. Contains the olfactory epithelium and olfactory bulbs.
  - Paranasal sinuses = Air-filled cavities located around the nasal cavity. Divided in to frontal sinuses, maxillary sinuses, ethmoid sinuses, and sphenoid sinuses.

3.2.2 Radiography and Computed Tomography (Fig. 3.5)

- Radiography primarily shows the bony structures of the nose, such as the nasal bones, and does not provide clear differentiation of the skin or soft tissue structures.
- On computed tomography, the skin and subcutaneous tissue appears as a thin, low-density layer on the surface of the nose. The subcutaneous tissue beneath the skin has slightly higher density than the skin but lower than bone.
- The cartilaginous structures of the nose, such as the septal cartilage and the alar cartilages, appear with intermediate density on computed tomography.
- For nasal bones, computed tomography provides excellent detail of the nasal bones and adjacent bony structures.

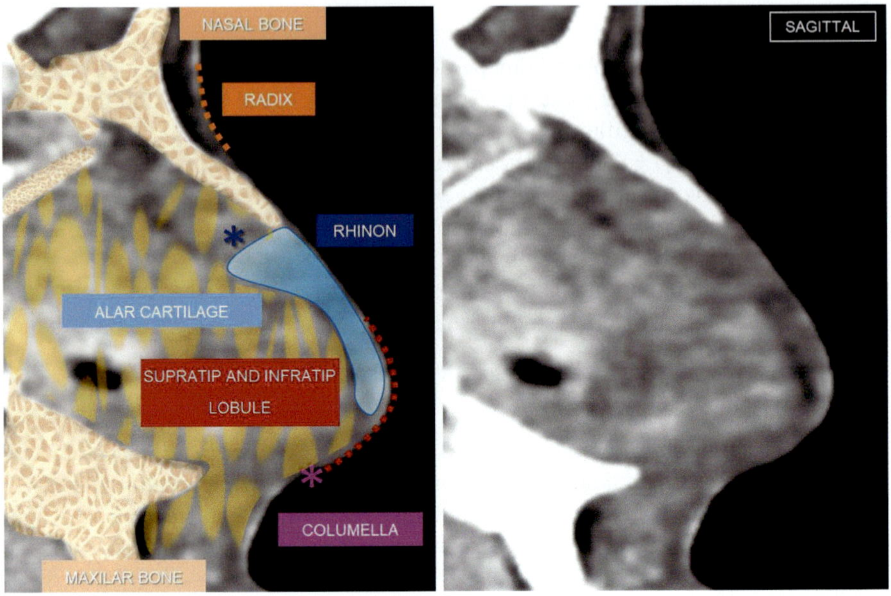

Fig. 3.5 The image is divided into two sections. The left side is a labeled diagram of nasal anatomy on sagittal view showing structures such as the nasal bone, radix, rhinon, alar cartilage, supratip and infratip lobule, columella, and maxillary bone. Each part is color-coded for clarity. The right side displays a sagittal CT scan of a nose, highlighting the same anatomical features for comparison (Philips Brilliance CT 64-slice)

3.2.3 Ultrasonography (Fig. 3.6) [9, 10]

- Skin:
  - The skin appears as a hyperechoic outer layer due to the reflection of ultrasound waves at the skin surface.
- Subcutaneous tissue:
  - Beneath the skin, the subcutaneous tissue appears hypoechoic, containing fat and connective tissue.
- Cartilage:
  - The nasal cartilage appears as a more hypoechoic structure compared to the subcutaneous tissue but less hypoechoic than the bone. Alar cartilages show a typical layered appearance of hypoechoic and echogenic bands. The septal cartilage shows a different and more homogeneous hypoechoic appearance.
- Nasal septum and turbinates:
  - Some of the soft tissue structures within the nasal cavity can be visualized, but the depth of penetration and clarity are limited by the presence of air and

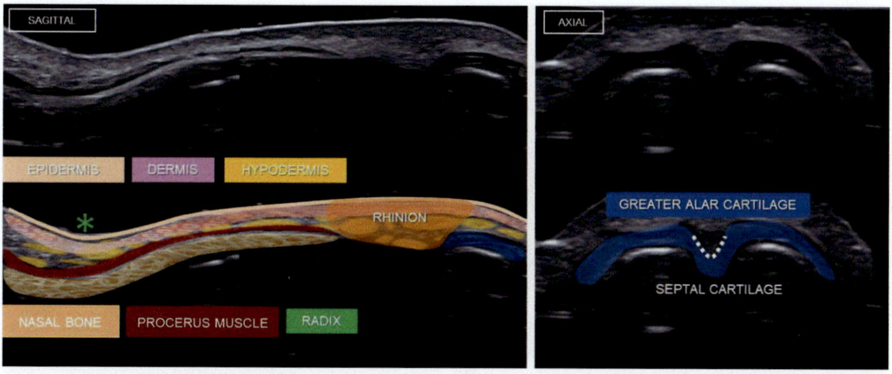

Fig. 3.6 The image shows two ultrasonographic scans of the nasal structure with 24 MHz probe. The left scan illustrates layers of the nose, including the epidermis, dermis, hypodermis, nasal bone, procerus muscle, radix, and rhinion. The right scan highlights the greater alar cartilage and septal cartilage. Each anatomical feature is color-coded for clarity (Aplio i800, Canon Medical Systems)

bone. On sagittal view, and ventral parts of the hypoechoic septal cartilage can be visualized in depth. On an axial view, it is possible to see both the greater cartilages and their fusion in the midline as well as parts of the caudal cartilaginous septum.

3.2.4 MRI (Fig. 3.7)

- Skin:
  - The skin appears as a thin, hyperintense line on T1-weighted images and shows variable intensity on T2-weighted images.
- Subcutaneous tissue:
  - The subcutaneous tissue beneath the skin shows intermediate to high signal intensity on T1-weighted images and higher intensity on T2-weighted images due to fat content.
- Cartilage:
  - Nasal cartilage shows intermediate signal intensity on both T1 and T2-weighted images, allowing for good differentiation from both the skin and the surrounding soft tissues.
- Nasal cavity:
  - MRI provides detailed visualization of the soft tissue structures within the nasal cavity, including the mucosa, turbinates, and septum. The differentiation between various soft tissues is excellent due to the high contrast resolution.

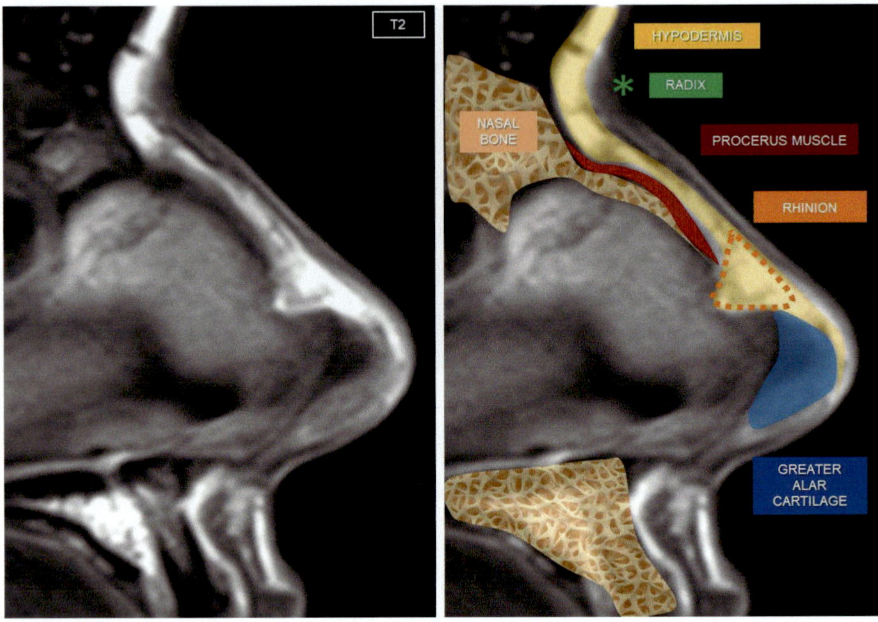

Fig. 3.7 The image shows a side-by-side sagittal MRI scan of a human nose on T2-weighted sequence. The left side displays the unannotated MRI image highlighting the nasal structure. The right side features the same MRI with labeled anatomical components. The annotations provide a detailed view of the nasal anatomy, with color-coded sections for clarity (Magnetom Prisma 3T MRI, Siemens)

3.3 Lips

3.3.1 Anatomy (Figs. 3.8 and 3.9) [1, 3–5]

The lips are composed of several components including the vermilion border and zone, philtrum, Cupid's bow, and labial commissures. Internally, the lips consist of the oral mucosa, labial glands, and the orbicularis oris muscle.

- External anatomy
  - Vermilion border: The distinct line where the lip's reddish portion (vermilion) meets the surrounding skin. It is a well-defined border that separates the pink mucosal part of the lip from the surrounding facial skin.
  - Vermilion zone: The pink or red area of the lips. This region is rich in blood vessels and has a different texture and color compared to the surrounding skin. It lacks the usual hair follicles and sweat glands.
  - Philtrum: The vertical groove in the middle of the upper lip. It extends from the nasal septum to the upper lip, contributing to the shape and appearance of the lips.

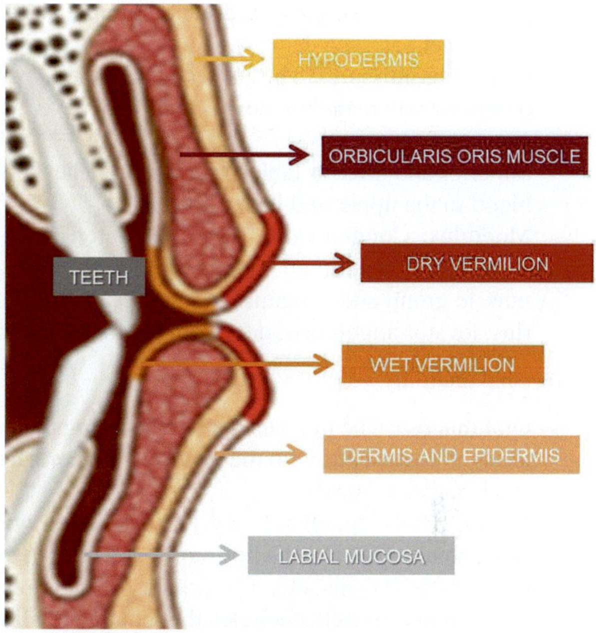

Fig. 3.8 Sagittal cross-sectional diagram of human lip anatomy with labeled parts. From top to bottom, the labels indicate: hypodermis, orbicularis oris muscle, teeth, dry vermilion, wet vermilion, dermis and epidermis, and labial mucosa. The image highlights the structural layers and components of the lip

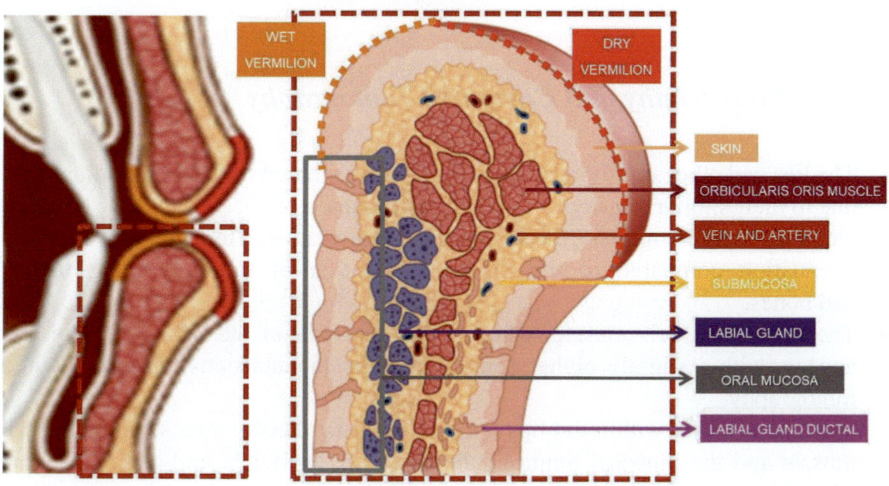

Fig. 3.9 Sagittal cross-sectional diagram of the lip showing detailed anatomy of the inferior lip. The image highlights the wet and dry vermilion areas. Key structures are labeled: skin, orbicularis oris muscle, veins and arteries, submucosa, labial gland, oral mucosa, and labial gland ductal. The diagram uses color coding to differentiate each component, providing a clear view of the lip's internal structure

  - Cupid's bow: The curved, double-humped shape of the upper lip's vermilion border.
  - Labial commissures: The corners where the upper and lower lips meet. These points are where the lips connect and can move, playing a role in facial expressions and speech.
  - Superior and inferior labial arteries: Branches of the facial artery that provide blood to the upper and lower lips.
  - Modiolus: Conglomerate of closely intertwined muscle and fibrous tissue located just lateral and superior to the angle of the mouth. This is a largest muscle group and contains six muscles: the orbicularis oris, buccinator, risorius, levator anguli oris, depressor anguli oris, and zygomaticus major.

- Internal anatomy
  - Oral mucosa: The mucous membrane lining the inner surface of the lips. This lining is continuous with the mucosa of the oral cavity and contains numerous small salivary glands.
  - Labial glands: Small salivary glands located within the lips, which secrete saliva that helps keep the lips moist, assisting in the initial stages of digestion.
  - Orbicularis oris muscle: The primary muscle responsible for lip movement. This circular muscle encircles the mouth and allows for the pouting, closing, and compression of the lips.

3.3.2 Radiography and Computed Tomography

- The lips and other soft tissues are not well-differentiated on standard radiographs due to their similar density to surrounding tissues.
- On computed tomography, the skin of the lips appears as a thin outer layer of low attenuation compared to the higher attenuation of the underlying tissues and bones.
- The orbicularis oris muscle, which forms the bulk of the lips, is visible and appears with a slightly higher density than the subcutaneous fat on computed tomography.
- Subcutaneous fat within the lips appears as a low-density area surrounding the muscle and the mucosal lining of the inner lips is visible and distinguishable from the outer skin on computed tomography.
- Minor salivary glands within the lips can sometimes be visualized as small areas of slightly different attenuation on computed tomography.

3.3.3 Ultrasonography (Fig. 3.10) [11]

- Skin:
  - The skin of the lips appears as a hyperechoic outer layer.
- Subcutaneous tissue:
  - Beneath the skin, the subcutaneous tissue appears hypoechoic, containing fat and connective tissue.
- Muscles:
  - The orbicularis oris muscle appears as a more hypoechoic structure compared to the skin and subcutaneous tissue but more echogenic than deeper structures. The orbicularis oris muscle occupies the entire width of the lips. It has no direct skeletal attachment, but merges with the modiolus.
- Vessels and glands:
  - Blood vessels and minor salivary glands can be visualized as anechoic tubular and small round structures, respectively.

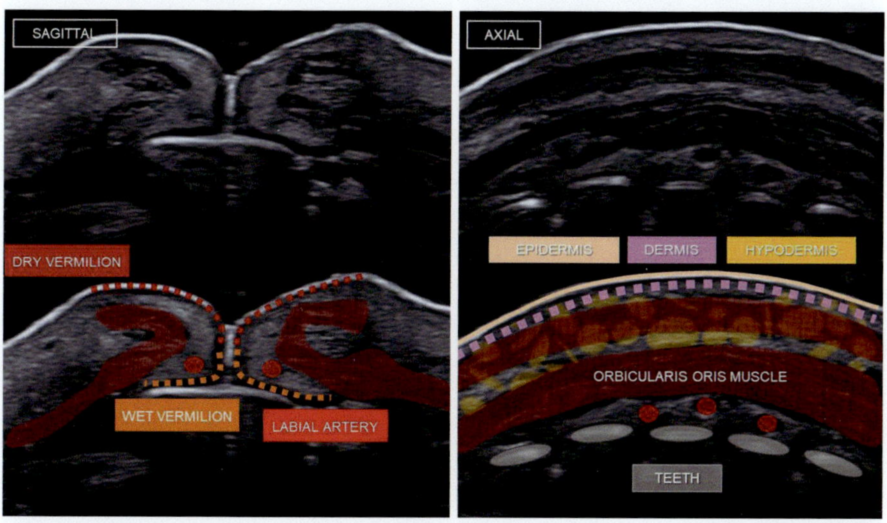

Fig. 3.10 The image shows two ultrasonographic scans of the lip with 24 MHz probe on sagittal and axial views. Each anatomical feature is color-coded for clarity (Aplio i800, Canon Medical Systems)

3.3.4 *MRI (Fig. 3.11) [12]*

- Skin:
  - The skin of the lips appears as a thin hyperintense line on T1-weighted images and shows variable intensity on T2-weighted images.
- Subcutaneous tissue:
  - The subcutaneous tissue appears with intermediate to high signal intensity on T1-weighted images and higher intensity on T2-weighted images due to fat content.
- Muscles:
  - The orbicularis oris muscle is clearly visible, showing intermediate signal intensity on both T1- and T2-weighted images.
- Mucosa:
  - The mucosal lining of the inner lips can be distinguished from the outer skin and shows intermediate to high signal intensity on MRI sequences.

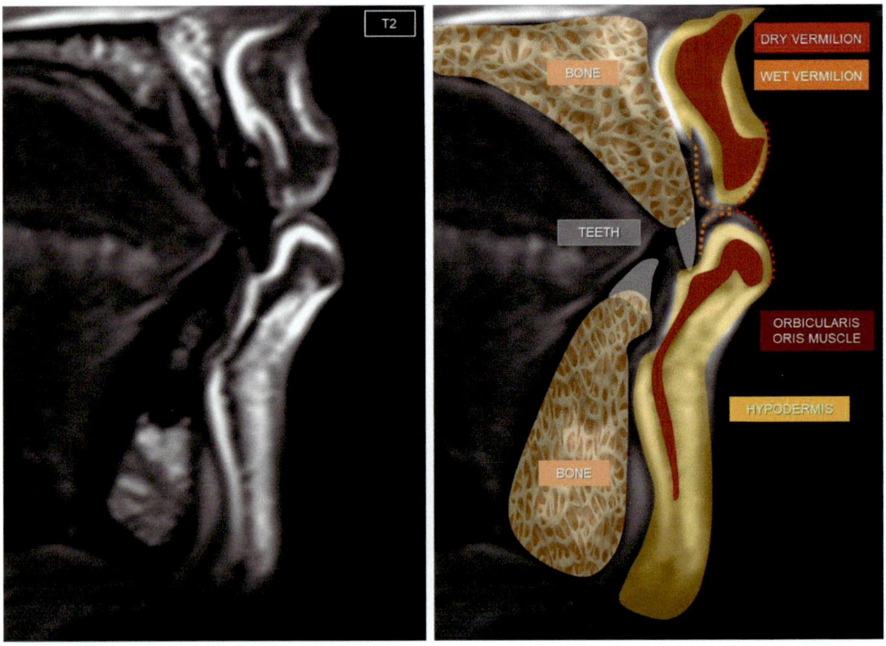

Fig. 3.11 The image is split into two sections. The left side shows a T2-weighted MRI scan of a human head in profile, highlighting the oral cavity. The right side is an annotated image, labeling structures such as bone, teeth, orbicularis oris muscle, hypodermis, and the dry and wet vermilion of the lips. The diagram provides a detailed view of the anatomical layers and their relationships (Magnetom Prisma 3T MRI, Siemens)

- Glands and vessels:
  - Minor salivary glands and blood vessels are visible, with glands appearing as small structures with intermediate signal intensity and vessels as voids due to flowing blood.

3.4 Eyes

3.4.1 Anatomy (Figs. 3.12 and 3.13) [2, 4, 5]

The components of the eye region anatomy include the epidermis, dermis, subcutaneous tissue, muscles, and associated structures. Here is a detailed description:

- Epidermis
  - The epidermis is the outermost layer of the skin and acts as a protective barrier against environmental factors.
  - The epidermis on the eye region presents the same histological appearance as the epidermis on the rest of the body.
- Dermis
  - The dermis on the eye region presents the same histological appearance as the dermis on the rest of the body.

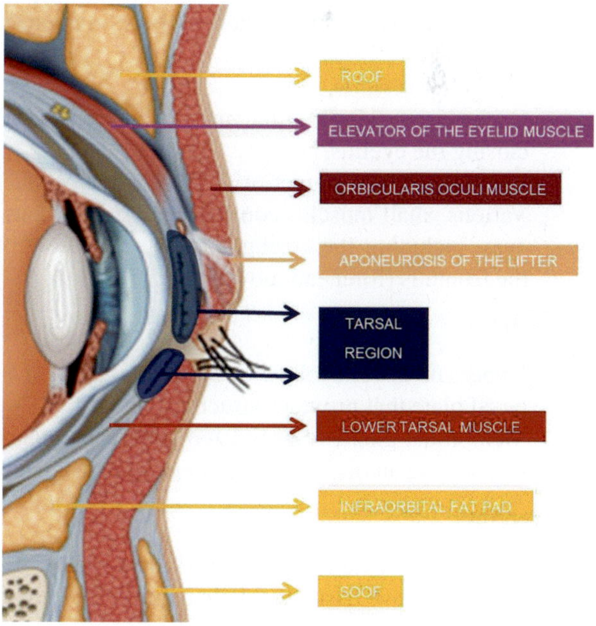

Fig. 3.12 Cross-sectional diagram of the human eye and surrounding structures, labeled with various components. From top to bottom, the labels are: retro-orbicularis oculi fat (ROOF), Elevator of the Eyelid Muscle, Orbicularis Oculi Muscle, Aponeurosis of the Lifter, Tarsal Region, Lower Tarsal Muscle, Infraorbital Fat Pad, and suborbicularis oculi fat (SOOF). Each label is color-coded and points to the corresponding anatomical part, illustrating the complex layers and muscles involved in eyelid function

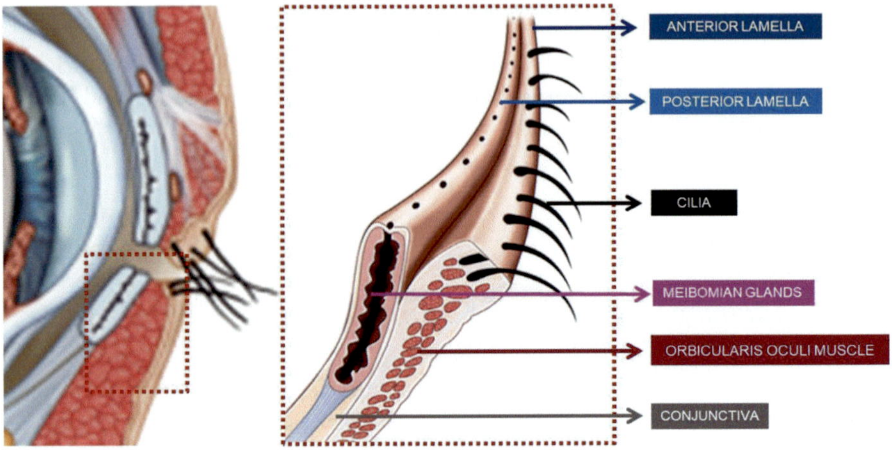

Fig. 3.13 The image is a detailed anatomical illustration of the eyelid focus on tarsal plate, highlighting its cross-sectional structure. On the left, a zoomed-out view of the eye shows the area of focus. The right side features a close-up of the eyelid, labeled with key components: the anterior lamella, posterior lamella, cilia, meibomian glands, orbicularis oculi muscle, and conjunctiva. Each part is marked with arrows and color-coded labels, providing a clear view of the eyelid's anatomy and its various layers and structures

- Subcutaneous tissue
  - The subcutaneous tissue lies beneath the dermis and acts as a cushion and insulator.
  - The subcutaneous tissue on the eye region presents the same histological appearance as the subcutaneous tissue on the rest of the body.
- Muscles
  - Orbicularis oculi: Ringlike muscle that encircles the eye and is responsible for closing the eyelids.
  - Levator palpebrae superioris: Muscle that elevates the upper eyelid.
  - Various small muscles control facial expressions and movements around the eyes, including the corrugator supercilii (controls eyebrow movement) and the frontalis (forehead movement).
- Eyelids
  - Upper and lower eyelids: Composed of skin, muscle, connective tissue, and a tarsal plate that provides structural integrity.
  - Meibomian glands: Specialized sebaceous glands located within the eyelids that secrete an oily substance to prevent tear evaporation.
- Eyebrows
  - The eyebrows are composed of skin and hair follicles, with underlying muscle and connective tissue that help control their movement.

- Lacrimal apparatus
  - Includes the lacrimal glands and ducts that help drain tears into the nasal cavity.
- Conjunctiva
  - A thin, transparent membrane that covers the sclera and lines the inside of the eyelids, providing lubrication and protection.

3.4.2 Radiography and Computed Tomography (Fig. 3.14)

- Radiography is not typically used to visualize the skin and soft tissue structures of the eye region.
- Computed tomography.
  - Skin and subcutaneous tissue:

    The skin appears as a thin, low-density layer on the surface of the eye region. The subcutaneous tissue beneath the skin has slightly higher density than the skin but lower than bone.
  - Muscles:

    The extraocular muscles are well visualized and appear with intermediate density.

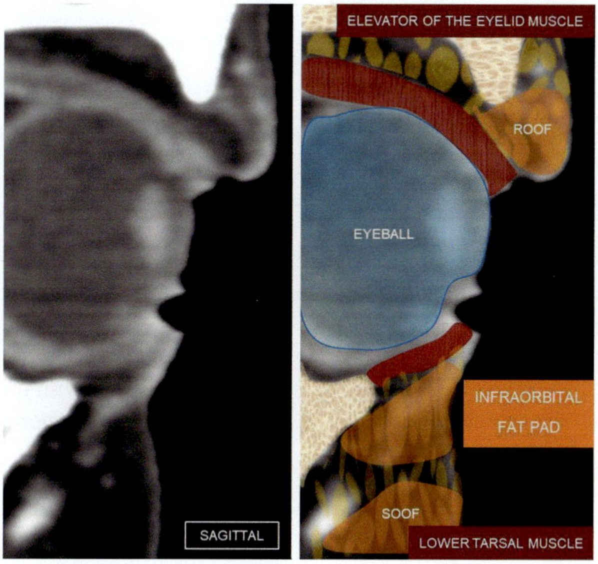

Fig. 3.14 The image is divided into two sections. The left side shows a grayscale sagittal CT scan of the eye region. The right side is a color-coded anatomical image, highlighting different structures. The diagram provides a detailed view of the eye's anatomical components (Philips Brilliance CT 64-slice)

– Orbital fat:

The orbital fat appears as a low-density area surrounding the eyeball and muscles, providing a clear contrast with the denser bony structures.

– Eye:

The globe of the eye is well visualized, with the vitreous body appearing as a low-density area and the lens as a higher density structure.

– Lacrimal gland:

The lacrimal gland can be seen in the superolateral aspect of the orbit as a structure with intermediate density.

– Bony structures:

Detailed images of the orbital bones and surrounding facial skeleton are provided.

3.4.3 Ultrasonography (Figs. 3.15 and 3.16) [13–15]

- Ultrasonography of the periorbital region should be performed with the system's output power reduced to approximately 75–80%, given the anatomical proximity to the globe and the need to minimize acoustic energy exposure to ocular structures.
- Skin:
  - The skin appears as a hyperechoic outer layer.
- Subcutaneous tissue:
  - Beneath the skin, the subcutaneous tissue appears hypoechoic, containing fat and connective tissue.
- Muscles:
  - The extraocular muscles appear as more hypoechoic structures compared to the skin and subcutaneous tissue but more echogenic than the orbital fat.
- Eye:
  - The globe of the eye is clearly visualized, with the vitreous body appearing as an anechoic area. The lens can be seen as a more hyperechoic structure.

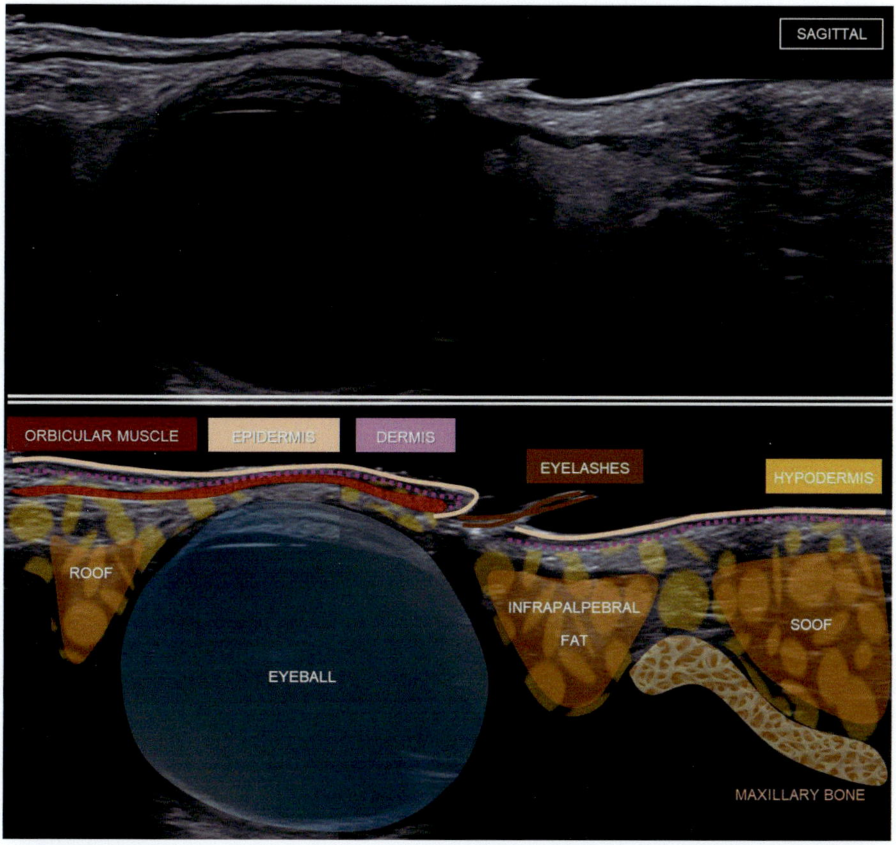

Fig. 3.15 The image consists of two parts: a sagittal ultrasonographic scan of an eye with 24 MHz probe and a labeled anatomical diagram. The top section shows a grayscale ultrassonographic image. The bottom section is a colorful cross-sectional diagram of the eye, labeled with parts such as the eyeball, orbital fat, dermis, epidermis, and skeletal muscle. The diagram highlights the layers and structures surrounding the eye, including the hypodermis and maxillary bone (Aplio i800, Canon Medical Systems)

- Optic nerve:
  - The optic nerve can be visualized as a hypoechoic tubular structure extending from the back of the globe.
- Lacrimal gland:
  - The lacrimal gland can sometimes be visualized as a hypoechoic structure in the superolateral aspect of the orbit.

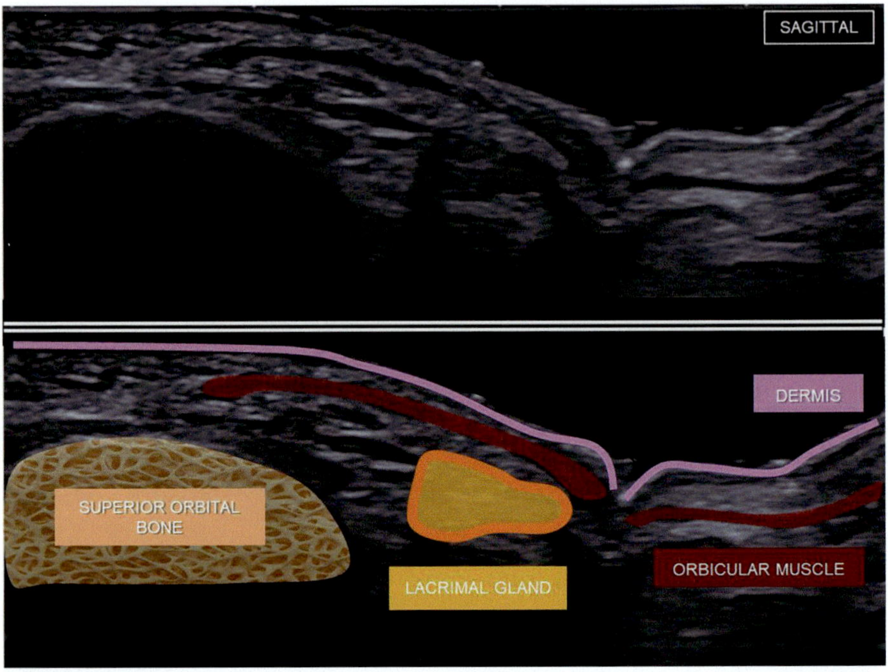

Fig. 3.16 An ultrasonographic image with 24 MHz probe in sagittal view showing anatomical structures of the eye region focus on lacrimal gland. The top part displays a grayscale ultrasonographic scan, while the bottom part includes labeled overlays (Aplio i800, Canon Medical Systems)

3.4.4 MRI (Fig. 3.17) [16]

- Skin:
  - The skin appears as a thin, hyperintense line on T1-weighted images and shows variable intensity on T2-weighted images.
- Subcutaneous tissue:
  - The subcutaneous tissue appears with intermediate to high signal intensity on T1-weighted images and higher intensity on T2-weighted images due to fat content.
- Muscles:
  - The extraocular muscles are clearly visible, showing intermediate signal intensity on both T1- and T2-weighted images.

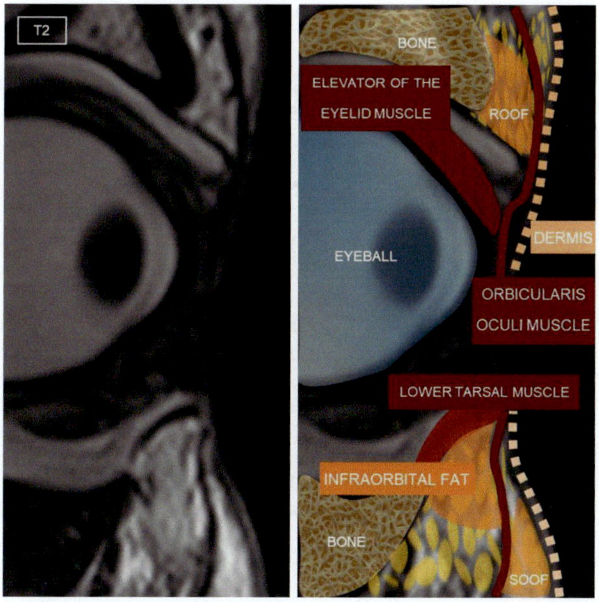

Fig. 3.17 The image shows a sagittal T2-weighted MRI scan of the eye region on the left and a detailed anatomical diagram on the right. The anatomical diagram labels various components: the eyeball, bone, elevator of the eyelid muscle, ROOF (retro-orbicularis oculi fat) dermis, orbicularis oculi muscle, lower tarsal muscle, infraorbital fat, and SOOF (suborbicularis oculi fat). The diagram uses color coding to differentiate the structures (Magnetom Prisma 3T MRI, Siemens)

- Orbital fat:
  - The orbital fat appears with high signal intensity on T1-weighted images and intermediate to high intensity on T2-weighted images.
- Eye:
  - The globe of the eye is well visualized, with the vitreous body showing low signal intensity on T1 and high on T2. The lens appears as a low-signal-intensity structure.
- Optic nerve:
  - The optic nerve is visible as a structure with intermediate signal intensity on T1 and high intensity on T2-weighted images.
- Lacrimal gland:
  - The lacrimal gland appears as a structure with intermediate signal intensity on T1-weighted images and higher intensity on T2-weighted images in the superolateral aspect of the orbit.

References

1. Elder DE, Elenitsas R, Murphy GF, Rosenbach M, Rubin AI, Seykora JT, et al. Lever's dermatopathology: histopathology of the skin. 12th ed. Lippincott Williams & Wilkins; 2022.
2. Patterson JW. Weedon's skin pathology. 6th ed. Elsevier; 2024.
3. Lindberg MR, Lamps LW. Diagnostic pathology: normal histology. 2nd ed. Elsevier; 2018.
4. Werner B. Biópsia de pele e seu estudo histológico: Por quê? Para quê? Como? Parte I. An Bras Dermatol. 2009;84:391–5.
5. Barnhill RL, Crowson AN, Magro CM, Piepkorn MW, Kutzner H, Desman GT. Barnhill's dermatopathology. 4th ed. McGraw Hill/Medical; 2019. https://dermatology.mhmedical.com/content.aspx?bookid=2802&sectionid=238125236.
6. Tsuno NSG, Tsuno MY, Coelho Neto CAF, Noujaim SE, Decnop M, Pacheco FT, et al. Imaging the external ear: practical approach to normal and pathologic conditions. RadioGraphics. 2022;42:522–40.
7. Wortsman X, Jemec GBE. Sonography of the ear pinna. J Ultrasound Med. 2008;27:761–70.
8. Jeffrey DR, Watt I. Imaging hyaline cartilage. Br J Radiol. 2003;76:777–87.
9. Earwaker J. Anatomic variants in sinonasal CT. Radiographics. 1993;13:381–415. https://doi.org/10.1148/radiographics.13.2.8460226.
10. Gossner J. Sonography of the nasal cartilage: technique and normal anatomy. J Ultrasound. 2014;17:317–4.
11. Greenall C, Drage N. Sebaceous carcinoma of the lip: comparing normal lip and cheek anatomy with the imaging features of a rare cutaneous malignancy. Ultrasound. 2015;23:126–9.
12. Som PM, Ng SA, Stuchen C, Tang CY, Lawson W, Laitman JT. The MR imaging identification of the facial muscles and the subcutaneous musculoaponeurotic system. Neurographics. 2012;2:35–43.
13. Tansatit T, Phumyoo T, Jitaree B, Sahraoui YME, Lee JH. Anatomical and ultrasound-based injections for sunken upper eyelid correction. J Cosmet Dermatol. 2020;19:346–52.
14. Wortsman X. Practical applications of ultrasound in dermatology. Clin Dermatol. 2021;39:605–23.
15. Wortsman X. Common applications of dermatologic sonography. J Ultrasound Med. 2012;31:97–111. https://doi.org/10.7863/jum.2012.31.1.97.
16. Dobbs NW, Budak MJ, White RD, Zealley IA. MR-eye: high-resolution microscopy coil MRI for the assessment of the orbit and periorbital structures, part 1: technique and anatomy. Am J Neuroradiol. 2020;41:947–50.

Chapter 4
Anatomy of Nail and Periungual Region: Clinical, Imaging, and Histological Aspects

Robertha Nakamura, Ludmila do Valle Vieira Gusmão, André da Silva Cartell, Carolina Ávila de Almeida, and Clarissa Canella Moraes do Carmo

The nail unit is a complex skin appendage situated on the dorsal surfaces of the fingertips and toes. It serves crucial roles in both protection and sensory perception, enhancing our daily functional abilities. This structure consists of several integral components: the nail plate, nail bed, nail matrix, and periungual folds. The nail plate, the visible

R. Nakamura
Institute of Dermatology Professor Rubem David Azulay, Rio de Janeiro, RJ, Brazil

Dermatology by the Brazilian Society of Dermatology, Rio de Janeiro, RJ, Brazil

Dermatology from the Federal University of Medicine at Rio de Janeiro, Rio de Janeiro, RJ, Brazil

Nail Study Center—Institute of Dermatology Professor Ruben David Azulay, Santa Casa da Misericórdia do Rio de Janeiro, Rio de Janeiro, RJ, Brazil

L. do Valle Vieira Gusmão
Marcilio Dias Naval Hospital, Dermatological Imaging Department of DASA - Rio de Janeiro, Rio de Janeiro, Brazil

A. da Silva Cartell
Adjunct Professor at Faculdade de Medicina da Universidade Federal do Rio Grande do Sul, Rio de Janeiro, Brazil

Dermatologist and Dermatopathologist in Private Practice, Rio de Janeiro, Brazil

C. Á. de Almeida
Faculty of Medicine of Valença—UniFaa, Valença, Brazil

Federal University of Rio de Janeiro—UFRJ, Rio de Janeiro, Brazil

C. Canella Moraes do Carmo (✉)
Fluminense Federal University—UFF, Rio de Janeiro, Brazil

Federal University of Rio de Janeiro—UFRJ, Rio de Janeiro, Brazil

Diagnóstico das Américas—DASA—RJ, Rio de Janeiro, Brazil

Biodesign Laboratory, DASA-PUC, Rio de Janeiro, Brazil

© The Author(s), under exclusive license to Springer Nature Switzerland AG 2025
C. Canella Moraes do Carmo (ed.), *Atlas of Diagnostic Imaging in Dermatology*, https://doi.org/10.1007/978-3-031-77987-9_4

part of the nail, is produced through ongoing cellular differentiation within the nail matrix and is firmly anchored to the nail bed by the surrounding folds, extending distally to form its free edge. A thorough understanding of the anatomy and terminology associated with the nail unit is essential for accurately recognizing and interpreting various conditions and changes affecting this area. This chapter offers a detailed overview of the nail unit anatomy, describing each of its constituent structures. It lays the foundation for visualizing these structures through imaging techniques, with a focus on ultrasonography and magnetic resonance imaging with surface coil.

4.1 Anatomy [1–3]

The nail unit is a complex skin appendage situated on the dorsal surface of the fingertips and toes, serving crucial protective and sensory roles. It comprises several key components: the nail plate, nail bed, nail matrix, and periungual folds.

The nail plate results from the ongoing cellular differentiation within the nail matrix, and is secured in place by the surrounding nail folds, firmly attached to the nail bed. It extends distally to form a free edge. Understanding the anatomy and terminology related to the nail unit is essential for recognizing and interpreting changes and conditions affecting this region.

4.1.1 Nail Unit [1, 3–5]

- Nail plate: This continuously growing, hardened, and semitransparent structure is composed of a modified and keratinized stratum corneum derived from epidermal cells. It covers the nail bed and matrix, forming the visible portion of the nail and extending distally to create a free edge.
- Lateral nail folds: These are cutaneous folds on the sides of the nail plate, defining its lateral borders. While they consist of normal skin, they lack pilosebaceous units. They provide cushioning for the lateral margins of the nail plate and contribute to its adhesion to the nail bed.
- Proximal nail fold: This fold is covered with epithelium on both its ventral and dorsal surfaces. Its free end forms the cuticle. The ventral surface of the proximal fold gives rise to the eponychium, with the proximal matrix located beneath. Together with the nail plate, the proximal fold protects the nail matrix.
- Eponychium: Located on the lower surface or ventral region of the proximal nail fold, the eponychium is a "nail pocket" featuring flat epidermis, a granular layer, and orthokeratosis. It is responsible for producing the cuticle.
- Cuticle: A thin, delicate epidermal layer extending from the proximal nail fold to the nail plate surface. Produced by the eponychium, it adheres firmly to the nail plate's dorsal surface and forms a protective barrier for the nail matrix.
- Nail matrix: This active structure, responsible for continuous nail plate production, constitutes 15–25% of the proximal tissue beneath the nail plate. The matrix

consists of germinal epithelium that keratinizes to form the dorsal and intermediate plates and contains melanocytes. The matrix can be divided into:

  - Dorsal or proximal matrix: Located below the proximal fold, responsible for forming the back of the nail plate.
  - Intermediate, germinal, or distal matrix: Positioned after the dorsal matrix, producing the majority of the nail plate.
  - Ventral matrix or nail bed: Starting at the lunula's edge and extending to the onychodermal band, this striated tissue represents 75–85% of the tissue beneath the nail plate. It is pinkish due to its vascular structure and assists in attaching the nail plate to the bed while aiding in its continuous movement.

- Lunula: A half-moon-shaped, convex edge of the intermediate or distal matrix visible through the nail plate. It contrasts with the adjacent nail bed's color and is most visible on the thumbs and hallux.
- Onychodermal band: A transverse stripe, measuring 1 to 1.5 mm, found in the distal region of the nail bed. It varies in color (pink, white, or brown) depending on skin color and represents the site of greatest nail plate adherence before physiological onycholysis, acting as a protective barrier.
- Hyponychium: A specialized structure crucial for physiological onycholysis, the separation of the nail plate from the nail bed. It is highly keratinized and forms a protective barrier, preventing foreign substances from entering beneath the nail plate.
- Distal groove: A demarcation zone between the subungual structures and surrounding skin, appearing as a skin ridge located distally in the hyponychium.
- Anterior and posterior ligaments: These strong, flexible collagen bands connect the nail to the bone, playing a crucial role in stabilizing the nail components and maintaining the structural integrity of the nail unit.

  - Anterior ligament: Located in the anterior or distal region, just below the onychodermal band.
  - Posterior ligament: Situated in the posterior or proximal region, where the proximal matrix begins.

- Enthesis: The point where tendons, ligaments, or joint capsules attach to bone. In the nail complex, this includes the extensor and flexor enthesis at the base of the distal phalanx.
- Distal interphalangeal joint: The joint located between the distal and middle phalanges of the fingers and toes (Figs. 4.1, 4.2, and 4.3).

4.1.2 Vascular Supply [1, 6, 7]

- The fingers receive their blood supply from four main arteries originating from the superficial and deep palmar arches, with two arteries on each side:

  - Dorsal arteries
  - Palmar (or plantar) arteries

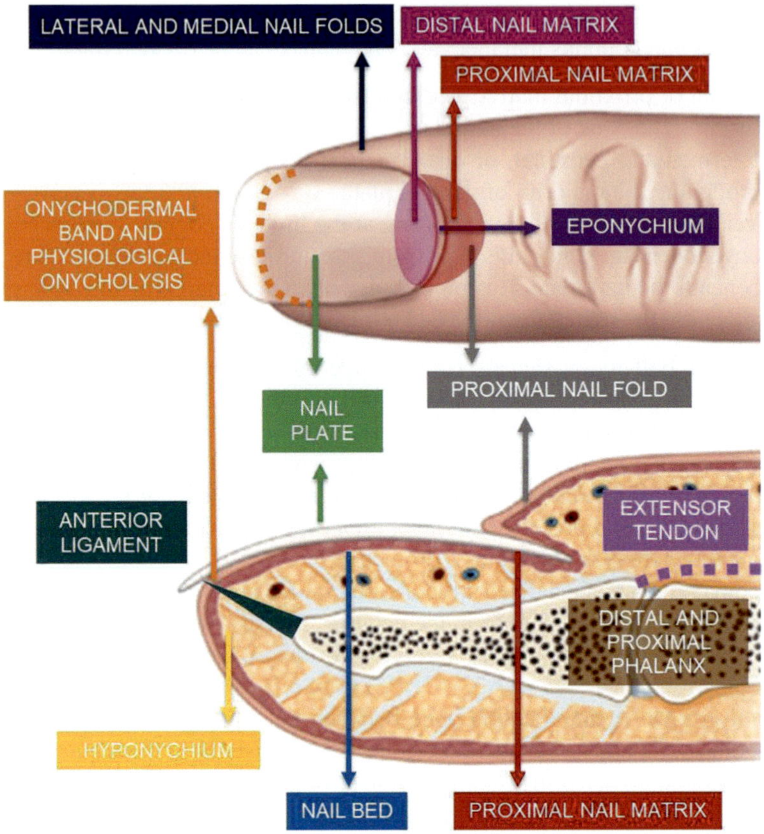

Fig. 4.1 Schematic representation with a detailed view of the nail unit components and surrounding tissues

   - These arteries extend toward the nail unit, situated in the distal finger region, and converge to form a superficial arcade just beyond the distal phalanx. This arterial network is crucial for supplying blood to the proximal nail fold and matrix.

- The subungual area is supplied by both proximal and distal subungual arcades. These arcades are formed through anastomoses between the palmar arcade and the superficial arcade, ensuring a comprehensive blood supply. Venous drainage from the finger is managed by both superficial and deep venous systems.
- The nail bed is richly vascularized and contains specialized structures known as glomus bodies. These neurovascular structures act as arteriovenous anastomoses, regulating peripheral capillary circulation, particularly in response to cold temperatures. The presence of glomus bodies highlights their essential role in regulating blood flow and maintaining nail health.

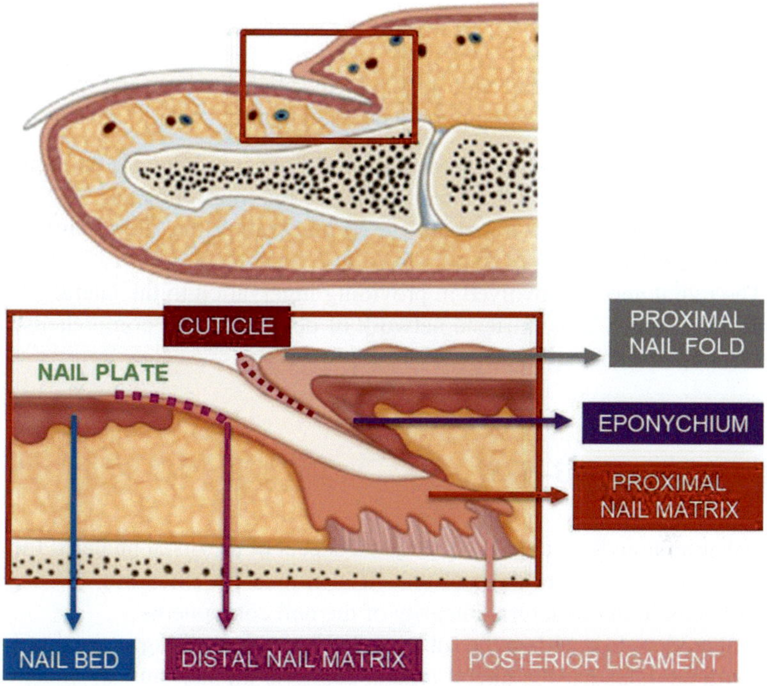

Fig. 4.2 Schematic representation with a detailed view of the nail matrix components

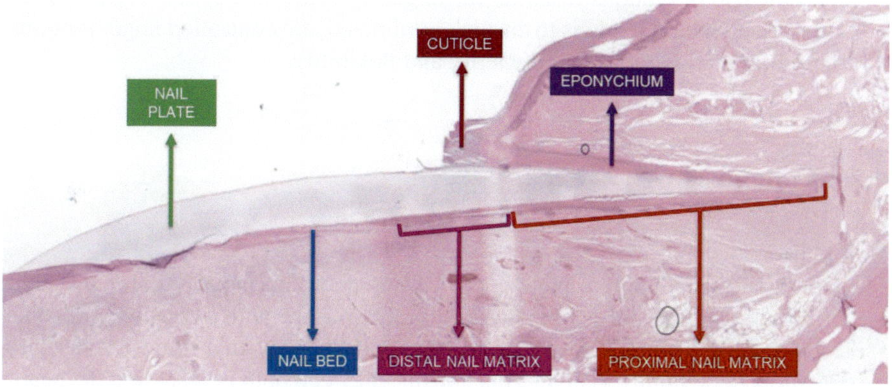

Fig. 4.3 Histological section of a human nail, labeled with key anatomical structures (x4)

4.1.3 Innervation [1]

- The innervation of the nail unit involves contributions from the median, ulnar, and radial nerves, encompassing both dorsal and palmar (or plantar) aspects.
  - The median nerve assumes the responsibility of supplying the nail unit for the first, second, third, and the lateral aspect of the fourth fingers.
  - The ulnar nerve plays a pivotal role in innervating the lateral portion of the fourth and fifth fingers.
  - The radial nerve is involved in providing innervation to the lateral portion of the first finger. This intricate network of nerves ensures comprehensive sensory input to the nail [1, 2, 4, 12].

4.1.4 Tendons [1, 3–5, 8]

- Extensor tendon: Positioned on the dorsal aspect of the distal phalanx, the extensor tendon is integral to the nail unit. It is crucial for extending the finger and helps maintain the structural integrity of the nail components.
- Lateral tendon: Located on the subungual sides and attaching to the distal region of the distal phalanx, the lateral tendon supports the nail unit by enhancing its stability and functionality.
- Flexor tendon: The flexor tendon, found on the palmar side of the finger, completes the trio of tendons essential for finger movement. It collaborates with the extensor and lateral tendons to ensure coordinated and controlled finger motions, contributing to overall finger dexterity and flexibility.

4.2 Onichoscopy [9–12]

Nail plate

- Smooth surface: The nail plate is typically smooth and evenly colored. Under dermoscopy, it appears as a relatively uniform surface with a consistent sheen.
- Translucency: The nail plate has a slight translucency that allows underlying structures to be faintly visible. This translucency can help in assessing the health of the nail.

Lunula or distal nail matrix (visible region of the matrix)

- Visible crescent: The lunula, the white crescent-shaped area at the base of the nail, is visible under dermoscopy as a slightly opaque, lighter area compared to the rest of the nail plate. It's usually well-defined and extends from the cuticle area.

Nail bed

- Pinkish color: The nail bed beneath the nail plate appears pinkish due to the underlying vascular structures. This color can vary slightly among individuals but should be relatively uniform and free from discoloration.
- Subungual capillaries: Small, fine capillaries in the nail bed can be seen as a delicate network of red lines or dots. In normal conditions, these capillaries are not overly prominent or irregular.

Cuticle

- Well-defined border: The cuticle, which is the thin layer of skin at the base of the nail, appears as a smooth, slightly darker line. It separates the nail plate from the surrounding skin and provides a clear boundary under dermoscopy.

Proximal nail matrix

- No direct visualization: While the proximal nail matrix (the area responsible for nail growth) itself is not directly visible, its health indirectly affects the appearance of the nail plate. Normal nail growth patterns and smooth nail plate surfaces suggest a healthy matrix.

Nail folds

- Normal contour: The lateral nail folds (the skin on the sides of the nail) should appear smooth and without significant changes or irregularities. The proximal nail fold is level with the cuticle and in its normal state shows no signs of inflammation or swelling.

Subungual structures

- Absence of abnormalities: Under dermoscopy, the area beneath the nail plate, the hyponychial region, should appear clear of any abnormal pigmentation, streaks, or lesions. Normal findings include a clean, unblemished appearance (Fig. 4.4).

4.3 Imaging Methods [13]

High-frequency ultrasonography is increasingly becoming the preferred initial method for assessing nail lesions. Computed tomography and plain radiography are now typically reserved for cases where bone involvement is suspected or evident.

Magnetic resonance imaging with surface coils is also emerging as a favored technique for evaluating nail lesions due to its high resolution, excellent contrast, and ability to distinguish various components of the lesion, thus simplifying diagnosis.

Recent advancements in 3D reconstruction from 3T MRI images have significantly improved the visualization and understanding of the extent of nail lesions. Isotropic sequences from 3T MRI can be used for 3D reconstruction, enabling virtual navigation and 3D printing of the model.

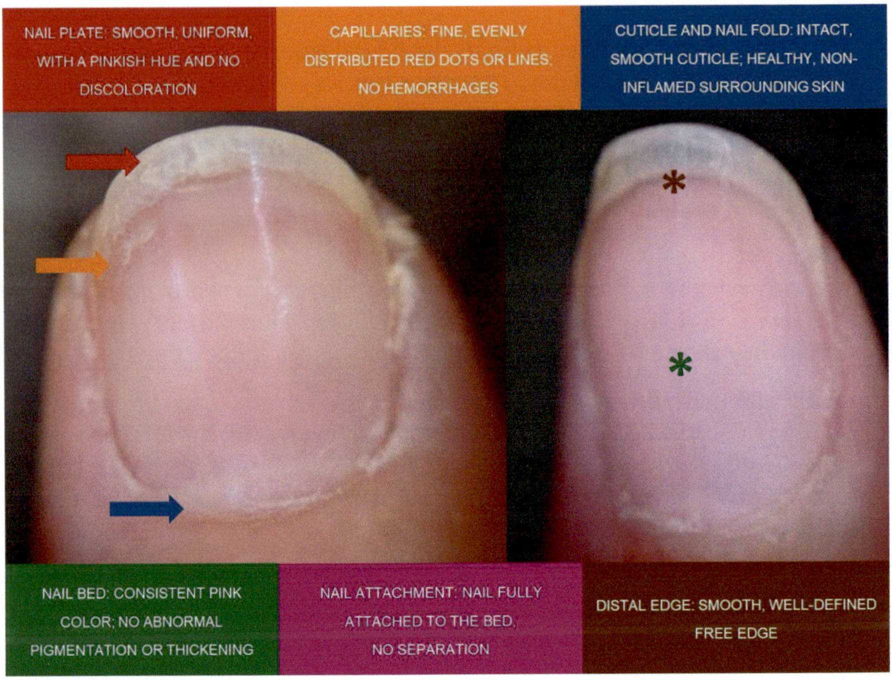

Fig. 4.4 Onichoscopy findings of the normal nail unit (x10)

4.3.1 Radiography and Computed Tomography [13, 14]

- Radiography provides clear images of bone structures, which is particularly important for evaluating inflammatory lesions like psoriatic nails and traumatic lesions with underlying fractures.
- It offers limited soft tissue detail and produces 2D images, which may not fully capture the complexity of certain anatomical structures.
- Computed tomography (CT) provides detailed cross-sectional images and highly detailed images of bones and blood vessels; however, it is not an ideal method for analyzing soft tissue related to the nail complex.
- Anatomy:
  - Distal phalanx: The terminal bone of the finger or toe, clearly visible on radiographs. It features a consistently dense cortical outline and a prominent distal portion on the dorsal side, where the anterior ligament attaches. It also contains a recess for the arterial distal arcade of the nail.
  - Nail plate: Often seen faintly on radiographs as a thin, linear structure that overlays the distal phalanx.

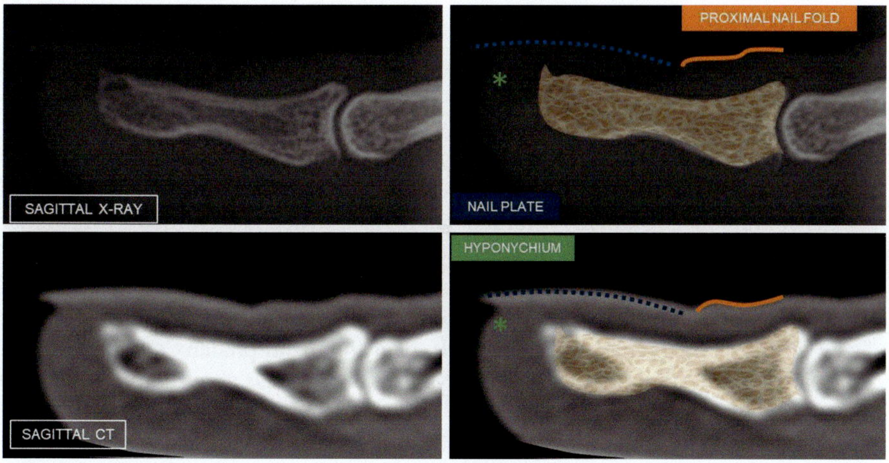

Fig. 4.5 Imaging aspects of the normal nail unit on radiography and sagittal reconstructed computed tomography (Philips Duo Diagnost R&F Room Digital RF and Tomo System and Philips Brilliance CT 64-slice)

– Proximal and lateral nail folds: Skin folds that frame and protect the edges of the nail plate. On radiographs, they appear as soft tissue outlines surrounding the nail plate.
– Hyponychium: Situated beneath the free edge of the nail plate, it is visible on radiographs as soft tissue at the distal end of the nail bed (Fig. 4.5).

4.3.2 Ultrasonography [2, 15, 16]

- Ultrasonography is a real-time, noninvasive technique that has become widely used for evaluating nail unit lesions with a high-frequency probe (18–24 MHz).
- For accurate imaging, both axial and sagittal planes of the nail should be obtained, with a generous amount of gel used to ensure clear visualization.
- A high-frequency 33 MHz probe is ideal for analyzing the nail plate's structure and detecting any lesions.
- Occasionally, it may be necessary to use markers to identify very small lesions. Typically, a needle or toothpick is placed over the lesion detected during the physical examination to aid in accurately locating the area during ultrasound imaging.
- In addition to examining the nail unit structures, it is crucial to also assess the distal interphalangeal joint, as well as the extensor and flexor tendon entheses.

- Anatomy:
  - Nail plates: Seen as hyperechoic, parallel structures separated by a thin hypoechoic line, known as the interplate space. This trilaminar structure is characterized by the varying density of keratin along the plates.
  - Nail Bed: Located deep to the nail plate and superficial to the bone, it appears hypoechoic, becoming slightly hyperechoic in its proximal portion. This area is continuous proximally with the nail matrix, which is identified by its higher echogenicity and position beneath the eponychium and proximal nail fold. The nail bed is highly vascularized, receiving blood from the ulnar and radial arteries. On power or color Doppler, vascularity is evident in the proximal two-thirds of the nail bed, especially near the distal phalanx's cortical bone. Normal flow does not extend to the ventral plate unless abnormalities increase vascularity or vessel dilation.
  - Proximal nail fold: This skin fold covering the proximal part of the nail appears as a hypoechoic soft tissue structure overlying the proximal nail matrix.
  - Eponychium: A small band of epidermis extending from the proximal nail fold onto the nail plate, appearing as a thin, echogenic line.
  - Hyponychium: Thickened skin under the free edge of the nail, visible as a hypoechoic area distal to the nail bed.
  - Distal phalanx: Displays a hyperechoic and smooth bone cortex. It is the site where the extensor tendon attaches and shows continuity between the nail matrix and tendon insertion, which is important for assessing disease or inflammation spread.
  - Extensor tendon enthesis: Appears as a hyperechoic structure with a fibrillar pattern due to the parallel arrangement of collagen fibers. At the enthesis, there may be a slight hypoechoic area representing the transition between the tendon and bone, where the tendon fibers blend with fibrocartilage.
  - Distal interphalangeal joint:
    - Joint space: Visualized as a hypoechoic space between the distal end of the middle phalanx and the proximal end of the distal phalanx, potentially filled with synovial fluid, which also appears hypoechoic.
    - Articular cartilage: Appears as a thin, anechoic layer adjacent to the bone surfaces.
    - Bone surfaces: The distal end of the middle phalanx and the proximal end of the distal phalanx are seen as continuous, hyperechoic lines.
    - Synovium and joint capsule: Surrounding the joint as a thin, hypoechoic layer encasing the joint space (Fig. 4.6).

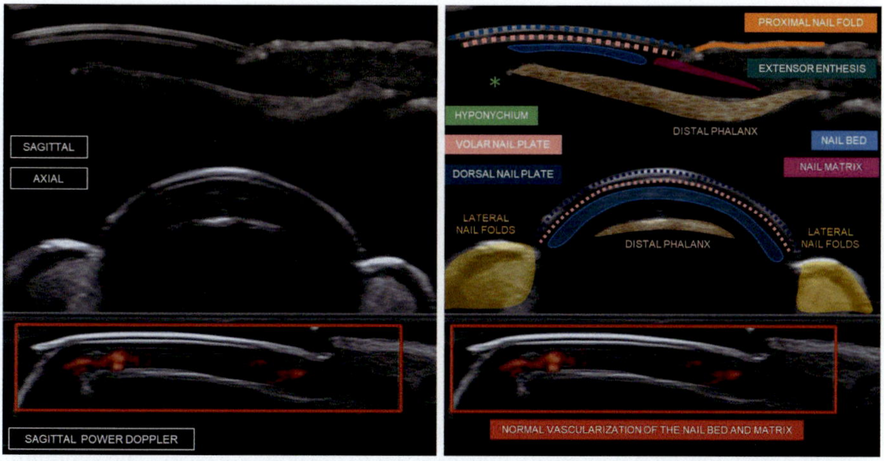

Fig. 4.6 Imaging aspects of the normal nail unit on sagittal and axial ultrasonography with 24 MHz probe (Aplio i800, Canon Medical Systems)

4.3.3 MRI [17, 18]

- MRI examination of the nail unit requires the use of a surface coil and precise patient positioning within the machine.
- MRI is particularly useful for detecting lesions in the nail bed and matrix. However, the nail plates themselves are not clearly visible on MRI, except for their superficial aspects. To improve visualization, a combination of gel and gadolinium can be applied around the finger.
- Anatomy:
  - Nail plate: Typically appears as a low signal intensity structure on T1-weighted images due to its dense, keratinized composition. When gel and gadolinium are used, the superficial portions of the nail plate may be more visible.
  - Nail bed: Shows up as a low to intermediate signal intensity structure on both T1-weighted and T2-weighted images. Located beneath the nail plate and continuous with the surrounding soft tissues, it may display slight hyperintensity on T2-weighted images due to its vascularity and fluid content.
  - Nail matrix: Appears as a region of increased signal intensity on T2-weighted images, reflecting its higher water content and vascularity.
  - Proximal nail fold: This skin fold covering the proximal part of the nail appears as a low signal intensity structure on T1-weighted images and is slightly hyperintense on T2-weighted images due to the presence of soft tissue and underlying vascular structures.

- Eponychium: The small band of epidermis extending from the proximal nail fold onto the nail plate is visible as a thin, low signal intensity line on T1-weighted images and may appear slightly hyperintense on T2-weighted images.
- Hyponychium: Located under the free edge of the nail plate, it appears as a low to intermediate signal intensity area on MRI.
- Distal phalanx: The distal phalanx is seen as a high signal intensity structure on T1-weighted images due to its bone marrow and appears hypointense on T2-weighted images. The cortical bone is hypointense across all sequences.
- Extensor tendon enthesis: The extensor tendon and its enthesis are visualized as low signal intensity structures on both T1- and T2-weighted images.
- Distal interphalangeal joint: The joint space appears as a low signal intensity area on T1-weighted images and may show slight hyperintensity on T2-weighted images due to synovial fluid. The articular cartilage is visualized as a thin, low signal intensity line adjacent to the bone surfaces. The synovium and joint capsule surrounding the joint space appear as low to intermediate signal intensity layers (Figs. 4.7, 4.8, and 4.9).

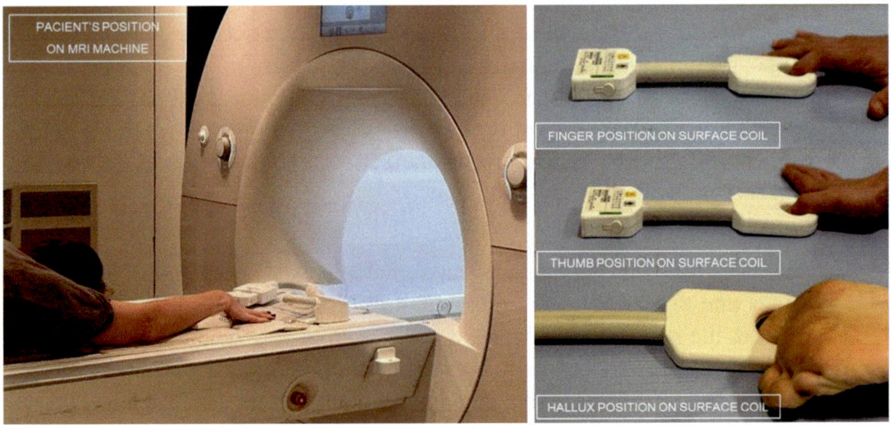

Fig. 4.7 Technique and position of the nail unit on MRI with surface coil (Magnetom Prisma 3T MRI, Siemens)

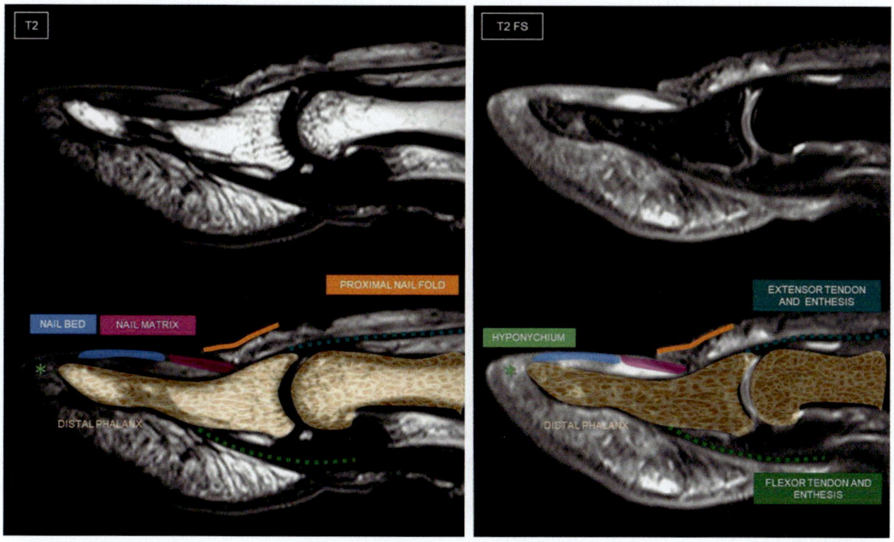

Fig. 4.8 Imaging aspects of the normal nail unit on MRI with surface coil on sagittal T2 FS and T2-weighted sequences (Magnetom Prisma 3T MRI, Siemens)

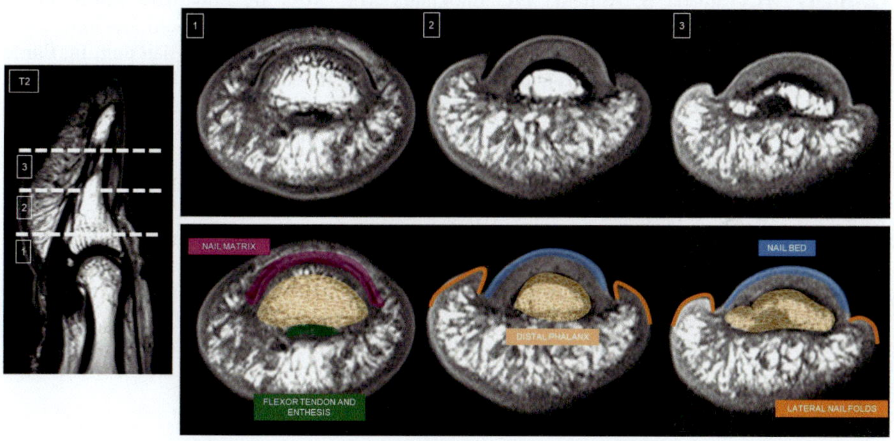

Fig. 4.9 Imaging aspects of the normal nail unit on MRI with surface coil on sagittal T2 and axial T1-weighted sequences (Magnetom Prisma 3T MRI, Siemens)

References

1. De Berker D. Nail anatomy. Clin Dermatol. 2013;31:509–15. https://doi.org/10.1016/j.clindermatol.2013.06.006.
2. Rodriguez-Takeuchi SY, Villota V, Renjifo M. Anatomy and pathology of the nail and subungual space: imaging evaluation of benign lesions. Clin Imaging. 2018;52:356–64. https://doi.org/10.1016/j.clinimag.2018.09.002.
3. Cammas C, Carmès S, Brunelli F, Dumontier C. Surgical anatomy of the nail. Hand Surg Rehabil. 2024;43:101644.
4. Zook EG. Anatomy and physiology of the perionychium. Hand Clin. 2002;18:553–9.
5. Fleckman P. Anatomy and physiology of the nail. Dermatol Clin. 1985;3:373–81.
6. Tan RES, Lahiri A. Vascular anatomy of the hand in relation to flaps. Hand Clin. 2020;36:1–8.
7. Miletin J, Sukop A, Baca V, Kachlik D. Arterial supply of the thumb: systemic review. Clin Anat. 2017;30:963–73.
8. Palomo-López P, Losa-Iglesias ME, Becerro-de-Bengoa-Vallejo R, Rodríguez-Sanz D, Calvo-Lobo C, Murillo-González J, et al. Anatomic and histological features of the extensor digitorum longus tendon insertion in the proximal nail matrix of the second toe. Diagnostics. 2020;10:147.
9. Nirmal B. Dermatoscopy: physics and principles. Indian J Dermatopathol Diagn Dermatol. 2017;4:27.
10. Solish D, Weinberg T, Murray C. Surface anatomy of the nail for the dermatologist. J Cutan Med Surg. 2016;20:467–9.
11. Ronger S, Touzet S, Ligeron C, Balme B, Viallard AM, Barrut D, et al. Dermoscopic examination of nail pigmentation. Arch Dermatol. 2002;138:1327.
12. Hirata SH, Yamada S, Almeida FA, Enokihara MY, Rosa IP, Enokihara MMS, et al. Dermoscopic examination of the nail bed and matrix. Int J Dermatol. 2006;45:28–30.
13. Thomas L, Vaudaine M, Wortsman X, Jemec GBE, Drapé JL. Imaging the nail unit. In: Baran & Dawber's diseases of the nails and their management. 4th ed. Wiley; 2012. p. 101–82.
14. Wortsman X, Jemec GBE, Villani A. Ultrasound and other imaging methods. Baran & Dawber's diseases of the nails and their management. Chichester: John Wiley & Sons; 2018. p. 140–74. https://doi.org/10.1002/9781119323396.ch5.
15. Berritto D, Iacobellis F, Rossi C, Reginelli A, Cappabianca S, Grassi R. Ultra high-frequency ultrasound: new capabilities for nail anatomy exploration. J Dermatol. 2017;44:43–6.
16. Wortsman X. Concepts, role, and advances on nail imaging. Dermatol Clin. 2021;39:337–50.
17. Soscia E, Sirignano C, Catalano O, Atteno M, Costa L, Caso F, et al. New developments in magnetic resonance imaging of the nail unit. J Rheumatol. 2012;39:49–53.
18. Mundada P, Becker M, Lenoir V, Stefanelli S, Rougemont A-L, Beaulieu JY, et al. High resolution MRI of nail tumors and tumor-like conditions. Eur J Radiol. 2019;112:93–105.

Part II
Scalp

Chapter 5
Clinical, Imaging, and Histological Findings in Inflammatory Lesions of the Scalp

Maria Carolina Zafra Páez, Carolina Ávila de Almeida, André da Silva Cartell, Ana Leticia Boff, Ximena Wortsman, Clarissa Canella Moraes do Carmo, and Bruna Duque-Estrada

Inflammatory lesions of the scalp encompass a wide array of dermatological conditions that can significantly impact patients' quality of life. These conditions often present with symptoms such as itching, pain, and visible discomfort, and can lead to psychological distress due to their prominent and visible nature. Understanding the etiology, epidemiology, clinical presentation, and advanced diagnostic techniques of these lesions is crucial for effective management and treatment. This chapter delves into the intricacies of inflammatory scalp conditions, focusing on psoriasis, one of the most prevalent and challenging disorders in dermatology.

M. C. Z. Páez
Zafra Dermatology Private Clinic, Rio de Janeiro, Brazil

BCM Dermatologia Especializada, Private Practice, Rio de Janeiro, Rio de Janeiro, Brazil

C. Á. de Almeida
Faculty of Medicine of Valença—UniFaa, Valença, Brazil

Federal University of Rio de Janeiro—UFRJ, Rio de Janeiro, Brazil

A. da Silva Cartell
Adjunct Professor at Faculdade de Medicina da Universidade Federal do Rio Grande do Sul, Rio de Janeiro, Brazil

Dermatologist and Dermatopathologist in Private Practice, Rio de Janeiro, Brazil

A. L. Boff
Santa Casa Hospital, Porto Alegre, RS, Brazil

Dermathopathologist Private Practice, Clinica Dermapat, Porto Alegre, RS, Brazil

X. Wortsman
Faculty of Medicine, Department of Dermatology, Universidad de Chile, Santiago, Chile

Department of Dermatology, School of Medicine, Pontificia Universidad Catolica de Chile, Santiago, Chile

Department of Dermatology and Cutaneous Surgery, Miller School of Medicine, University of Miami, Miami, FL, USA

Institute for Diagnostic Imaging and Research of the Skin and Soft Tissues, Santiago, Chile

© The Author(s), under exclusive license to Springer Nature Switzerland AG 2025

C. Canella Moraes do Carmo (ed.), *Atlas of Diagnostic Imaging in Dermatology*,
https://doi.org/10.1007/978-3-031-77987-9_5

5.1 Psoriasis

5.1.1 Definition [1]

- Psoriasis is a common immune-mediated chronic, systemic inflammatory condition, affecting the skin and other organ systems, in a variety of clinical manifestations.
- The scalp is the most commonly affected region in psoriasis, involved in about 80% of the cases, and may be an indicator of psoriatic arthritis. Psoriasis of the scalp is considered a high-impact site, which can have an increased negative impact on quality of life, regardless of disease extension.

5.1.2 Epidemiology [2]

- It affects children and adults worldwide, with an estimated prevalence of 2%.
- It occurs equally in men and women.
- The peak ages for the onset are between 30–39 years and between 50–69 years.

5.1.3 Clinical Presentation [3]

- Psoriasis of the scalp tends to appear as erythematous, thick, crusted plaques with an overlying powdery and silvery scale. Pruritus may be nonexistent to severe.
- Other commonly affected sites include beard, ears, on extensor surfaces, elbows, knees, sacrum, and nails.
- The Koebner phenomenon refers to the development of skin lesions at sites of trauma.
- Auspitz sign: The Auspitz sign refers to the visualization of pinpoint bleeding after removal of scale overlying a psoriatic plaque - the so called Brocq's methodical curettage (Fig. 5.1).

C. Canella Moraes do Carmo (✉)
Fluminense Federal University—UFF, Rio de Janeiro, Brazil

Federal University of Rio de Janeiro—UFRJ, Rio de Janeiro, Brazil

Diagnóstico das Américas—DASA—RJ, Rio de Janeiro, Brazil

Biodesign Laboratory, DASA-PUC, Rio de Janeiro, Brazil

B. Duque-Estrada
BCM Dermatologia Especializada, Private Practice, Rio de Janeiro, Rio de Janeiro, Brazil

Universidade Federal de São Paulo, São Paulo, Brazil

Hair Diseases Department, Instituto de Dermatologia Prof. Rubem David Azulay – Santa Casa da Misericórdia do Rio de Janeiro, Rio de Janeiro, Brazil

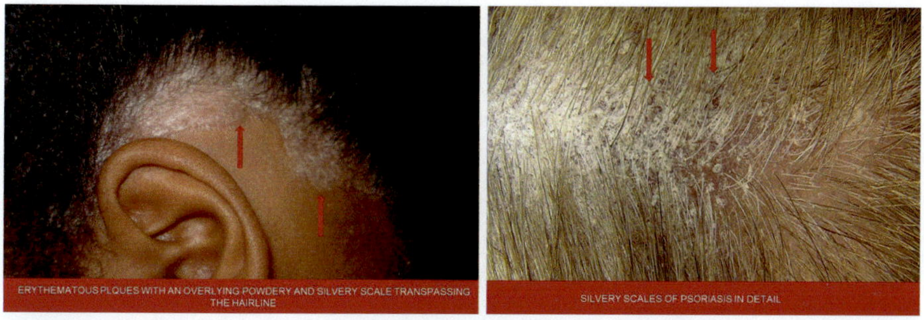

Fig. 5.1 Clinical photograph of a patient presenting with scalp psoriasis

5.1.4 Trichoscopy [4–6]

- The vascular patterns of scalp psoriasis are the most typical features and may present as:
  - Multiple red dots at low magnification (×10–20), in a linear or circular arrangement. At higher magnifications (×40 or more), they are seen as glomerular vessels.
  - Lace-like vessels arranged in circles or in lines, which represent twisted vessels.
  - Extravasations, or punctate hemorrhage, indicate high disease activity and may occur spontaneously or be triggered by scratching, as seen in Auspitz sign.
  - Pink background all around the plaque.
- White perifollicular scaling, either diffuse or patchy in distribution (Fig. 5.2).

5.1.5 Histopathology (Fig. 5.3) [7–9]

- Scalp psoriasis has several similarities to other forms of psoriasis, except that it is similar to seborrheic dermatitis. A clue to differential diagnosis may be the reduction or absence of sebaceous glands in psoriasis, although it has bee described in seborrheic dermatitis and atopic dermatitis.
- Histopathological aspects:
  - Focal or confluent parakeratosis; may alternate with lamellar hyperkeratosis.
  - Focal or diffuse hypogranulosis/agranulosis; although psoriasis is a disease of the interadnexal epithelium, sparing the follicular ostia, in scalp psoriasis, parakeratosis can involve the edges of the hair infundibulum, mimicking seborrheic dermatitis.
  - Regular acanthosis, characteristically without spongiosis.

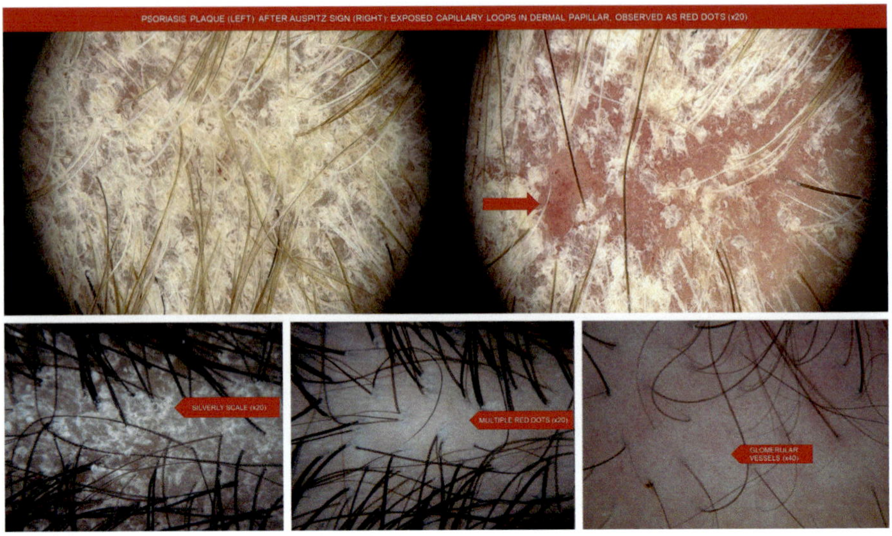

Fig. 5.2 Trichoscopic image of the scalp in a patient with scalp psoriasis (x20 and x40) (Courtesy of Dr Leonardo Abraham)

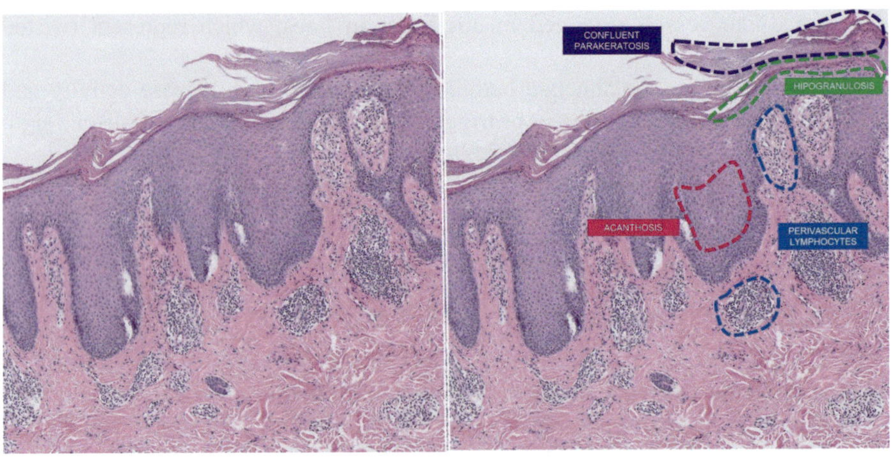

Fig. 5.3 Histological findings of scalp psoriasis (H&E x4)

– Viable neutrophils may or may not be present at the top of the parakeratosis mounds, forming subcorneal collections called Munro's microabscesses; if they are in an intraepidermal location and associated with spongiosis, usually in the upper third of the epiderma, they are called Kogoj's spongiform pustules; despite the predominance of neutrophils, lymphocytes may be present, especially in the early phase; Munro's microabscesses are more common in recent lesions.

- Extremely regular and downward growth of the interpapillary cones with bulbous due to the tendency of cones to melt with clubbing in the more developed lesions.
- Increase in the number of basal and suprabasal mitoses due to increased cell replication.
- Keratinocytes appear more immature, exhibiting a basaloid aspect, reduced eosinophilia, and increased cellularity due to a smaller cell diameter.
- Suprapapillary atrophy with upward elongation and narrowing of the dermal papillae is the cause of Auspitz's sign. Exposure of dilated vessels in the dermal papilla are ruptured during Brocq's methodical curettage. Suprapapillary atrophy greater than two-thirds of the thickness of the epidermis is characteristic of psoriasis; the papilla is elongated but usually retains its diameter, resembling the columns of the Parthenon.
- Dilation and tortuosity of the superficial dermal vessels, with the most important histopathological sign, being the most precocious.
- Superficial mononuclear inflammatory infiltrate usually discrete.

• Focal hemorrhage in the derma papillary (nonspecific) especially in eruptive lesions, which may be mistaken for Gibert's pityriasis rosea.

  - Apart from the pustular form, spongiosis is absent or discrete, usually restricted to the lower third of the epiderma, unlike eczema.

5.1.6 Ultrasonography (Fig. 5.4) [10]

• Increased skin thickness

  - Affected psoriasis plaques exhibit significantly increased skin thickness.

• Decreased echo-intensity

  - Lower echo-intensity observed in psoriasis plaques compared to adjacent healthy skin.

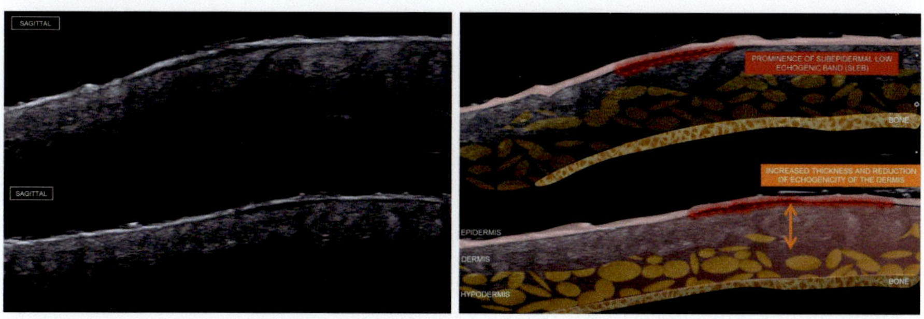

Fig. 5.4 Ultrasonographic findings of scalp psoriasis with a 24 MHz probe (Aplio i800, Canon Medical Systems)

- Epidermal changes
  - Increased epidermal thickness due to keratinocyte proliferation and desquamation.
- SLEB (subepidermal low echogenic band)
  - Increased SLEB in psoriasis lesions, indicating a higher degree of inflammation.
  - SLEB variation may also reflect acanthosis. It is characteristic, but not specific of psoriasis.
- Dermal changes:
  - Increased thickness of the papillary dermis due to inflammation, edema, and variations in vascularity.
  - Increased dermal component due to leukocyte infiltration and epidermal acanthosis.
- Skin edema:
  - Presence of edema leads to restructuring of the dermis, increasing density between collagen fibers and decreasing skin consistency.

5.2 Scalp Dermatomyositis

5.2.1 Definition [11–13]

- Dermatomyositis (DM) is a chronic autoimmune connective tissue disease that may present with a spectrum of cutaneous lesions, muscle weakness, and systemic manifestations.
- Cutaneous involvement of the scalp is a common manifestation of dermatomyositis (DM), occurring in up to 57–82% of affected adults. It is increasingly recognized as a distinct dermatologic subset of DM.
- Concurrent muscle involvement may or may not be present.
- SDM predominantly is characterized by dermatitis, alopecia, pruritus, and/or burning. Scalp symptoms are often severe, debilitating, and recalcitrant to standard DM therapies.

5.2.2 Epidemiology [11–13]

- DM has an estimated incidence of 1–10 cases per million inhabitants annually, with higher prevalence in women (2:1 ratio).

- SDM may be underdiagnosed due to overlapping features with other dermatologic conditions such as psoriasis or seborrheic dermatitis.

5.2.3 Clinical Presentation (Fig. 5.5) [11–13]

- Common findings include:
  - Erythema (100% of SDM cases)
  - Non-scarring alopecia (87.5%)
  - Pruritus (70.8%)
  - Poikiloderma (51.6%)
  - Erythemato-squamous plaques (83.3%)
- May coexist with other signs of active systemic disease or be the sole manifestation.
- In children, disease onset may be abrupt, with scalp involvement occasionally preceding muscular symptoms.

5.2.4 Trichoscopy (Fig. 5.6) [12]

- Major trichoscopic features:
  - Enlarged, tortuous, and arborizing vessels (capillaries) (71.4%)
  - Peripilar casts (57.1%)

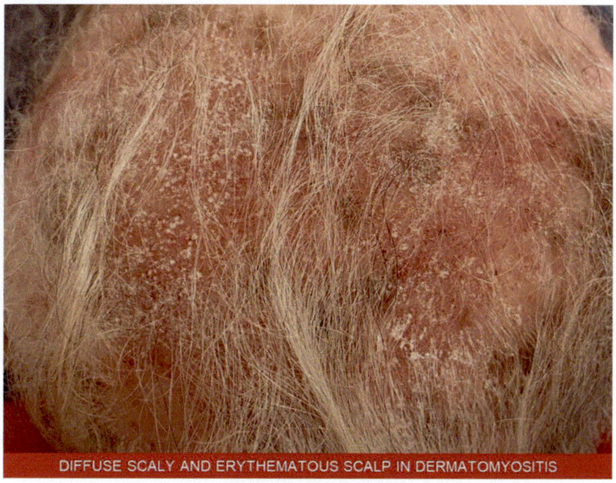

Fig. 5.5 Clinical photograph of a patient presenting with scalp dermatomyositis (Courtesy of Dr. Ana Luisa Sampaio)

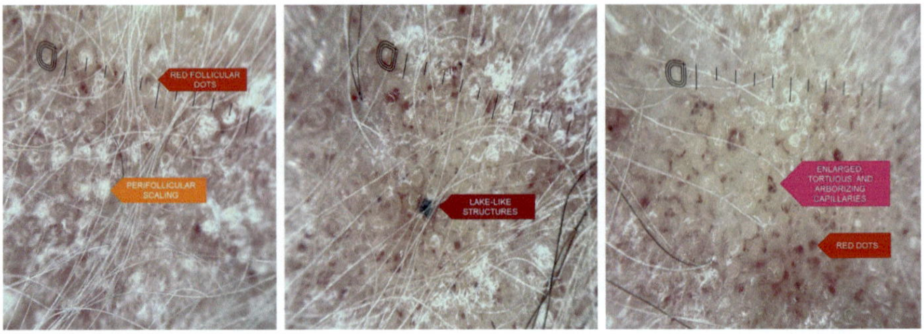

Fig. 5.6 Trichoscopic image of the scalp in a patient with dermatomyositis (×10) (Courtesy of Dr. Ana Luisa Sampaio)

- Minor trichoscopic features:
  - Bushy vessels—similar to capillaries observed in the proximal nail fold (<50%)
  - Vascular lake-like structures—ectatic vascular structures with red blood cells (14.3%)
  - Interfollicular scaling (50%)
  - Tufting (3 or more hairs emerging together in the same follicular ostia)
  - Perifollicular or interfollicular pigmentation
- Trichoscopy findings often mirror nailfold capillaroscopy—capillary loss and enlarged bushy capillaries (70%).

5.2.5 Histopathology [14–16]

- Interface dermatitis with:
  - Epidermal atrophy
  - Dilated capillaries
  - Mucin deposition
  - Partial or zonal thickening of the basement membrane zone
  - Acrosyringeal hypergranulosis and hyperkeratosis
  - Features resembling lupus erythematosus, but generally less intense
- Presence of eosinophils helps distinguishing dermatomyositis from lupus erythematosus.
- Scalp involvement typically shows:
  - A non-scarring pattern on horizontal histological sections
  - Findings consistent with chronic telogen effluvium
  - Preserved follicular structure
  - Reduced follicular density
- In young patients, calcinosis cutis may also be observed.

5.2.6 *Ultrasonography (Fig. 5.7) [17, 18]*

Allows evaluation of lesion extent, activity, and chronicity. It is also useful for monitoring treatment response and guiding early intervention to prevent long-term sequelae.

- Acute Phase:
  - Thickened epidermis with increased echogenicity, due to edema in the upper dermis and significant vacuolar interface changes.
  - Dermal thickening with reduced echogenicity, reflecting edema, and inflammatory infiltration.
  - Prominent subepidermal low echogenic band (SLEB), representing banded hypoechoic areas in the superficial dermis related to capillary dilation and perivascular edema.
  - Hypoechoic areas in the subcutaneous fat caused by edema and inflammatory infiltration.
  - Perifollicular hypoechogenicity with increased power Doppler signal, consistent with perifolliculitis.
  - On power Doppler imaging, increased dermal and subcutaneous vascularity is observed, reflecting hyperemia.
- Chronic Phase:
  - Epidermal atrophy with reduced thickness and echogenicity.
  - Increased dermal echogenicity and loss of normal skin architecture, secondary to fibrosis.
  - Progressive follicular dropout and fibrosis in long-standing disease.
  - On power Doppler imaging, reduced dermal and subcutaneous vascularity is seen due to decreased perfusion, ischemia, and microinfarcts.
  - In late disease, intradermal hyperechoic foci with posterior acoustic shadowing may be present, indicating calcium deposition (calcinosis).

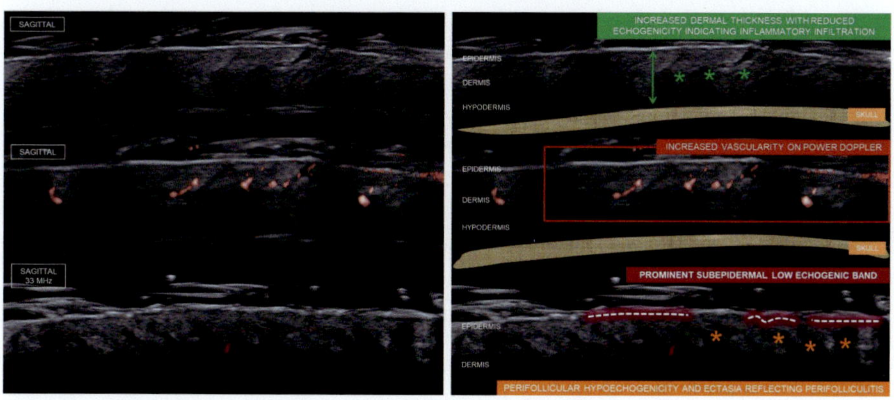

Fig. 5.7 Ultrasonographic findings of scalp dermatomyositis with a 24 MHz probe (Aplio i800, Canon Medical Systems)

5.3 Scalp Morphea

5.3.1 Definition [19]

- Scalp morphea, particularly in the form of linear scleroderma *en coup de sabre* (LSCS), is a localized subtype of scleroderma of the scalp and forehead, characterized by linear sclerotic patches of the skin with fibrosis of the subcutaneous tissue.
- LSCS may extend to deeper tissues including muscle, bone, ocular involvement, and even the central nervous system, potentially leading to significant morbidity if untreated.

5.3.2 Epidemiology [19]

- LSCS is the most common subtype of morphea affecting the scalp.
- Typically presents in children and adolescents, with mean onset at 13.6 years.
- A male predominance (2:1) is noted, though adult-onset cases are also documented.
- It is a rare condition, with unclear prevalence. In early phases, it is often misdiagnosed as alopecia areata, discoid lupus, lichen planopilaris, or other scalp conditions.

5.3.3 Clinical Presentation (Fig. 5.8) [19]

- The classic linear scleroderma (LSCS) demonstrates a well-defined, linear atrophic patch of alopecia on the frontoparietal or frontotemporal scalp, along Blaschko's lines.
- In addition to the classic presentation, other unusual presentations have been described, such as a linear patch resembling a bruise in a patient with dark skin phototypes, two lines on the same side or on either sides, three lines on the same side, and annular, patchy involvement of the vertex and occiput.
- In early stages, the lesion may show erythema or hyperpigmentation.
- Without intervention, the natural course includes progressive scarring alopecia and tissue atrophy.
- Deep tissue involvement may cause muscle wasting, bony remodeling, and neurological symptoms in advanced cases.

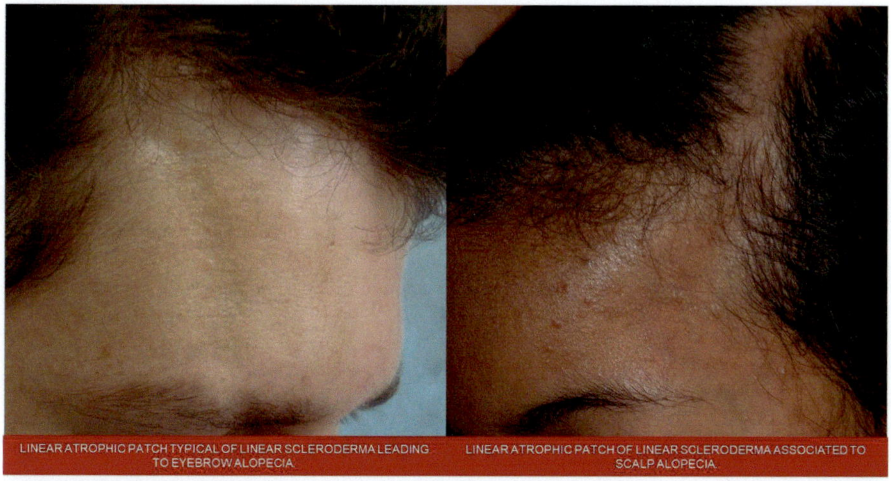

Fig. 5.8 Clinical photograph of a patient presenting with scalp morphea

5.3.4 Trichoscopy (Fig. 5.9) [20]

- Trichoscopic findings may not be specific of LSCS but correlates with dermal, vascular, and sclerotic involvement of the disease.
- Loss of follicular openings over a whitish background—a clue to underlying dermal fibrosis.
- Scattered black dots, broken hairs, and pili torti—suggesting increased hair shaft fragility and perifollicular fibrosis.
- Thick linear and branching tortuous vessels observed at the periphery of lesions—similar to discoid lupus and dermatomyositis.

5.3.5 Histopathology (Fig. 5.10) [21, 22]

- Scarring alopecia pattern, with:
  - Sclerosis of the dermis
  - Reduced number of follicular units
- Cross-sectional and vertical biopsy sections typically show:
  - Dense dermal fibrosis (sclerosis)
  - Marked atrophy of eccrine glands
  - Absence of sebaceous glands
  - Replacement of adipose tissue by collagenous tissue

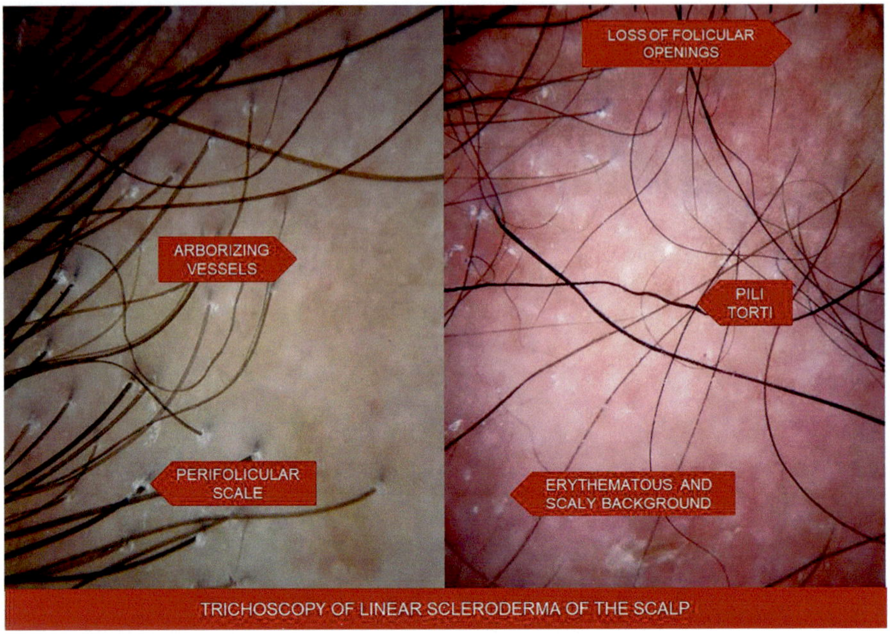

Fig. 5.9 Trichoscopic image of the scalp in a patient with morphea (×20)

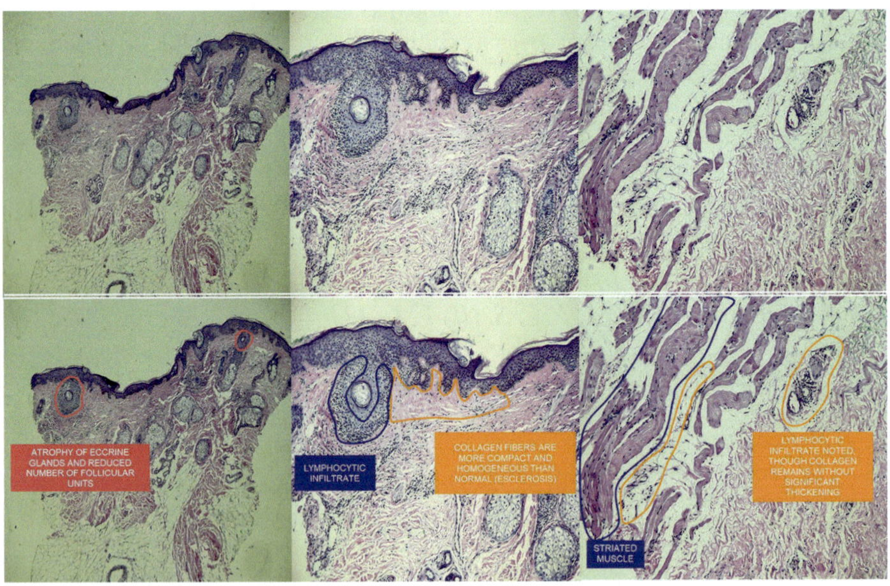

Fig. 5.10 Histological findings of scalp morphea (H&E ×40 and ×100)

- The erector pili muscle is generally preserved.
- Perineural inflammatory infiltrates may be present, including:
  - Lymphocytes
  - Plasma cells (occasionally observed)

5.3.6 Ultrasonography (Fig. 5.11) [19, 23]

- High-frequency ultrasound can evaluate the activity of the disease, as it is highly sensitive (up to 100%) and specific (98.8%) in distinguishing active and inactive lesions, compared to the gold-standard histological findings.
- Early inflammatory phase:
  - Hypoechogenicity of the dermis
  - A mild subepidermal low echogenic band (SLEB) may sometimes be observed due to edema.
  - Loss of the dermal–hypodermal interface and altered subcutaneous vascularity.
  - Decreased follicular density and loss of visible follicles in the affected area.
  - Power Doppler may demonstrate increased blood flow, indicating active inflammation.
- Sclerotic phase:
  - Indeterminate thickness of skin layers.

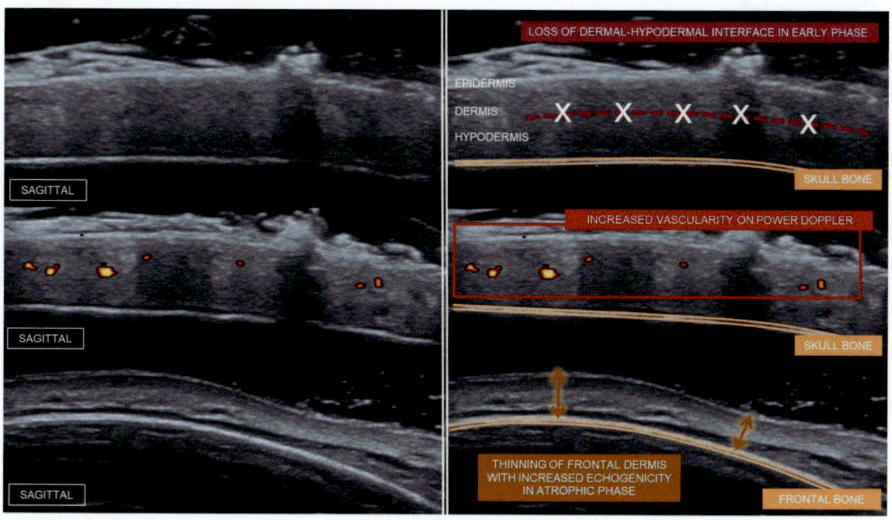

Fig. 5.11 Ultrasonographic findings of scalp morphea with a 22 MHz probe (HM70 EVO—Samsung Healthcare Global)

  - Hyperechoic and heterogeneous subcutaneous fat.
  - Increased echogenicity due to the greater collagen content in the dermis, hypodermis, and sometimes superficial intramuscular hyperechogenicity.
  - Blood flow signal is attenuated on power Doppler imaging.
- Sclerodermatous skin in atrophic phase:
  - Thinning of the dermis, subcutaneous layer may disappear and visible depressions may be present in severe cases.
  - The subepidermal low echogenic band may be absent or reduced in late-stage lesions due to fibrosis.
  - Hyperechoic and heterogeneous subcutaneous fat, consistent with fibrotic replacement and disorganized accumulation of collagen.
  - Thinning of the subcutaneous fat layer and even loss of fat planes, reflecting advanced fibrosis.
  - Associated scarring alopecia and follicular ectasia are common in long-standing disease.
  - Reduced or absent vascularity in sclerotic areas, especially in later stages.

5.4 Scalp Seborrheic Dermatitis (SSD)

5.4.1 Definition [24]

- Scalp seborrheic dermatitis (SSD) is a chronic, relapsing inflammatory skin disorder predominantly affecting sebaceous gland-rich areas, such as the scalp, face, and upper trunk.
- The etiology is multifactorial, and it is closely related with the presence of Malassezia sp.
- Though benign, SSD significantly affects quality of life and may contribute to microinflammation, potentially worsening both telogen effluvium and androgenetic alopecia.

5.4.2 Epidemiology [24]

- Affects approximately 1–3% of the general population, but subclinical forms may be present in up to 15–20%.
- Age Groups:
  - Infants: Common during the first 3 months of life, usually self-limited.
  - Adolescents and adults: Peaks during puberty and adulthood due to increased sebaceous gland activity

- Older adults: Another prevalence peak, possibly due to decreased skin barrier function.

- Slight male predominance, possibly linked to hormonal influences on sebaceous glands.
- Occurs across all ethnicities, but scalp involvement may present differently based on hair type and grooming practices.
- Environmental triggers such as humidity, cold weather, and reduced sun exposure may exacerbate the condition.
- Higher prevalence is observed in immunosuppressed individuals (e.g., HIV/AIDS, Parkinson's disease, depression, anxiety, immunosuppression, or chronic illnesses).

5.4.3 Clinical Presentation (Fig. 5.12) [24]

- Presents with greasy, yellowish, or white scales, erythema, pruritus, and burning sensation, particularly in areas with high sebaceous activity. It is clinically characterized by scaling on an erythematous base, sometimes accompanied by seborrhea, or dry scalp.
- Pityriasis capitis or dandruff is a variant of SD. It is a chronic disease restricted to the scalp, involving flaking skin without inflammation signs and pruritus.
- In infants, lesions often appear as adherent yellow scales and crusts, usually non-pruritic, resembling pseudotinea amiantacea.
- May coexist with or exacerbate other hair and scalp disorders, such as androgenetic alopecia.
- As SDD can vary greatly in severity and extent, the differential diagnosis may include several other scaling conditions, such as psoriasis, tinea capitis, atopic dermatitis, contact dermatitis, dermatomyositis, pemphigus vulgaris, diffuse lichen planopilaris, and discoid lupus erythematosus.

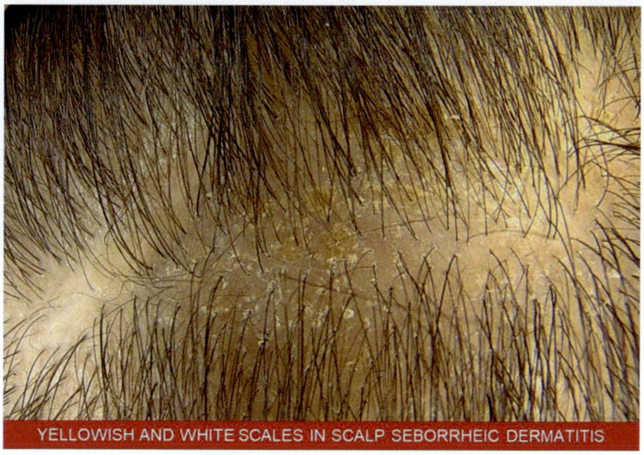

Fig. 5.12 Clinical photograph of a patient presenting with scalp seborrheic dermatitis

- Wood's lamp, trichoscopy, UV-trichoscopy, and mycological tests (KOH, culture) are extremely helpful for distinguishing SSD from fungal or scarring conditions.

5.4.4 *Trichoscopy (Fig. 5.13) [24]*

- Trichoscopy should first be performed without immersion fluid to evaluate scaling and superficial structures, followed by examination with immersion fluid to visualize deeper structures, such as vascular patterns.
- Classic findings include:
  - Perifollicular scaling (diffuse or clustered) (46%): white color dominating over yellow/oily scaling
  - Peripilar casts
  - Erythematous background with multicomponent vascular patterns: arborizing red vessels, twisted red loop, glomerular vessels, comma vessels, serpentine vessels
- New descriptive patterns (observed in higher magnifications):
  - Dandelion vascular conglomerate: yellow dot surrounded by glomerular and comma vessels
  - Cherry blossom pattern: conglomerate of arborizing vessels with multiple glomerular and comma vessels surrounding them

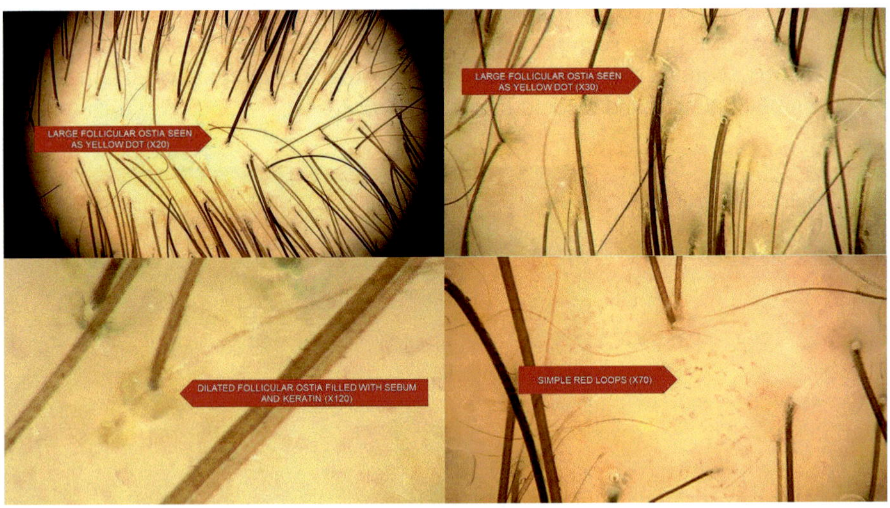

Fig. 5.13 Trichoscopic image of the scalp in a patient with scalp seborrheic dermatitis (×20, ×30, ×120 and ×70)

– Intrafollicular oily material: accumulation of sebum and keratin within the follicular ostia

5.4.5 *Histopathology (Fig. 5.14) [25, 26]*

- Microscopic findings include:
  - Spongiotic dermatitis in the early stages
  - Progression to a psoriasiform pattern in chronic stages
  - Regular acanthosis
  - Parakeratosis adjacent to the follicular ostia, often with intracorneal neutrophils
  - Non-specific superficial chronic inflammatory infiltrate
- Reduction of sebaceous gland size may also be observed and represent a finding originally described in scalp psoriasis, but also seen in seborrheic dermatitis.

5.4.6 *Ultrasonography (Fig. 5.15) [27, 28]*

- The epidermis may appear slightly thickened or irregular, particularly in chronic cases.
- A prominent subepidermal low echogenic band (SLEB) is commonly observed, indicating active inflammation and dermal edema.
- Mild to moderate increase in dermal thickening is present due to inflammation.

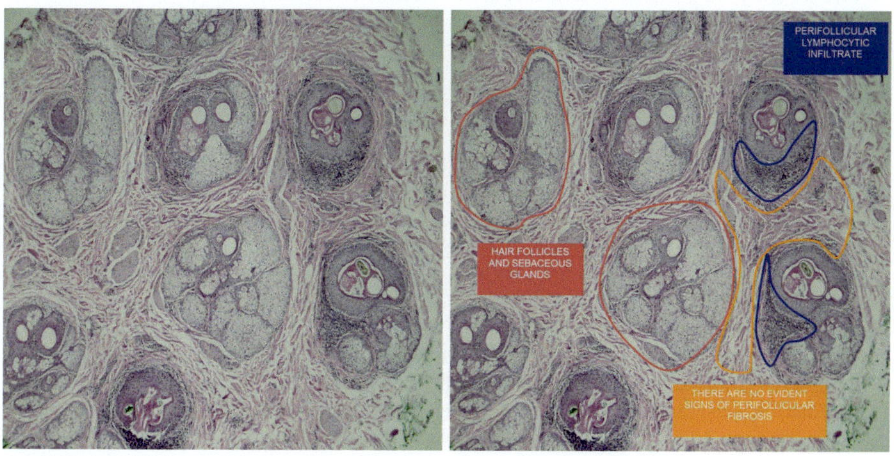

Fig. 5.14 Histological findings of scalp seborrheic dermatitis (H&E ×40)

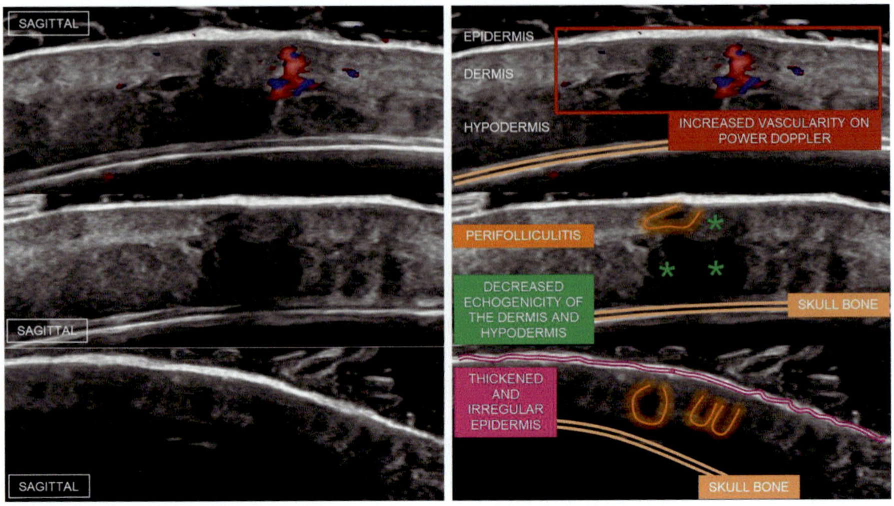

Fig. 5.15 Ultrasonographic findings of scalp seborrheic dermatitis with a 22 MHz probe (HM70 EVO—Samsung Healthcare Global)

- Decreased echogenicity of the dermis, reflecting edema and inflammatory infiltration.
- Perifollicular hypoechogenicity, consistent with inflammatory infiltration or perifolliculitis, leading to dilated hair follicles.
- In some cases, mild perifollicular vascularization may be seen. Indeed, enlarged hair follicles are eventually observed in some patients.
- Increased vascularity on power Doppler imaging is noted in the dermis and superficial subcutaneous tissue, especially in active lesions.
- The subcutaneous tissue typically maintains normal architecture, though mild edema may be present in more severe or chronic forms.

References

1. Castelino M, Eyre S, Barton A. Psoriasis and psoriatic arthritis. In: The microbiome in rheumatic diseases and infection. Springer; 2018. p. 239–50.
2. Parisi R, Symmons DPM, Griffiths CEM, Ashcroft DM. Global epidemiology of psoriasis: a systematic review of incidence and prevalence. J Invest Dermatol. 2013;133:377–85.
3. Griffiths CEM, Armstrong AW, Gudjonsson JE, Barker JNWN. Psoriasis. Lancet. 2021;397:1301–15.
4. Miteva M, Tosti A. Hair and scalp dermatoscopy. J Am Acad Dermatol. 2012;67:1040–8.
5. Kim G-W, Jung H-J, Ko H-C, Kim M-B, Lee W-J, Lee S-J, et al. Dermoscopy can be useful in differentiating scalp psoriasis from seborrhoeic dermatitis. Br J Dermatol. 2011;164:652.
6. Golinska J, Sar-Pomian M, Rudnicka L. Diagnostic accuracy of trichoscopy in inflammatory scalp diseases: a systematic review. Dermatology. 2022;238:412–21.
7. Werner B, Brenner FM, Böer A. Histopathologic study of scalp psoriasis: peculiar features including sebaceous gland atrophy. Am J Dermatopathol. 2008;30:93–100.

8. Hall BJ, Hall JC, Cockerell CJ, Affolter K, Alvarez P. Diagnostic pathology: nonneoplastic dermatopathology. Elsevier; 2017.
9. Patterson JW. Weedon's skin pathology. 6th ed. Elsevier; 2024.
10. Şomlea M, Boca A, Pop A, Ilieş R, Vesa S, Buzoianu A, et al. High-frequency ultrasonography of psoriatic skin: a non-invasive technique in the evaluation of the entire skin of patients with psoriasis: a pilot study. Exp Ther Med. 2019;18:4981.
11. Kolla AM, Liu L, Shaw K, Shapiro J, Femia A, Lo SK. A narrative review of therapies for scalp dermatomyositis. Dermatol Ther. 2021;34(6):e15138. https://doi.org/10.1111/dth.15138. Epub 2021 Sep 30
12. Golińska J, Sar-Pomian M, Rudnicka L. Diagnostic accuracy of trichoscopy in inflammatory scalp diseases: a systematic review. Dermatology. 2022;238(3):412–21. https://doi.org/10.1159/000517516. Epub 2021 Jul 15
13. Chai K, Zhu R, Luo F, Shi Y, Liu M, Xiao Y, Xiao R. Updated role of high-frequency ultrasound in assessing dermatological manifestations in autoimmune skin diseases. Acta Derm Venereol. 2022;102:adv00765.
14. Jasso-Olivares J, Diaz-Gonzalez JM, Miteva M. Horizontal and vertical sections of scalp biopsy specimens from dermatomyositis patients with scalp involvement. J Am Acad Dermatol. 2018;78(6):1178–84. https://doi.org/10.1016/j.jaad.2018.01.031. Epub 2018 Jan 31
15. Sanchez II, Herrera HO, Elsensohn A, Lee BA, Kraus CN. Dermatomyositis with eosinophils. Dermatopathology (Basel). 2023;10(4):310–7. https://doi.org/10.3390/dermatopathology10040039. PMID: 38131900; PMCID: PMC10742320
16. Rathore U, Gupta L. Scalp calcinosis in juvenile dermatomyositis. Rheumatology (Oxford). 2021;60(3):1569. https://doi.org/10.1093/rheumatology/keaa566.
17. Sudoł-Szopińska I, Jacques T, Gietka P, Cotton A. Imaging in dermatomyositis in adults and children. J Ultrason. 2020;20:e36–42. https://doi.org/10.15557/JoU.2020.0007. Piotr Gietka, Anne Cotten Review Cite as:
18. Jasso-Olivares JC, Tosti A, Miteva M, Domínguez-Cherit J, Díaz-González JM. Clinical and dermoscopic features of the scalp in 31 patients with dermatomyositis. Skin Appendage Disord. 2017;3(3):119–24. https://doi.org/10.1159/000464469. Epub 2017 Mar 29. PMID: 28879187; PMCID: PMC5582479
19. Chai K, Zhu R, Luo F, Shi Y, Liu M, Xiao Y, Xiao R. Updated role of high-frequency ultrasound in assessing dermatological manifestations in autoimmune skin diseases. Acta Derm Venereol. 2022;24(102):adv00765. https://doi.org/10.2340/actadv.v102.1969. PMID: 36000997; PMCID: PMC9558316.ela (já esta na dermatomiosite)
20. Saceda-Corralo D, Tosti A. Trichoscopic features of linear morphea on the scalp. Skin Appendage Disord. 2018;4(1):31–3. https://doi.org/10.1159/000478022. Epub 2017 Jul 12. PMID: 29457011; PMCID: PMC5806185
21. Goh C, Biswas A, Goldberg LJ. Alopecia with perineural lymphocytes: a clue to linear scleroderma en coup de sabre. J Cutan Pathol. 2012;39(5):518–20. https://doi.org/10.1111/j.1600-0560.2012.01889.x.
22. Pierre-Louis M, Sperling LC, Wilke MS, Hordinsky MK. Distinctive histopathologic findings in linear morphea (en coup de sabre) alopecia. J Cutan Pathol. 2013;40(6):580–4. https://doi.org/10.1111/cup.12124. Epub 2013 Mar 18
23. Khorasanizadeh F, Kalantari Y, Etesami I. Role of imaging in morphea assessment: a review of the literature. Skin Res Technol. 2023;29:e13410. https://doi.org/10.1111/srt.13410.
24. Ruiz-Arriaga LF, Arenas R, Vega-Sánchez DC, Asz-Sigall D, Martínez-Velazco MA. Seborrheic dermatitis: three novel trichoscopic signs and its correlation to Malassezia sp. colonization. Skin Appendage Disord. 2019;5(5):288–92. https://doi.org/10.1159/000497782. Epub 2019 Jun 28. PMID: 31559252; PMCID: PMC6751444
25. Park JH, Park YJ, Kim SK, Kwon JE, Kang HY, Lee ES, Choi JH, Kim YC. Histopathological differential diagnosis of psoriasis and seborrheic dermatitis of the scalp. Ann Dermatol. 2016;28(4):427–32. https://doi.org/10.5021/ad.2016.28.4.427. Epub 2016 Jul 26. PMID: 27489423; PMCID: PMC4969470

26. Zengin S, Guthrie J, Zoumberos N, Hamza M, Shalin SC. Sebaceous gland atrophy due to seborrheic dermatitis in a patient with alopecia: a potential pitfall. J Cutan Pathol. 2024;51(7):513–7. https://doi.org/10.1111/cup.14623. Epub 2024 Apr 13
27. Leroy AK, Cortez de Almeida RF, Obadia DL, Frattini S, Melo DF. Scalp seborrheic dermatitis: what we know so far. Skin Appendage Disord. 2023;9(3):160–4. https://doi.org/10.1159/000529854. Epub 2023 Apr 5. PMID: 37325288; PMCID: PMC10264915
28. Zheng X, Wu C, Jin H, Liu J, Wang H. Investigation of using very high-frequency ultrasound in the differential diagnosis of early-stage pemphigus vulgaris vs seborrheic dermatitis. Skin Res Technol. 2020;26(4):476–81. https://doi.org/10.1111/srt.12836. Epub 2020 Jan 13. PMID: 31930604; PMCID: PMC7496295.

Chapter 6
Clinical, Imaging, and Histological Findings in Tumoral Lesions of the Scalp

Maria Carolina Zafra Páez, André da Silva Cartell, Ana Leticia Boff, Davi Berardo Porciuncula, Mariana Franco Ferraz Santino, Simone Guarçoni, Carolina Ávila de Almeida, Clarissa Canella Moraes do Carmo, and Bruna Duque-Estrada

Tumoral lesions of the scalp present a unique diagnostic challenge due to their clinical and morphological diversity. While clinical examination and trichoscopy offer valuable initial insights, they often fall short in differentiating between benign and malignant entities or distinguishing scalp tumors. In such cases, radiologic imaging and histopathological evaluation become indispensable, providing definitive structural and cellular-level information. The integration of these modalities not only enhances diagnostic accuracy but also guides appropriate management and surgical planning. High-quality imaging (clinical, trichoscopic, radiologic, and histological)

Supplementary Information The online version contains supplementary material available at https://doi.org/10.1007/978-3-031-77987-9_6.

M. C. Z. Páez
Zafra Dermatology Private Clinic, Rio de Janeiro, Brazil

BCM Dermatologia Especializada, Private Practice, Rio de Janeiro, Brazil

A. da Silva Cartell
Adjunct Professor at Faculdade de Medicina da Universidade Federal do Rio Grande do Sul, Rio de Janeiro, Brazil

Dermatologist and Dermatopathologist in Private Practice, Rio de Janeiro, Brazil

A. L. Boff
Santa Casa Hospital, Porto Alegre, RS, Brazil

Dermathopathologist Private Practice, Clinica Dermapat, Porto Alegre, RS, Brazil

D. B. Porciuncula
Pathologist in Private Practice – Diagnósticos da América – DASA, Rio de Janeiro, Brazil

M. F. F. Santino
Dermatology Division, Universidade Federal do Rio de Janeiro—UFRJ, Rio de Janeiro, Brazil

Hospital São Vicente de Paulo and Hospital Copa D'or, Rio de Janeiro, RJ, Brazil

© The Author(s), under exclusive license to Springer Nature Switzerland AG 2025

C. Canella Moraes do Carmo (ed.), *Atlas of Diagnostic Imaging in Dermatology*, https://doi.org/10.1007/978-3-031-77987-9_6

plays a crucial role in bridging diagnostic gaps, especially when surface-level assessments are inconclusive. This comprehensive, image-guided approach is essential for effective evaluation of scalp tumors, ensuring timely and precise diagnosis.

6.1 Pilomatricoma

6.1.1 *Definition [1]*

- Pilomatricoma, also known as calcifying epithelioma of Malherbe, is a benign cutaneous adnexal tumor that arises from hair follicle matrix cells.

6.1.2 *Epidemiology [1, 2]*

- Pilomatricomas can occur at any age, with no sex predilection, and exhibit a bimodal distribution, being most common in children and adults over 50.
- Approximately 50% of cases occur on the head and neck.

6.1.3 *Clinical Presentation (Fig. 6.1) [1, 3]*

- Firm, papules or nodules with skin-colored, white or bluish color.
- The lesion has a firm to stone-hard consistency, and a lobular shape on palpation. Most lesions are smaller than 3 cm, but giant lesions up to 15 cm have been reported.

S. Guarçoni
Clinica ALTA - DASA, Rio de Janeiro, Brazil

C. Á. de Almeida
Faculty of Medicine of Valença—UniFaa, Valença, Brazil

Federal University of Rio de Janeiro—UFRJ, Rio de Janeiro, Brazil

C. Canella Moraes do Carmo (✉)
Fluminense Federal University—UFF, Rio de Janeiro, Brazil

Federal University of Rio de Janeiro—UFRJ, Rio de Janeiro, Brazil

Diagnóstico das Américas—DASA—RJ, Rio de Janeiro, Brazil

Biodesign Laboratory, DASA-PUC, Rio de Janeiro, Brazil

B. Duque-Estrada
BCM Dermatologia Especializada, Private Practice, Rio de Janeiro, Brazil

Universidade Federal de São Paulo, São Paulo, Brazil

Hair Diseases Department, Instituto de Dermatologia Professor Rubem David Azulay – Santa Casa da Misericórdia do Rio de Janeiro, Rio de Janeiro, Brazil

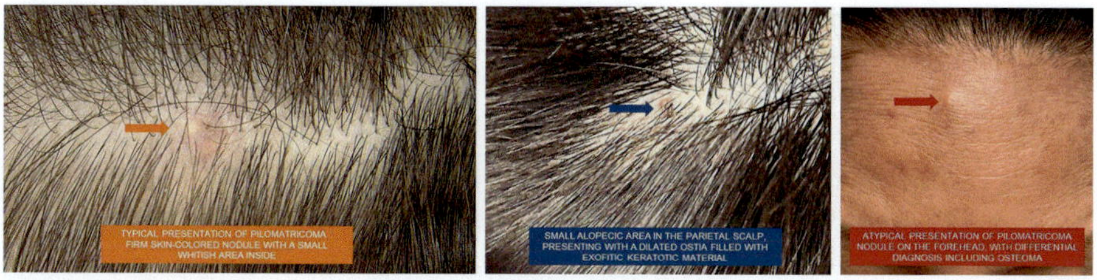

Fig. 6.1 Clinical photograph of a patient with a pilomatricoma

- Transepidermal elimination (perforation) sometimes occurs with extrusion of calcified or ossified portions of the neoplasm, making the clinical diagnosis easier. Although, in small lesions, transepidermal elimination may be misdiagnosed as a dilated pore of Winer, or epidermoid cyst. Rare clinical types of pilomatricomas characterized by anetodermic or keloid-like appearance were described.
- Differential diagnosis include epidermoid cysts, lipomas, or even malignant tumors, making accurate diagnosis challenging.

6.1.4 Dermoscopy (Fig. 6.2) [3, 4]

- Pilomatricomas typically present as pigmented nodules, being single or multiple colors, ranging from blue to red or yellow. The typical presentation has yellowish-white structureless areas, which correspond to calcification or keratin masses beneath the skin.
- White streaks, shiny linear structures, indicate fibrosis.
- Irregular linear vessels, and hairpin-like vessels raise suspicion for a tumoral process when observed with other features.
- A pinkish background may be observed, specially when inflammation is present.
- Trichoscopic features are often non-specific, and surface clues may not be sufficient to distinguish it from other lesions.

6.1.5 Histopatology (Fig. 6.3) [1, 5]

- Pilomatricoma, also know as Pilomatrixoma or later calcifying epithelioma of Malherbe is a benign adnexal neoplasm derived from the matrix of the hair follicle. This neoplasm evolve with time and have been classified into four histopathologic stages: early, fully developed, early regressive, and late regressive.
- Histopathological findings
  - A dermal tumor well circumscribed by fibrosis with a rounded, smooth silhouette, resembling a solid-cystic lesion on macroscopic examination.

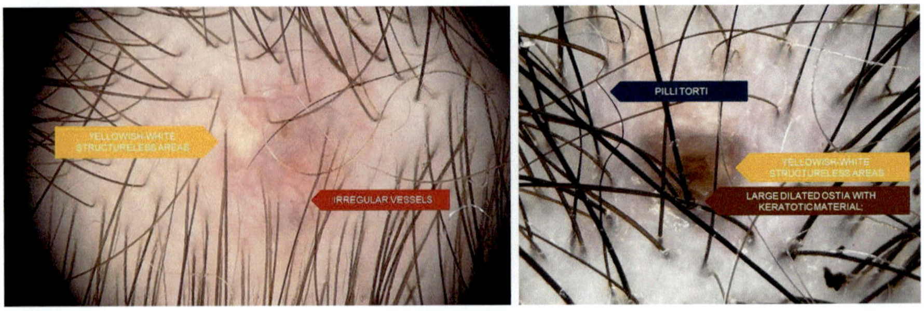

Fig. 6.2 Dermoscopy of a patient with a pilomatricoma (×20)

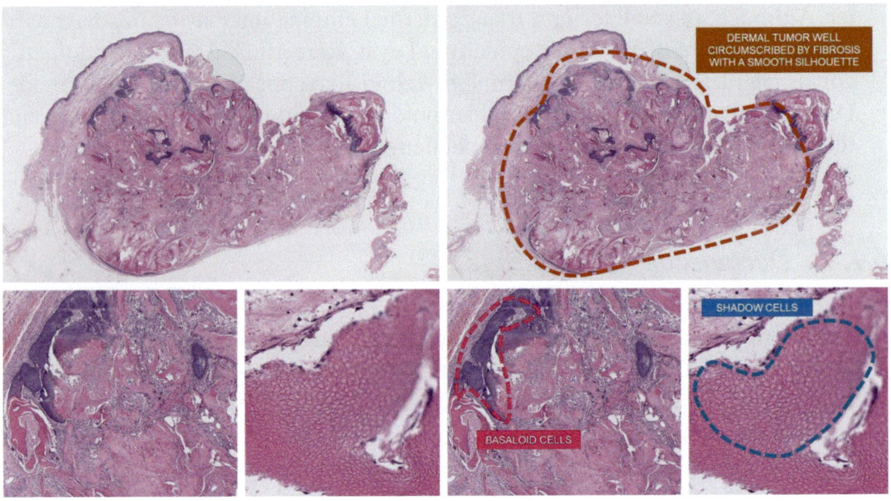

Fig. 6.3 Histological findings of a pilomatricoma (H&E ×4 and ×10)

- Presence of a biphasic population with basaloid cells located in the periphery, and shadow cells more centrally, corresponding to the grouping of eosinophilic squamous cells devoid of a nucleus. Between the two, there may be intermediate or transitional cells.
- Unlike the brisk mitotic figures found in basaloid cells, none are seen in shadow cells.
- In the late phase, keratinous debris, shadow cells, calcification, or even ossification may be the only histological signs observed. Incidence of calcification ranges from 69% to 85%.
- In response to extruded keratin, calcified or cellular debris, the surrounding dermis often shows a granulomatous foreign-body inflammatory reaction.
- There may rarely be expression of melanin in the pigmented pilomatricoma.
- Exceptionally, there may be a perforating variant with extrusion of calcified material through epidermal channels.

- Pilomatrical carcinoma is a rare, locally aggressive malignant adnexal tumor derived from hair matrix cells, which arises de novo, but can also develop from long-standing or recurrent pilomatricomas. Pilomatrical carcinoma is usually ulcerated, poorly circumscribed cellular, and infiltrative tumor. Numerous mitosis and tumor necrosis are often present.

- Immunochemistry
  - Cytoplasmic and nuclear for Beta-catenin is strongly positive in vast majority of cases.
  - Nuclear staining for cyclin-D in basaloid cells.
  - Keratins 5, 14, and 17 often positive in Pilomatrical carcinomas, but negative in benign pilomatricoma.

6.1.6 Radiography and Computed Tomography [6, 7]

- Plain X-ray films show nonspecific calcification in the majority of lesions, with some potentially being completely calcified.

6.1.7 Ultrasonography (Figs. 6.4 and 6.5) [6]

- Pilomatricoma typically shows distinctive features on high-frequency ultrasonography, which can help differentiate it from other subcutaneous lesions as epidermoid cyst, lipomas, dermatofibromas, and trichilemmal cyst.

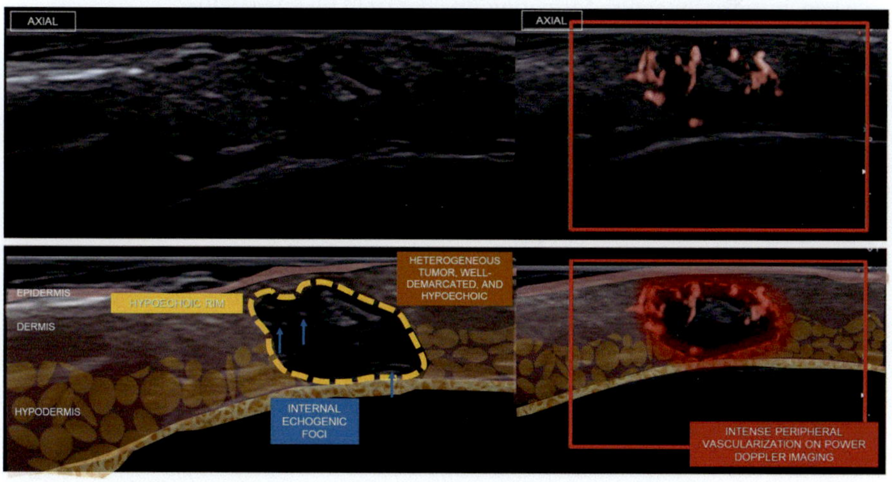

Fig. 6.4 Ultrasonographic findings of a pilomatricoma with a 24 MHz probe (Aplio i800, Canon Medical Systems)

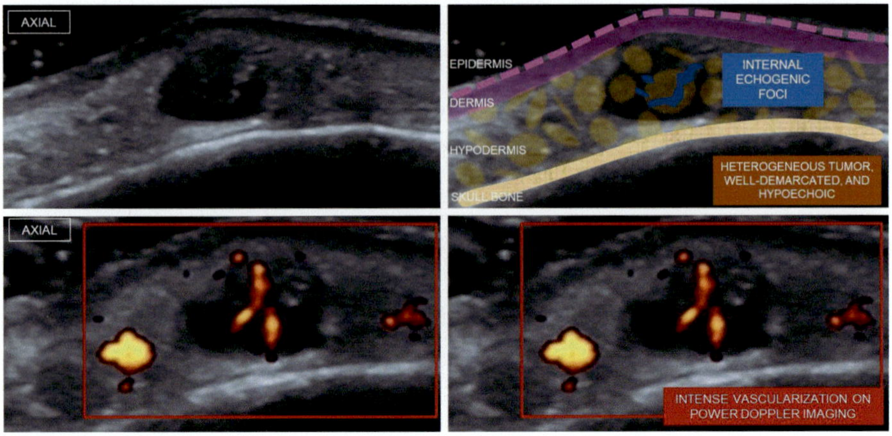

Fig. 6.5 Ultrasonographic findings of a pilomatricoma with a 22 MHz probe (MX7 Portable Ultrasound, Mindray)

- Heterogeneous tumors, well-demarcated, and hypoechoic, located between the deep dermis and subcutaneous tissue.
- Mostly arranged in a regular shape (oval or round), while a few were irregular in shape.
- The most common features are internal echogenic foci, hypoechoic rim, posterior shadowing, and peritumoral hyperechogenicity.
- In pilomatricoma, calcification may present in three distinct patterns: scattered dots, clumps, and arc-like structures.
- Posterior enhancement is observed only in the early and fully developed stages, when cystic architecture formation was detected histologically.
- At power Doppler examination, most lesions exhibited vascularity either peripheral or with a peripheral component.

6.1.8 MRI (Fig. 6.6) [6]

- The majority are isointense to skeletal muscle and show heterogeneous signal on STIR images, with regions of increased and decreased signal intensity.
- Upon injection of gadolinium-based contrast, enhancement is predominantly peripheral.
- The lesion does not show restricted diffusion on DWI sequences, as it does not demonstrate hypercellularity.

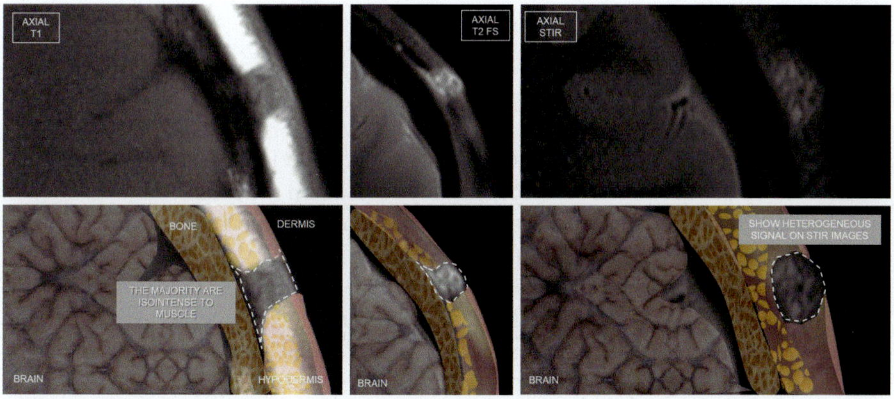

Fig. 6.6 MRI findings of pilomatricoma in T1, T2 FS-weighted, and STIR sequences (Magnetom Prisma 3T MRI, Siemens)

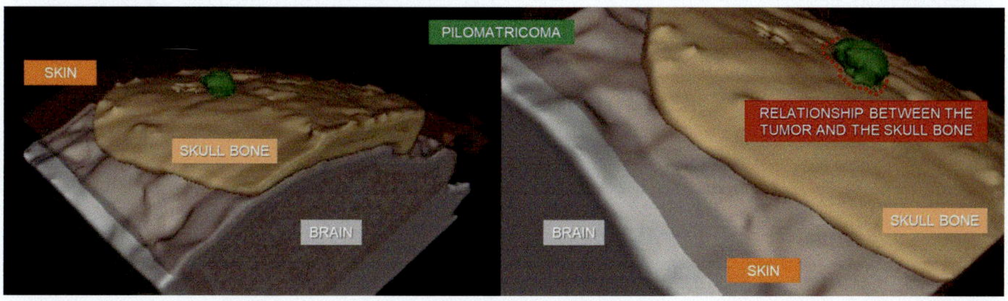

Fig. 6.7 3D virtual findings of a pilomatricoma after images segmentation of MRI isotropic images for surgical planning

6.1.9 3D Images (Fig. 6.7; Video 6.1)

- Most useful on small lesions or recurrent difficult cases.
- Allow the visualization of the extension of the lesion, enabling to assess the severity and relation with adjacent structures, especially the the galea aponeurotica.
- Contribute to more precise surgical interventions, assessing the exact location and depth of the tumor relative to critical anatomical landmarks such as the skull and vascular structures.
- Detailed assessment of the lesion's internal structure and components.
- Biomodels can be used and allows the creation of physical replicas of the affected area, offering representations that aid in surgical planning and patient education.

6.2 Trichilemmal Cyst

6.2.1 *Definition [8]*

- A cyst derived from the root sheath of the hair follicle, containing keratin and breakdown products. It is most commonly located on the scalp.
- Common intrdermal or subcutaneous cysts, also known as pilar cysts.
- Affects less than 10% of the population.
- Most commonly found on the head, particularly the scalp.
- Filled with keratin, arises from the stratified squamous epithelium similar to the outer root sheath of hair follicles, at the level of the isthmus.
- In less than 3% of trichilemmal cysts, proliferating cells in single or multiple foci grow into a Proliferating Trichilemmal Tumour (PTT), which is categorized into three groups: benign, locally aggressive, and malignant.
- Malignant proliferating trichilemmal tumor (MPTT) is a rare, malignant adnexal neoplasm that arises from a proliferating trichilemmal tumour. Typically presents as a rapidly enlarging, firm or ulcerated nodule on the scalp, most frequently in elderly women. Clinically, it may mimic squamous cell carcinoma.

6.2.2 *Epidemiology [8]*

- More common in young individuals.
- Occur more frequently in women than in men.
- No known racial predilection.
- May be inherited as an autosomal dominant trait.
- Familial cases often present with multiple lesions, and occur in younger patients.

6.2.3 *Clinical Presentation (Fig. 6.8) [8]*

- They present clinically as firm, smooth and mobile nodules. Multiple trichilemmal cysts occur in approximately 30–70% of cases, especially in familial cases.
- Very slow growth rate, taking several years to reach a large size.
- Most commonly found on the head, particularly the scalp. Predominantly found on the scalp, only occasionally on the face, trunk, groin and extremities.
- The overlying skin is normal, without erythema or ulceration (unless inflamed or secondarily infected). No central punctum is observed (unlike epidermoid cysts).
- Clinical differential diagnosis include epidermoid cyst, lipoma, dermoid cyst, proliferating trichilemmal tumor, non-ulcerated trichilemmal carcinoma, and cutaneous metastasis. Since all these lesions may present as subcutaneous nod-

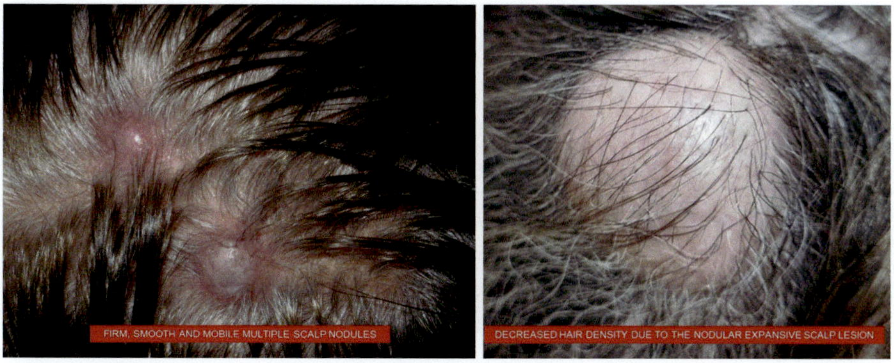

Fig. 6.8 Clinical photograph of a patient with a trichilemmal cyst

ules without distinctive surface skin changes, imaging techniques play a crucial role in aiding diagnosis prior to surgical excision.

6.2.4 Dermoscopy (Fig. 6.9) [9, 10]

- Arborising or branching blood vessels.
- Pinkish-yellow or homogeneous yellowish-white background.
- Whitish Structureless Areas.
- Peripheral erythematous halo.
- Pinkish-yellow or homogeneous yellowish-white background: the multiple shades of yellow corresponds to keratin mass from trichilemmal keratinization.
- Absence of pore sign.
- Blue pigmentation (Tyndall effect of keratin).

6.2.5 Histopathology (Fig. 6.10) [5]

- Trichilemmal cyst - also known as pilar cyst or isthmus-cathagen cyst - is the second most common type of cutaneous cyst overall and the most common cystic lesion found on the scalp. It is a benign skin lesion originating from the outer hair root sheath of the hair follicle.
- Histopathological findings
  - Circumscribed cyst located in dermis or subcutaneous tissue.
  - Epithelial proliferation within the dermis. Biopsy samples usually contain only the cyst.

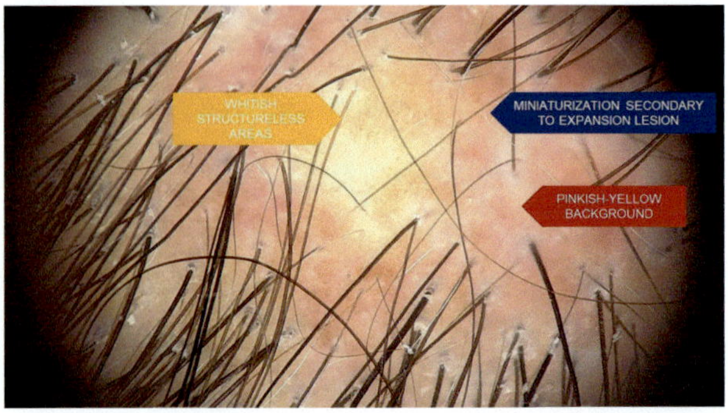

Fig. 6.9 Dermoscopy of a patient with a trichilemmal cyst (x20)

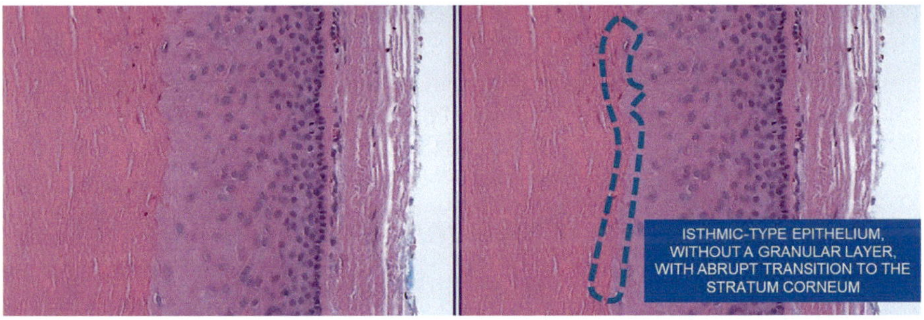

Fig. 6.10 Histological findings of a trichilemmal cyst (H&E x20)

- Isthmic-type coating epithelium, characterized by the absence of a granular layer, and an abrupt transition to the stratum corneum. The cyst is filled with dense eosinophilic corneum material, the typical trichilemmal keratinization.
- Great tendency to dystrophic calcification.
- Due to the highly compacted keratinous material, the lesion may not appear cystic and can instead resemble a solid, hyaline nodule.

6.2.6 Radiography and Computed Tomography

- Trichilemmal cysts typically exhibit soft tissue attenuation on imaging and may demonstrate speckled calcifications, along with areas of increased density attributed to cholesterol crystals and compact keratin.

6.2.7 *Ultrasonography (Fig. 6.11) [11]*

- Well-defined, hypoechoic lesions located within the subcutaneous soft tissues, often exhibiting internal calcification and posterior acoustic enhancement.
- Power Doppler ultrasonography typically reveals an absence of vascularization.

6.2.8 *MRI (Fig. 6.12) [11]*

- Trichilemmal cysts typically appear isointense or hyperintense compared to brain parenchyma in T1-weighted sequences.

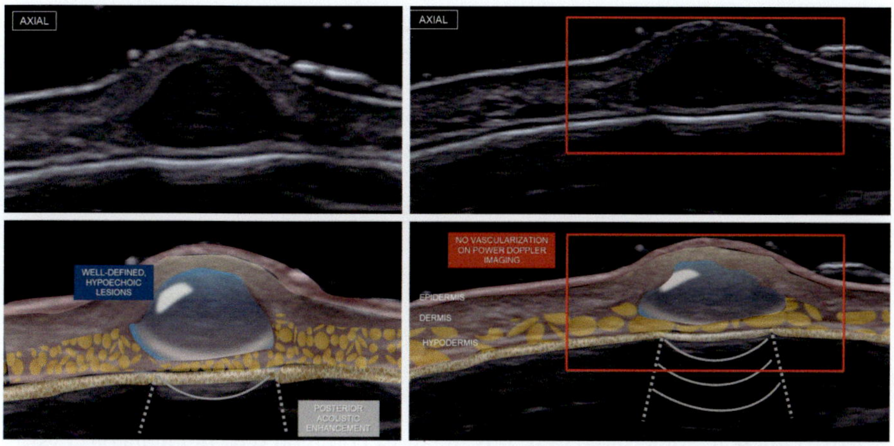

Fig. 6.11 Ultrasonographic findings of trichilemmal cyst with a 24 MHz probe (Aplio i800, Canon Medical Systems)

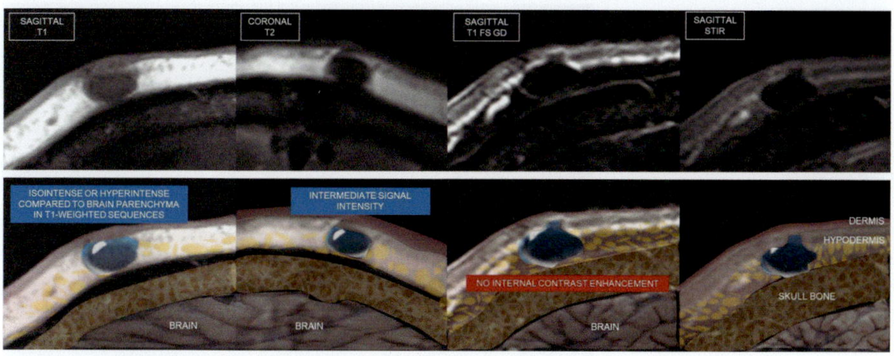

Fig. 6.12 MRI findings of a trichilemmal cyst in T1, T2 FS-weighted, and STIR sequences (Magnetom Prisma 3T MRI, Siemens)

- Internal contrast enhancement is absent.
- In T2-weighted sequences, they commonly exhibit intermediate signal intensity, often with accompanying linear or reticular hypointensity suggestive of calcification.

6.2.9 3D Images (Fig. 6.13; Video 6.2)

- Particularly valuable for small or recurrent lesions that pose diagnostic challenges, allowing the assessment of the lesion's internal structure and components.
- Provides a detailed view of the lesion's extent, helping evaluate its severity and relationship with surrounding structures, notably the galea and sometimes the root sheath of the hair follicle.
- Enhances the accuracy of surgical procedures by offering clear insights into the lesion's characteristics, specially the relation with the galea subaponeurotica and the cortical bone.
- Biomodels can be utilized to create tangible replicas of the affected area, which facilitate surgical planning and improve patient education through realistic visualizations.

6.3 Infundibular Cyst

6.3.1 Definition [12]

- Also called an epidermoid cyst, it is the most common type of cutaneous cyst.
- Epidermoid cysts originate from the follicular infundibulum.

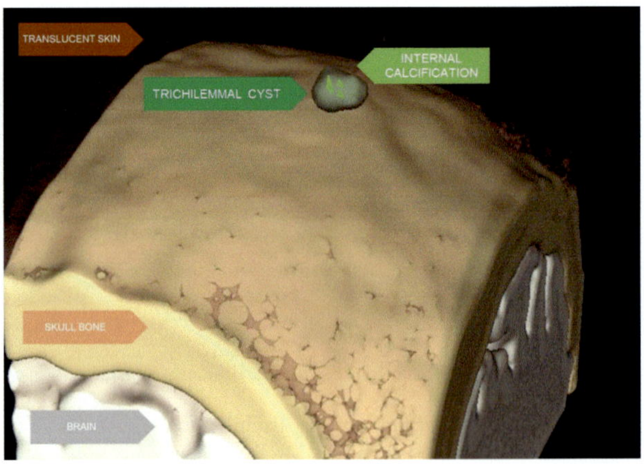

Fig. 6.13 3D virtual findings of a trichilemmal cyst after images segmentation of MRI isotropic sequences for surgical planning

- Epidermal inclusion cysts may arise following trauma that disrupts the skin's continuity, leading to the implantation and proliferation of epidermal keratinocytes within the dermis. They can also develop secondary to bullous dermatoses, particularly in conditions such as porphyria.

6.3.2 Epidemiology [12]

- More common in men than in women, with a ratio of 2:1.
- More frequently in patients in their 20s to 40s.

6.3.3 Clinical Presentation (Fig. 6.14) [13]

- It can occur anywhere on the body and typically presents as an asymptomatic, skin-colored dermal nodule, often with a clinically visible central punctum.
- The size ranges from a few millimeters to several centimeters in diameter.

6.3.4 Dermoscopy (Fig. 6.15) [13]

- The most characteristic finding which helps in the diagnosis is the punctum – a dilated yellow-brown-black dot representing the follicular ostium from which the cyst originates.
- Yellowish-white structureless areas: represent keratin-filled content within the cyst.
- Overlying Telangiectatic or Linear Vessels are observed, particularly, when the cyst is inflamed.

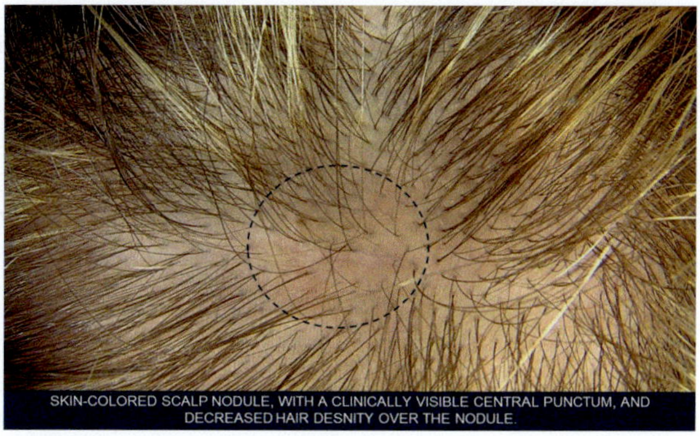

Fig. 6.14 Clinical photograph of a patient with an infundibular cyst

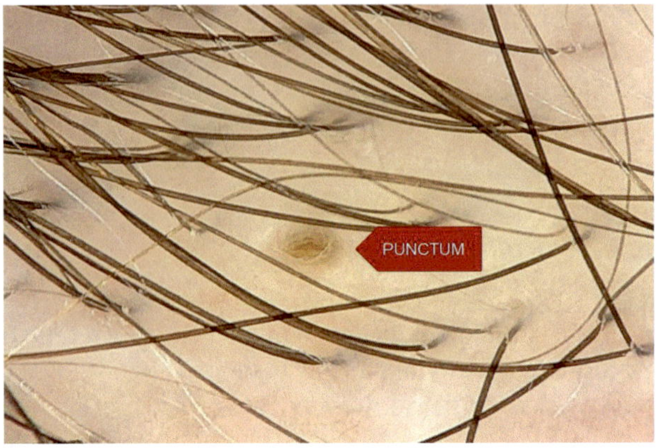

Fig. 6.15 Dermoscopy of a patient with an infundibular cyst (x20)

- Decrease or absence of hair follicles over the lesion may be observed, due to compression by the cystic mass.

6.3.5 Histopathology (Fig. 6.16) [14]

- Cystic epithelial proliferation is located entirely in the dermal or subcutaneous adipose tissue.
- The cyst is lined by epithelium resembling the interadnexal epidermis, characterized by a preserved granular layer and loosely arranged lamellar corneal material, which histologically has been likened to 'seagulls flocking on the beach.'
- As the lesion enlarges, the lining epithelium becomes increasingly flattened, often making it difficult to distinguish the epithelial layers.
- Absence of adnexal structures around the cyst wall, differentiating it from dermoid cyst.
- When the cyst ruptures, the lesion may become surrounded by acute suppurative inflammation and/or chronic inflammattry response, often accompanied by dystrophic calcification, and foreign body granuloma in reaction to corneal lamellae.
- Surrounding fibrosis – or total replacement of the cyst by a fibrotic nodule – characterizes the late phase of the lesion.

6.3.6 Radiography and Computed Tomography [15]

- Radiography may occasionally reveal soft tissue masses with areas of increased density. Although radiographs have limited value in the assessment of epidermoid cysts, they can be useful in detecting associated bone involvement or when the cyst contains calcifications within the soft tissues.

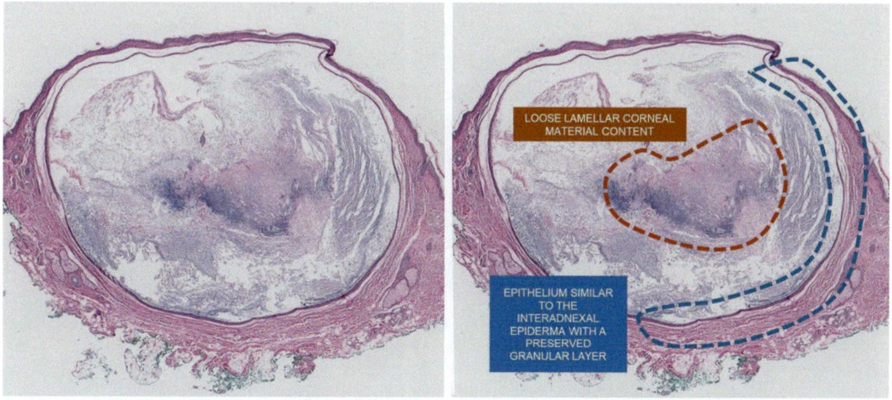

Fig. 6.16 Histological findings of an infundibular cyst (H&E x4)

- Epidermoid cysts related to bones may appear as well-demarcated intradiploic osteolytic lesions with smooth sclerotic margins on radiographs. These lesions often lead to remodeling and expansion of cortical bone.
- CT plays an essential role in diagnosing epidermoid cysts. It confirms the diagnosis of large epidermoid cysts effectively.
- On CT, epidermoid cysts appear as a well-encapsulated mass with heterogeneous densities. The majority of epidermoid cysts are hypodense and not enhanced with contrast material, as cystic contents are normally filled with debris, keratin, water, and lipids.
- An atypical hyperdense appearance on CT scans may be attributed to the presence of abundant calcification, as well as high concentrations of albumin, iron, copper, or proteinaceous material within the cyst.

6.3.7 Ultrasonography (Fig. 6.17) [15]

- Typical features of cysts, but can appear as either cystic or solid.
- Cysts have a round to oval structure.
- They are well-circumscribed and avascular on power Doppler.
- Hyperechoic with slight or absent posterior acoustic enhancement.
- Located in the dermis and subcutaneous tissue.
- Show phenomena of dorsal acoustic amplification and lateral shadowing.

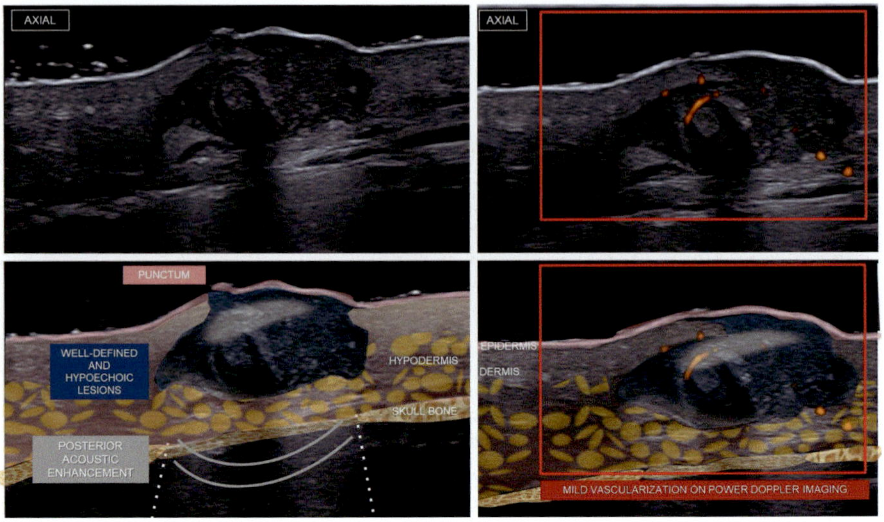

Fig. 6.17 Ultrasonographic findings of infundibular cyst with a 24 MHz probe (Aplio i800, Canon Medical Systems)

6.3.8 MRI (Fig. 6.18) [15]

- On T1-weighted MRI, the tumor showed slightly high signal intensity in some cases and iso-signal intensity in others.
- T2-weighted images consistently showed high signal intensity.
- Irregular low signal intensity areas were observed on both T1 and T2-weighted images.
- No enhancement was seen inside the tumors.
- DWI (diffusion-weighted imaging) high signal intensities and low ADC (apparent diffusion coefficient) values.

6.3.9 3D Images (Fig. 6.19; Video 6.3)

- Especially effective for addressing small or recurring lesions that are difficult to diagnose.
- Offers a comprehensive view of the lesion's size and its interaction with nearby structures, such as the galea and occasionally the follicular infundibulum Indeed the relationship and distance with the cortical bone can be assessed.
- Improves surgical precision by providing detailed information about the lesion's features and also components

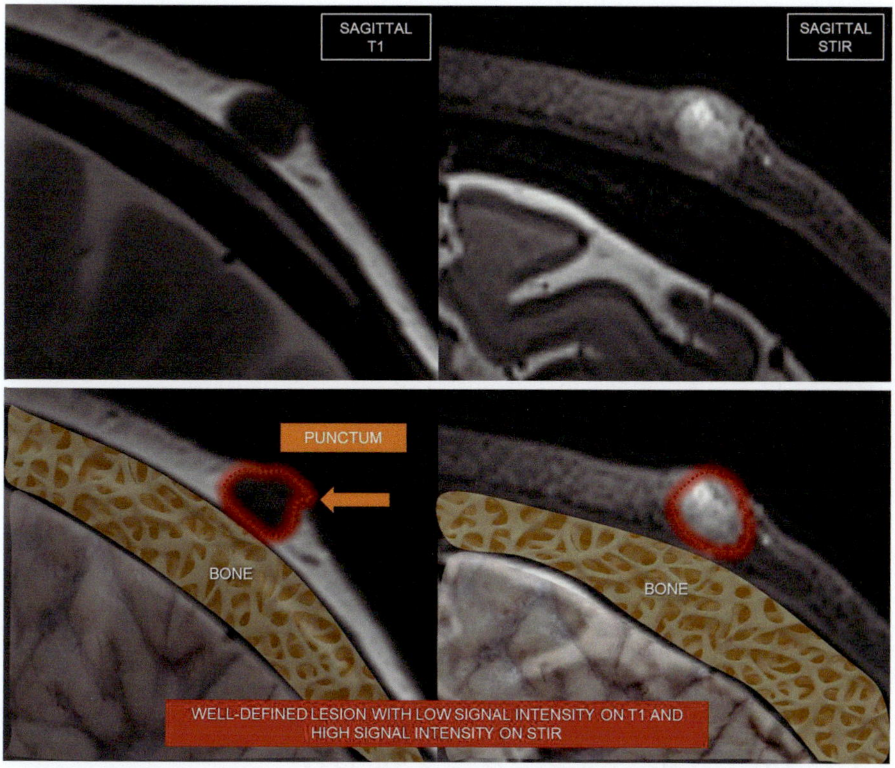

Fig. 6.18 MRI findings of an infundibular cyst in T1-weighted and STIR sequences (Magnetom Prisma 3T MRI, Siemens)

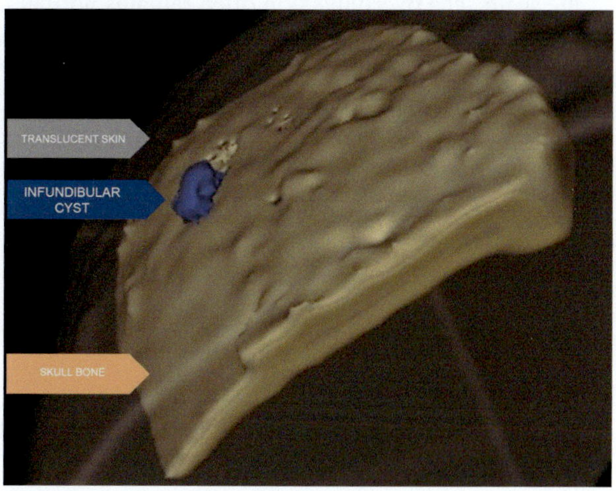

Fig. 6.19 3D virtual findings of an infundibular cyst after images segmentation of MRI isotropic sequences for surgical planning

- Allows the use of biomodels to produce physical replicas of the affected area, aiding in surgical preparation and enhancing patient understanding with realistic representations.

6.4 Lipoma

6.4.1 *Definition [16]*

- The most common mesenchymal tumors of the human body.
- A lipoma is a benign tumor composed of mature adipocytes (fat cells), typically located in the subcutaneous layer.

6.4.2 *Epidemiology [16]*

- Adults between 40 and 60 years, with a slight male predominance.
- Solitary lipomas are more common than multiple lipomas. Familial multiple lipomatosis is a rare inherited condition, usually autosomal dominant.

6.4.3 *Clinical Presentation (Fig. 6.20) [16]*

- Soft, painless subcutaneous nodules ranging in size from 1 to >10 cm.
- The lipoma may appear as a smooth, skin-colored, or slightly elevated area on the scalp. The overlying skin often remains normal in texture and appearance.
- They occur most frequently on the trunk and upper extremities and can be round, oval, or multilobulated.
- Frequently, patients may have more than one lipoma.
- Lipomas can occur on any part of the body and usually develop superficially in the subcutaneous tissue. Rarely, they may involve fascia or deeper muscular planes.

6.4.4 *Trichoscopy (Fig. 6.21) [17]*

- Overlying skin usually appears intact, with normal follicular openings and no signs of epidermal disruption. Rarely, a diffuse yellowish hue may be visible under trichoscopy due to the presence of underlying adipose tissue.

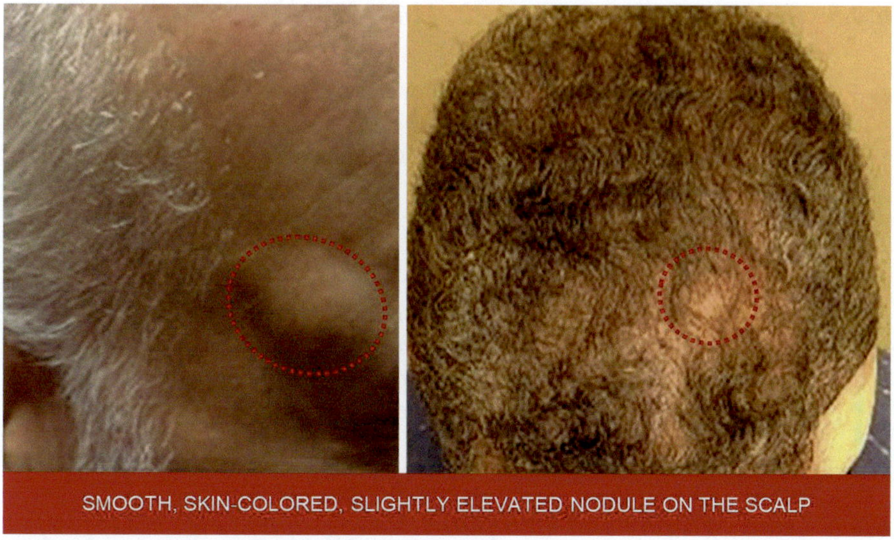

Fig. 6.20 Clinical photograph of patients with subgaleal lipoma

Fig. 6.21 Trichoscopy of a patient with a subgaleal lipoma (x20)

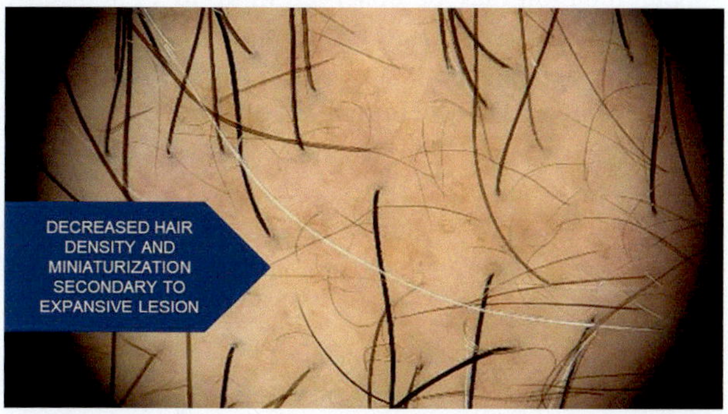

- Fine, linear blood vessels (telangiectasias) may be observed on the surface, though this is less common.
- Unlike cysts or tumors that compress follicles, lipomas usually do not displace or distort hair follicles.
- Trichoscopy is not a reliable diagnostic tool for lipomas because they are deep, subcutaneous lesions that do not alter the superficial epidermis or hair follicle architecture in a characteristic way. While trichoscopy is highly useful for evaluating hair disorders and superficial skin lesions, it offers limited information about deeper soft tissue masses such as lipomas.

6.4.5 *Histopathology (Fig. 6.22) [16–18]*

- Proliferation of normal-looking lobules or bundles of adipocytes with minimal variation in adipocyte size.
- The lesion is usually located in the subcutaneous adipose tissue. While most lipomas are deep-seated, there are superficial variants—such as superficial lipomatous nevus—as well as deeper forms that may extend into muscle or fascia.
- The tumor is surrounded by a thin capsule of connective tissue.
- It may present myxoid alterations (degenerations), hemorrhage, adipose necrosis, dystrophic calcification, cavitation or fibrosis.
- Variants: superficial adipose nevus, fibrolipoma, myxolipoma, angiolipoma (often painful, differentiating from other forms), intramuscular, spindle cell lipoma, pleomorphic cell lipoma, and lipomatosis.

6.4.6 *Radiography and Computed Tomography (Fig. 6.23) [19]*

- Large lipomas are recognizable as low-density areas causing a mass effect.
- Calcification may be observed in up to 11% of cases, with a higher association with well-differentiated liposarcoma.
- Classic appearance is a circumscribed, homogeneously low-density mass ranging from -120 to 65 Hounsfield units on computed tomography.

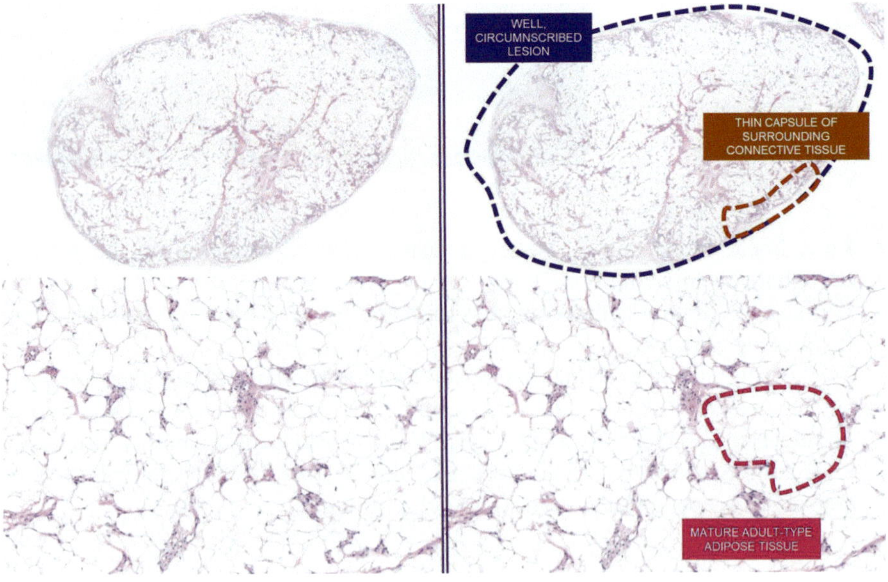

Fig. 6.22 Histological findings of a subgaleal angiolipoma (H&E x4 and ×20)

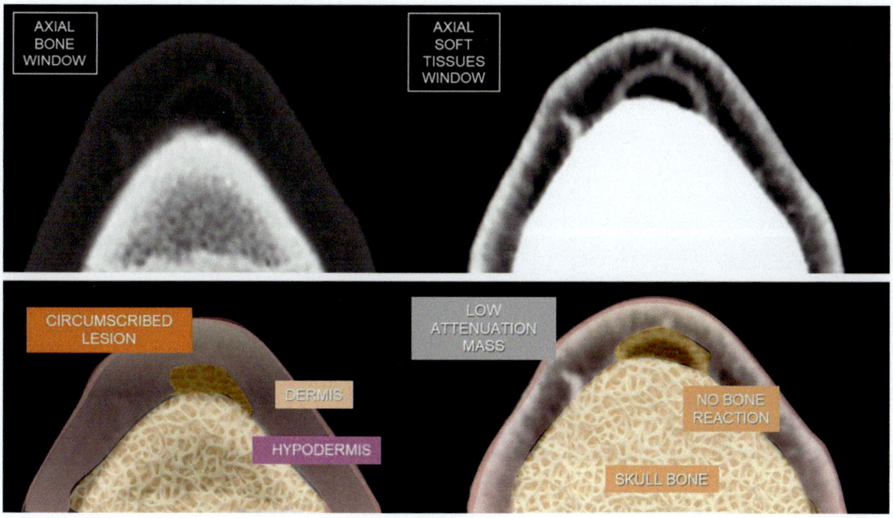

Fig. 6.23 Imaging findings of a subgaleal lipoma on axial CT (Philips Brilliance CT 64-slice)

6.4.7 Ultrasonography (Fig. 6.24) [19]

- Ultrasound is a valuable, non-invasive tool for evaluating subcutaneous soft tissue masses as lipomas. It helps assess the lesion's size, shape, echotexture, vascularity, and relationship to surrounding structures. The lesion may present as soft masses with varying echogenicity:
  - Hyperechoic: 20–52%
  - Isoechoic: 28–60%
  - Hypoechoic: 20%
  - Identifying the capsule of encapsulated lipomas can be challenging on ultrasonography.
- Characteristics include:
  - Absence of acoustic shadowing
  - Minimal or absent power Doppler flow
  - Suspicion for liposarcoma increases with:
  - Heterogeneous echotexture
  - Presence of more than minimal power Doppler flow

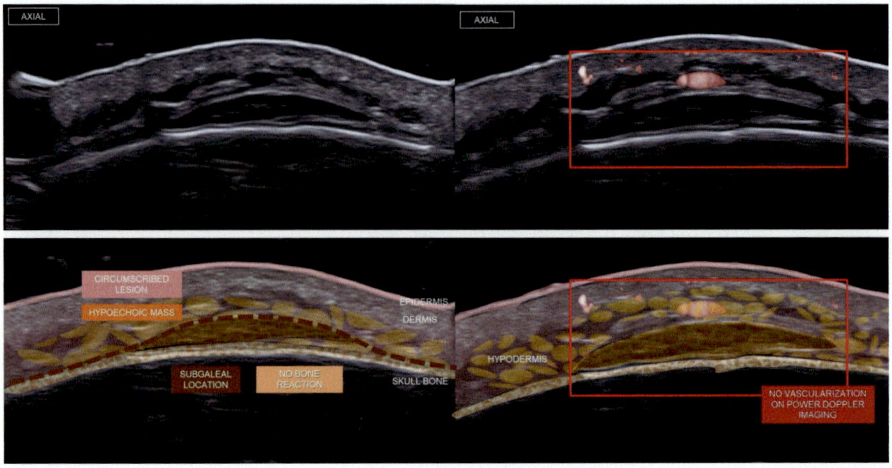

Fig. 6.24 Ultrasonographic findings of a subgaleal lipoma with a 24 MHz probe (Aplio i800, Canon Medical Systems)

6.4.8 MRI [19]

- Characteristic appearance is an encapsulated lesion isointense to subcutaneous fat on all sequences.
- Intramuscular lipomas may insinuate within skeletal muscle, unlike liposarcoma.
- Thin internal septa are common in imaged lipomas; usually do not enhance.
- Marked enhancement seen in well-differentiated liposarcomas.
- Thick and nodular septa present in some lipomas, making them indistinguishable from liposarcoma.

6.4.9 3D Images (Fig. 6.25; Video 6.4)

- Particularly useful for evaluating small or recurring lesions that are challenging to diagnose.
- Provides an in-depth view of the lesion's dimensions and its relationship with surrounding structures, including the galea and cortical bone, assessing if any periosteal reaction is present.
- Enhances surgical accuracy by delivering precise details about the lesion's characteristics, allowing for clear differentiation between benign and potentially malignant variants. While benign lipomas typically appear as well-defined, smaller lesions with homogeneous components, malignant forms often present with larger volumes, heterogeneous appearance, and multiple septations.

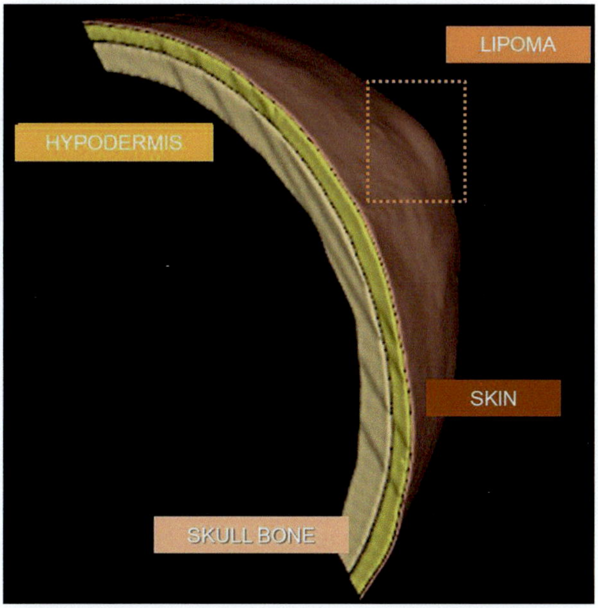

Fig. 6.25 3D virtual findings of a subgaleal lipoma after images segmentation of MRI isotropic sequences for surgical planning

- Facilitates the creation of biomodels that generate physical replicas of the affected area, supporting both surgical planning and patient education with accurate, three-dimensional visualizations.

6.5 Osteoma

6.5.1 Definition [20, 21]

- Osteoma is a common benign tumor primarily composed of well-differentiated compact or cancellous bone.
- It is slow-growing and osteogenic, often arising from the outer table of the skull, and is often found incidentally on imaging.
- Osteomas are usually asymptomatic, but depending on their size and location, they can cause obstruction, pain, or cosmetic deformity.

6.5.2 Epidemiology [21]

- Predominantly affects men in their fifth and sixth decades of life.
- It is the most frequent benign bone tumor in adults.

6.5.3 Clinical Presentation (Fig. 6.26) [20]

- Typically asymptomatic and solitary.
- Can be sessile or pedunculated; when arising from the inner table, it may mimic ossified meningiomas but lacks soft tissue components and enhancement.
- Multiple osteomas may indicate Gardner syndrome, characterized by colonic polyposis and other benign tumors.

6.5.4 Histopathology [18]

- Composed of dense lamellar or cancellous bone.
- The tissue structure is highly organized, consistent with the benign nature of the tumor.
- Osteomas are classified into two main histologic types: Compact (ivory) Osteoma, which resembles cortical bone, and Cancellous (trabecular) osteoma, that resembles medullary bone.

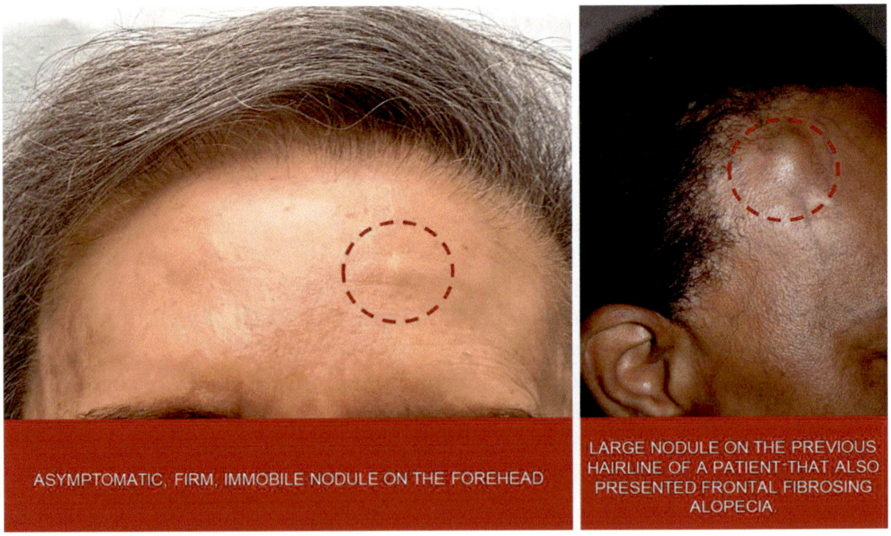

Fig. 6.26 Clinical photograph of osteomas

6.5.5 Radiography and Computed Tomography (Fig. 6.27) [21]

- Radiography and CT are useful for detection and monitoring of superficial or accessible lesions. Osteomas appear as well-defined, homogeneously sclerotic radiopaque lesions.
- Typically located juxtacortically, these lesions are round or oval and do not involve the sutures.

6.5.6 Ultrasonography (Fig. 6.28) [22, 23]

- Well-defined and hyperechoic lesions due to their dense and calcified nature in continuity with the skull bone.
- Posterior acoustic shadowing due to the attenuation of sound waves as they pass through the dense and calcified material.
- Do not show blood flow on power Doppler imaging.

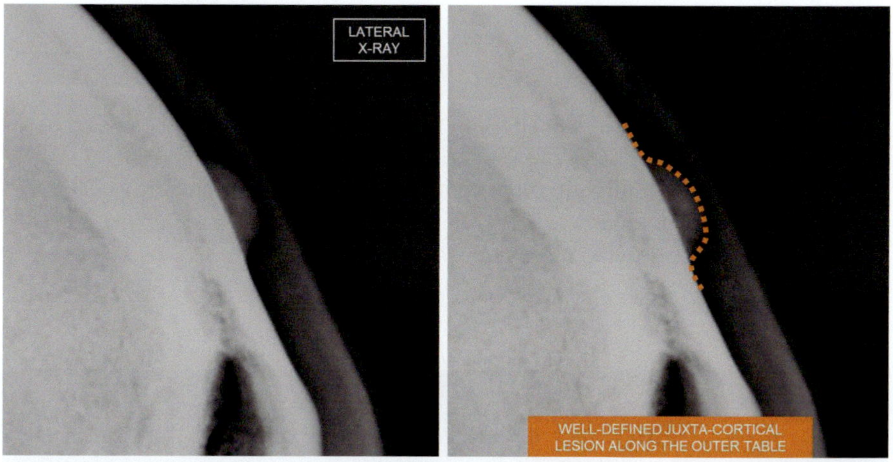

Fig. 6.27 Radiographic findings of osteoma (Philips Duo Diagnost R&F Room Digital RF and Tomo System)

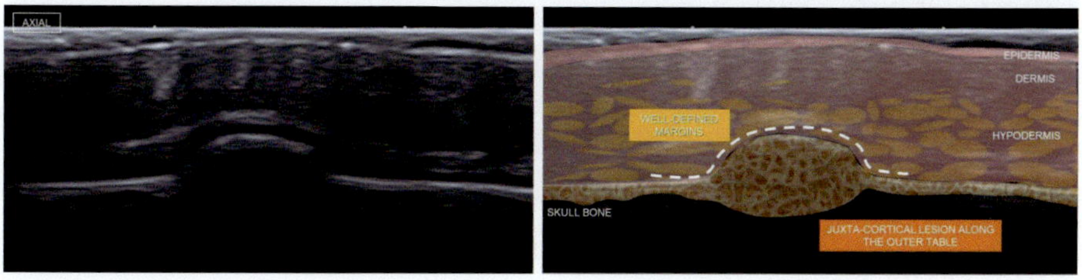

Fig. 6.28 Ultrasonographic findings of osteoma with a 24 MHz probe (Aplio i800, Canon Medical Systems)

6.5.7 MRI (Fig. 6.29)

- Exhibits homogeneous low signal intensity on T1-weighted images.
- T2-weighted images can vary depending on the proportions of compact and cancellous bone within the lesion.
- Osteomas do not enhance with contrast.

6.6 Dermoid Cyst

6.6.1 Definition [24]

- A benign congenital tumor originating from ectodermal and mesodermal tissues.
- Surrounded by keratinizing squamous cells and typically contains adnexal structures like hair follicles, sweat glands, and sebaceous glands.

6.6.2 Epidemiology [24]

- Approximately 70% found in children 5 years old or younger, but can also occur in adults.
- Gender distribution: Slightly more common in females (34 females vs. 28 males in a sample of 62 patients).
- Prevalence in age groups

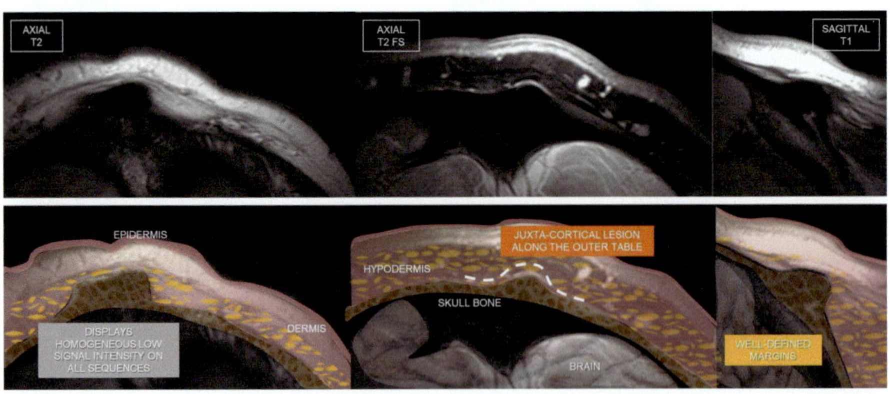

Fig. 6.29 MRI findings of an osteoma in T1, T2 FS, and T2-weighted sequences (Magnetom Avanto 1.5T MRI, Siemens)

- 0–5 years: 52%
- 6–10 years: 3%
- 11–16 years: 8%
- 17 years and older: 37%

6.6.3 Clinical Findings (Figs. 6.30 and 6.31) [24]

- Typically presents as a palpable mass, often in the periorbital lateral eyebrow area.
- Symptoms
  - 30% of patients showed symptoms since birth.
  - 32% reported a change in tumor size, and few having a history of trauma.
  - 5% had a local infection.
- Location of lesions
  - Periorbital region: Most common (84% of cases)
  - Medial brow
  - Lateral brow
  - Ear: Preauricular, retroauricular
  - Nose: Nasal dorsum
  - Scalp: Occipital region
  - Other areas: Chin, cheek
- Dermoid cysts can lead to serious neurological complications, such as encephalomeningitis and seizures, particularly if they extend intracranially and rupture.

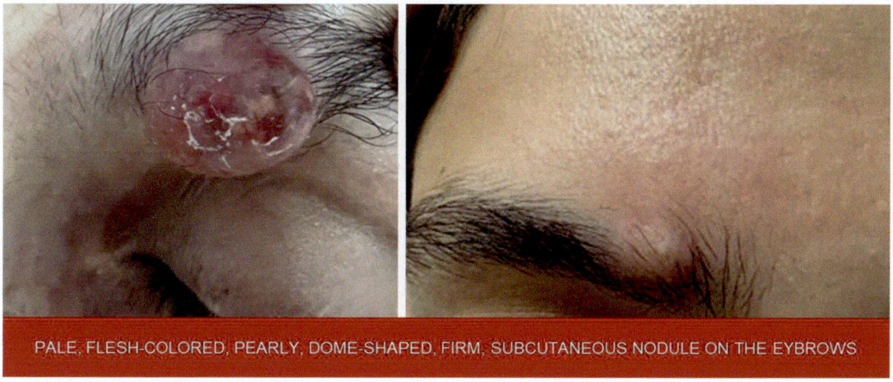

Fig. 6.30 Clinical photograph of dermoid cysts (Image courtesy of Dr. Andre Luíz Vairo Donda—Rio de Janeiro, Brazil)

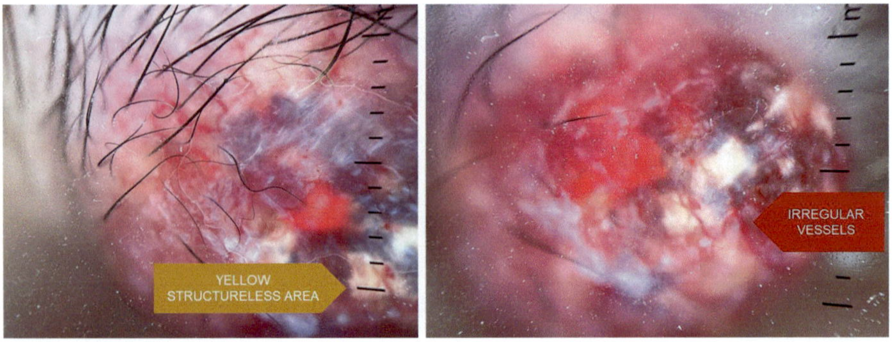

Fig. 6.31 Dermoscopic findings of a dermoid cyst (x20) (Image courtesy of Dr. Andre Luíz Vairo Donda—Rio de Janeiro, Brazil)

6.6.4 Trichoscopy

There are no descriptions in the literature of the ultrasonographic findings of dermoid tumors; however, based on the authors' experience, the following features can be observed:

- Dilated vessels and capillaries.
- While not specific to dermoid cysts, the presence of hair within the cyst can be a helpful finding, especially when combined with other features.
- Large yellow dots or dilated follicular ostia can be seen in dermoid cysts, indicating the presence of keratin or sebum within the follicular openings.

6.6.5 Histopathology [18]

- Congenital cyst occurring in midline areas and embryonic fusion lines.
- Cystic epithelial proliferation in the derma or subcutaneous adipose tissue.
- The lining epithelium is similar to the interadnexal epiderma with a preserved granular layer and a loose lamellar corneal material content, resembling seagulls flocking on the beach, and may also contain fragments of hair shaft.
- Unlike the epidermal cyst, it exhibits multiple hair follicles adhered and opening directly into the cystic cavity and, sometimes, associated sebaceous glands.

6.6.6 Radiography and Computed Tomography [25]

- Typically, well-defined hypodense masses (-20 to -140 HU), similar to fat tissue density.

- Rarely can be hyperdense, reflecting high protein content, saponification of lipid, or keratinized debris with microcalcification.

6.6.7 Ultrasonography (Fig. 6.32) [25]

- Hypoechoic masses with scattered echogenic foci, no internal vascularity on power Doppler.
- Echogenic foci correlate with keratin debris on microscopic examination.

6.6.8 MRI (Fig. 6.33) [25]

- Usually hyperintense on T1-weighted images and variable on T2-weighted images.
- Presence of a "fat" density or signal intensity is due to internal composition like cholesterol, not adipose tissue.
- "Sack of marbles" appearance due to multiple fat globules in the cyst.
- Enhancement of mural nodules reported, pathologic explanation unknown.

6.6.9 3D Images

- Especially beneficial for assessing small or recurrent lesions that are difficult to identify.

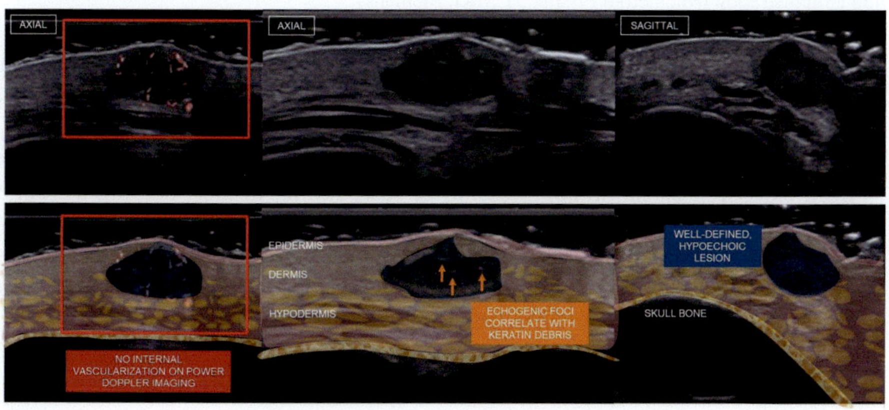

Fig. 6.32 Ultrasonographic findings of dermoid cyst with a 24 MHz probe (Aplio i800, Canon Medical Systems)

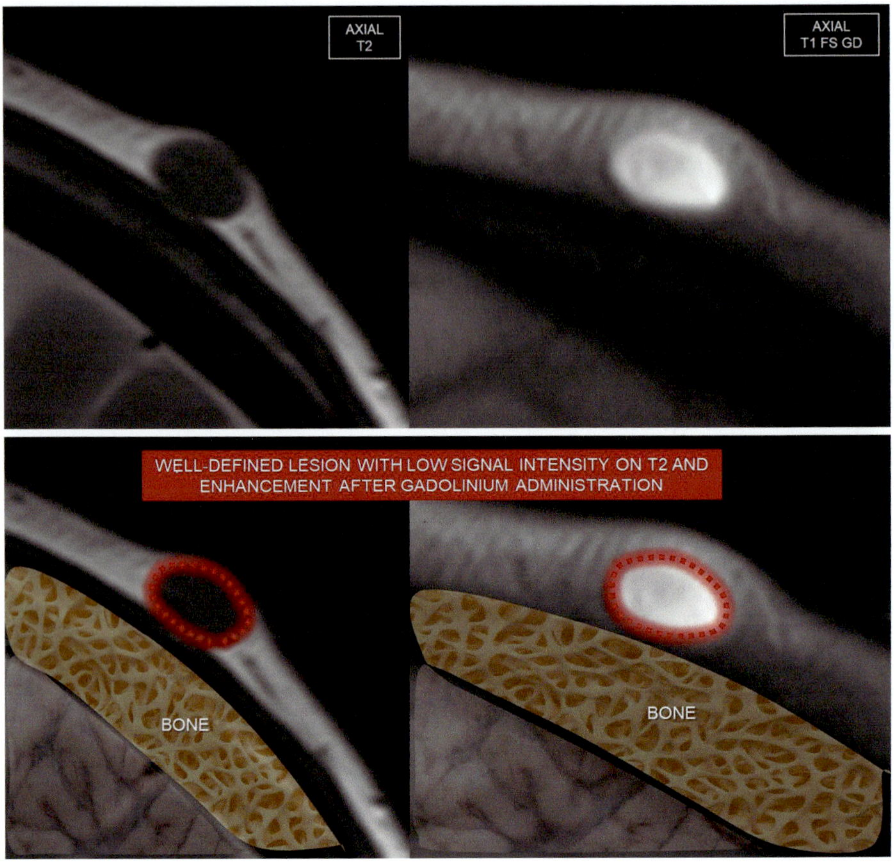

Fig. 6.33 MRI findings of a dermoid cyst in T2 FS and T1 FS-weighted sequences after gadolinium administration (Magnetom Prisma 3T MRI, Siemens)

- By offering a high-resolution, volumetric perspective, it enhances the assessment of lesion size, shape, and its relationship with adjacent structures such as the galea.
- This advanced visualization is especially useful in cases where the cyst exhibits deep extension or subtle compression of surrounding tissues, helping to refine surgical strategies and minimize complications.
- Enables the development of biomodels that create physical replicas of the affected area, aiding in surgical planning and enhancing patient education through realistic, three-dimensional representations.

References

1. Jones CD, Ho W, Robertson BF, Gunn E, Morley S. Pilomatrixoma: a comprehensive review of the literature. Am J Dermatopathol. 2018;40:631–41.
2. Hernández-Núñez A, Nájera Botello L, Romero Maté A, Martínez-Sánchez C, Utrera Busquets M, Calderón Komáromy A, et al. Estudio retrospectivo de pilomatricomas: 261 tumores en 239 pacientes. Actas Dermosifiliogr. 2014;105:699–705.
3. Bulman JC, Ulualp SO, Rajaram V, Koral K. Pilomatricoma of childhood: a common pathologic diagnosis yet a rare radiologic one. Am J Roentgenol. 2016;206:182–8.
4. Ayhan E, Ertugay O, Gundogdu R. Three different dermoscopic view of three new cases with pilomatrixoma. Int J Trichology. 2014;6:21. https://doi.org/10.4103/0974-7753.136753.
5. Liersch J, von Köckritz A, Schaller J. Dermatopathology 101. Part 2—skin tumors. J Dtsch Dermatol Ges. 2017;15:906–29.
6. Li L, Xu J, Wang S, Yang J. Ultra-high-frequency ultrasound in the evaluation of paediatric pilomatricoma based on the histopathologic classification. Front Med (Lausanne). 2021;8:673861.
7. Rothman D. Giant Pilomatrixoma (Malherbe calcifying Epithelioma). Arch Surg. 1976;111:86.
8. Al Aboud DM, Naga Yarrarapu SS, Patel BC. Pilar cyst continuing education activity. StatPearls Publishing; 2024. https://www.ncbi.nlm.nih.gov/books/NBK534209/.
9. Miyachi H, Togawa Y, Yamamoto Y, Oguma R, Suehiro K, Matsue H. Proliferating trichilemmal tumour: a comparison of dermoscopic, ultrasonographic and histopathological features. Eur J Dermatol. 2016;26:400–2.
10. Rudnicka L, Olszewska M, Waskiel A, Rakowska A. Trichoscopy in hair shaft disorders. Dermatol Clin. 2018;36:421–30.
11. He P, Cui L, Wang J, Zhao B, Chen W, Xu Y. Trichilemmal cyst: clinical and sonographic features. J Ultrasound Med. 2019;38:91–6.
12. Zito PM, Scharf R. Epidermoid cyst. StatPearls Publishing; 2024.
13. Ghigliotti G, Cinotti E, Parodi A. Usefulness of dermoscopy for the diagnosis of epidermal cyst: the 'pore' sign. Clin Exp Dermatol. 2014;39:649–50.
14. López-Ríos F, Rodríguez-Peralto JL, Castaño E, Benito A. Squamous cell carcinoma arising in a cutaneous epidermal cyst. Am J Dermatopathol. 1999;21:174–7.
15. Hoang VT, Trinh CT, Nguyen CH, Chansomphou V, Chansomphou V, Tran TTT. Overview of epidermoid cyst. Eur J Radiol Open. 2019;6:291–301.
16. Kolb L, Naga Yarrarapu SS, Atif Ameer M, Rosario-Collazo JA. Lipoma. StatPearls Publishing; 2023. https://www.ncbi.nlm.nih.gov/books/NBK507906/?report=printable.
17. Johnson CN, Ha AS, Chen E, Davidson D. Lipomatous soft-tissue tumors. J Am Acad Orthop Surg. 2018;26:779–88.
18. Calonje E, Lazar AJ, Luzar B. Diagnostic atlas of cutaneous mesenchymal neoplasia. Elsevier; 2020. https://linkinghub.elsevier.com/retrieve/pii/C20100684550.
19. Burt AM, Huang BK. Imaging review of lipomatous musculoskeletal lesions. SICOT J. 2017;3:34.
20. Khodarahmi I, Alizai H, Chalian M, Alaia EF, Burke CJ, Slasky SE, et al. Imaging spectrum of calvarial abnormalities. Radiographics. 2021;41:1144–63.
21. Gomez CK, Schiffman SR, Bhatt AA. Radiological review of skull lesions. Insights Imaging. 2018;9:857–82.
22. Lucas VS, Burk RS, Creehan S, Grap MJ. Utility of high-frequency ultrasound. Plast Surg Nurs. 2014;34:34–8.
23. Bhatt K, Tambe S, Jerajani H, Dhurat R. Utility of high-frequency ultrasonography in the diagnosis of benign and malignant skin tumors. Indian J Dermatol Venereol Leprol. 2017;83:162.
24. Choi JS, Bae YC, Lee JW, Bin KG. Dermoid cysts: epidemiology and diagnostic approach based on clinical experiences. Arch Plast Surg. 2018;45:512–6.

25. Chung BM, Kim WT, Park CK, Kim MA. Dermoid cyst in the subcutaneous tissues of the back: a rare case with multimodal imaging and pathologic correlation. Radiol Case Rep. 2021;16:1127–32.
26. Neto MPS, Assis BR, Andrade GR. Sebaceous nevus of Jadassohn: review and clinical-surgical approach. An Bras Dermatol. 2022;97:628–36.
27. Wortsman X, Ferreira-Wortsman C, Corredoira Y. Ultrasound imaging of nevus sebaceous of Jadassohn. J Ultrasound Med. 2021;40:407–15. https://doi.org/10.1002/jum.15405.

Chapter 7
Clinical, Imaging, and Histological Findings in Alopecias

Bruna Barroso Gonçalves, Maria Carolina Zafra Páez, Ana Leticia Boff, André da Silva Cartell, Carolina Ávila de Almeida, Davi Berardo Porciuncula, Ximena Wortsman, Clarissa Canella Moraes do Carmo, and Bruna Duque-Estrada

In recent years, advancements in imaging technologies have revolutionized our understanding and management of inflammatory scalp conditions, including various forms of alopecia. These techniques offer unparalleled insights into the underlying pathophysiology of these complex disorders, facilitating more accurate diagnoses and tailored treatments. This chapter delves into the cutting-edge imaging modalities used to visualize and assess inflammatory lesions of the scalp. Through high-resolution ultrasonography, magnetic resonance imaging with surface coil, and dermoscopy, we explore how these techniques enhance the differentiation of alopecia types, monitor disease progression, and evaluate the efficacy of therapeutic

B. B. Gonçalves
Hair Diseases Department, Instituto de Dermatologia Professor Rubem David Azulay – Santa Casa de Misericórdia do Rio de Janeiro, Rio de Janeiro, Brazil

M. C. Z. Páez
Zafra Dermatology Private Clinic, Rio de Janeiro, Brazil

BCM Dermatologia Especializada, Private Practice, Rio de Janeiro, Brazil

A. L. Boff
Santa Casa Hospital, Porto Alegre, RS, Brazil

Dermathopathologist Private Practice, Clinica Dermapat, Porto Alegre, RS, Porto Alegre, RS, Brazil

A. da Silva Cartell
Adjunct Professor at Faculdade de Medicina da Universidade Federal do Rio Grande do Sul, Rio de Janeiro, Brazil

Dermatologist and Dermatopathologist in Private Practice, Rio de Janeiro, Brazil

C. Á. de Almeida
Faculty of Medicine of Valença—UniFaa, Valença, Brazil

Federal University of Rio de Janeiro—UFRJ, Rio de Janeiro, Brazil

D. B. Porciuncula
Pathologist in Private Practice – Diagnósticos da América – DASA, Rio de Janeiro, Brazil

© The Author(s), under exclusive license to Springer Nature Switzerland AG 2025

C. Canella Moraes do Carmo (ed.), *Atlas of Diagnostic Imaging in Dermatology*,
https://doi.org/10.1007/978-3-031-77987-9_7

interventions. As we navigate through these imaging techniques, we will uncover their potential to bridge gaps in clinical practice and contribute to more personalized and effective management strategies for patients suffering from scalp inflammation.

7.1 Cicatricial Alopecias

7.1.1 Lupus Erythematosus

7.1.1.1 Definition [1]

- Several patterns of hair loss can occur in lupus erythematosus (LE). Alopecias occurring with LE may be non-scarring or scarring, and they may be considered LE-specific or non-LE-specific.
- Alopecias are considered LE-specific when they exhibit LE-specific features on histology, and include discoid LE (DLE), diffuse or patchy hair loss in acute LE (ALE), subacute cutaneous LE (SCLE), and rarely tumid LE.
- Alopecia is also common in chronic cutaneous lupus erythematosus (CLE), especially in discoid lupus erythematosus, which may be scarring and permanent. Scalp involvement occurs in 60–80% of patients with DLE.
- Lupus Panniculitis or Profundus (LP) is a rare subtype of CLE, associated with non-scarring and scarring alopecia. It has been reported to cause alopecia along Blaschko's lines (Linear and annular lupus panniculitis of the scalp).
- Tumid Lupus Erythematosus (TLE) is a subtype of CLE, with non-scarring patchy hair loss.

X. Wortsman
Faculty of Medicine, Department of Dermatology, Universidad de Chile, Santiago, Chile

Department of Dermatology, School of Medicine, Pontificia Universidad Catolica de Chile, Santiago, Chile

Department of Dermatology and Cutaneous Surgery, Miller School of Medicine, University of Miami, Miami, FL, USA

Institute for Diagnostic Imaging and Research of the Skin and Soft Tissues, Santiago, Chile

C. Canella Moraes do Carmo (✉)
Fluminense Federal University—UFF, Rio de Janeiro, Brazil

Federal University of Rio de Janeiro—UFRJ, Rio de Janeiro, Brazil

Diagnóstico das Américas—DASA—RJ, Rio de Janeiro, Brazil

Biodesign Laboratory, DASA-PUC, Rio de Janeiro, Brazil

B. Duque-Estrada
BCM Dermatologia Especializada, Private Practice, Rio de Janeiro, Brazil

Universidade Federal de São Paulo, São Paulo, Brazil

Hair Diseases Department, Instituto de Dermatologia Professor Rubem David Azulay – Santa Casa da Misericórdia do Rio de Janeiro, Rio de Janeiro, Brazil

- Alopecia in subacute cutaneous LE is less frequent and usually non-scarring.
- Hair loss has been noted in up to 85% of patients with systemic lupus erythematosus (SLE).The latest validated Systemic Lupus International Collaborating Clinics Classification Criteria (SLICCCC) includes non-scarring alopecia as a criterion. Therefore, recognising the aetiology of hair loss in the setting of LE is crucial in classifying a patient to have systemic disease. Non-scarring alopecia od SLE may present as diffuse, patchy, or "lupus-hair" pattern. "Lupus hair" in SLE is a poorly characterized entity and may be a form of telogen effluvium.
- Other non-scarring types of hair loss not specific of LE (in which histology fails to show LE-features), include telogen effluvium, alopecia areata, and anagen effluvium, which have a myriad of causes which include disease flares, drugs and stress in the setting of LE.
- Lupus classification and detailed descriptions of subtypes are covered in chapter 13. In this chapter, we will illustrate the most important features of lupus erythematosus in the scalp, such as discoid lupus, lupus panicullitis, and tumid lupus.

7.1.2 Discoid Lupus Erythematosus

7.1.2.1 Epidemiology [2]

- Discoid lupus erythematosus is a subtype of Chronic Lupus Erythematosus. While scalp discoid lupus erythematous is more frequently observed in women, both sexes have an equal tendency to develop scarring alopecia from this condition.
- The typical age of onset is between 20 and 40 years.
- Most prevalent among African-Americans.

7.1.2.2 Clinical Presentation (Fig. 7.1) [2]

- Though DLE lesions are non-scarring in early stages, they can progress towards permanent scarring and result in irreversible hair loss.
- Discoid lupus erythematosus is characterized by several distinct features:
  - Erythematous to violaceous scaly papules and plaques with follicular plugging, hypo- and hyperpigmentation, variable atrophy, and telangiectasia.

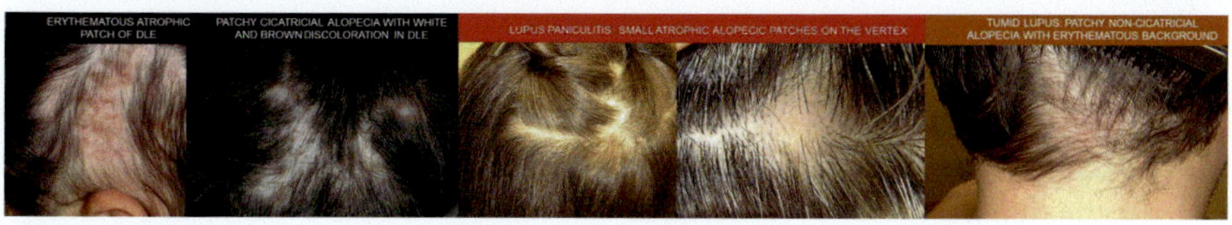

Fig. 7.1 Clinical pictures of discoid lupus erythematosus, lupus paniculitis, and tumid lupus

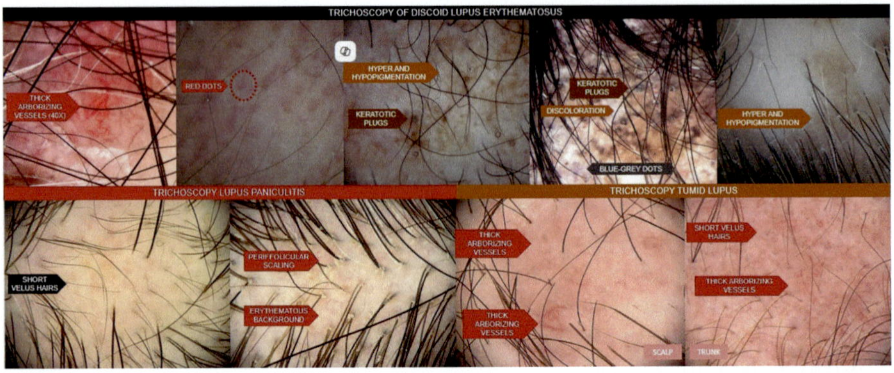

Fig. 7.2 Trichoscopy of discoid lupus erythematosus, lupus panniculitis, and tumid lupus (x40 and x20)

- Brown patches without atrophy or scarring have been reported. Specially in single lesions, it may be misdiagnosed as melanocytic lesions.
- Lesions may be pruritic, tender, or burning.

7.1.2.3 Trichoscopy (Fig. 7.2) [3, 4]

- Keratotic Plugs (follicular hyperkeratosis): the most characteristic sign of DLE
- Thick arborizing vessels: large, branching vessels in interfollicular areas
- Red dots or globules: present in early disease, represent dilated capillaries in active disease, surrounding the follicular ostium
- Perifollicular and interfollicular scaling: common in active lesions
- Loss of follicular openings and white structureless areas: represent cicatricial fibrotic zones lacking follicular units
- Pigmentary changes: brown discoloration as post-inflammatory hyperpigmention
- Blue-grey dots in a speckled pattern: observed in dark skin phototypes and represent pigment incontinence in the dermis. Blue-white veil-like features correspond to the combination of epidermal hyperkeratosis and prominent pigment incontinence.

7.1.2.4 Histopathology (Fig. 7.3) [1, 2]

- The morphologic alterations in non-cicatricial lupus alopecia resemble milder forms of those seen in the scarring phase of the disease, which are as follows:
  - Vacuolar interface damage of the dermoepidermal junction and follicular epithelium.
  - Epidermal atrophy and the presence of dermal melanophages indicate prior interface damage.

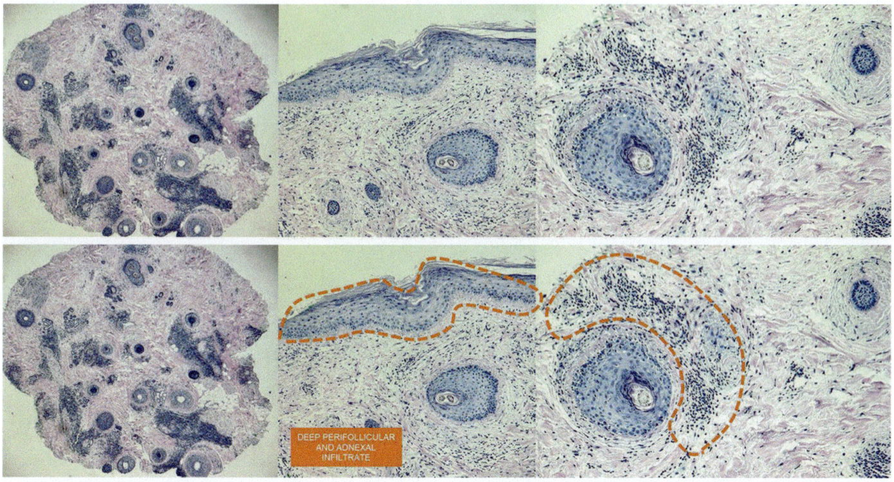

Fig. 7.3 Histological findings of discoid lupus erythematosus of the scalp (H&E x10)

- Lymphocytic infiltrate in superficial, deep, peribulbar, and perieccrine periphery; sometimes leading to miniaturized hairs and increase in telogen count.
- Interstitial mucin is present.
- Increased in telogen or catagen hair follicles, decreased follicular density, and preserved sebaceous glands.

- In DLE, additional findings include follicular infundibula plugged by keratin; thickened membrane involving the follicular epithelium; pigment incontinence and absent sebaceous glands. Furthermore, pathology in horizontal sections may show 2 patterns of inflammation in DLE: (1) Alopecia Areata-like, with deep perifollicular inflammation and (2) Lichen Planopilaris-like, with lamelar fibrosis and moderate perifollicular lymphocytic inflammation at the isthmus and infundibular level.

7.1.2.5 Ultrasonography (Figs. 7.4 and 7.5) [5, 6]

- Diffuse dermal hypoechogenicity correlates with the presence of a diffuse inflammatory infiltrate typical of all Lupus subtypes. Along with loss of dermo-hypodermal differentiation, which refers to the typical deep dermal inflammatory process, including hair follicles and sweat glands, those features differentiate DLE from Lichen Planopilaris, the typical perifollicular disease.
- Inflammatory changes and hyperemia (increased blood flow on power Doppler) are observed along the involved and surrounding subcutaneous adipose layer.
- Hair follicles are observed in the upper dermis, instead of hypodermis (compatible with telogen/catagen cycling).

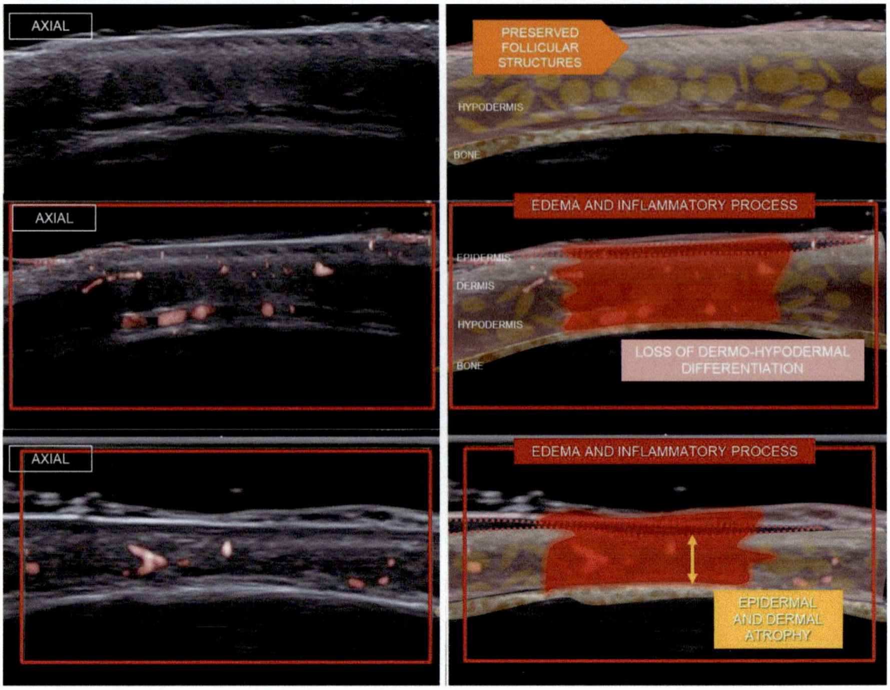

Fig. 7.4 Ultrasonographic findings of discoid lupus erythematosus of the scalp with a 24 MHz probe (Aplio i800, Canon Medical Systems)

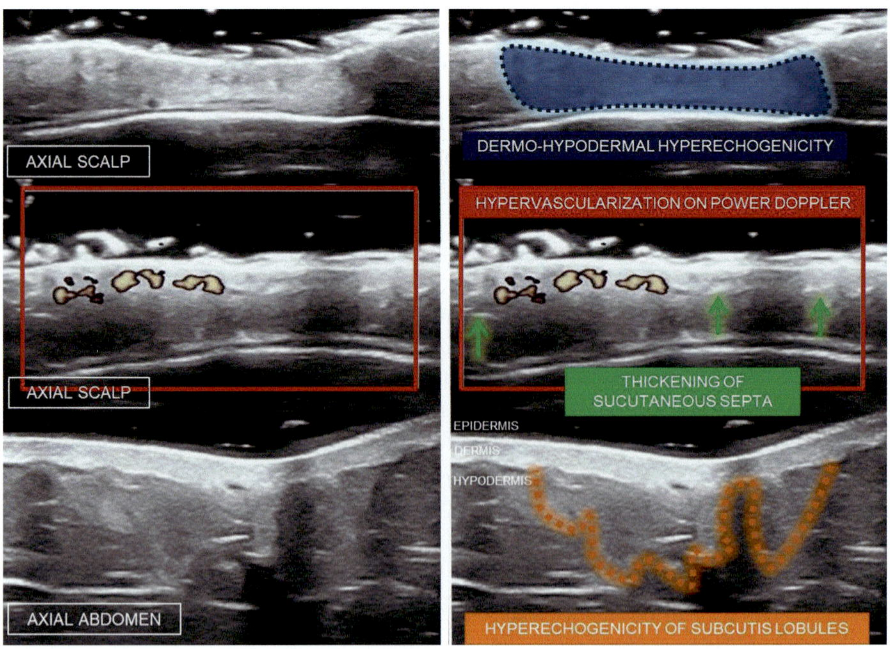

Fig. 7.5 Ultrasonographic findings of Lupus Panniculitis of the scalp with a 24 MHz probe (Aplio i800, Canon Medical Systems)

- Follicular widening is prominent in the upper part of the hair follicle in DLE, compatible with keratotic plugs observed clinically and under trichoscopy.
- The ultrasonographic differential diagnosis with other types of alopecia can be found in Table 7.1.

7.1.3 Lupus Erythematosus Panniculitis or Profundus (LEP)

7.1.3.1 Definition

- Rare variant within the spectrum of CLE which may produce both non-scarring and scarring alopecia.
- When the inflammation is confined to the lower layers of the skin and affects only the lower portion of the hair follicle (the follicular bulbs), the stem cells of the hair follicle are preserved; therefore, the hair loss is non-scarring.
- Although rare in LEP, if the inflammation affects the dermis surrounding the bulge of the follicle, permanent hair loss and irreversible alopecia may develop.

7.1.3.2 Clinical Presentation

- Clinically, LEP of the scalp may present as atrophic or depressed, tender, slightly erythematous alopecic patches, sometimes with overlying ulceration.
- It has been reported to cause alopecia along Blaschko's lines in East Asian men and that subtype is termed Linear and annular lupus panniculitis of the scalp (LALPS).
- It bears a better prognosis and is less frequently associated with SLE.
- The images are presented alongside those of lupus DLE and TEL in Fig. 7.1 for didactic and comparative purposes.

7.1.3.3 Trichoscopy

- Large yellow dots, black dots, short vellus hairs, thick arborizing vessels, and diffuse erythema of the interfollicular areas have been described.
- The images are presented alongside those of lupus DLE and TEL in Fig. 7.2 for didactic and comparative purposes.

7.1.3.4 Histopathology

- Histopathological evaluation shows predominantly lymphocytic infiltration of the subcutaneous lobules (lobular panniculitis) and deep dermis.
- Mucinosis, and hyalinization of the fat.

7.1.3.5 Ultrasonography

- Loss of dermo-hypodermal differentiation.
- Inflammatory changes of the dermis with increased blood flow on power Doppler.
- Thickening of septa and increased echogenicity of subcutaneous lobules.
- The images are presented alongside those of lupus DLE and TEL in Fig. 7.5 for didactic and comparative purposes.

7.1.4 Tumid Lupus Erythematosus (TEL)

7.1.4.1 Definition

- Tumid LE is a subtype of Chronic Cutaneous Lupus Erythematosus (CCLCE).
- Has been reported in rare cases to affect the scalp resulting in non- scarring, patchy hair loss.

7.1.4.2 Clinical presentation

- Clinically tumid LE is characterized by erythematous, indurated papules and plaques with no superficial changes.
- The images are presented alongside those of lupus DLE and LEP in Fig. 7.1 for didactic and comparative purposes.

7.1.4.3 Trichoscopy

- It provides limited information, revealing prominent arborizing blood vessels overlying an erythematous background, and decreased hair density, without scaling, ulceration, or atrophy.
- As specific clinical findings and trichoscopy features are often lacking, skin biopsy and histological examination are typically required to confirm the diagnosis.
- In cases of non-scarring alopecia, a biopsy is crucial for differentiating TLE from other forms of alopecia, like alopecia areata.
- The images are presented alongside those of lupus DLE and LEP in Fig. 7.2 for didactic and comparative purposes.

7.1.4.4 Histopathology

- Histopathological evaluation shows no interface dermatitis but significant mucin infiltration in the deep dermis.

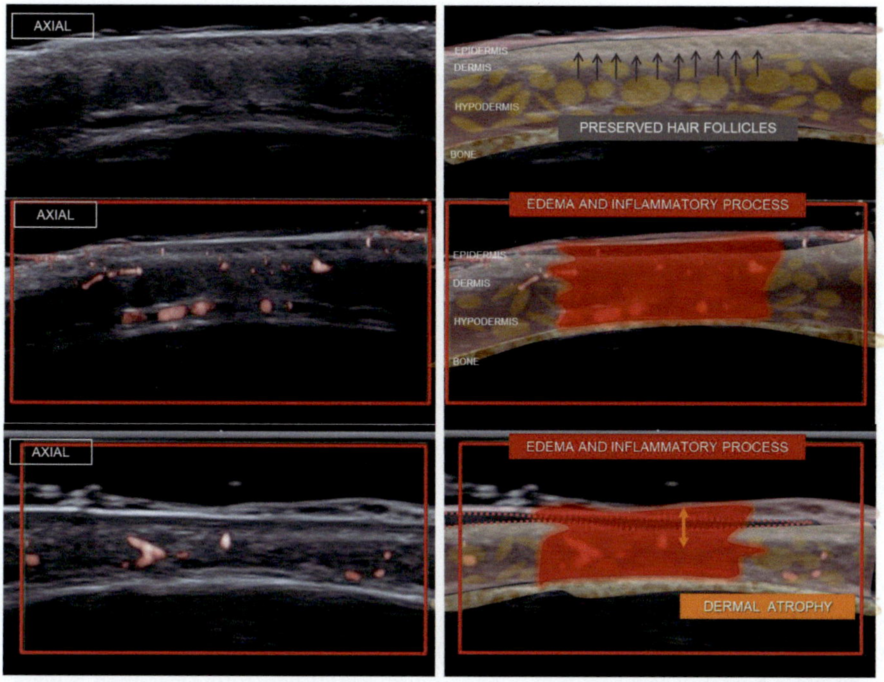

Fig. 7.6 Ultrasonographic findings of tumid lupus erythematosus of the scalp with a 24 MHz probe (Aplio i800, Canon Medical Systems)

7.1.4.5 Ultrasonography

- Loss of dermo-hypodermal differentiation.
- Inflammatory changes of the dermis with increased blood flow on power Doppler.
- Thickening of septa and increased echogenicity of subcutaneous lobules.
- The images are presented alongside those of lupus DLE and LEP in Fig. 7.6 for didactic and comparative purposes.

7.1.5 Classic Lichen Planopilaris

7.1.5.1 Definition [7]

- Primary lymphocytic cicatricial alopecia, which leads to permanent hair loss due to destruction of the hair follicle, particularly the stem cell–rich bulge area.
- Characterized by patchy or diffuse permanent hair loss.
- Typically affects the vertex or parietal scalp.
- A T-cell-mediated autoimmune attack to follicular antigens leads to inflammation and cicatricial alopecia.

7.1.5.2 Epidemiology [7]

- Rare condition with a relapsing and slowly progressive course.
- Increased prevalence of thyroid disorders, especially hypothyroidism.
- A higher occurrence of seborrheic dermatitis is observed in affected patients.
- Co-occurrence with lichen planus of the skin, nails, or mucous membranes ranges from 8.75% to 30%.

  Often idiopathic, but may be associated with:

- Autoimmune diseases.
- Certain medications (e.g., immune checkpoint inhibitors).
- Genetic predisposition.

7.1.5.3 Clinical Presentation (Fig. 7.7) [7]

- Presents as single or multiple scarring alopecic patches on the vertex and parietal scalp.
- Symptoms include intense pruritus, burning, and scalp tenderness.
- Symptoms often worsened by sweating, friction, stress, or UV light exposure.
- Active disease indicated by perifollicular erythema, perifollicular scaling and a positive hair pull test yielding anagen hairs. Small hair tufts (less than 5 hairs) may be observed in cicatricial areas.
- Alopecic patches become whitish and atrophic with a complete loss of follicular orifices.

7.1.5.4 Trichoscopy (Fig. 7.8) [3, 4]

- Reveals perifollicular pink-red erythema.
- Presence of perifollicular scaling and peripilar casts.

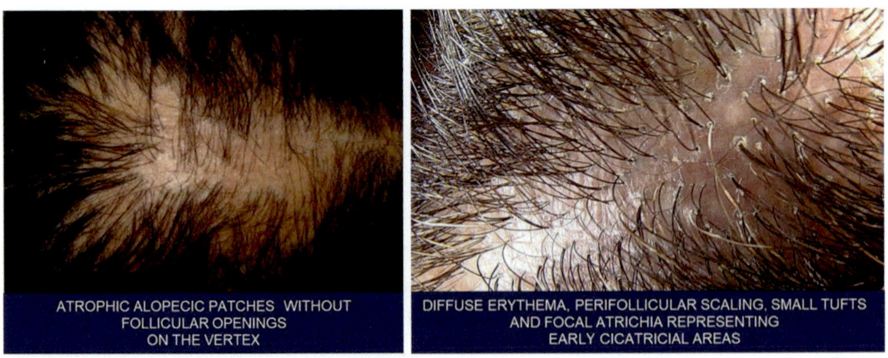

Fig. 7.7 Clinical picture of a patient presenting classic lichen planopilaris on the scalp

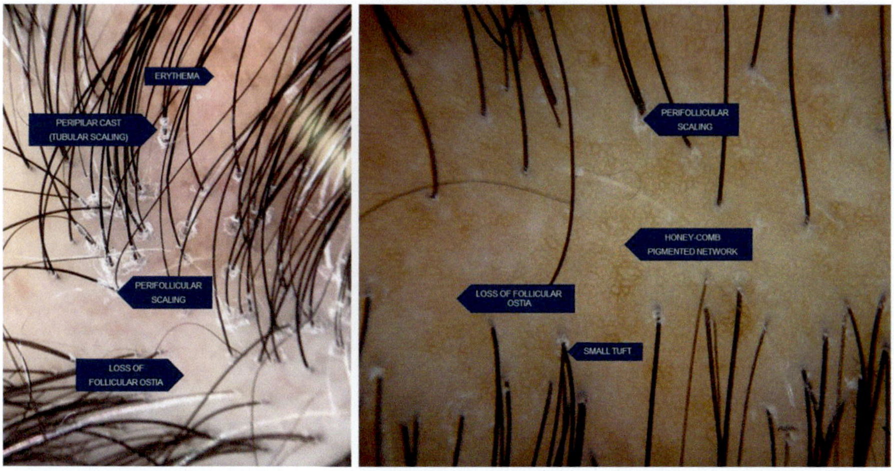

Fig. 7.8 Trichoscopy of classic lichen planopilaris (x40)

- Interfollicular irregular white dots in a irregular distribution
- Perifollicular blue-gray dots in a targeted pattern.
- Small tufts (less than 5 hairs emerging together from the same follicular ostia) represent early concentric lammelar fibrosis around hair follicles. The absence of follicular orifices represent late stage cicatricial areas.

7.1.5.5 Histopathology (Fig. 7.9) [7]

- Hyperkeratosis, acanthosis, hypergranulosis, interface lichenoid pattern, with vacuolar damage and apoptotic cells may be observed in the follicular epitthelium, typically affecting the infundibular and isthmic regions.
- The inflamed follicles then develop concentric lamellar fibrosis, with the classic backing-away of inflammatory cells, artifactual cleft between epithelium and stroma.
- Despite its relation to lichen planus, the classic epidermal involvement is seen in less than a third of cases, with atrophy, pigment incontinence and saw-tooth irregularity being much more frequent.
- Disease progression follows the cicatricial pathway, with consumption of pilosebaceous units and copious fibrosis.

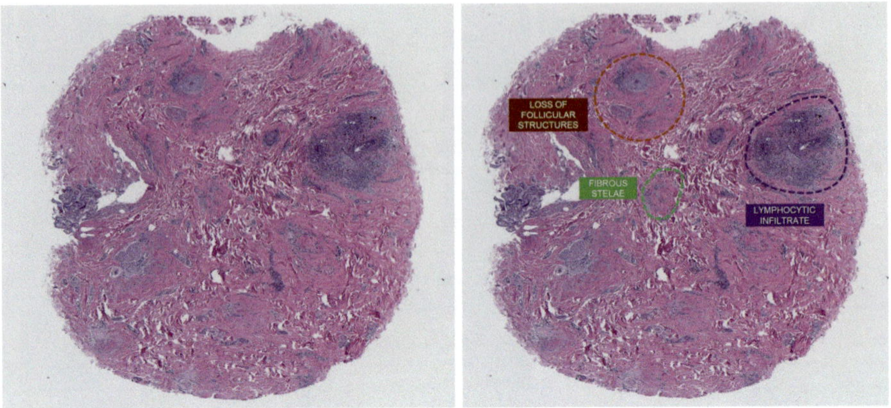

Fig. 7.9 Histological findings of classic lichen planopilaris of the scalp

7.1.5.6 Ultrasonography (Figs. 7.10, 7.11 and 7.12) [8]

Ultrasonographic findings in LPP with a 20–24 MHz probe:

- A hypoechogenic fusiform band is typically seen in the dermis due to the active inflammatory process (?).
- The thickness of this hypoechogenic zone often corresponds to the areas of greatest perifollicular inflammatory infiltrate.
- Hypoechoic perifollicular widening of hair follicles anchored normally in the dermo-hypodermal junction, although with an irregular distribution is also characteristic of LPP. Indeed, it's an important finding to differentiate from DLE, in which hair follicles are anchored in the upper dermis (telogen/catagen phases).
- Increased vascularization around follicular structures on Doppler corresponds to the inflammatory process.
- A varied degree of abscence of follicles is observed in cicatricial areas.

Ultrasonographic findings in LPP with a 70 MHz probe [9]:

- Active areas
  - Perifollicular hypoechogenicity in mid-dermis that might reflect ongoing inflammation around the bulge region.
  - Disrupted morphology of the upper portions of the hair follicles, suggesting significant edema, or destruction of the upper follicles.

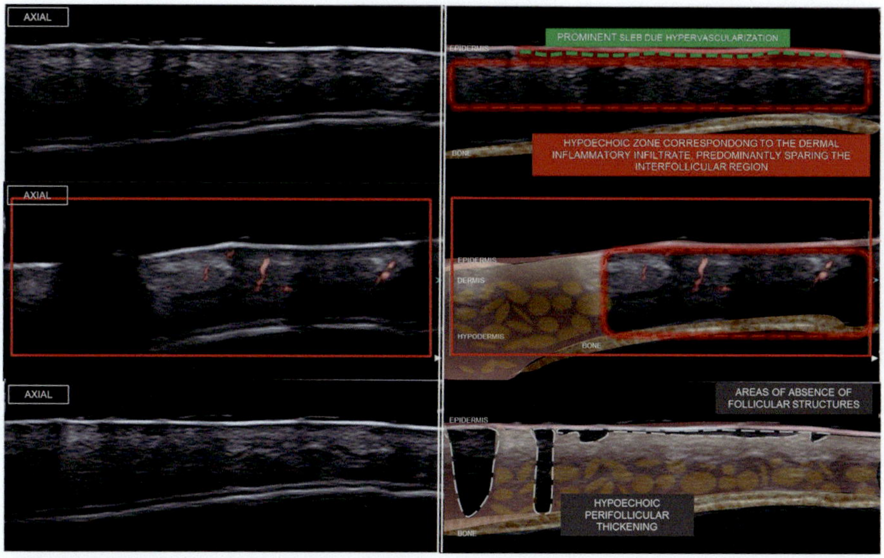

Fig. 7.10 Ultrasonographic findings of classic lichen planopilaris of the scalp with a 24 MHz probe (Aplio i800, Canon Medical Systems)

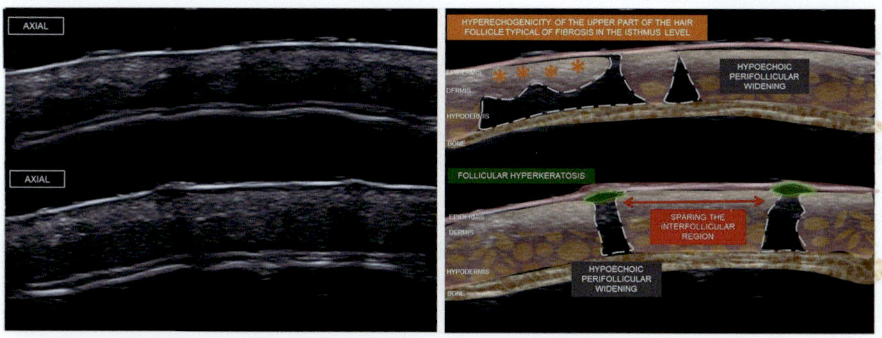

Fig. 7.11 Ultrasonographic findings of classic lichen planopilaris of the scalp with a 24 MHz probe (Aplio i800, Canon Medical Systems)

- Cicatricial areas
  - Homogeneous dermis without follicular structures.

The ultrasonographic differential diagnosis with other types of alopecia can be found in Table 7.1.

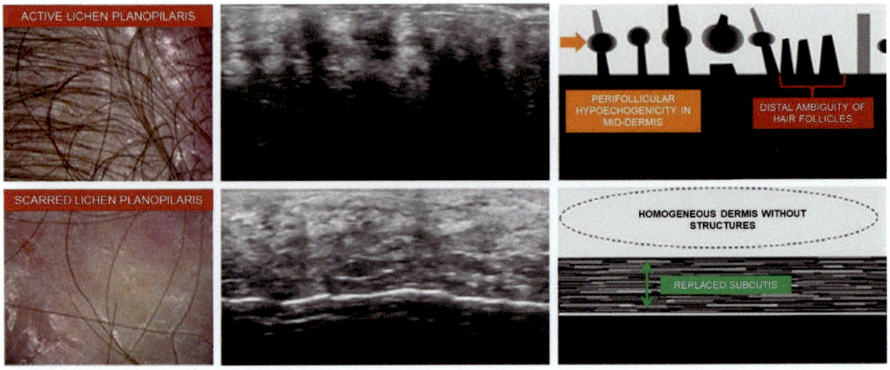

Fig. 7.12 Ultrasonographic findings of lichen planopilaris with a 70 MHz probe (Reprinted from Journal of Dermatological Science, 102 (2021), Kinoshita-Ise M, Ohyama M, Ramjist JM, Foster FS, Yang VXD, Sachdeva M, Sade S, Shear NH. Ultra high-frequency ultrasound with seventy-MHz transducer in hair disorders: Development of a novel noninvasive diagnostic methodology, 167–174, Copyright (2025), with permission from Elsevier)

7.1.6 Frontal Fibrosing Alopecia (FFA)

7.1.6.1 Definition [10]

- Primary cicatricial alopecia.
- Characterized by progressive recession of the frontotemporal hairline.

7.1.6.2 Epidemiology [10, 11]

- Significant increase in incidence in recent years.
- Predominantly seen in postmenopausal women.
- Also reported in men and premenopausal women.

7.1.6.3 Clinical Presentation (Fig. 7.13) [10]

- Progressive, recession of the frontal hairline.
- Alopecia of the eyebrows is reported in up to 70–90% of patients with frontal fibrosing alopecia (FFA). It is often bilateral but may be patchy and reversible in early stages, and can precede frontal hairline recession by up to 10 years.
- Body hair loss, facial papules, depression of the frontal veins, lichen planus pigmentosus, or preauricular wrinkles are also observed.

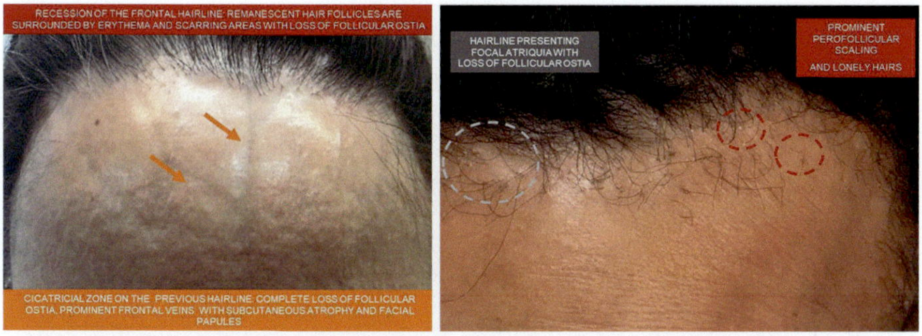

Fig. 7.13 Clinical picture of a patient frontal fibrosing alopecia

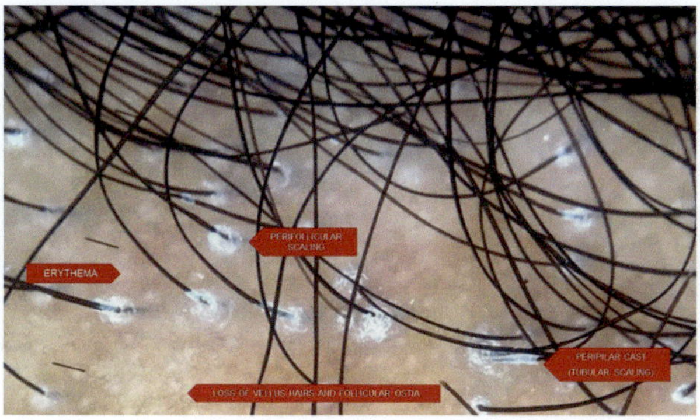

Fig. 7.14 Trichoscopy of a patient presenting frontal fibrosing alopecia (x60)

7.1.6.4 Trichoscopy (Fig. 7.14) [12] of the Frontal Hairline

- Reduction or loss of vellus hairs and loss of follicular openings.
- Perifollicular erythema.
- Perifollicular scaling and peripilar casts.
- Pili torti, ingrown hairs and broken hairs may be observed in areas with active disease.

7.1.6.5 Histopathology (Fig. 7.15) [10]

- Lymphocytic infiltrate primarily involves the infundibular and isthmic portions of the hair follicle, typically less dense than in lichen planopilaris.
- There is vacuolar degeneration of the follicular epithelium, with prominent apoptotic keratinocytes.
- Concentric lamellar fibrosis is observed, often affecting intermediate and miniaturized follicles as well.
- As disease progresses, there is loss of pilosebaceous units, formation of fibrous stellae, and dermal fibrosis, reflecting permanent scarring.

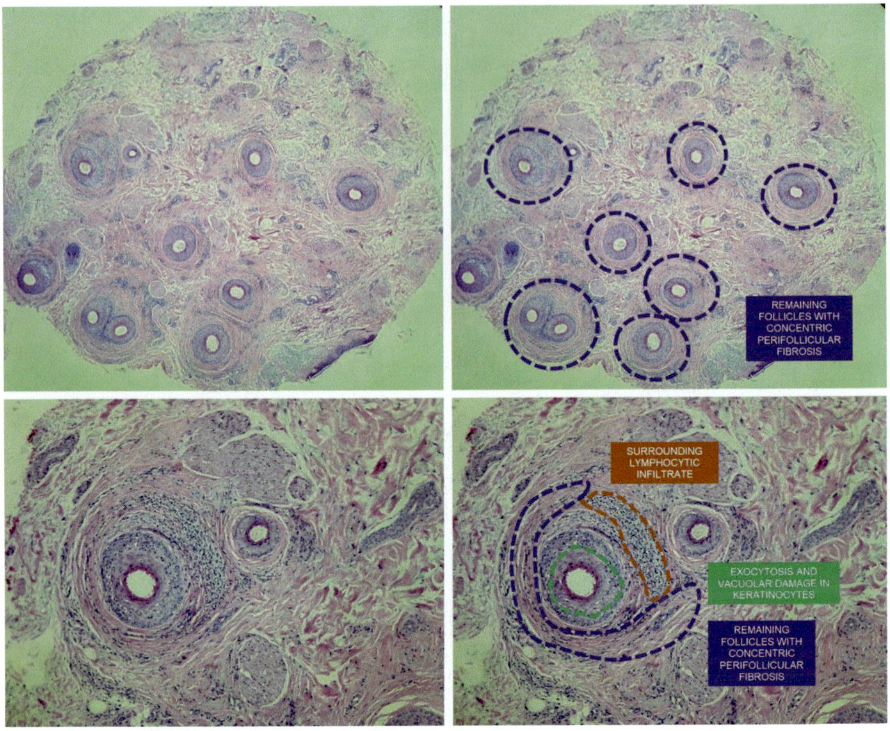

Fig. 7.15 Histological findings of frontal fibrosing alopecia (H&E x4 and x10)

7.1.6.6 Ultrasonography (Figs. 7.16 and 7.17) [13]

Ultrasonographic findings in FFA with a 20–24 MHz probe:

- Irregular thickening of the hair follicles: Hypoechoic perifollicular widening, or decrease in hair follicle diameter, as well as elongated hyperechoic structures extending vertically from dermis to hypodermis.
- Dermal and subcutaneous inflammation typically appears as hypoechogenicity in the dermis and hyperechogenicity in the subcutaneous tissue.
- Increased vascular diameter and higher blood flow showed by Power Doppler, especially in the hairline region.
- In cicatricial areas, absence of follicles is characteristic.
- Ultrasound could play a relevant role in the early evaluation of subclinical signs such as perifollicular inflammation and skin thickness, even in areas apparently clinically unaffected.

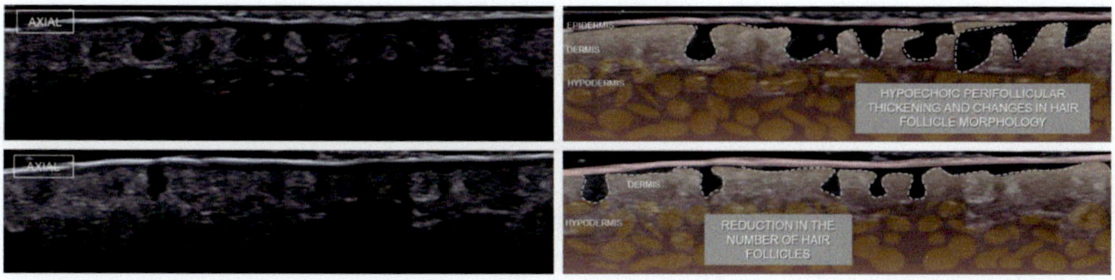

Fig. 7.16 Ultrasonographic findings of frontal fibrosing alopecia with a 24 MHz probe (Aplio i800, Canon Medical Systems)

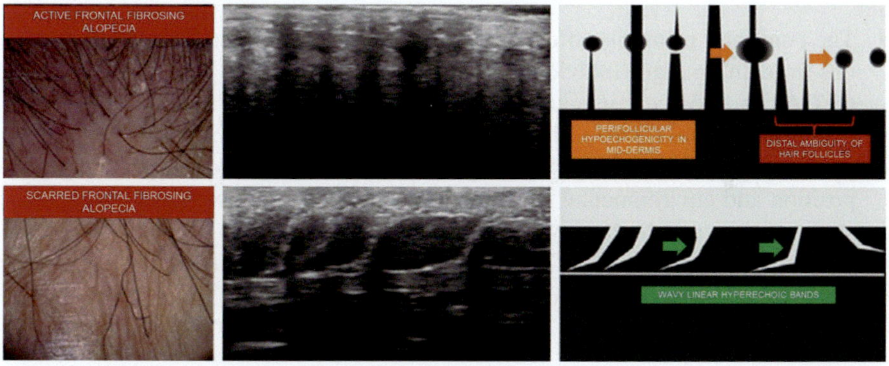

Fig. 7.17 Ultrasonographic findings of frontal fibrosing alopecia with a 70 MHz probe (Reprinted from Journal of Dermatological Science, 102 (2021), Kinoshita-Ise M, Ohyama M, Ramjist JM, Foster FS, Yang VXD, Sachdeva M, Sade S, Shear NH. Ultra high-frequency ultrasound with seventy-MHz transducer in hair disorders: Development of a novel noninvasive diagnostic methodology, 167–174, Copyright (2025), with permission from Elsevier)

Ultrasonographic findings in FFA with a 70 MHz probe [9]:

- Active areas
  - Perifollicular hypoechogenicity in mid-dermis
  - Disrupted morphology of the upper portions of the hair follicles in the majority of cases
- Cicatricial lesions
  - Homogeneous dermis without distinguishable structures
  - Wavy linear hyperechoic bands (ondulating, bright echogenic lines) observed in the subcutaneous fat layer

The ultrasonographic differential diagnosis with other types of alopecia can be found in Table 7.1.

7.1.7 Central Centrifugal Cicatricial Alopecia (CCCA)

7.1.7.1 Definition [14, 15]

- Central centrifugal cicatricial alopecia (CCCA).
- Is characterized by progressive hair loss starting at the crown or vertex of the scalp and extending outward in a centrifugal pattern. The condition leads to permanent hair loss due to the destruction of hair follicles and subsequent scarring.

7.1.7.2 Epidemiology [14]

- The condition primarily affects middle-aged and older women but can also be observed in younger individuals. While women are more frequently affected, CCCA can also occur in men.
- The pathophysiology of CCCA is not yet fully understood; however, emerging evidence suggests a role for fibroproliferative processes driven by genetic predisposition and environmental triggers, such as chemical relaxers, heat-based hair straightening, and certain styling practices.
- A hereditary association in CCCA suggested an autosomal dominant inheritance of CCCA in some families.

7.1.7.3 Clinical Presentation (Fig. 7.18) [15]

- CCCA typically begins with a patchy of thinning hair loss at the vertex of the scalp. Over time, this area expands in a centrifugal manner, leading to a larger area of baldness.
- Patients may experience itching, tenderness, or a burning sensation in the affected area, although some may be asymptomatic.

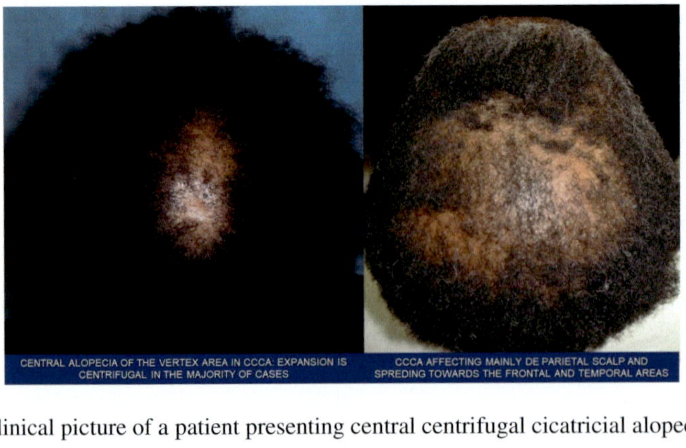

Fig. 7.18 Clinical picture of a patient presenting central centrifugal cicatricial alopecia

- As the condition progresses, scarring occurs, resulting in permanent. The scalp in the affected area may appear smooth, shiny, and devoid of hair follicles.
- Early stages of CCCA may show signs of inflammation, including erythema (redness) and perifollicular scaling. As the disease progresses, these signs may diminish, leaving behind areas of scarring alopecia.

7.1.7.4 Trichoscopy (Fig. 7.19) [16]

- Loss of follicular openings in cicatricial areas.
- White dots represent fibrotic (scarred) hair follicles and are a hallmark of CCCA.
- Perifollicular erythema and scaling.
- In less advanced cases, there may be a mixture of thin, miniaturized, and broken hair shafts.

7.1.7.5 Histopathology [14]

- The predisposing feature of CCCA is premature desquamation of the inner root sheath of most follicles, both affected and seemingly normal ones, leaving the hair shaft bare and susceptible to inflammation:
  - Isthmic lymphocytic inflammation, interface follicular damage, eccentric epithelial atrophy, and lamellar fibrosis.
  - Progressive disease leads to follicular fusion, dropout, granulomatous reaction to stromal shafts, consumption of pilosebaceous units, and dermal fibrosis.

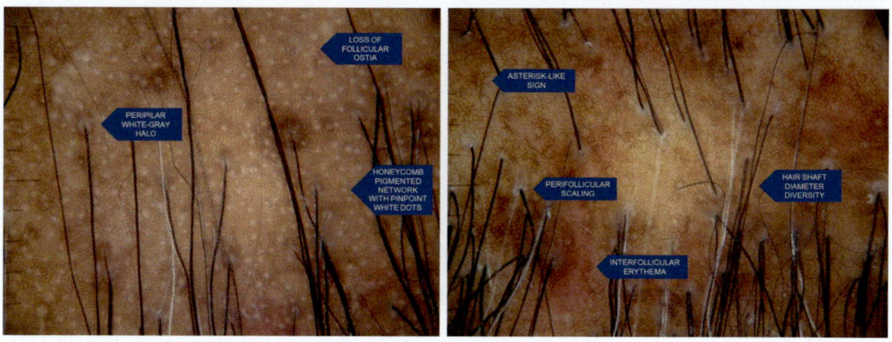

Fig. 7.19 Trichoscopy of a patient presenting central centrifugal cicatricial alopecia (x40)

7.1.7.6 Ultrasonography (Figs. 7.20 and 7.21)

Ultrasonographic findings in CCCA with a 20–24 MHz probe:

- Dermis often appears thickened, reflecting fibrosis and scarring. In the affected areas, there is a marked reduction in the number of visible hair follicles.
- Echogenicity patterns vary depending on disease stage:
  - Early phase: Heterogeneous echogenicity of dermis due to active inflammation.
  - Late stage: Uniform hyperechogenicity (hyperechoic bands or foci within the dermis) represents fibrotic replacement of normal follicular structures.
- Subcutaneous fat layer may exhibit thinning or increased echogenicity, depending on the degree of associated inflammation and scarring.
- Power Doppler: Reduction in blood flow may be noted in affected areas, reflecting loss of vascular structures secondary to fibrosis.

Ultrasonographic findings in CCCA with a 70 MHz probe:

- Uniform hypoechoic dermis lacking distinguishable structures [9]

The ultrasonographic differential diagnosis with other types of alopecia can be found in Table 7.1.

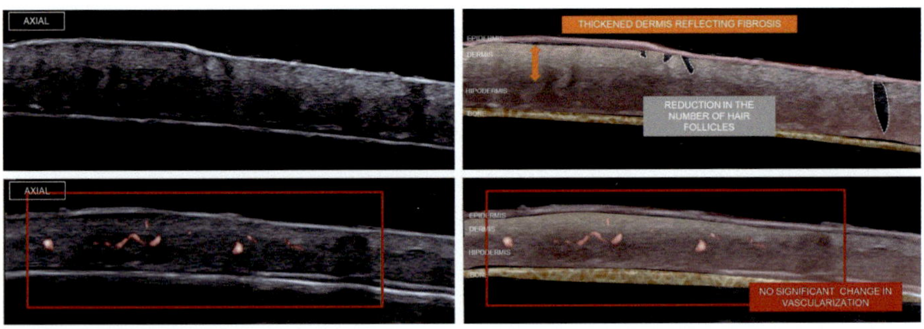

Fig. 7.20 Ultrasonographic findings of central centrifugal cicatricial alopecia with a 24 MHz probe (Aplio i800, Canon Medical Systems)

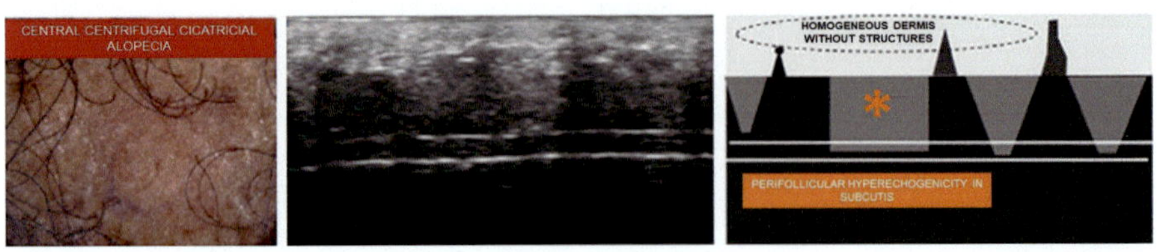

Fig. 7.21 Ultrasonographic findings of central centrifugal cicatricial alopecia with a 70 MHz probe (Reprinted from Journal of Dermatological Science, 102 (2021), Kinoshita-Ise M, Ohyama M, Ramjist JM, Foster FS, Yang VXD, Sachdeva M, Sade S, Shear NH. Ultra high-frequency ultrasound with seventy-MHz transducer in hair disorders: Development of a novel noninvasive diagnostic methodology, 167–174, Copyright (2025), with permission from Elsevier)

7.1.8 Mucinous Alopecia

7.1.8.1 Definition [17]

- Mucinous alopecia is a rare condition characterized by hair loss associated with mucin (glycosaminoglycan) deposition within the hair follicle epithelium and sebaceous glands.
- The condition involves the accumulation of mucin in the outer root sheath and sebaceous glands, which leads to follicular disruption, inflammation, and non-scarring or scarring alopecia, depending on the stage.

7.1.8.2 Epidemiology [17]

- Mucinous alopecia is relatively uncommon and can occur in both adults and children.
- It can occur at any age but is more frequently observed in middle-aged and older adults. There is no significant gender predilection, though some reports suggest a slight male predominance.
- Secondary mucinous alopecia is often linked with underlying systemic conditions, such as lupus erythematosus, and more frequently, with cutaneous T-cell Lymphoma.

7.1.8.3 Clinical Presentation (Fig. 7.22) [17]

- The condition typically presents with well-circumscribed, erythematous, or flesh-colored plaques or patches of hair loss. The affected areas due to the accumulation of mucin.
- Hair loss within the lesions can be partial or complete, depending on the extent of follicular damage.
- The lesions are usually asymptomatic, though some patients may report mild itching or tenderness in the affected areas.
- The condition can be chronic and progressive, especially when associated with underlying malignancies. Spontaneous resolution can occur, particularly in primary cases.

7.1.8.4 Trichoscopy (Fig. 7.23) [3, 17]

- Keratotic plugs.
- Follicular openings, representing the mucinous deposits within the follicles.
- In severe cases.

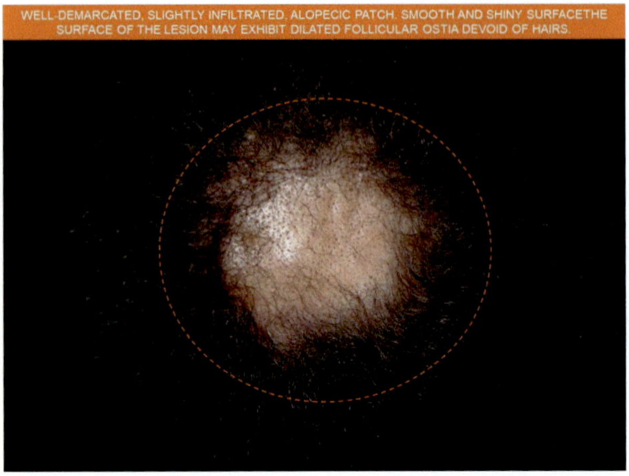

Fig. 7.22 Clinical picture of a patient presenting mucinous alopecia

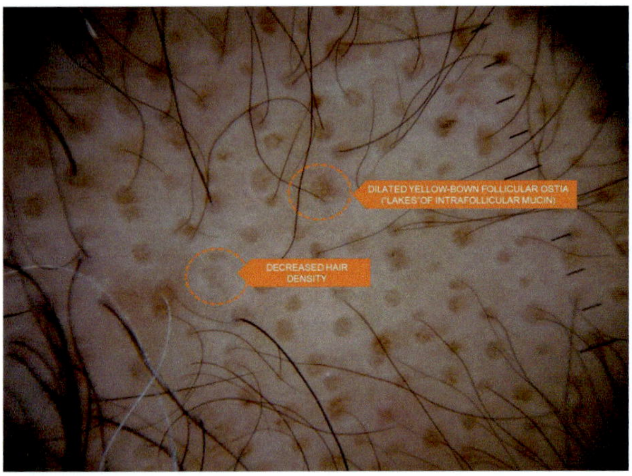

Fig. 7.23 Trichoscopy of a patient presenting mucinous alopecia (x20)

7.1.8.5 Histopathology (Fig. 7.24) [18]

- The infundibulum and isthmus regions show mucin infiltrating and splaying the epithelial follicular cells apart, with pool formation and variable mixed inflammatory cells surrounding the area and in a perivascular pattern. Alcian blue stain aids in this identification.
- Lymphocytes exocytosis is a common occurrence, with epidermotropism, atypia, and papilar fibrosis present in cases related to T-cell lymphomas.

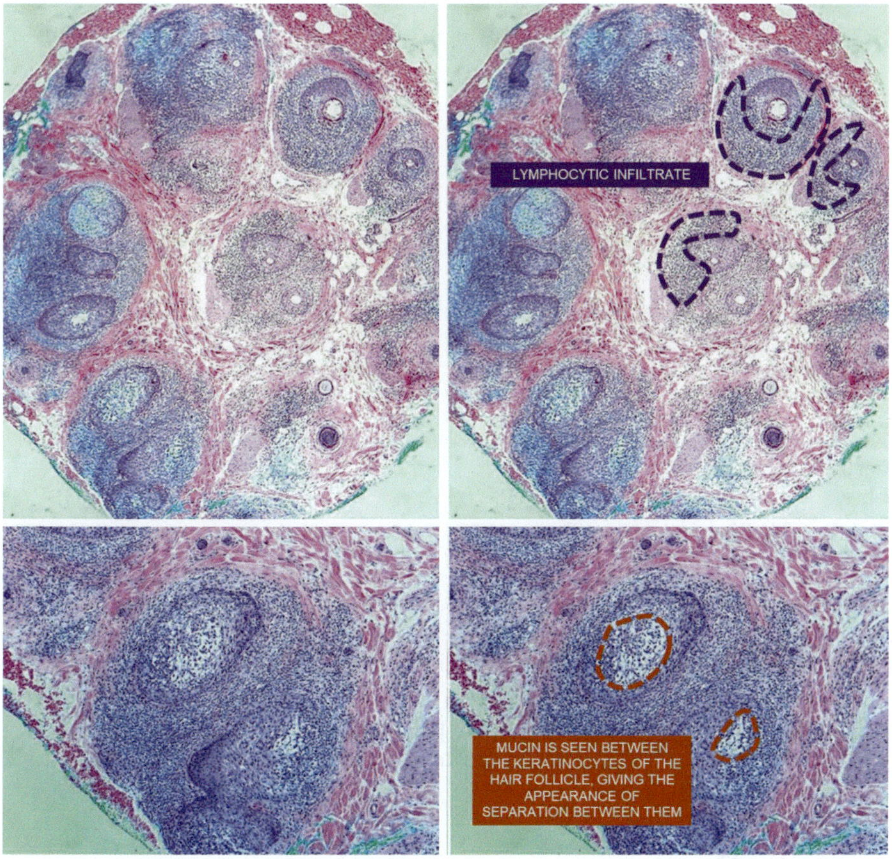

Fig. 7.24 Histological findings of mucinous alopecia (H&E x10)

7.1.8.6 Ultrasonography (Fig. 7.25)

- The presence of mucin in the dermis and around hair follicles can appear as hypoechoic areas on ultrasonography. These areas correspond to the gelatinous mucin deposits that are characteristic of the condition.
- The affected areas of the scalp may show thickened dermis due to the accumulation of mucin and associated inflammation in the dermal layer.
- In cases where hair follicles are severely affected, there may be a noticeable reduction in the visibility of hair follicles on ultrasonography. This correlates with the clinical presentation of alopecia.
- Unlike some other types of inflammatory alopecia, mucinous alopecia may not show significant changes in blood flow or vascularity on power Doppler ultrasonography, as the condition primarily affects the follicles and sebaceous glands.
- The ultrasonographic differential diagnosis with other types of alopecia can be found in Table 7.1.

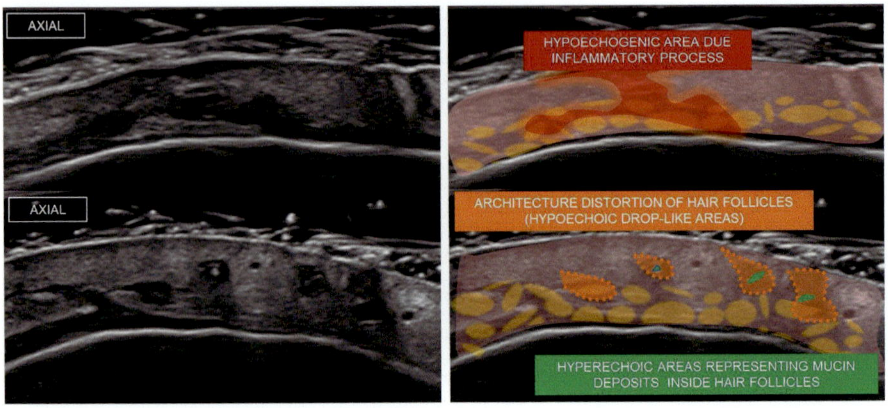

Fig. 7.25 Ultrasonographic findings of mucinous alopecia with a 24 MHz probe (Aplio i800, Canon Medical Systems)

7.1.9 Folliculitis Decalvans [19, 20]

7.1.9.1 Definition [20]

- Chronic inflammatory condition targeting hair follicles
- Leads to scarring alopecia
- Characterized by pustules, crusts, and patchy hair loss
- Results in permanent hair loss in affected areas which is diagnosed in up to 2.8% of patients with hair loss

7.1.9.2 Epidemiology [20]

- Relatively rare condition, which is diagnosed in up to 2.8% of patients with hair loss.
- Affects both men and women, predominantly young and middle-aged adults
- Slight male predominance
- More frequent in African Americans compared to Caucasians
- Accounts for approximately 11% of primary cicatricial alopecia cases

7.1.9.3 Clinical Presentation (Fig. 7.26)

- Primarily involves the vertex and occipital areas of the scalp.
- Initial presentation includes erythematous follicular papules.
- Development of scarred areas and follicular pustules is characteristic.
- Livid to bright erythema and yellow-gray scales around follicles.
- Follicular hyperkeratosis, erosions, and hemorrhagic crusts may be present.

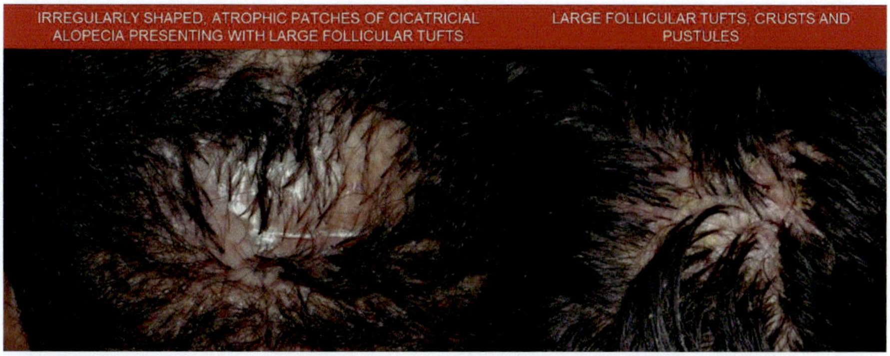

Fig. 7.26 Clinical picture of a patient presenting folliculitis decalvans of the scalp

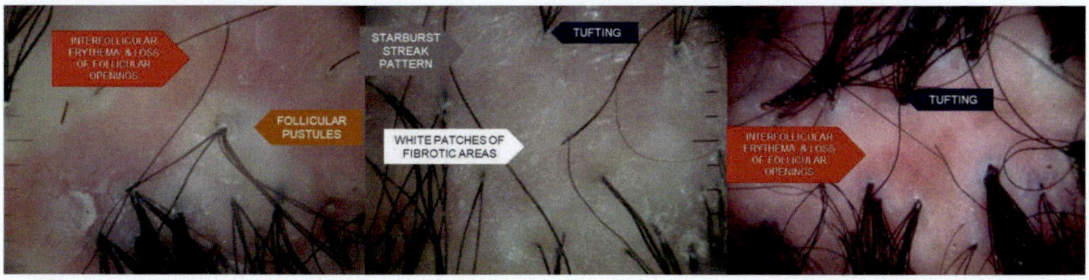

Fig. 7.27 Trichoscopy of a patient presenting folliculitis decalvans of the scalp (x40)

- Symptoms include pain, itching, burning, and occasional spontaneous bleeding.
- Chronic disease progression leads to irregularly shaped, atrophic patches of cicatricial alopecia.
- Tufted folliculitis, characterized by multiple hairs emerging from a single follicular ostia, is common.

7.1.9.4 Trichoscopy (Fig. 7.27) [21]

- Tufted hairs: more than 5 hair shafts emerging from a single dilated follicular ostia. It's the most characteristic sign of FD and a consequence of intense perifollicular fibrosis and fusion of follicular structures.
- Reveals perifollicular pustules and crusting.
- Noticeable lack of follicular openings in scarred areas.
- Other signs include perifollicular scaling and erythema.
- Dermoscopic examination often shows multiple hairs (5–20) emerging from a single dilated follicular orifice.

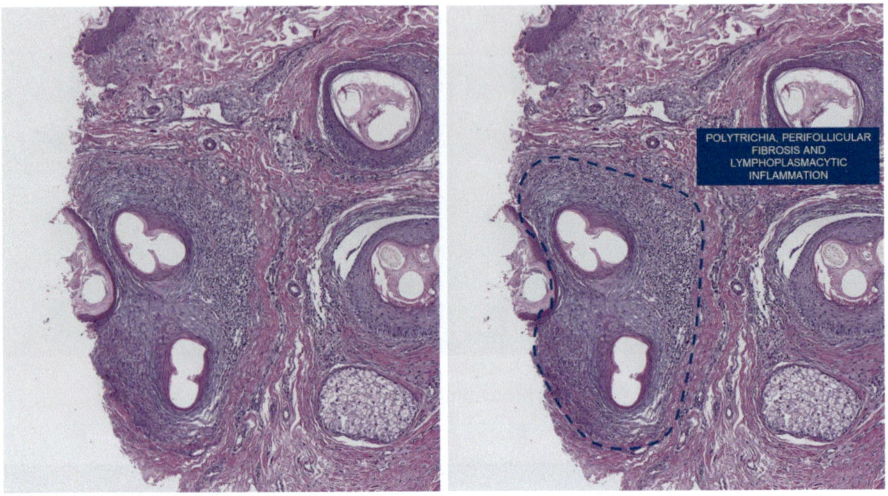

Fig. 7.28 Histological findings of folliculitis decalvans of the scalp (H&E x10)

7.1.9.5 Histopathology (Fig. 7.28) [22]

- Perifollicular lymphoplasmacytic, neutrophilic and pustular inflammation, most notable in the isthmus and lower infundibulum with lamellar fibrosis, loss of sebaceous glands.
- Follicular destruction with asymmetrical atrophy of the epithelium, "naked" dermal shafts, engulfed by a granulomatous inflammation, perifollicular fibrosis may lead to depressed and fused follicular infundibula, leading to polytrichia (tufting of more than 5 hairs).
- Stable and late-stage disease may have a predominantly lymphoplasmacytic profile to the infiltrate.

7.1.9.6 Ultrasonography (Figs. 7.29 and 7.30) [23]

Ultrasonographic findings in folliculitis decalvans with a 24 MHz probe:

- Vertical hypoechoic dilated and distorted follicular structures represent fused hair follicles.
- Dilated follicular structures may present with internal debris.
- Hypoechoic or anechoic fluid collections in the upper dermis represent "pus lakes."
- Hyperechoic fibrotic bands and architectural distortion in the dermis are observed in cicatricial areas.
- Power Doppler: Increased vascularity in inflammatory areas.

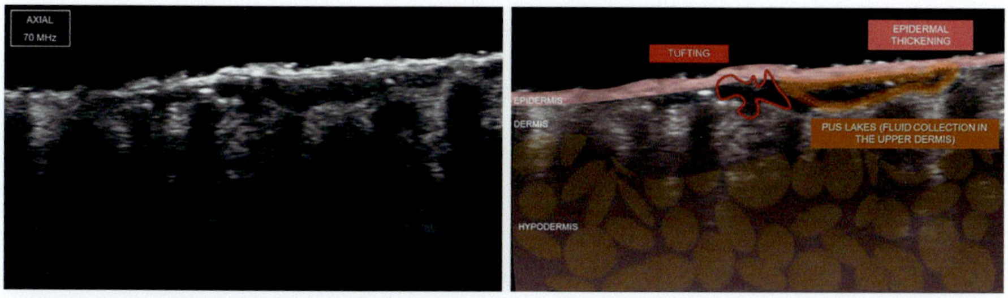

Fig. 7.29 Ultrasonographic findings of folliculitis decalvans with a 24 MHz probe (Aplio i800, Canon Medical Systems)

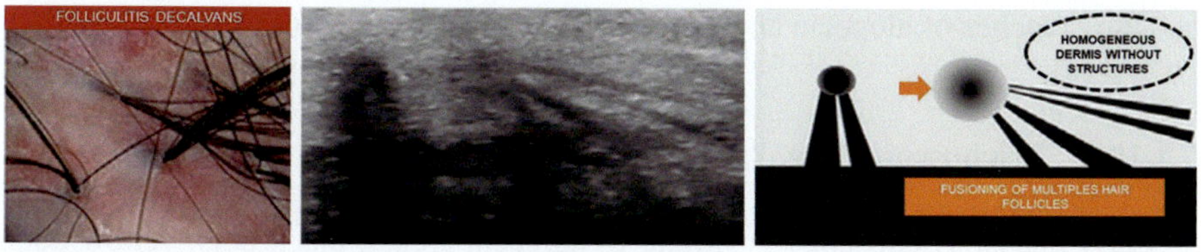

Fig. 7.30 Ultrasonographic findings of folliculitis decalvans with a 70 MHz probe (Reprinted from Journal of Dermatological Science, 102 (2021), Kinoshita-Ise M, Ohyama M, Ramjist JM, Foster FS, Yang VXD, Sachdeva M, Sade S, Shear NH. Ultra high-frequency ultrasound with seventy-MHz transducer in hair disorders: Development of a novel noninvasive diagnostic methodology, 167–174, Copyright (2025), with permission from Elsevier)

Ultrasonographic findings in folliculitis decalvans with a 70 MHz probe:

- The most characteristic finding is the fusion of adjacent hair follicles (tufted hairs), represented by coalescent hypoechoic linear structures in the dermis, resembling a comet shape [9]

The ultrasonographic differential diagnosis with other types of alopecia can be found in Table 7.1.

7.1.10 *Dissecting Cellulitis of the Scalp*

7.1.10.1 Definition [24]

- Dissecting cellulitis of the scalp (DCS), also known as perifolliculitis capitis abscedens et suffodiens, is a rare, chronic, progressive and relapsing inflammatory condition that primarily affects the scalp's hair follicles of young afro-descendent men.

7.1.10.2 Epidemiology [25]

- It is more frequent in young Afro-descendent men in the vertex and occipital area.
- The typical age of onset is between 20 and 40 years.

7.1.10.3 Clinical Presentation (Fig. 7.31) [26]

- Severe inflammation; presence of pustules, nodules, and abscesses with inter-communicating sinus tract in abscess phase.
- Fibrotic cicatricial phase: Presence of scarring and permanent alopecia, with shiny patches of alopecia and cutaneous clefts with hair tufts.

7.1.10.4 Trichoscopy (Fig. 7.32) [3, 4]

- Early phase: Trichoscopy is similar to alopecia areata: black dots, yellow dots, and broken hairs.

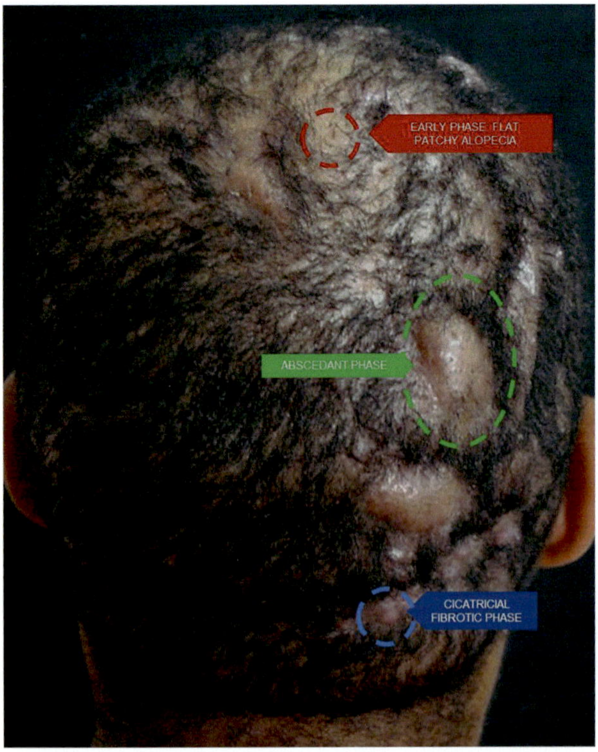

Fig. 7.31 Clinical picture of a patient presenting dissecting cellulitis of the scalp

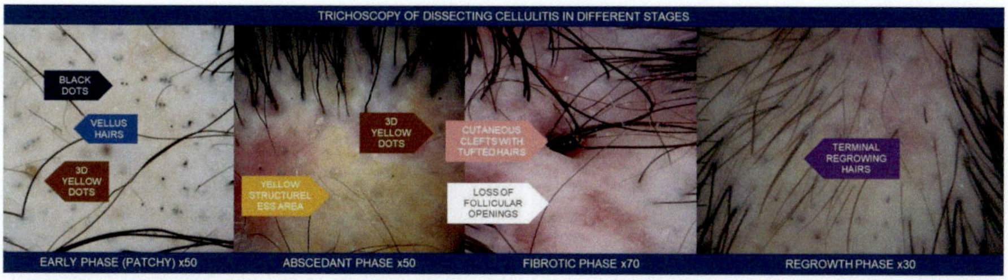

Fig. 7.32 TricDhigoistec oo pteyx toof adqiusisecting cellulitis of the scalp (x30, x50 and x70) (Coutesy of Dr Rodrigo Pirmez and Leonardo Spagnol-Abraham)

- Abscedant phase: Three-dimensional yellow dots with a "soap bubble"-like appearance; yellow structureless areas duelakes of exudate around hair follicles.
- Tissue fibrosis with lack of follicular openings and cutaneous clefts with emerging hair tufts.

7.1.10.5 Histopathology [25]

- Moderately dense chronic and acute interstitial and perifollicular inflammation mainly in the deep reticular dermis and subcutaneous tissue, often making follicles shift into the catagen/telogen phase, without—initially—sebaceous glands loss.
- The deep peribulbar inflammatory infiltrate in early phases resembles that observed in alopecia areata, thereby accounting for the similar trichoscopic features noted in both conditions.
- As the disease progresses and the keratotic debris gathers, infundibula dilate, the dermis relate granulation tissue and the inflammation leads to abscess, inflammatory sinus, and true epithelium injury.
- A biopsy should be ideally obtained from the border of the lesion, in order not to be regarded as "abscess," should it be taken from one the fluctuant nodules.

7.1.10.6 Ultrasonography (Figs. 7.33 and 7.34) [27]

Ultrasonographic findings in dissecting cellulitis with a 24 MHz probe:

- Well-demarcated hypoechoic or anechoic fluid-filled cavities within the dermis or subcutaneous tissue, which represent abscesses or inflammatory nodules. Internal echoes are observed if debris or pus is present.
- Pseudocystic structures identified by hypoechoic lesions lacking true epithelial lining represent ruptured follicles or sterile inflammatory cavities.
- Increased vascularity on power Doppler around active lesions indicates ongoing inflammation or superimposed infection.

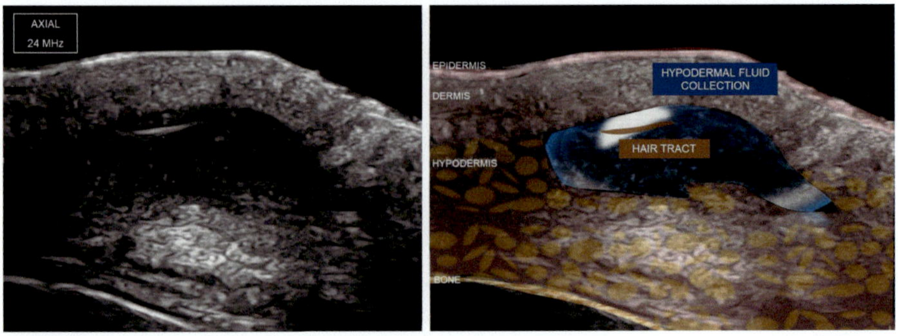

Fig. 7.33 Ultrasonographic findings of dissecting cellulitis with a 24 MHz probe (Aplio i800, Canon Medical Systems)

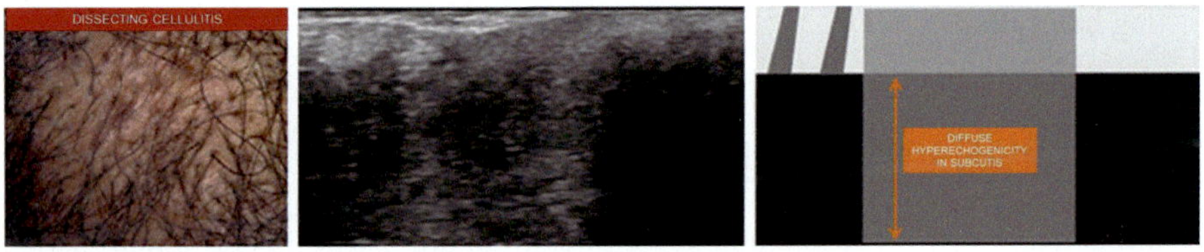

Fig. 7.34 Ultrasonographic findings of dissecting cellulitis with a 70 MHz probe (Reprinted from Journal of Dermatological Science, 102 (2021), Kinoshita-Ise M, Ohyama M, Ramjist JM, Foster FS, Yang VXD, Sachdeva M, Sade S, Shear NH. Ultra high-frequency ultrasound with seventy-MHz transducer in hair disorders: Development of a novel noninvasive diagnostic methodology, 167–174, Copyright (2025), with permission from Elsevier)

- Sinus tracts appear as interconnected, tubular hypoechoic structures extending horizontally or obliquely within the dermis and subcutaneous tissue. It may contain fluid or debris and can be seen tracking between adjacent nodules.
- Loss of normal follicular structure characterized by disruption of the hyperechoic linear parallel structures, which represent hair follicles. Advanced cases show absence of follicular units, consistent with cicatricial alopecia.
- Thickened hyperechoic dermis due to fibrosis and chronic inflammation. It may be associated with posterior acoustic attenuation.

Ultrasonographic findings in dissecting cellulitis with a 70 MHz probe:

- Diffuse increased echogenicity within the subcutaneous tissue, with a well-defined border demarcating the inflamed region, which served as a useful guide for intralesional steroid injection [9]

The ultrasonographic differential diagnosis with other types of alopecia can be found in Table 7.1.

7.1.11 Folliculitis Keloidalis

7.1.11.1 Definition [28]

- Folliculitis keloidalis, also known as acne keloidalis, is a condition that primarily affects the occipital scalp.
- It is characterized by the formation of keloid-like scars resulting from chronic inflammation of hair follicles.

7.1.11.2 Epidemiology [28]

- This disorder predominantly affects young African American males, individuals being more susceptible to its development.
- The male-to-female ratio is approximately 20:1 within affected age groups.

7.1.11.3 Clinical Presentation (Fig. 7.35) [29, 30]

- Acne keloidalis nuchae initially presents as firm, dome-shaped, inflammatory papules and pustules localized at the nape of the neck.

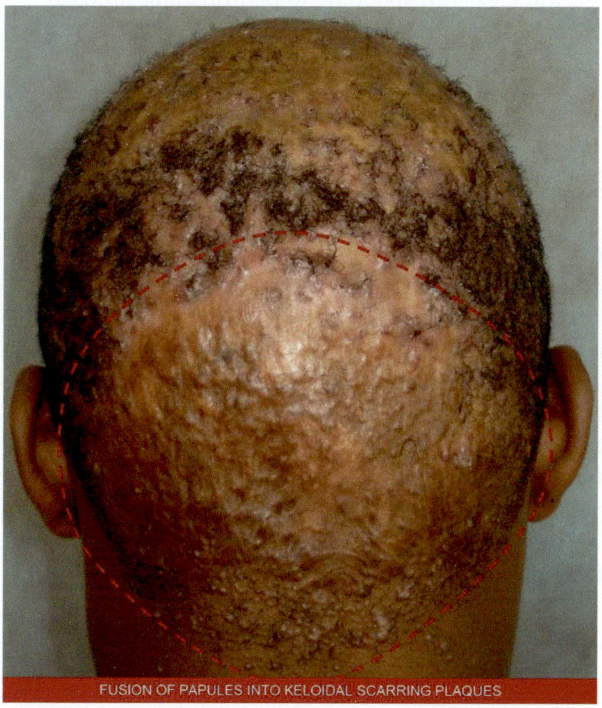

Fig. 7.35 Clinical picture of a patient presenting folliculitis keloidalis of the scalp

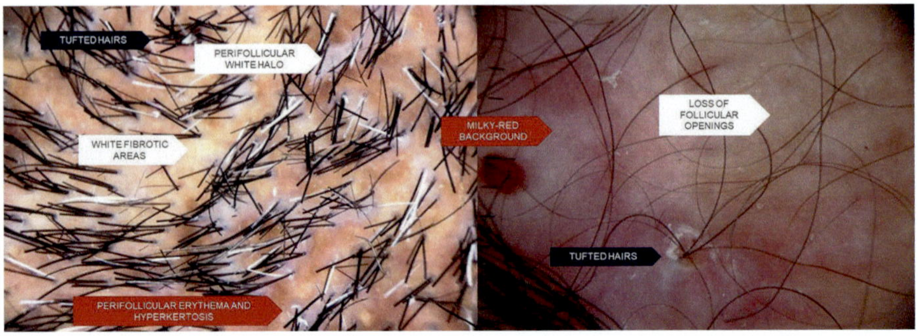

Fig. 7.36 Trichoscopy of Folliculitis Keloidalis (x20 and x50)

- Over time, fibrosis ensues, resulting in the coalescence of these papules into keloidal scarring plaques.
- Scarring is typically evident at the time of medical evaluation and manifests as keloidal papules, plaques, or nodules.

7.1.11.4 Trichoscopy (Fig. 7.36) [30]

- In early stages, dermoscopy shows perifollicular pustules and a white halo surrounding hair follicles corresponding to perifollicular fibrosis.
- In advanced stages, dermoscopy typically reveals the presence of tufted hairs.
- Dilated follicular ostia can be seen in early lesions but is most common in advanced stages.

7.1.11.5 Histopathology (Fig. 7.37) [29, 31]

- Inflammatory lymphocytic-mediated cicatricial alopecia.
- Perifollicular lymphoplasmacytic inflammation, most notable in the isthmus and lower infundibulum with lamellar fibrosis and loss of sebaceous glands.
- Follicular destruction with asymmetrical atrophy of the epithelium, “naked” dermal shafts, engulfed by a granulomatous inflammation, polytrichia, premature desquamation of the inner root sheath.
- This marked inflammation acts as a trigger to bacterial secondary infection, fibrosis and the “keloidal” moniker.

7.1.11.6 Ultrasonography (Fig. 7.38) [31]

Ultrasonographic findings in folliculitis keloidalis with a 20–24 MHz probe:

- Full-thickness cutaneous inflammation is visualized, associated with dilated and distorced hair follicles.

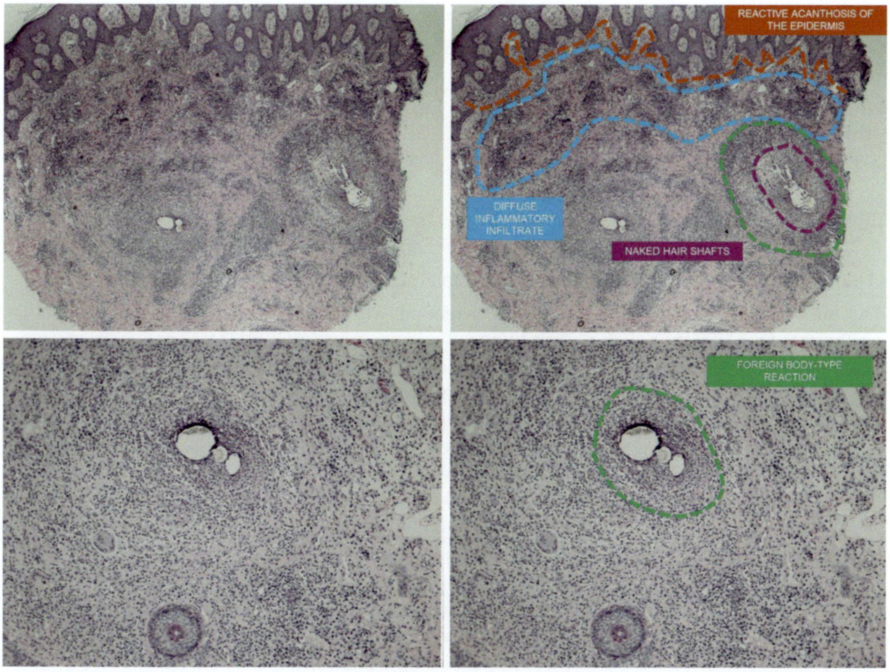

Fig. 7.37 Histological findings of folliculitis keloidalis of the scalp

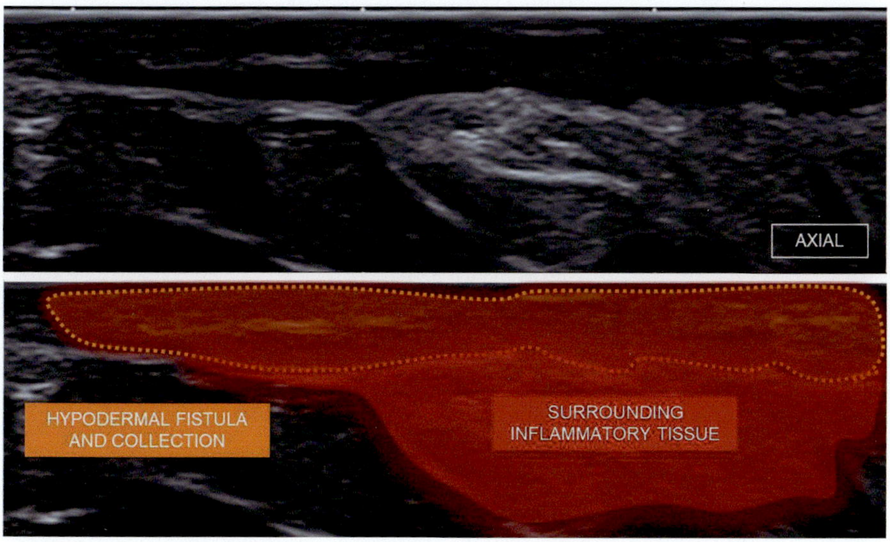

Fig. 7.38 Ultrasonographic findings of folliculitis keloidalis with a 24 MHz probe (Aplio i800, Canon Medical Systems)

- Hypoechoic fistulous tracts may be seen connecting inflamed areas.
- Ovoid-shaped hypoechoic areas represent keloid lesions.

The ultrasonographic differential diagnosis with other types of alopecia can be found in Table 7.1.

Table 7.1 Ultrasonographic findings and differential diagnosis in cicatricial alopecias

Alopecia type	Appropriate probe (MHz)	Ultrasonographic features
Discoid lupus erythematosus	20–24 33 70	Follicular widening with dilated infundibulum and irregular distribution Hair follicles observed in the upper dermis Diffuse dermal hypoechogenicity Loss of dermal-hypodermal differentiation Increased blood in dermis and hypodermis on power Doppler in active lesions Abscense of hair follicles, diffuse hypoechogenicity and decreased blood flow in late cicatricial areas
Tumid lupus erythematosus	20–24 33 70	Preserved epidermis and dermo-epidermal junction Hair follicles in regular distribution Diffuse hyperechogenicity in the dermis, hypodermis and loss of dermo-hypodermal differentiation Increased blood flow in dermis and subcutaneous on Power Doppler
Lupus panniculitis	20–24 33 70	Preserved epidermis and dermo-epidermal junction Hair follicles in regular distribution Diffuse hyperechogenicity in the dermis, hypodermis and loss of dermo-hypodermal differentiation Increased echogenicity of subcutaneous lobules and septal thickening Increased blood flow in dermis and subcutaneous on Power Doppler
Lichen planopilaris	20–24 70	Perifollicular hypoechogenicity Hypoechoic perifollicular widening Irregular distribution of hair follicles Dermal hypoechogenicity, predominantly sparing the interfollicular dermis A hypoechogenic fusiform band is typically seen in the dermis Homogeneous hyperechogenic dermis in cicatricial areas
Frontal fibrosing alopecia	20–24 70	Irregular thickening and widening of lower follicles with a serrated appearance Narrowing of the upper follicle associated with hyperechogenic upper dermis Dilated infundibulum and fusioning of hair follicles (small tufts) Elongated hyperechoic strands from dermis to hypodermis Dermal hypoechogenicity and subcutaneous hyperechogenicity Increased vascular diameter and blood flow on Power Doppler Absence of follicles in cicatricial areas

(continued)

Table 7.1 (continued)

Alopecia type	Appropriate probe (MHz)	Ultrasonographic features
Central centrifugal cicatricial alopecia	24 70	Thickened, hypoechoic dermis with reduction in the number of visible hair follicles Uniform hyperechogenicity in late stages Fibrotic bands Low power Doppler vascularity
Mucinous alopecia	20–24	Hypoechoic areas reflect mucin deposits in dermis and around follicles Dermal thickening due to mucin accumulation and inflammation Reduced follicle visibility No significant vascular changes on Power Doppler
Folliculitis decalvans	70	Hypoechoic or anechoic "pus lakes" in upper dermis Vertical hypoechoic distorted follicles indicating fused follicles Dilated follicles may contain internal debris Hyperechoic fibrotic bands and dermal distortion in scars Power Doppler shows increased vascularity
Dissecting cellulitis	16–18 20–24	Well-defined hypoechoic or anechoic cavities indicate abscesses Pseudocystic lesions suggest ruptured follicles or sterile cavities Sinus tracts appear as tubular hypoechoic structures with possible debris Power Doppler shows increased vascularity Loss of hyperechoic follicular lines indicates cicatricial alopecia Thickened hyperechoic dermis due to fibrosis and chronic inflammation
Folliculitis keloidalis	16–18 20–24	Full-thickness cutaneous inflammation with dilated and distorted follicles Hypoechoic fistulous tracts connecting inflamed regions Ovoid hypoechoic areas correspond to keloid lesions

7.2 Non-cicatricial Alopecias

7.2.1 Alopecia Areata

7.2.1.1 Definition [32]

- A chronic, immune-mediated disorder that targets anagen hair follicles and causes nonscarring hair loss.

7.2.1.2 Epidemiology [33]

- The estimated prevalence is approximately with a lifetime risk of approximately 2%.
- Affects children and adults with no sex predilection.

7.2.1.3 Clinical Presentation (Fig. 7.39) [33]

- Patchy alopecia, which manifests as smooth, circular, discrete areas of complete hair loss that develop over a period of a few weeks, is the most common clinical variant.
- AA can also affect other areas, such as the beard, eyebrows, eyelashes.
- In a minority of patients, patchy alopecia progresses to alopecia totalis or alopecia universalis.

7.2.1.4 Trichoscopy (Fig. 7.40) [34]

- Yellow dots in a large amount is characteristic in both, acute and chronic disease.
- Broken hairs, black dots, Pohl-Pinkus constrictions, monilethrix-like hairs, exclamation mark hairs, coudability hairs are found in active phase.
- Short regrowing hairs and circular or pigtail hairs as signs of hair regrowth.

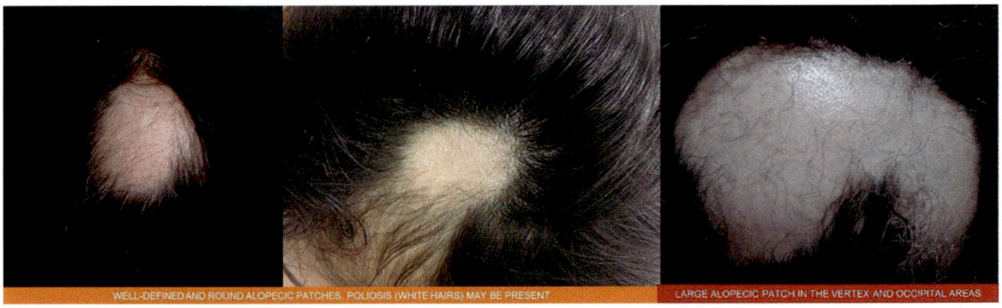

Fig. 7.39 Clinical picture of a patient presenting areata alopecia

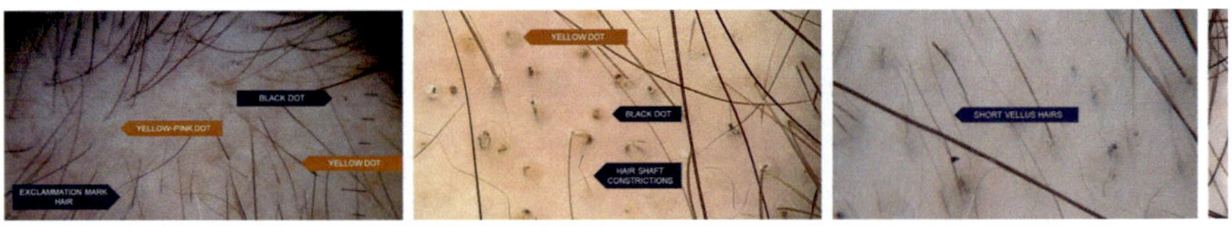

Fig. 7.40 Trichoscopy of a patient presenting areata alopecia (x20, x50 and x30)

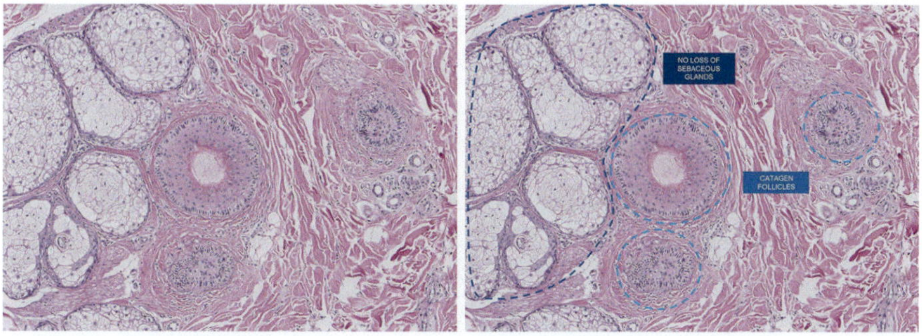

Fig. 7.41 Histological findings of areata alopecia (H&E x10)

7.2.1.5 Histopathology (Fig. 7.41) [32, 33]

- Initial Early and active disease show normal number of hair follicles, with a peribulbar mononuclear infiltrate ("swarm of bees") around anlagen hairs and some eosinophils. Plasma cells, however, are not an important component.
- The exocytosis of inflammatory cells produces edema, cytoplasmic vacuolation, and apoptosis of matrix and suprabulbar follicular epithelium, leading to miniaturization.
- Follicles subsequently shift to the catagen/telogen phase, habitually exceeding 50% of the total count, and inflammation tends to subside.
- Pigment clumps are therefore identified in the epithelium, papilla, fibrous stella, or infundibulum.
- Repeated injury causes dystrophy of hair formation, leaving cornified, irregular, and progressive smaller shafts and, with subsequent catagen/telogen period, turning into nanogen hairs of chronic alopecia areata.

7.2.1.6 Ultrasonography (Figs. 7.42 and 7.43) [35–37]

Ultrasonographic findings in alopecia areata with a 20–24 MHz probe:

- Follicular structures show increased echogenicity and widening in all alopecia areata phases.
- Acute phase
  - Follicular structures have well-defined borders and widened distal ends.
  - Drop-like shaped follicles are seen in the deeper dermal layers. This finding is related to the inflammatory infiltrate at the bulbar level that occurs in the acute phase of the disease.
  - Increased echogenicity in dermis and hypodermis.

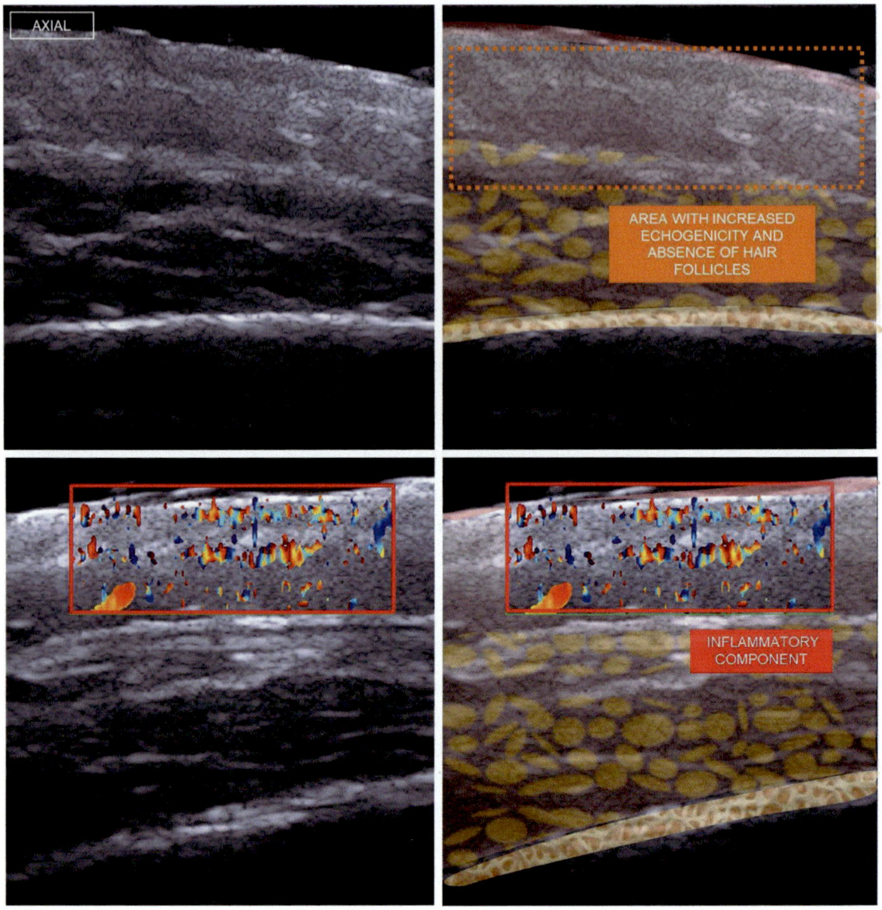

Fig. 7.42 Ultrasonographic findings of alopecia areata with a 22 MHz probe (My Lab Touch, Esaote)

- Subacute phase
  - Fewer follicular structures are present, with less distinct borders.
  - Some follicles still show widened distal ends, though in lower numbers.
- Regrowth phase
  - Follicular structures vary in width, appear elongated, and often have widened distal parts.
  - Follicles are located at different dermal depths, with some extending into the subcutaneous tissue. Decreased number of hair follicles may be detected.

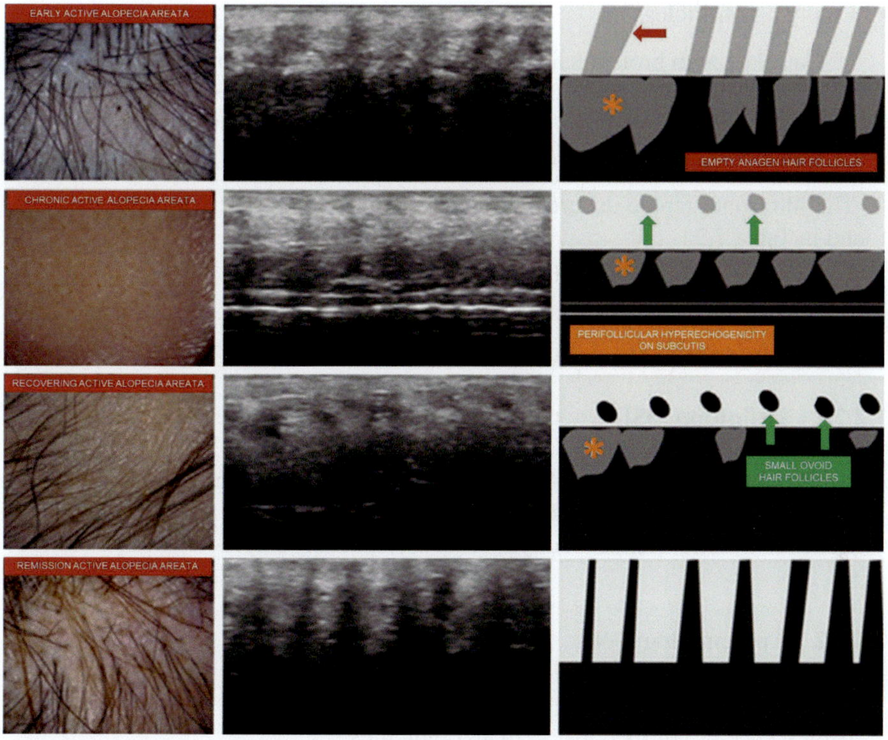

Fig. 7.43 Ultrasonographic findings of alopecia areata with a 70 MHz probe (Reprinted from Journal of Dermatological Science, 102 (2021), Kinoshita-Ise M, Ohyama M, Ramjist JM, Foster FS, Yang VXD, Sachdeva M, Sade S, Shear NH. Ultra high-frequency ultrasound with seventy-MHz transducer in hair disorders: Development of a novel noninvasive diagnostic methodology, 167–174, Copyright (2025), with permission from Elsevier)

Descriptive ultrasonographic features in alopecia areata with a 70 MHz probe [9]:

- Small ovoid hair follicles
  - Prominent in chronic alopecia areata.
  - Associated with yellow dots on trichoscopy.
  - May represent nanogen, telogen hair follicles, or emerging vellus hairs.
  - Hair follicles on recovering lesions appear more hypoechoic than on chronic lesions, indicating growing vellus hair shafts.
- Perifollicular hyperechogenicity in subcutis
  - Associated with the typical inflammation in the lower part of the hair follicle in alopecia areata.

- Empty hair follicles
  - Correlate with broken hairs and black dots on trichoscopy.
  - Appear more echogenic than normal anagen hair follicles.
  - Show a distinct boundary between the follicle and subcutis.
  - Common in active disease.

The ultrasonographic differential diagnosis with other types of alopecia can be found in Table 7.2.

7.2.2 Androgenetic Alopecia

7.2.2.1 Definition [38]

- Androgenetic alopecia (AGA) is a genetically determined, progressive non-scarring alopecia characterized by gradual miniaturization of hair follicles in a patterned distribution, influenced by androgens, especially dihydrotestosterone (DHT).

7.2.2.2 Epidemiology [38]

- It affects 50% of women and 80% of men, with onset mostly occurring during adolescence or perimenopause in all ethnicities.

7.2.2.3 Clinical Presentation (Fig. 7.44) [39]

- Androgenetic alopecia manifests as a gradual and predictable hair loss pattern usually after puberty.
- In men, it typically begins with bitemporal thinning of the frontal scalp followed by involvement of the vertex.
- In women, hair thinning is more diffuse, often concentrated on the crown of the scalp while retaining the frontal hairline.

7.2.2.4 Trichoscopy (Fig. 7.45) [3]

- Hair shaft diameter diversity >20% is diagnostic of AGA
- Increased proportion of single hair units and yellow dots (empty hair follicles that accumulate sebum)
- Peripilar sign: brownish halos around follicles, reflecting inflammation and melanin incontinence. This sign appears in early stages of AGA.

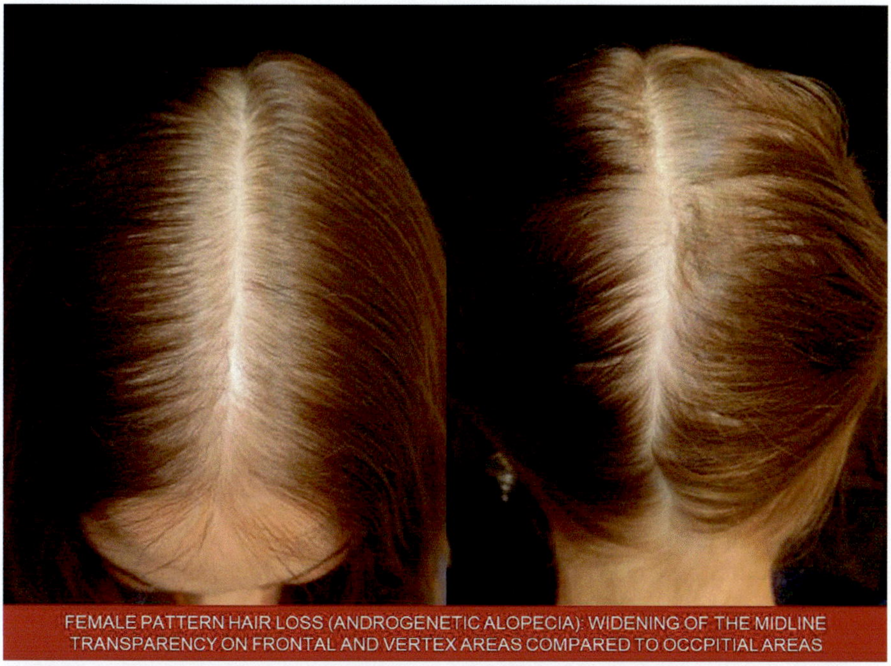

Fig. 7.44 Clinical picture of a patient presenting androgenetic alopecia

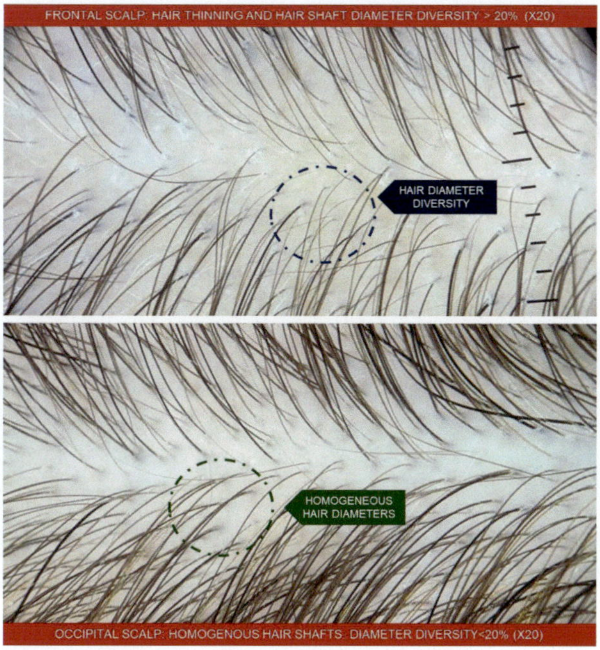

Fig. 7.45 Trichoscopy of a patient presenting androgenetic alopecia (x20)

7.2.2.5 Histopathology (Fig. 7.46)

- Progressive shortening of anagen cycle, leading to increasing numbers of telogen follicles (15–20%), miniaturization with follicular bulbs in the mid dermis and fibrous tissue (streamer or stela) left behind (<6–7:1).
- Hais shafts smaller than the inner root sheath diameter or <0.06 mm.
- Follicular units of assorted sizes (anisotrichosis).
- Inflammation is reported to be mild at most and not the driving mechanism of disease. Sebaceous glands are preserved.

7.2.2.6 Ultrasonography (Figs. 7.47 and 7.48) [37, 40]

Ultrasonographic findings in androgenetic alopecia with a 20–24 MHz probe:

- Hair follicles are thinner in frontal, parietal and vertex regions compared to occipital region.
- Anisocoria (hair diameter diversity) is the hallmark of AGA. Hair follicles are found at different levels of depth: unaffected terminal follicles in anagen reach the

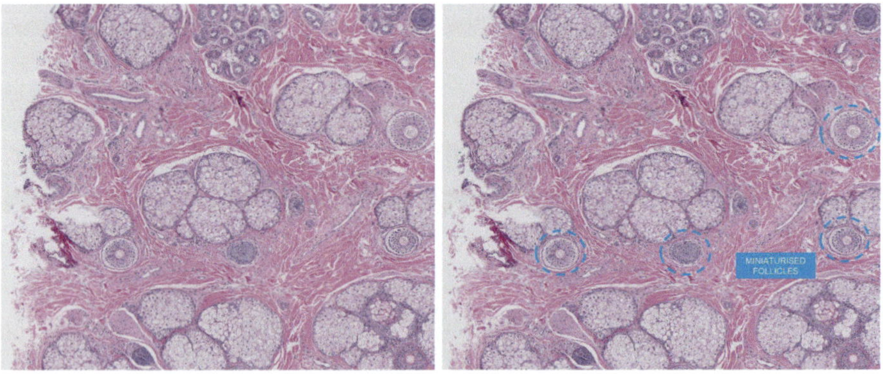

Fig. 7.46 Histological findings of androgenetic alopecia (H&E x10)

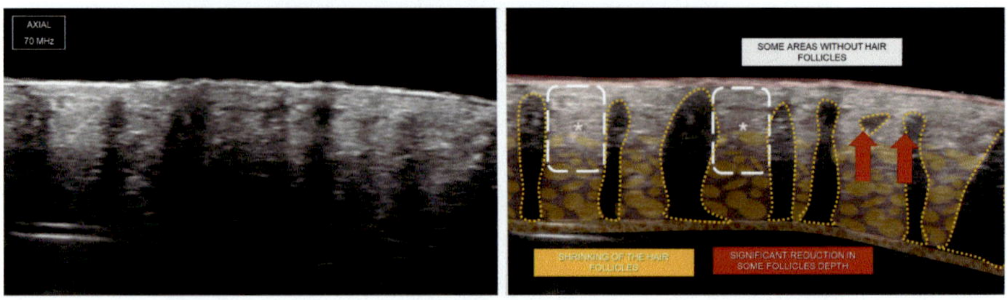

Fig. 7.47 Ultrasonographic findings of androgenetic alopecia with a 70 MHz probe (Vevo MD, FUJIFILM VisualSonics, Amsterdam)

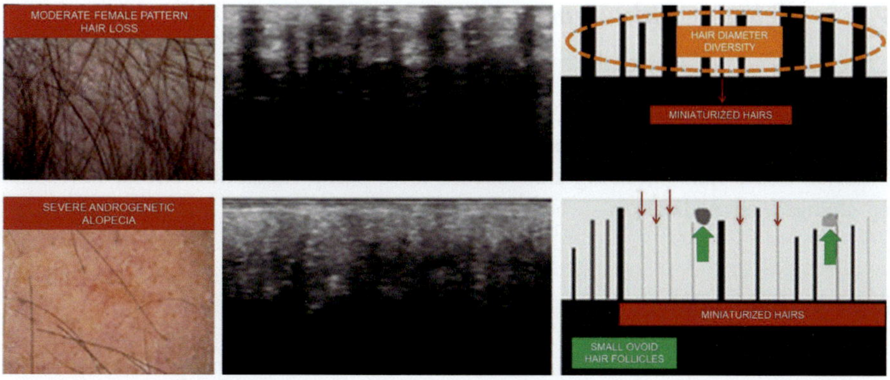

Fig. 7.48 Ultrasonographic findings of female pattern hair loss and androgenetic alopecia with a 70 MHz probe (Reprinted from Journal of Dermatological Science, 102 (2021), Kinoshita-Ise M, Ohyama M, Ramjist JM, Foster FS, Yang VXD, Sachdeva M, Sade S, Shear NH. Ultra high-frequency ultrasound with seventy-MHz transducer in hair disorders: Development of a novel noninvasive diagnostic methodology, 167–174, Copyright (2025), with permission from Elsevier)

deep dermis or dermohypodermal border, in contrast with miniaturized follicles of smaller diameter and length (sometimes with ovoid morphology) reaching only the superficial dermis.
- A limitation of current ultrasound equipment lies in its failure to differentiate follicles that comprise a multifollicular unit (3-4 follicles in the same unit), which subsequently affects the ability of the technique to identify androgenetic alopecia in its earliest stages, since follicular units of a single non-miniaturized follicle could be considered as normal.
- In some cases of late-stage AGA, ultra-high frequency probes can show a tendency for the shafts to be bilaminar rather than trilaminar, presumably due to the substitution of the terminal hairs with medulla by amedullary vellus hairs.
- No significant difference in overall dermal thickness.

Most common ultrasonographic findings in female pattern hair loss and androgenetic alopecia with a 70 MHz probe [9]:

- Anisocoria: hair diameter diversity, or Miniaturized hairs
  - Most frequent finding.
  - Multiple miniaturized hairs with varying degrees of reduction in moderate lesions.
  - Pronounced miniaturization in severe lesions. It also affects nearly all hairs, leading to uniform follicular thinning.
- Small ovoid hair follicles in the upper and mid dermis.

The ultrasonographic differential diagnosis with other types of alopecia can be found in Table 7.2.

7.2.3 Telogen Effluvium

7.2.3.1 Definition [41]

- Telogen effluvium is a form of nonscarring alopecia characterized by diffuse, often acute hair shedding that occurs after some metabolic stress, hormonal changes, or medication.

7.2.3.2 Epidemiology [42]

- Common condition that can affect individuals of any age, gender, or racial background
- Many adults experience an episode of telogen effluvium at some point in their lifetime.
- Women tend to be more susceptible.

7.2.3.3 Clinical Presentation (Fig. 7.49) [37, 43]

- Diffuse hair shedding, usually without other symptoms and with a relatively abrupt onset.
- Generally, hair loss occurs 2–3 months after the trigger exposure, and may last from weeks to several months, depending on the time exposed to the trigger point.

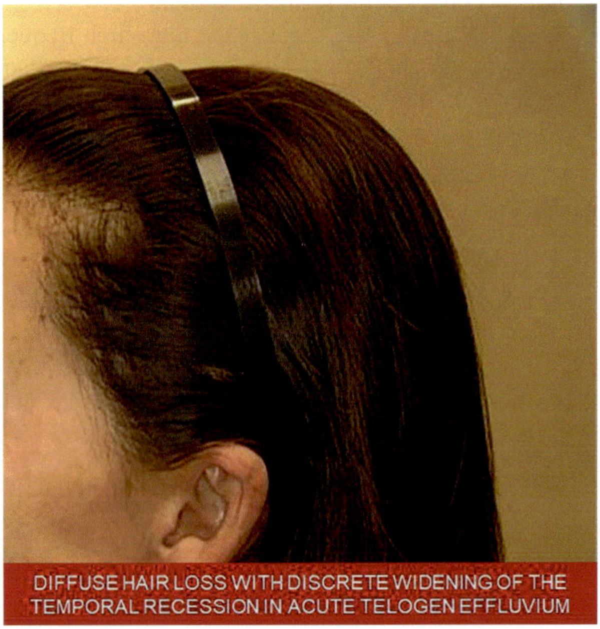

Fig. 7.49 Clinical picture of a patient presenting telogen effluvium

- Hair loss is typically diffuse, affecting the entire scalp rather than being localized to specific areas. Patients may notice increased shedding especially when washing or brushing their hair, and even on their pillow or.
- Despite increased shedding, overall hair density may remain intact, though some patients may experience visible thinning, especially on the crown, fronto-temporal hairline and "ponytail" diameter.
- Telogen effluvium is a non-scarring form of hair loss, meaning there is no permanent damage to the hair follicles or scalp. There is also typically no visible inflammation or redness of the scalp. Telogen effluvium is generally a self-limiting and reversible condition. Once the triggering factor is removed, hair growth usually resumes within 3–6 months.
- The examination of the scalp may show a positive pull test of telogen hairs during the shedding phase, and short regrowing terminal hairs mainly in the frontal and bitemporal areas, although may be present in all scalp areas.

7.2.3.4 Trichoscopy (Fig. 7.50) [26, 34]

- Trichoscopy alone has limited diagnostic value. It is important to exclude other differential diagnosis, as AGA and diffuse Alopecia Areata.
- Short regrowing hairs may be observed in all scalp areas.
- Unlike androgenetic alopecia, where variation in hair shaft diameter (miniaturization) is common, telogen effluvium typically shows uniform hair shaft diameters, with no significant miniaturization of hair follicles.
- The vascular pattern in telogen effluvium usually appears normal, with no significant increase in blood vessels or telangiectasias (small, dilated blood vessels).
- There are generally no associated findings on the scalp; however, it is important to consider that telogen effluvium may coexist with other scalp conditions, particularly the most common ones such as androgenetic alopecia and frontal fibrosing alopecia. Therefore, trichoscopy may occasionally reveal features of more than one disorder.

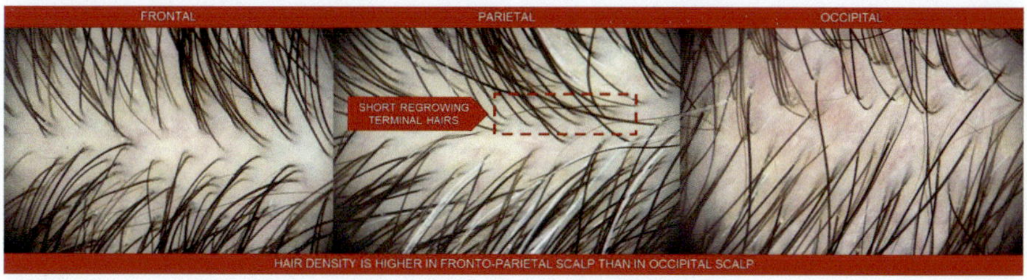

Fig. 7.50 Trichoscopy of a patient presenting telogen effluvium (x20)

7.2.3.5 Histopathology (Fig. 7.51)

- Overall normal total follicular count, more than 20% of hair in the catagen and telogen phase, usually not exceeding 50% with and fibrous stela in the deep dermis and subcutis.
- Counts between 15% and 20% can be suspicious, but not diagnostic.
- Miniaturization and inflammation are not a feature.

7.2.3.6 Ultrasonography (Figs. 7.52 and 7.53) [37]

Ultrasonographic findings in telogen effluvium with a 20–24 MHz probe:

- Reduced number of visible hair shafts, though follicles remain structurally intact and undamaged.
- Occasionally, there may be slightly increased echogenicity around follicular openings due to a higher proportion of telogen hairs.

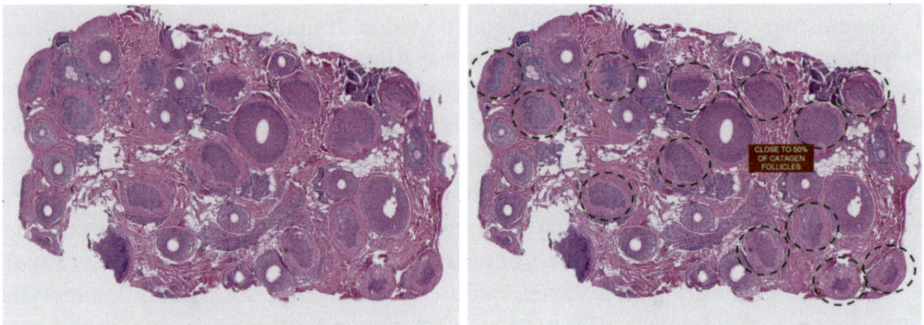

Fig. 7.51 Histological findings of telogen effluvium (H&E x10)

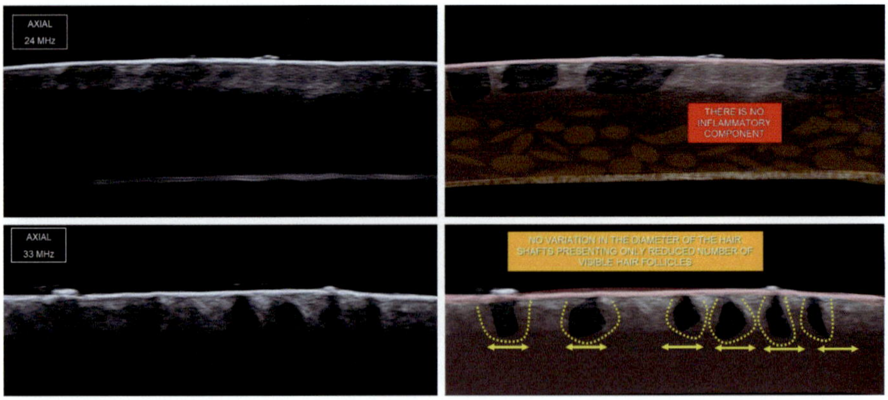

Fig. 7.52 Ultrasonographic findings of telogen effluvium with 24 and 33 MHz probes (Aplio i800, Canon Medical Systems)

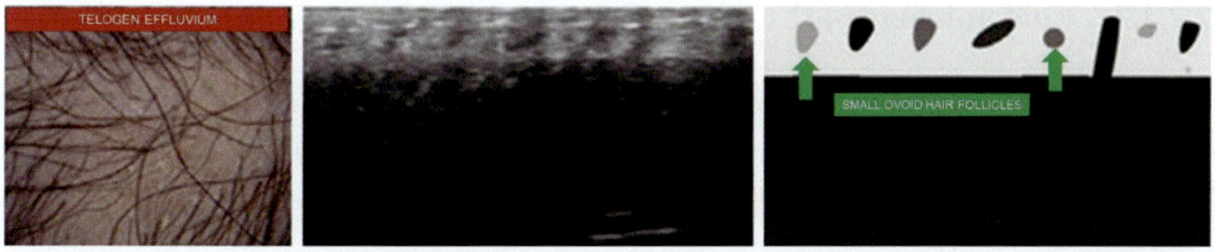

Fig. 7.53 Ultrasonographic findings of telogen effluvium with a 70 MHz probe (Reprinted from Journal of Dermatological Science, 102 (2021), Kinoshita-Ise M, Ohyama M, Ramjist JM, Foster FS, Yang VXD, Sachdeva M, Sade S, Shear NH. Ultra high-frequency ultrasound with seventy-MHz transducer in hair disorders: Development of a novel noninvasive diagnostic methodology, 167–174, Copyright (2025), with permission from Elsevier)

- Dermis and ***subcutaneous fat layer typically appears normal in thickness, unlike scarring alopecias.
- Absence of fibrosis, with uniform dermis and subcutaneous fat layer echogenicity and no hyperechoic areas.
- Power Doppler shows normal vascularity, reflecting minimal or absent inflammation.

Most common ultrasonographic findings in telogen effluvium with a 70 MHz probe [9]:

- Multiple "small ovoid hair follicles" with variable echogenicities
- Indicates telogen hair follicles with or without hair shafts

The ultrasonographic differential diagnosis with other types of alopecia can be found in Table 7.2.

7.2.4 Trichotillomania

7.2.4.1 Definition [44]

- Trichotillomania, also known as hair-pulling disorder, is a psychiatric condition characterized by the repetitive urge to pull out one's own hair, leading to noticeable hair loss.
- It is considered an impulse control disorder, and the behavior is often preceded by an increasing sense of tension or anxiety, followed by a sense of relief or gratification after pulling out the hair.

7.2.4.2 Epidemiology [44]

- Trichotillomania affects approximately 1–2% of the population. It is more common in females than males, with a female-to-male ratio of about 10:1 in adults.
- The disorder typically begins in childhood or adolescence, with the average onset around ages 10–13.
- It is often associated with other psychiatric disorders such as anxiety, depression, and obsessive–compulsive disorder (OCD).

7.2.4.3 Clinical Presentation (Fig. 7.54) [45]

- The most noticeable symptom is patchy hair loss in areas where the hair is easy to reach, such as the scalp, eyebrows, and eyelashes. The hair loss is often asymmetric and irregularly shaped.
- Patients may engage in hair-pulling during periods of stress, boredom, or relaxation. The act is usually performed in private, and some patients may attempt to hide the behavior.
- The affected areas might show signs of irritation, scarring, or secondary infections due to repeated trauma.
- Patients often experience significant distress and embarrassment about their appearance, leading to social withdrawal and difficulties in personal and professional relationships.

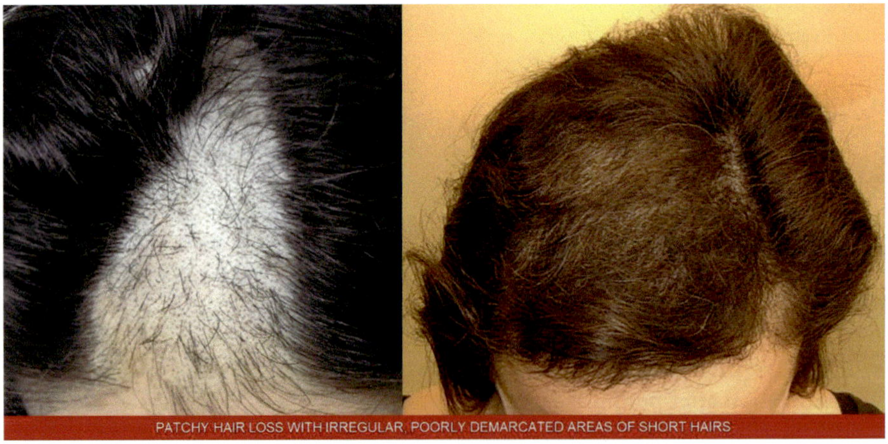

Fig. 7.54 Clinical picture of a patient presenting trichotillomania

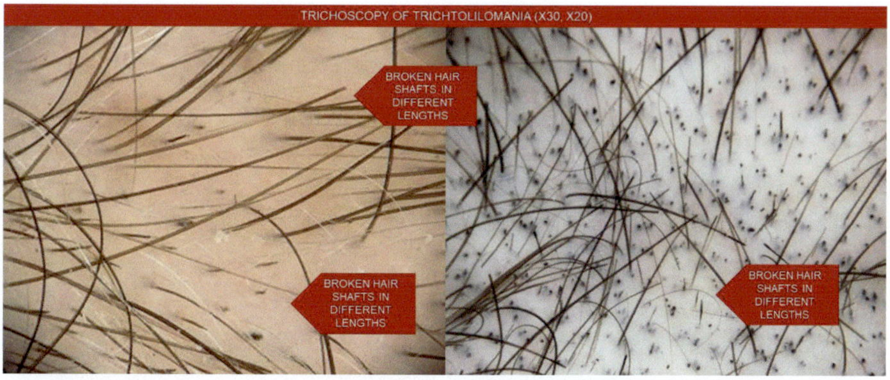

Fig. 7.55 Trichoscopy of a patient presenting trichotillomania (x30 and x20)

7.2.4.4 Trichoscopy (Fig. 7.55) [44, 45]

- One of the hallmark features is the presence of hairs broken at different lengths. These broken hairs often have blunt or frayed ends.
- Black dots representing hair fragments within the follicles, a result of incomplete hair pulling.
- Although more commonly associated with alopecia areata, exclamation mark hairs may be seen in trichotillomania and are characterized by tapering near the scalp.
- Also known as "tulip hairs," these have a V-shaped split at the distal end, indicative of hair shaft damage due to pulling.
- Areas with reduced hair density and empty follicles are common, reflecting the repetitive nature of the hair-pulling behavior.
- Small hemorrhagic spots around the hair follicles may be observed due to the trauma inflicted during hair pulling.

7.2.4.5 Histopathology (Fig. 7.56) [44, 45]

- The distinguishing feature is distortion of the follicular anatomy, which is a result of hair avulsion.
- Collapsing of the inner root sheath with fragmented, damaged and often no hair shaft.
- Pigments remnants ("casts") displaced cortical cells and intrafollicular hemorrhage.
- The traumatized follicular epithelium produces abnormally pigmented and reduced diameter shafts—trichomalacia.
- Forced removal of hairs also promotes a variable shift to catagen/telogen phase, a helpful although not specific detail.

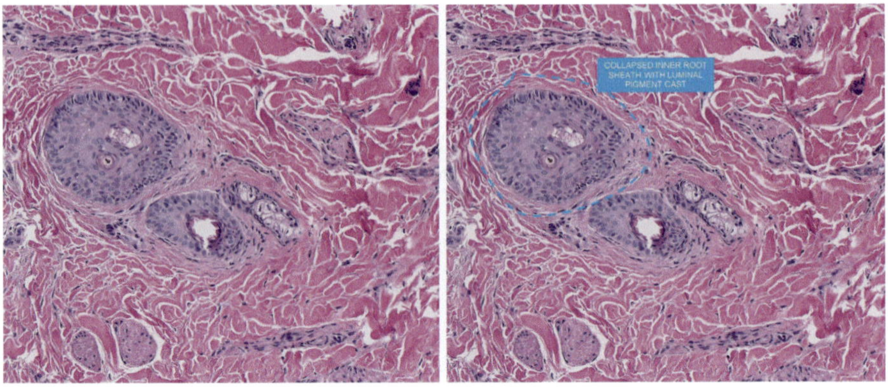

Fig. 7.56 Histological findings of trichotillomania (H&E x20)

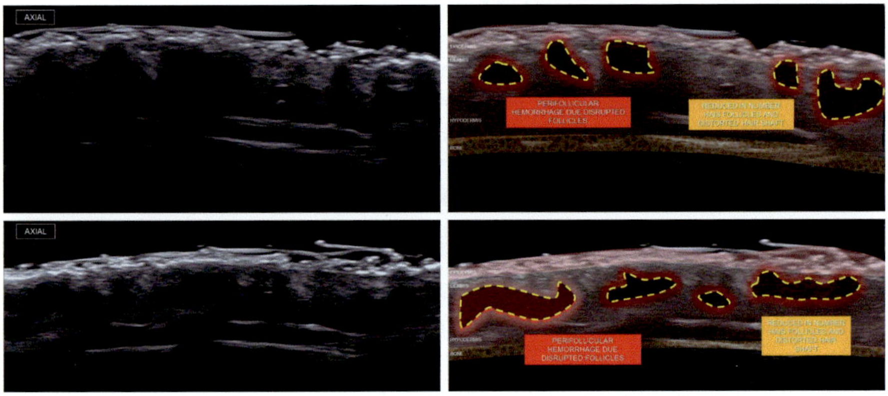

Fig. 7.57 Ultrasonographic findings of trichotillomania with a 24 MHz probe (Aplio i800, Canon Medical Systems)

7.2.4.6 Ultrasonography (Fig. 7.57) [37]

- The echogenicity of the scalp in trichotillomania may be mixed, reflecting a combination of intact areas, regions of inflammation, and trauma-induced changes. This variability helps distinguish it from other types of hair loss. Areas with continuous trauma from pulling may appear as localized hypoechoic areas of dermal thickening.
- Mechanical trauma of hair pulling may lead to distorted, reduced, or complete abscent hair follicles. Increase in hair follicle thickness has been described, associated with perifollicular inflammatory changes and fibrosis.
- In some cases, power Doppler ultrasonography may reveal mild increased vascularity in the affected areas, reflecting localized inflammation. However, this is typically not as prominent as in more inflammatory conditions.
- Unlike scarring alopecias, trichotillomania usually does not show significant fibrotic changes. The lack of hyperechoic bands or widespread dermal thickening is consistent with the non-scarring nature of the condition.

- The subcutaneous fat layer generally appears normal on ultrasonography, as trichotillomania primarily affects the hair follicles and dermis without significantly altering the deeper layers.
- In Trichotheiromania – the compulsive rubbing or scratching the hair and scalp – it is possible to identify some dermal hypoechogenicity and increased vascularization on Doppler, presumably a consequence of inflammation due to continued scratching.
- The ultrasonographic differential diagnosis with other types of alopecia can be found in Table 7.2.

7.2.5 Pressure-Induced Alopecia

7.2.5.1 Definition [46]

- Pressure-induced alopecias are group of scarring and nonscarring alopecias that occur after an ischemic obstruction of capillaries that leads to circumscribed areas of hair loss. Initially described after prolonged surgeries or immobilization, alopecia occurs after sustained external pressure to the skin, mainly in scalp prominences (e.g., prolonged hospitalization, surgical procedures, use of headgear, "television alopecia"). Alopecia induced by cosmetic procedures has been reported with increased frequency in literature and predominantly emerges from pressure exerted by the volume of injectables. It is important to differentiate pressure-induced alopecia by external volume of cosmetic procedures from vascular occlusion-induced alopecia because they represent distinct entities.

7.2.5.2 Epidemiology [46]

- More commonly seen in adults, rarely in children.
- Reported after prolonged surgical procedures (cardiothoracic, gynecological, reconstructive, genitourinary, and neurosurgical) and prolonged ICU stays.
- Also reported after application of electroencephalogram (EEG) electrodes, orthodontic headgear, and cervical collars, and cosmetic injectables applied on the temporal areas.

7.2.5.3 Clinical Presentation (Fig. 7.58) [46, 47]

- Alopecic patches develop in areas where external pressure was applied. The scalp prominences, particularly the occipital and vertex areas are the most frequently affected sites.
- Erythema, swelling, and tenderness are the most common symptoms ; however, alopecia might be the sole manifestation. Crusts and ulceration are associated with a worse outcome and a higher risk of scarring alopecia.

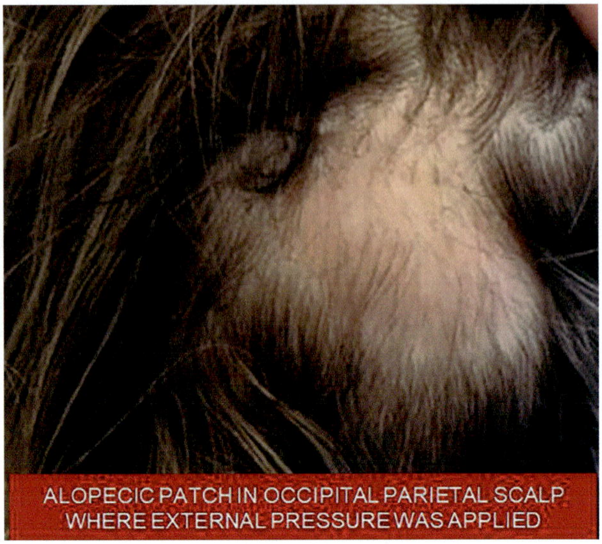

Fig. 7.58 Clinical picture of a patient presenting pressure-induced alopecia (Image courtesy of Dr. Yanna Barros)

7.2.5.4 Trichoscopy (Fig. 7.59) [46–48]

- Trichoscopy is considered nonspecific, although may help with clues to the diagnosis. Most trichoscopic features in acute phase are typical of anagen effluvium: Broken hairs, black dots, exclamation mark, yellow dots, peri and inter follicular erythema, vellus hairs and upright regrowing hairs.
- (H&E x0) Comedone-like black dots are a unique trichoscopic feature of pressure alopecia.
- Hair regrows in most cases, but prognosis depends on ischemia severity and timely treatment with reperfusion therapies or mobilization. Treatment of hair loss is usually not necessary because the disease in most cases is self-limited and reversible.

7.2.5.5 Histopathology [46, 48]

- Early stage (acute changes)
  - Follicular degeneration
    - The hair follicles show signs of degeneration, with loss of the normal architecture.
    - This degeneration is due to ischemia and mechanical pressure, leading to impaired hair follicle function.

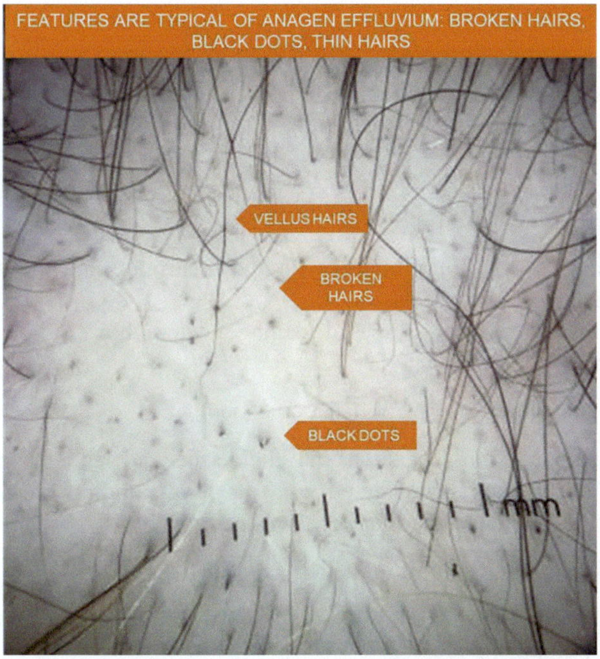

Fig. 7.59 Trichoscopy of pressure-induced alopecia (x20) (Image courtesy of Dr. Yanna Barros)

- Catagen and telogen predominance
  - There is a noticeable increase in hair follicles in the catagen (regression) or telogen (resting) phases.
  - These phases are characterized by the cessation of active hair growth, leading to hair shedding.
- Ischemic changes
  - Evidence of ischemic damage, including necrosis of follicular keratinocytes and endothelial cells.
  - Prolonged pressure causes reduced blood flow, leading to ischemia and subsequent tissue damage.

- Intermediate stage (subacute changes)
  - Follicular miniaturization:
    - Hair follicles become smaller and produce finer, thinner hairs.
    - This is a response to chronic pressure and reduced blood supply, leading to diminished hair follicle activity.

- Perifollicular fibrosis:
    - Fibrosis, or scarring, occurs around the hair follicles.
    - Perifollicular fibrosis indicates a chronic process, contributing to the irreversible loss of hair follicles.

- Late stage (chronic changes)
  - Complete follicular atrophy
    - Hair follicles may undergo complete atrophy and disappear, leaving behind fibrotic tracts.
    - This is the final stage of damage where hair follicles are permanently lost.
  - Dermal and subcutaneous fibrosis
    - Extensive fibrosis extends into the dermis and subcutaneous tissues.
    - This fibrosis is associated with the long-standing pressure and ischemia, leading to permanent alopecia.
  - Sparse inflammatory infiltrate
    - A mild, often chronic inflammatory infiltrate, predominantly lymphocytic, may be present.
    - The inflammation is usually mild and reflects the chronic nature of the condition rather than an active inflammatory process.

7.2.5.6 Ultrasonography (Fig. 7.60) [47]

- Prolonged pressure can cause localized hypoechoic areas in the dermis and subcutaneous tissue. These areas reflect edema, tissue compression, and potential ischemia resulting from sustained pressure on the scalp.
- The echogenicity in the affected regions may be mixed, reflecting a combination of tissue edema, early fibrosis, and reduced follicular density. This variability helps in assessing the severity and stage of the condition.
- Ultrasonography may reveal a reduction or absence of visible hair follicles in the affected areas. The hair follicles in these regions may be damaged or atrophied due to the mechanical stress and reduced blood supply.
- In cases where the pressure-induced alopecia has led to permanent hair loss, ultrasonography might show hyperechoic streaks or bands indicating early fibrotic changes or scarring within the dermis.
- Power Doppler ultrasonography may demonstrate reduced vascularity in the affected areas due to impaired blood flow from the sustained pressure. This finding correlates with the ischemic changes observed in pressure-induced alopecia.
- The ultrasonographic differential diagnosis with other types of alopecia can be found in Table 7.2.

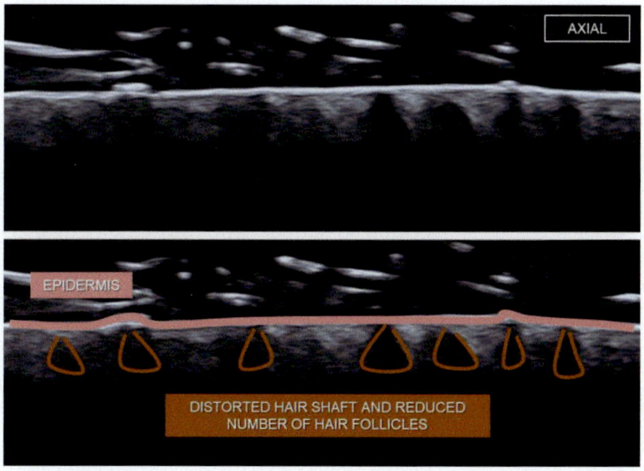

Fig. 7.60 Ultrasonographic findings of pressure-induced alopecia with a 24 MHz probe (Aplio i800, Canon Medical Systems)

Table 7.2 Ultrasonographic findings and differential diagnosis in non-cicatricial alopecias

Alopecia type	Appropriate probe (MHz)	Ultrasonographic features
Alopecia areata	24 70	Follicles widened and echogenic in all phases Acute phase: Well-defined, drop-like deep follicles, dermal hyperechogenicity , small ovoid follicles Subacute phase: Fewer, blurred follicles, occasional distal widening Regrowth phase: Elongated, variable-depth follicles, reduced count
Androgenetic alopecia	24 70	Unchanged dermal thickness Thinner hair follicles in frontal, parietal, and vertex regions versus occipital Anisotrichosis (hair diameter variability) Follicles vary in depth: terminal in deep dermis; miniaturized in superficial dermis Ovoid, shallow follicles suggest miniaturization Late-stage may show bilaminar shafts replacing trilaminar terminal hairs
Telogen effluvium	24 70	Dermis and subcutaneous fat layer with normal thickness No fibrosis and uniform echogenicity without hyperechoic areas Reduced number of visible hair shafts, follicles remain intact Mild perifollicular echogenicity (increased telogen hairs) Normal vascularity on Power Doppler

(continued)

Table 7.2 (continued)

Alopecia type	Appropriate probe (MHz)	Ultrasonographic features
Trichotillomania	20–24	Distorted, reduced, or absent hair follicles due to traction Follicular thickening with perifollicular inflammation and fibrosis Mixed scalp echogenicity from trauma and inflammation Localized dermal hypoechogenicity in areas of chronic pulling Normal subcutaneous fat layer Power Doppler may show mild increased vascularity In trichotheiromania: dermal hypoechogenicity and Doppler hyperemia from scratching
Pressure-induced alopecia	20–24	Localized hypoechoic areas from edema, compression, and ischemia Mixed echogenicity from edema, early fibrosis, and low follicular density Reduced or absent visible hair follicles due to damage or atrophy Hyperechoic bands may appear in chronic or scarring cases Power Doppler shows reduced vascularity in affected areas

References

1. Fijałkowska A, Kądziela M, Żebrowska A. The spectrum of cutaneous manifestations in lupus erythematosus: a comprehensive review. J Clin Med. 2024;13:2419.
2. Concha JSS, Werth VP. Alopecias in lupus erythematosus. Lupus Sci Med. 2018;5:e000291. https://doi.org/10.1136/lupus-2018-000291.
3. Rudnicka L, Rakowska A, Olszewska M. Trichoscopy. Dermatol Clin. 2013;31:29–41.
4. Rudnicka L, Olszewska M, Waśkiel A, Rakowska A. Trichoscopy in hair shaft disorders. Dermatol Clin. 2018;36:421–30.
5. Kimball H, Kimball D, Siroy A, Tuna IS, Boyce BJ, Albayram MS. Novel diagnostic imaging features of facial lupus panniculitis: ultrasound, CT, and MR imaging with histopathology correlate. Clin Imaging. 2019;58:177–81.
6. Giavedoni P, Podlipnik S, Fuertes de Vega I, Iranzo P, Mascaró JM. High-frequency ultrasound to assess activity in connective tissue panniculitis. J Clin Med. 2021;10:4516.
7. Svigos K, Yin L, Fried L, Lo Sicco K, Shapiro J. A practical approach to the diagnosis and management of classic lichen Planopilaris. Am J Clin Dermatol. 2021;22:681–92.
8. Ianoşi S, Forsea A, Lupu M, Ilie M, Zurac S, Boda D, et al. Role of modern imaging techniques for the in vivo diagnosis of lichen planus (review). Exp Ther Med. 2019;17:1052–60.
9. Kinoshita-Ise M, et al. Ultra high-frequency ultrasound with seventy-MHz transducer in hair disorders: development of a novel noninvasive diagnostic methodology. J Dermatol Sci. 2021;102(3):167–76.
10. Kerkemeyer KLS, Eisman S, Bhoyrul B, Pinczewski J, Sinclair RD. Frontal fibrosing alopecia. Clin Dermatol. 2021;39:183–93.
11. Kossard S. Postmenopausal frontal fibrosing alopecia: scarring alopecia in a pattern distribution. Arch Dermatol. 1994;130:770–4. https://doi.org/10.1001/archderm.1994.01690060100013.
12. Golińska J, Sar-Pomian M, Rudnicka L. Diagnostic accuracy of Trichoscopy in inflammatory scalp diseases: a systematic review. Dermatology. 2022;238:412–21.

13. Porriño-Bustamante ML, Fernández-Pugnaire MA, Castellote-Caballero L, Arias-Santiago S. Colour Doppler ultrasound study in patients with frontal fibrosing alopecia. Skin Res Technol. 2021;27:709–14.
14. Lawson CN, Bakayoko A, Callender VD. Central centrifugal cicatricial alopecia. Dermatol Clin. 2021;39:389–405.
15. Heath. Central centrifugal cicatricial alopecia. J Fam Pract. 2022;71:71.
16. Miteva M, Tosti A. Central centrifugal cicatricial alopecia presenting with irregular patchy alopecia on the lateral and posterior scalp. Skin Appendage Disord. 2015;1:1–5.
17. Khalil J, Kurban M, Abbas O. Follicular mucinosis: a review. Int J Dermatol. 2021;60:159–65.
18. LaSenna C, Miteva M. Special stains and immunohistochemical stains in hair pathology. Am J Dermatopathol. 2016;38:327–37.
19. Tberg IO, Oon H, Ang K, Lzolibani BAA, Erry J, Hapiro S. Dermatologic therapy folliculitis decalvans. Dermatol Ther. 2008;21:238–44.
20. Sarkis A, Cortez de Almeida RF, Lemes LR, Obadia DL, Machado CJ, Müller-Ramos P, et al. Folliculitis decalvans in women: a retrospective multicentre study of 150 patients. J Eur Acad Dermatol Venereol. 2024;38:38.
21. Saceda-Corralo D, Moreno-Arrones OM, Rodrigues-Barata R, Rubio-Lombraña M, Mir-Bonafé JF, Morales-Raya C, et al. Trichoscopy activity scale for folliculitis decalvans. J Eur Acad Dermatol Venereol. 2020;34:e55.
22. Larrondo J, McMichael AJ. Scarring alopecia. Dermatol Clin. 2023;41:519–37.
23. Wortsman X, Wortsman J, Matsuoka L, Saavedra T, Mardones F, Saavedra D, et al. Sonography in pathologies of scalp and hair. Br J Radiol. 2012;85:647–55.
24. Melo DF, Lemes LR, Pirmez R, Duque-Estrada B. Trichoscopic stages of dissecting cellulitis: a potential complementary tool to clinical assessment. An Bras Dermatol. 2020;95:514–7.
25. Lee C, Chen W, Hsu C, Weng T, Lee JY, Yang C. Dissecting folliculitis (dissecting cellulitis) of the scalp: a 66-patient case series and proposal of classification. J Dtsch Dermatol Ges. 2018;16:1219–26.
26. Vañó-Galván S, Saceda-Corralo D, Blume-Peytavi U, Cucchía J, Dlova NC, Gavazzoni Dias MFR, et al. Frequency of the types of alopecia at twenty-two specialist hair clinics: a multicenter study. Skin Appendage Disord. 2019;5:309–15.
27. Cataldo-Cerda K, Wortsman X. Dissecting cellulitis of the scalp early diagnosed by color doppler ultrasound. Int J Trichol. 2017;9:147–8.
28. Rigopoulos D, Stamatios G, Ioannides D. Primary scarring alopecias. In: Current problems in dermatology. S. Karger AG; 2015. p. 76–86. https://karger.com/books/book/229/chapter/5157826.
29. Al Aboud DM, Badri T. Acne keloidalis nuchae continuing education activity. StatPearls Publishing; 2024. https://www.ncbi.nlm.nih.gov/books/NBK459135/.
30. Chouk C, Litaiem N, Jones M, Zeglaoui F. Acne keloidalis nuchae: clinical and dermoscopic features. BMJ Case Rep. 2017;2017:bcr2017222222.
31. Chambert J, Lihoreau T, Joly S, Chatelain B, Sandoz P, Humbert P, et al. Multimodal investigation of a keloid scar by combining mechanical tests in vivo with diverse imaging techniques. J Mech Behav Biomed Mater. 2019;99:206–15.
32. Alkhalifah A, Alsantali A, Wang E, McElwee KJ, Shapiro J. Alopecia areata update. J Am Acad Dermatol. 2010;62:177–88.
33. Strazzulla LC, Wang EHC, Avila L, Lo Sicco K, Brinster N, Christiano AM, et al. Alopecia areata. J Am Acad Dermatol. 2018;78:1–12.
34. Pirmez R. The dermatoscope in the hair clinic: trichoscopy of scarring and nonscarring alopecia. J Am Acad Dermatol. 2023;89:S9–15.
35. Ávila de Almeida C, Guarçoni S, Leverone A, Nakamura R, Marchiori E, Canella C. Characterization of a glomus tumor using 33-MHz ultrasound and superb microvascular imaging, vol. 27. Skin Res Technol; 2021. p. 466–8.

36. Mikiel D, Polańska A, Żaba R, Adamski Z, Dańczak-Pazdrowska A. Usefulness of high-frequency ultrasonography in the assessment of alopecia areata—comparison of ultrasound images with trichoscopic images. Postepy Dermatol Alergol. 2022;39:132–40.
37. Rodríguez-Cuadrado FJ, Martínez-Mera C, Roustan-Gullón G, Alfageme-Roldán F. Trichosonography: ultrasound of alopecias and hair disorders. J Ultrasound. 2025:28(1):137–50.
38. de Lacharrière O, Deloche C, Misciali C, Piraccini BM, Vincenzi C, Bastien P, et al. Hair diameter diversity: a clinical sign reflecting the follicle miniaturization. Arch Dermatol. 2001;137:641–6.
39. Gan DCC, Sinclair RD. Prevalence of male and female pattern hair loss in Maryborough. J Investig Dermatol Symp Proc. 2005;10:184–9.
40. Wortsman X, Guerrero R, Wortsman J. Hair morphology in androgenetic alopecia. J Ultrasound Med. 2014;33:1265–72.
41. Asghar F, Shamim N, Farooque U, Sheikh H, Aqeel R. Telogen effluvium: a review of the literature. Cureus. 2020;12:e8320.
42. Elizabeth Hughes C, Syed HA, Saleh D. Telogen effluvium continuing education activity. StatPearls Publishing; 2024. https://www.ncbi.nlm.nih.gov/books/NBK430848/?report=printable.
43. Seyfi S, Alijanpour R, Aryanian Z, Ezoji K, Mahmoudi M. Prevalence of telogen effluvium hair loss in COVID-19 patients and its relationship with disease severity. J Med Life. 2022;15:631–4.
44. Pereyra AD, Saadabadi A. Trichotillomania. StatPearls Publishing; 2024.
45. Grant JE, Chamberlain SR. Trichotillomania. Am J Psychiatry. 2016;173:868–74.
46. Corona-Rodarte E, Cano-Aguilar LE, Baldassarri-Ortego LF, Tosti A, Asz-Sigall D. Dermatological perspectives on pressure alopecias: a call for awareness. J Am Acad Dermatol. 2024;90:e133–4.
47. Corona-Rodarte E, Cano-Aguilar LE, Baldassarri-Ortego LF, Tosti A, Asz-Sigall D. Pressure alopecias: A review. J Am Acad Dermatol. 2024;90(1):125–32.
48. Neema S, Vashisht D, Yadav A, Sinha A, Radhakrishnan S. Trichoscopy of pressure-induced alopecia and alopecia areata: a comparative study. Int J Trichology. 2022;14:17. https://doi.org/10.4103/ijt.ijt_46_20.

Further Reading

Desai K, Miteva M. Recent insight on the management of lupus erythematosus alopecia. Clin Cosmet Investig Dermatol. 2021;14:333–47.

Chapter 8
Clinical, Imaging, and Histological Findings in Infectious Lesions of the Scalp

Lara Franceschetto Milleri, Maria Carolina Zafra Páez, Manuela Boleira Sieiro Guimarães, André da Silva Cartell, Carolina Ávila de Almeida, Clarissa Canella Moraes do Carmo, and Bruna Duque-Estrada

This chapter delves into the complex world of scalp infections, focusing on three key conditions: myiasis, tinea capitis, and herpes zoster. Each of these infections can cause distinctive symptoms and require tailored approaches for effective management. Understanding the role of imaging modalities, particularly ultrasonography, is crucial in the diagnosis and treatment planning for these conditions. Ultrasonography offers a noninvasive and detailed view of the scalp's structural changes, aiding in the accurate identification and differentiation of infectious lesions. By exploring the diagnostic imaging techniques and their application in identifying myiasis, tinea capitis, and herpes zoster, this chapter aims to enhance the clinician's ability to effectively address these scalp infections and improve patient outcomes.

L. F. Milleri
BCM Dermatologia Especializada – Private Practice, Rio de Janeiro, Brazil

M. C. Z. Páez
Zafra Dermatology Private Clinic, Rio de Janeiro, Brazil

BCM Dermatologia Especializada, Private Practice, Rio de Janeiro, Brazil

M. B. S. Guimarães
Dermatology Department, Policlinica geral do Rio de Janeiro, Castelo, RJ, Brazil

A. da Silva Cartell
Adjunct Professor at Faculdade de Medicina da Universidade Federal do Rio Grande do Sul, Rio de Janeiro, Brazil

Dermatologist and Dermatopathologist in Private Practice, Rio de Janeiro, Brazil

C. Á. de Almeida
Faculty of Medicine of Valença—UniFaa, Valença, Brazil

Federal University of Rio de Janeiro—UFRJ, Rio de Janeiro, Brazil

© The Author(s), under exclusive license to Springer Nature Switzerland AG 2025

C. Canella Moraes do Carmo (ed.), *Atlas of Diagnostic Imaging in Dermatology*,
https://doi.org/10.1007/978-3-031-77987-9_8

8.1 Tinea Capitis and Kerion Celsi

8.1.1 Definition [1]

- Tinea capitis is a fungal infection of the scalp, most prevalent in children.
- Tinea capitis can be caused by various dermatophytes, primarily from the genera *Trichophyton* and *Microsporum*. Common pathogens include *Trichophyton tonsurans* and *Microsporum canis*.
- Kerion Celsi is a painful, purulent inflammatory mass on the scalp resulting from an intense immune response to a dermatophyte infection of hair follicles.
- Kerion is often associated with zoophilic dermatophytes.

8.1.2 Epidemiology [1]

- Tinea capitis most commonly affects children aged 3–7 years. It is rare in infants and adults.
- Gender predilection varies among studies, with some showing no preference, others reporting a higher prevalence in boys, and some indicating the highest prevalence among African-American girls.
- Short hair is associated with higher incidence due to easier fungal spore access to the scalp.
- Rural populations have a higher risk of developing kerion compared to suburban populations, possibly due to more frequent contact with animals.

8.1.3 Clinical Presentation (Fig. 8.1) [1]

- Characterized by scaling, patchy alopecia, broken and hypopigmented hairs.
- Inflammatory Kerion: a tender, boggy plaque, with pustules, crusting and purulent discharge, often misdiagnosed as bascteial abscess. Hairl loss may be temporary seen.

C. Canella Moraes do Carmo (✉)
Fluminense Federal University—UFF, Rio de Janeiro, Brazil

Federal University of Rio de Janeiro—UFRJ, Rio de Janeiro, Brazil

Diagnóstico das Américas—DASA—RJ, Rio de Janeiro, Brazil

Biodesign Laboratory, DASA-PUC, Rio de Janeiro, Brazil

B. Duque-Estrada
BCM Dermatologia Especializada, Private Practice, Rio de Janeiro, Brazil

Universidade Federal de São Paulo, São Paulo, Brazil

Hair Diseases Department, Instituto de Dermatologia Professor Rubem David Azulay – Santa Casa da Misericórdia do Rio de Janeiro, Rio de Janeiro, Brazil

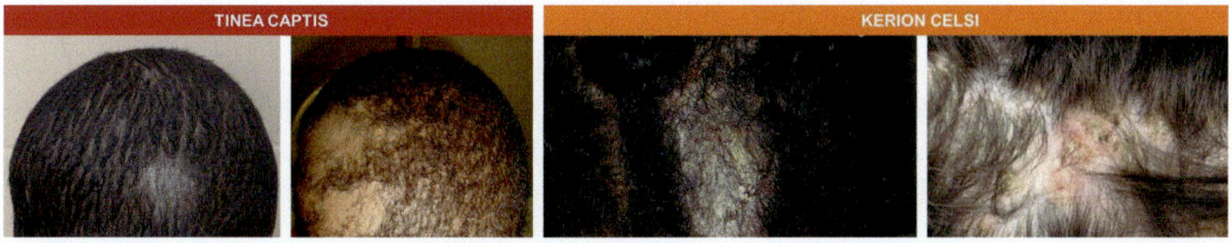

Fig. 8.1 Clinical photograph of patient with Kerion Celsi (Courtesy from Dr. Leonardo Spagnol Abraham)

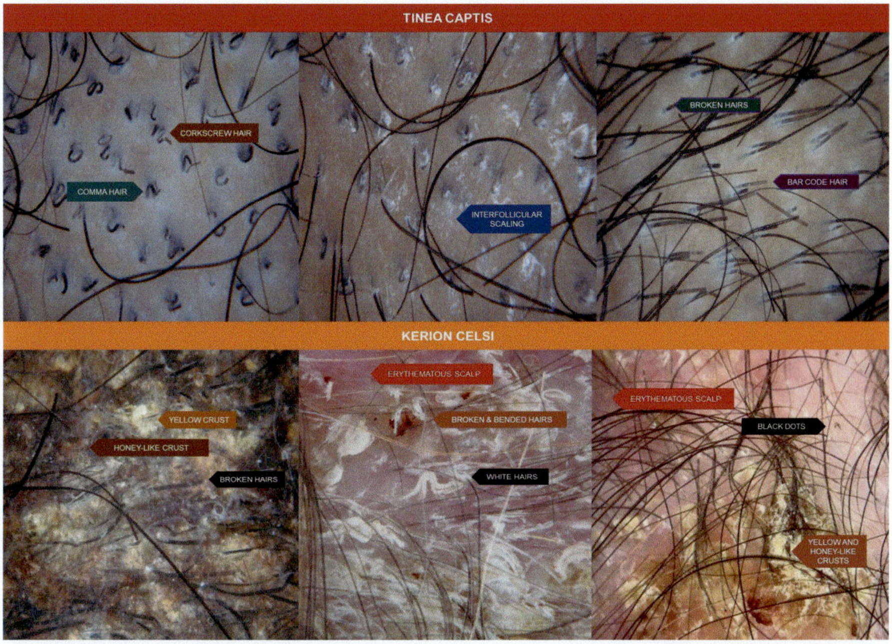

Fig. 8.2 Trichoscopy of tinea capitis (x20 and x50 with and without immersion fluid) (Courtesy from Dr. Leonardo Spagnol Abraham)

- Non-inflammatory Kerion: characterized by a patchy alopecia, with diffuse scaling or cicatricial. Regional lymphoadenopathy may occur.

8.1.4 Trichoscopy (Fig. 8.2) [2]

Characteristic trichoscopic features of tinea capitis include:

- Comma hairs (short C-shaped hairs).
- Corkscrew hairs (Twisted hairs).
- Morse code-like hairs (bar code hairs).
- Zigzag hairs (Bent hairs with sharp angles).

- Bent hairs (Bent without shortening).
- Block hairs and i-Hairs (Short hairs with transverse ends).
- Common but nonspecific features (broken hairs, black dots, diffuse scaling, perifollicular scaling, casts, trichorrexis nodosa).
- Species-Specific Clues:
  - Microsporum: Morse code-like hairs, zigzag hairs, bent hairs, and diffuse scaling.
  - Trichophyton: Corkscrew hairs.

8.1.5 Histopathology (Fig. 8.3) [1, 2]

- Endothrix and ectothrix infections are characterized by numerous fungal spores, and occasionally hyphae, located within (endothrix) or outside (ectothrix) the hair shaft, easily identified by Periodic acid–Schiff (PAS) staining.

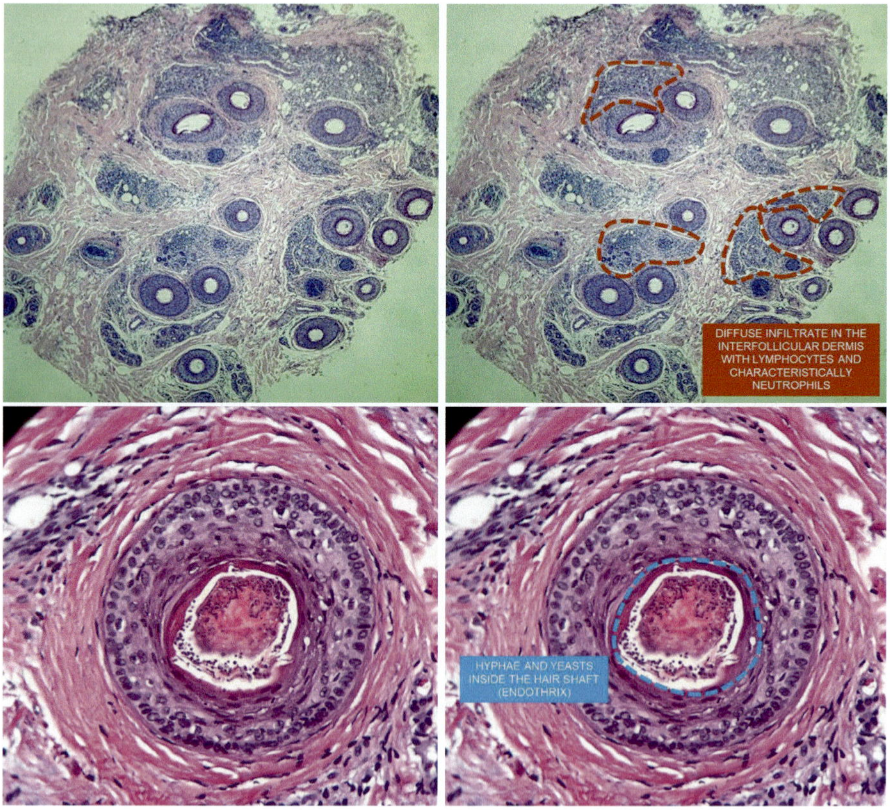

Fig. 8.3 Histological findings of tinea capitis

- Perifollicular fibrosis and mixed inflammatory infiltrate involving affected follicles—sometimes in a markedly brisk pattern—are observed, along with a corneal leukofibrinoid crust overlying the lesion.
- Highly inflamed variants can lead to edematous nodules and plaques, suppurative content, follicular destruction, granulomatous response, and subsequent cicatricial alopecia (Kerion).
- In other cases, it could have a dissecting cellulitis pattern.

8.1.6 *Ultrasonography (Fig. 8.4)*

- Ultrasonography reveals areas of low echogenicity within the scalp caused by edema, which appears as hypoechoic regions.
- The presence of fistulous tracts extending to hair follicles is indicative of infection and inflammation.
- Disrupted areas on the ultrasonography reflect the scarring process occurring within the scalp.
- Ultrasonography can detect retroauricular lymphadenopathy, which correlates with the clinical signs of infection and inflammation in patients with kerion celsi and Tinea Capitis.

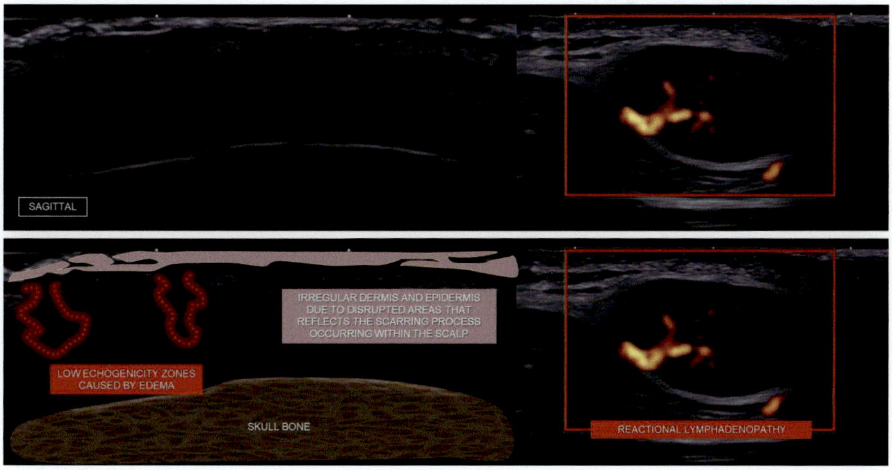

Fig. 8.4 Ultrasonographic findings of Kerion Celsi with a 24 MHz probe (Aplio i800, Canon Medical Systems)

8.2 Myiasis

8.2.1 *Definition [3]*

- Myiasis is a parasitic infestation caused by fly larvae.
- It is typically classified into two types: furuncular and cavitary.
- Furuncular myiasis is commonly associated with the *Dermatobia hominis* fly and usually affects the skin.

8.2.2 *Epidemiology [3]*

- Furuncular myiasis is a prevalent condition in tropical regions, particularly in rural areas of tropical America.
- The condition occurs when fly eggs are transported to the skin by phoretic insects, such as mosquitoes.
- These eggs penetrate the skin through hair follicles or bite perforations and develop into larvae within the subcutaneous tissue.

8.2.3 *Clinical Presentation (Fig. 8.5) [3]*

- Clinically, furuncular myiasis presents as an erythematous, painful nodule with a central orifice that secretes a serous fluid.
- This condition is often mistaken for abscessed lesions.
- Secondary bacterial infections may complicate the primary infestation, necessitating prompt detection and treatment.

8.2.4 *Trichoscopy (Fig. 8.6) [4]*

- The anterior portion of the larva, where the respiratory spiracles are located, can be seen through the cavity orifice. The larva shows recurrent movements toward the surface to breathe.
- When the orifice is occluded, the larva moves to the surface more frequently, facilitating identification.
- Observing a yellowish central structure with spikes around it, depending on the larva's size.
- Using polarized light equipment, although it might require longer observation times to detect larval movements.

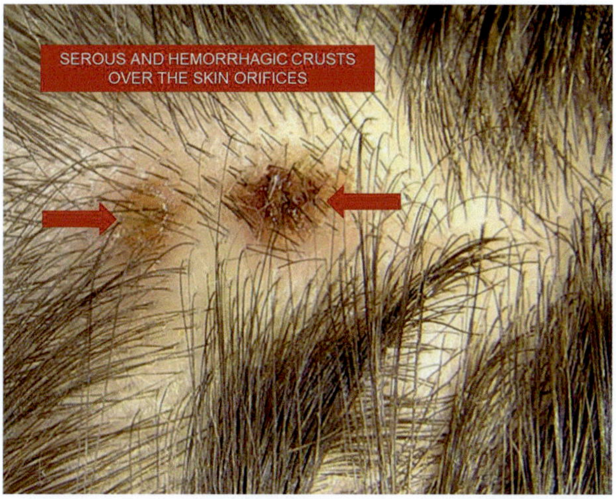

Fig. 8.5 Clinical photograph of patient with furuncular myiasis

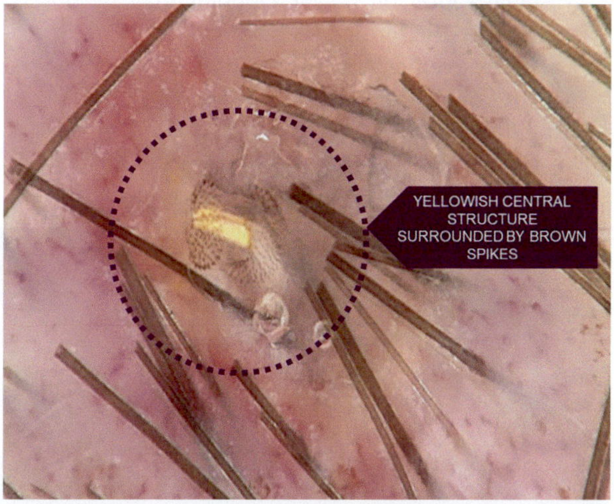

Fig. 8.6 Trichoscopy of a patient with furuncular myiasis (x120)

- Dermoscopy also assists in the treatment of furuncular myiasis. Occlusion of the orifice, for example, with adhesive tape, hinders the larva's ability to breathe, leading to its death. Observing the absence of respiratory movements through dermoscopy confirms the effectiveness of this treatment approach.

8.2.5 Histopathology [5]

- Primary or furunculoid and secondary myiasis. The larva can be seen during macroscopic examination.

- The exoskeleton of the larva consists of wavy chitinous cuticle with pigmented spines.
- Contained in the exoskeleton are the intestinal epithelium, striated muscle, and blood-filled luminal spaces.
- The surrounding tissue shows variably dense infiltration of neutrophils, lymphocytes, histiocytes, and eosinophils.

8.2.6 Ultrasonography (Fig. 8.7) [6–8]

- Hyperechoic area indicating the presence of the larva surrounding by hypoechoic rim.
- Sinus tract crossing through the dermis to the skin surface, representing the larval communication pore with the external environment.
- Hypoechoic area in superficial layers can represent the communication pore.
- Vascularization on power Doppler may be observed due to an inflammatory response to the foreign body.
- Larval movement can be observed and estimates the time since larval penetration.
- Bubbling sign:

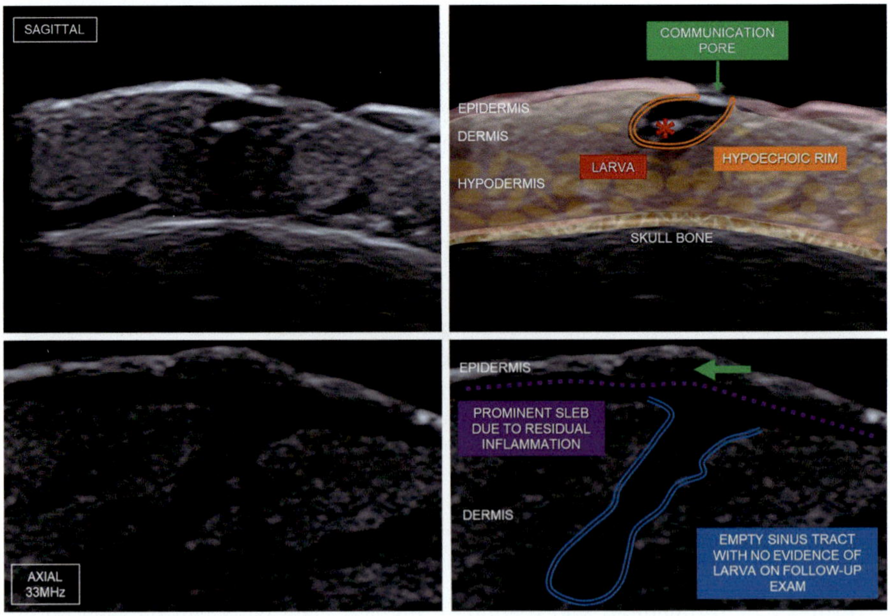

Fig. 8.7 Ultrasonographic findings of furuncular myiasis with a 24 MHz probe (Aplio i800, Canon Medical Systems)

- Observed during ultrasonography examination.
- Occurs when central pore of furuncular lesion is occluded with ultrasonography gel.
- Larval and fluid circulation within central core causes bubbling or fizzing appearance on ultrasonography screen.
- Indicates presence of live larva within lesion.

8.3 Herpes Zoster

8.3.1 Definition [9, 10]

- Herpes zoster, commonly known as shingles, is caused by the reactivation of the varicella zoster virus (VZV), a member of the Herpesviridae family.
- Varicella (chickenpox) is the primary disease caused by VZV, manifesting as a diffuse, contagious vesicular rash.
- Herpes zoster represents the reactivation of the dormant virus in the cranial nerve or sensory root ganglia, resulting in a painful vesicular eruption typically confined to a single dermatome.
- Scalp distribution: often follows the ophthalmic or maxillary branches of the trigeminal nerve.

8.3.2 Epidemiology [10, 11]

- Approximately 95% of the adult population in the western world has been exposed to VZV, putting them at risk for herpes zoster (HZ).
- In the United States, over one million new cases of HZ are diagnosed annually, with an incidence rate of 3 to 4 cases per 1000 persons.
- The lifetime risk of HZ is estimated to be as high as 30%, with about one-third of HZ patients developing post-herpetic neuralgia (PHN), a condition defined by dermatomal neuropathic pain persisting for at least 90 days after the onset of the zoster rash.
- The incidence of HZ is increasing, particularly among the elderly and immunocompromised populations.

8.3.3 Clinical Presentation (Fig. 8.8) [9, 10, 12]

- Herpes zoster typically presents with a painful, erythematous vesicular rash confined to a single dermatome.

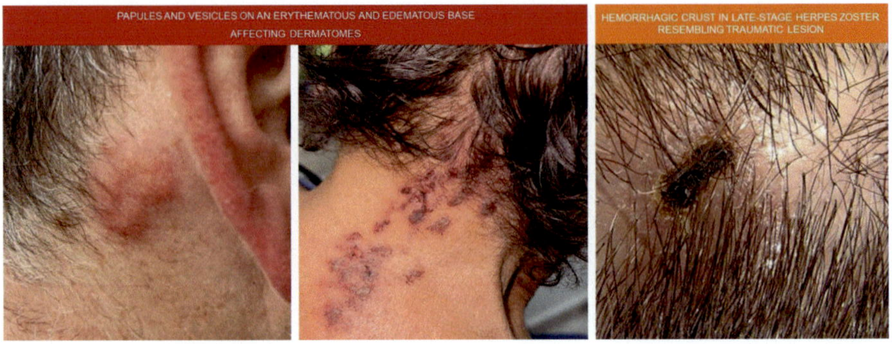

Fig. 8.8 Clinical photographs of herpes zoster (x20) (Courtesy from Dr. Felipe Aguinaga)

- Pain precedes rash: burning, tingling, or sharp pain may appear days before lesions.
- Usually, ir has a unilateral involvement.
- The condition may also present atypically, with manifestations such as zoster sine herpete (characterized by neuropathic pain without a rash) or bilateral herpes zoster (where lesions appear on both sides of the body).
- Complications can include post-herpetic neuralgia (PHN), herpes zoster ophthalmicus (affecting the eye), Ramsay-Hunt syndrome (affecting the facial nerve), and other neurological conditions, such as aseptic meningitis and transverse myelitis.
- Grouped vesicles on an erythematous base along a dermatomal distribution is the typical presentation, which evolve to crusting and scabbing. Alopecia (temporary or cicatricial) can develop due to crusting and scabbing in affected areas.

8.3.4 Trichoscopy (Fig. 8.9) [13]

- Dermoscopy is not typically a primary tool for diagnosing herpes zoster. Diagnosis is usually clinical, based on the distinctive rash and symptoms.
- Early herpes zoster lesions:
  - Multiple poly-lobular gray and brown globules.
  - Gray globules covered by a grayish veil-like structure with a gray rim.
  - Yellowish-orange structures surrounding the pigment globules.
  - Presence of red areas and scales.
  - Background is bright pink.

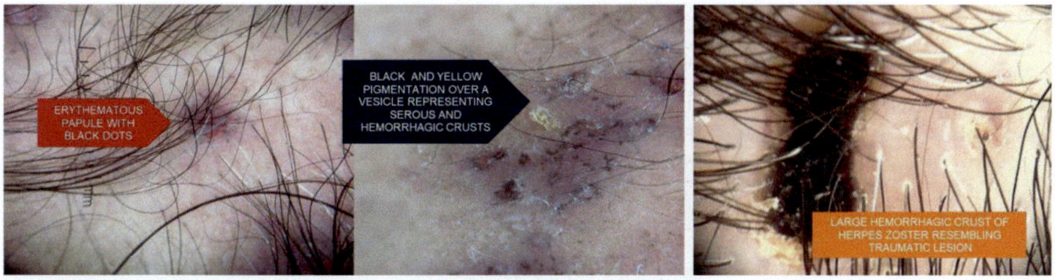

Fig. 8.9 Trichoscopy herpes zoster (x20) (Courtesy from Dr. Felipe Aguinaga)

- Late herpes zoster lesions:
  - Polylobular gray and brown structures surrounded by an erythematous zone, resembling a "solar eclipse" pattern.
  - Multiple brown and gray dots.
  - 'Crumpled fabric' appearance, describing the folding of the roof of flaccid bullae in late lesions.

8.3.5 Histopathology [14]

- Histopathology shows that the virus primarily affects epithelial cells. Infected epithelial cells exhibit acantholysis, nuclear clearing and nuclear enlargement, which have been termed ballooning degeneration.
- The acantholytic epithelial cells are termed Tzanck cells (not specific for herpes; refers to a free-floating epithelial cell in any intraepithelial vesicle). Nucleolar fragmentation occurs with condensation of chromatin around the periphery of the nucleus.
- Multinucleated, infected epithelial cells are formed when fusion occurs between adjacent cells. Intercellular edema develops and leads to the formation of an intraepithelial vesicle. Blister rupture and secondary pustulization often occur.

8.3.6 Ultrasonography (Fig. 8.10) [15]

- Ultrasonography can sometimes reveal thickening of the nerve root.
- Inflammatory changes of dermis and hypodermis characterized by dermal thickening with increased echogenicity. Power Doppler may occasionally reveal vascularization, reflecting an underlying inflammatory response.

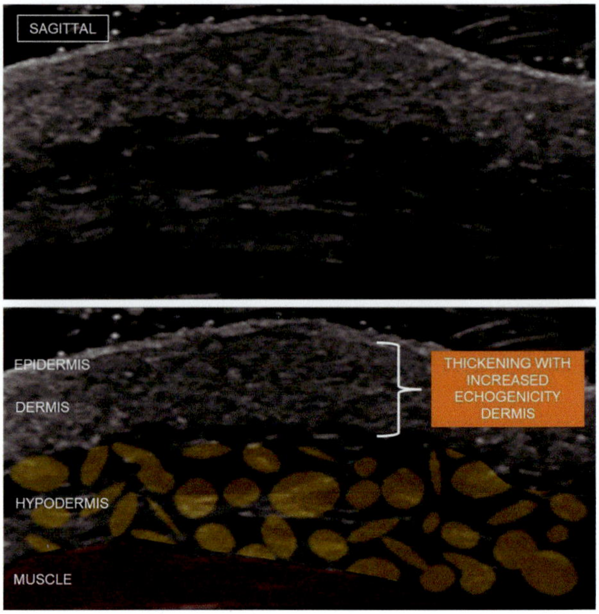

Fig. 8.10 Ultrasonographic findings of herpes zoster with a 24 MHz probe (Aplio i800, Canon Medical Systems)

References

1. John AM, Schwartz RA, Janniger CK. The kerion: an angry tinea capitis. Int J Dermatol. 2018;57:3–9.
2. Waskiel-Burnat A, Rakowska A, Sikora M, Ciechanowicz P, Olszewska M, Rudnicka L. Trichoscopy of tinea capitis: a systematic review. Dermatol Ther (Heidelb). 2020;10:43–52. https://doi.org/10.1007/s13555-019-00350-1.
3. Cardoso AEC, Cardoso AEO, Talhari C, Santos M. Update on parasitic dermatoses. An Bras Dermatol. 2020;95:1–14.
4. Bakos RM, Reinehr C, Escobar GF, Leite LL. Dermoscopy of skin infestations and infections (entomodermoscopy)—part I: dermatozoonoses and bacterial infections. An Bras Dermatol. 2021;96:735–45.
5. Hausdörfer-Scheiff S, Bourlond A, Pirard C. Histopathological aspects of Myiasis. Dermatology. 1993;186:298–300.
6. de Almeida CÁ, Nakamura R, Leverone A, Costa F, Estrada BD, Haui P, et al. Imaging features for the evaluation of skin and nail infections. Skeletal Radiol. 2024;53:2051. https://doi.org/10.1007/s00256-023-04557-4.
7. Papineni V, Dieu S, Rennie WJ. The human botfly “bubbling sign”: ultrasound features of cutaneous furuncular myiasis. Indian J Radiol Imaging. 2023;33:121–3. https://doi.org/10.1055/s-0042-1758203.
8. Jones CH, Leon M, Auerbach J, Portillo-Romero J. Ultrasound detection of human botfly Myiasis of the scalp: a case report. Cureus. 2020;12:e11905.
9. Schmader K. Herpes Zoster. Ann Intern Med. 2018;169:ITC17. https://doi.org/10.7326/AITC201808070.
10. Dayan RR, Peleg R. Herpes zoster–typical and atypical presentations. Postgrad Med. 2017;129:567–71.

11. John AR, Canaday DH. Herpes zoster in the older adult. Infect Dis Clin N Am. 2017;31:811–26.
12. Lautenschlager S. Herpes simplex und varizella-zoster-virus-infektionen. Ther Umsch. 2003;60:605–14.
13. Ankad BS, Koti VR, Lallas A. Dermoscopic differentiation of blister beetle dermatitis and herpes zoster: an observational study. Dermatol Pract Concept. 2022;12:e2022180.
14. Shah S, Singaraju S, Einstein A, Sharma A. Herpes zoster: a clinicocytopathological insight. J Oral Maxillofac Pathol. 2016;20:547.
15. Iguchi N, Mano T, Iwasa N, Kikutsuji N, Saito K, Sugie K. An ultrasonographic evaluation for the early detection of nerve root changes in herpes zoster-associated motor paresis. Intern Med. 2023;62:0039–22.

Chapter 9
Clinical, Imaging, and Histological Findings in Congenital Lesions of the Scalp

Maria Carolina Zafra Páez, André da Silva Cartell, Ana Leticia Boff, Carolina Ávila de Almeida, Clarissa Canella Moraes do Carmo, and Bruna Duque-Estrada

This chapter examines major congenital disorders of the scalp, including cutis verticis gyrata, aplasia cutis, and congenital triangular alopecia. These conditions, while relatively rare, can have significant implications for affected individuals, both functionally

M. C. Z. Páez
Zafra Dermatology Private Clinic, Rio de Janeiro, Brazil

BCM Dermatologia Especializada, Private Practice, Rio de Janeiro, Brazil

A. da Silva Cartell
Adjunct Professor at Faculdade de Medicina da Universidade Federal do Rio Grande do Sul, Rio de Janeiro, Brazil

Dermatologist and Dermatopathologist in Private Practice, Rio de Janeiro, Brazil

A. L. Boff
Santa Casa Hospital, Porto Alegre, RS, Brazil

Dermathopathologist Private Practice, Clinica Dermapat, Porto Alegre, RS, Porto Alegre, RS, Brazil

C. Á. de Almeida
Faculty of Medicine of Valença—UniFaa, Valença, Brazil

Federal University of Rio de Janeiro—UFRJ, Rio de Janeiro, Brazil

C. Canella Moraes do Carmo (✉)
Fluminense Federal University—UFF, Rio de Janeiro, Brazil

Federal University of Rio de Janeiro—UFRJ, Rio de Janeiro, Brazil

Diagnóstico das Américas—DASA—RJ, Rio de Janeiro, Brazil

Biodesign Laboratory, DASA-PUC, Rio de Janeiro, Brazil

B. Duque-Estrada
BCM Dermatologia Especializada, Private Practice, Rio de Janeiro, Brazil

Universidade Federal de São Paulo, São Paulo, Brazil

Hair Diseases Department, Instituto de Dermatologia Professor Rubem David Azulay – Santa Casa da Misericordia do Rio de Janeiro, Rio de Janeiro, Brazil

© The Author(s), under exclusive license to Springer Nature Switzerland AG 2025

C. Canella Moraes do Carmo (ed.), *Atlas of Diagnostic Imaging in Dermatology*,
https://doi.org/10.1007/978-3-031-77987-9_9

and aesthetically. To aid in the accurate diagnosis and management of these conditions, advanced imaging techniques such as scalp ultrasonography and magnetic resonance imaging (MRI) are invaluable. Scalp ultrasonography provides detailed, real-time insights into the superficial structures of the scalp, while MRI offers a comprehensive view of deeper tissues and abnormalities. By integrating these imaging modalities into the diagnostic process, this chapter aims to enhance understanding and facilitate more precise and effective treatment strategies for congenital scalp disorders.

9.1 Cutis Verticis Gyrata

9.1.1 Definition [1]

- A rare benign cutaneous disorder characterized by thickened, folded skin of the scalp, forming deep furrows and ridges, resembling the surface of the brain - cerebral sulci and gyri.

9.1.2 Epidemiology [1]

- Primary CVG typically manifests in postpubertal men under 30. In Primary essential CVG, there isn't underlying systemic disease, while in Primary non-essential CVG, it is associated with neurological or ophthalmologic disorders. This variant is called cutis verticis gyrata-intellectual disability.
- Reported prevalence is about 1:100,000 males and 0.026:100,000 females.
- Secondary CVG can occur at any age, with no gender predilection, and is associated to underlying causes such as: inflammatory dermatoses (e.g., psoriasis, eczema), neoplasms (e.g., lipomas, nevi, amyloidosis, plexiform neurofibroma), and endocrine disorders (e.g., acromegaly).

9.1.3 Clinical Presentation (Fig. 9.1) [2]

- Symmetric, redundant scalp folds that exhibit deep furrows and convolutions. The hypertrophy and folding of the skin produce the appearance of cerebral gyri.

9.1.4 Trichoscopy

- Normal follicular openings in most cases.
- Increased hair density in some areas (depending on associated conditions).

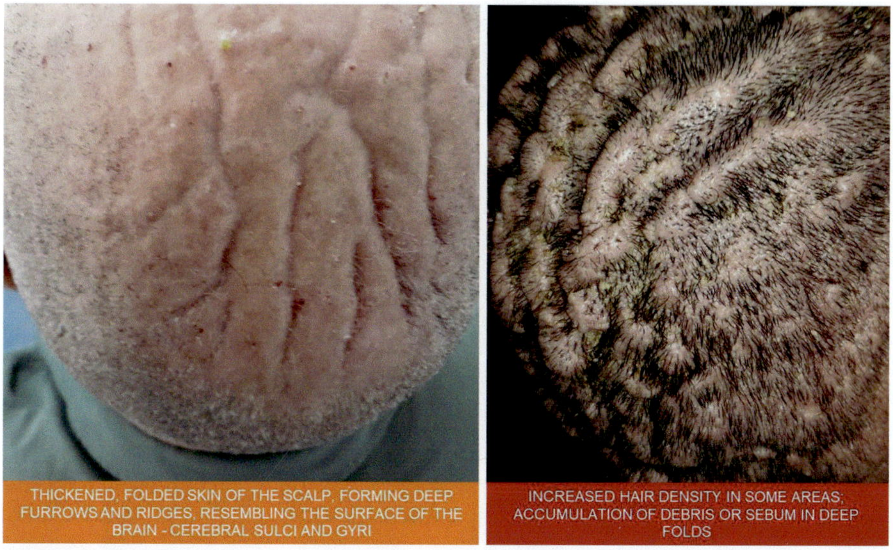

Fig. 9.1 Clinical photograph of two patients with cutis verticis gyrate (Images courtesy from Prof. Luna Azulay)

- Accumulation of debris or sebum in deep folds.
- Absence of scarring or inflammatory changes in primary forms.
- In secondary CVG, trichoscopic changes may reflect the underlying cause (e.g., psoriasis, folliculitis, seborrheic dermatitis).
- Dilated pores or comedones if associated with acne or sebaceous disorders.

9.1.5 Histopathology [1]

- Microscopic findings of cutis verticis gyrata are nonspecific, requiring differentiation from conditions such as acrochordon (fibroepithelial polyp), acanthosis nigricans, and lipoma.
- It may present with epithelial hyperplasia with variable acanthopapilomatosis, proliferation of cutaneous appendages, and thickening of dermal collagen. Without correlation with clinical aspects, the diagnosis may be unspecific.

9.1.6 Computed Tomography (Fig. 9.2) [3]

- Essential for assessing brain and orbital involvement in primary CVG.
- Scalp thickening with prominent ridges and furrows are observed.
- Skull is unaffected.

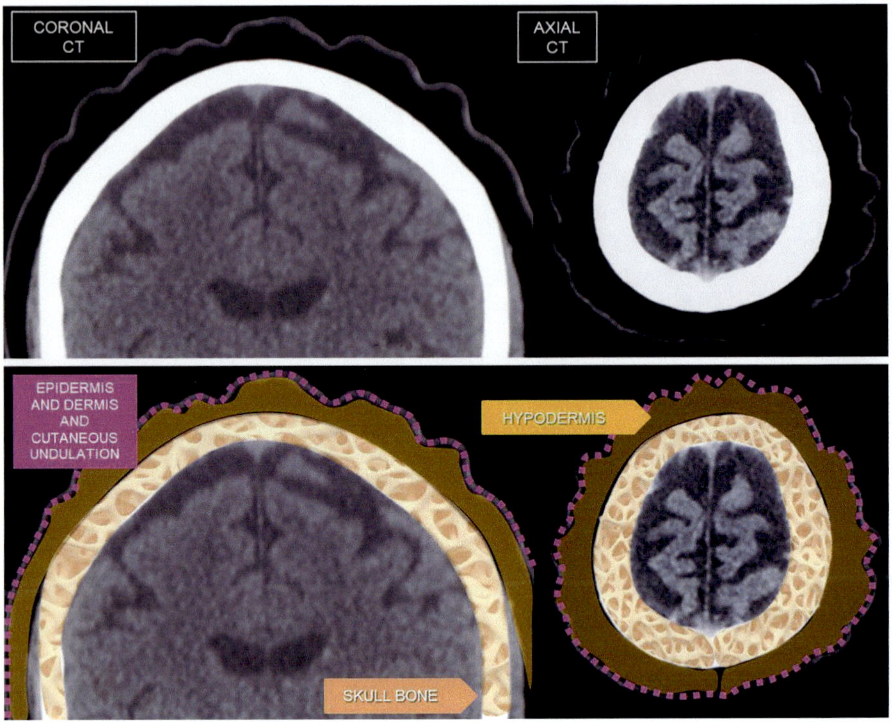

Fig. 9.2 Computed tomography findings of cutis verticis gyrate on coronal and axial reconstruction (Philips Brilliance CT 64-slice)

9.1.7 Ultrasonography (Fig. 9.3) [4]

- Dermal and hypodermal thickening that corresponded with the elevated clinical zones.
- Scalp folds with normal cutaneous thickness, showing undulation of the cutaneous layers in all cases.
- No significant dilation of the hair follicles was detected.

9.1.8 MRI [5]

- MRI reveals three scalp layers: epidermis, dermis, subcutaneous fat, galea, subgalea, and periosteum complex.
- Abnormal thickening of skin and subcutaneous tissues leads to scalp folds.
- Scalp thickening due to hyperplasia of connective tissues and fat.
- Better identified in coronal images.

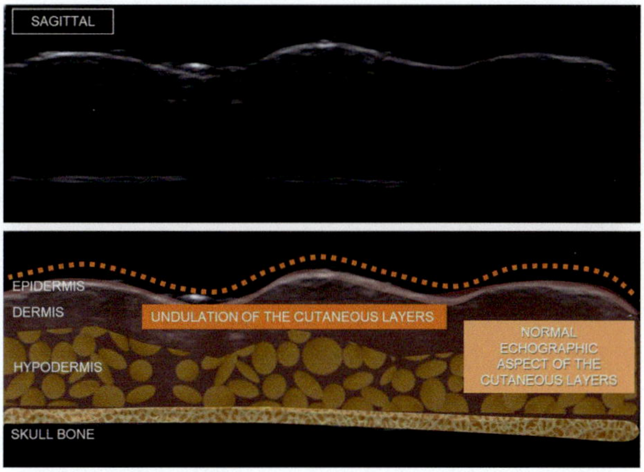

Fig. 9.3 Ultrasonographic findings of cutis verticis gyrata with a 24 MHz probe (Aplio i800, Canon Medical Systems)

9.2 Congenital Triangular Alopecia

9.2.1 Definition [6]

- Congenital triangular alopecia (CTA), also referred to as temporal triangular alopecia or Brauer nevus.
- A benign, asymptomatic, nonscarring and nonprogressive patchy hair loss.
- Typically affects the frontotemporal region of the scalp.
- The pattern of hair loss is traditionally described as triangular, oval, or lancet-shaped with apex toward to vertex.
- Can manifest at birth or develop later in life, but is often noted during infancy or childhood.

9.2.2 Epidemiology [6]

- There is no gender predilection.
- The incidence in the general population is estimated to be 0.11%.
- Present at birth or develop later in life.
- 79% of cases presented with unilateral hair loss.
- 18.5% of cases had bilateral involvement.
- 2.5% of cases involved occipital alopecia.
- Most cases reported in Caucasian patients, but also documented in Asians and African-Americans.

9.2.3 Clinical Presentation (Fig. 9.4) [7]

- Triangular or oval patch of alopecia in the temporal area, however it has been described in parietal, occipital and vertex areas.
- The area of involvement is usually only a few centimeters in diameter.
- Most cases are unilateral, though bilateral involvement may also occur.
- Fine vellus hairs are visible in the affected area with close inspection.

9.2.4 Trichoscopy (Fig. 9.5) [8]

- The most typical trichoscopic finding is the "carpet" of vellus hairs inside the alopecia patch, which may present length diversity.
- Empty follicular ostia, and white hairs are also described.
- Trichoscopy is specially important when a lesion of triangular alopecia presents in an unusual area of the scalp, or later in adulthood.

9.2.5 Histopathology [8]

- Microscopy is not highly specific, as both epidermis and dermis present a normal appearance. Hair count in cross-sections shows nosignificant changes, and the diagnosis is primarily made by clinical and trichoscopic findings.
- Occasionally, only vellus hairs may be present without any terminal hair.

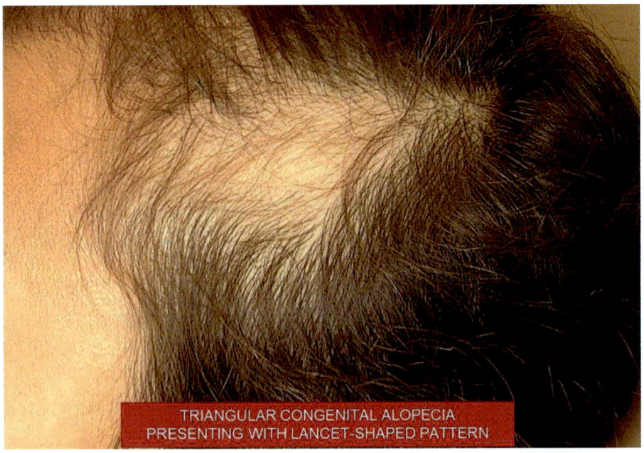

Fig. 9.4 Clinical photograph of patient with congenital triangular alopecia

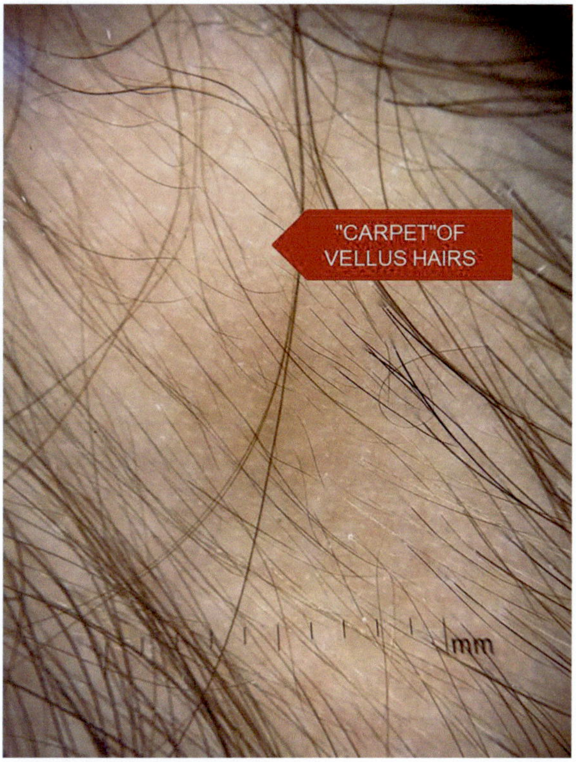

Fig. 9.5 Trichoscopy of a patient with congenital triangular alopecia (X20)

9.2.6 Ultrasonography (Fig. 9.6)

- Normal echographic appearances for both the epidermis and dermis.
- Follicles are present, although they may be less numerous.
- Sometimes only vellus follicles are observed, without any terminal hairs.

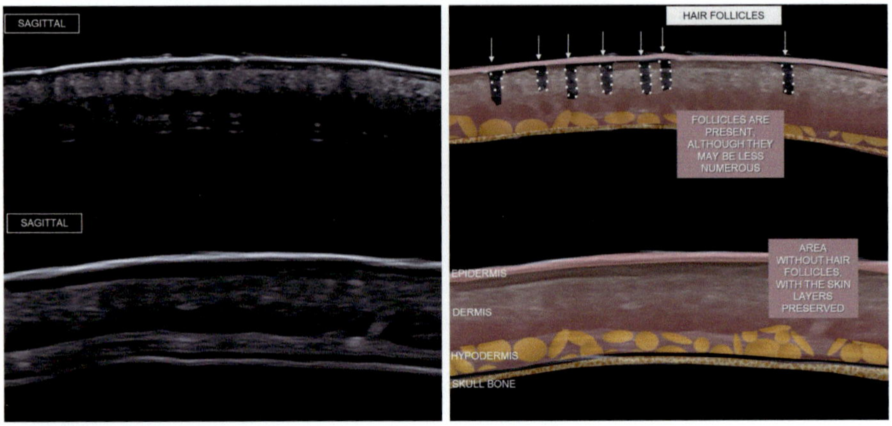

Fig. 9.6 Ultrasonographic findings of congenital triangular alopecia with a24 MHz probe (Aplio i800, Canon Medical Systems)

9.3 Aplasia Cutis

9.3.1 Definition [9]

- Aplasia Cutis is a rare congenital skin defect characterized by a focal or extensive absence of the epidermis, dermis, and occasionally subcutaneous tissue. The exact etiology of ACC is not well understood; however, it is likely due to impaired prenatal skin development.

9.3.2 Epidemiology [9]

- Rare congenital condition with an incidence of approximately 1 to 3 out of 10,000 births.
- No significant gender predilection has been reported.

9.3.3 Clinical Presentation (Fig. 9.7) [10, 11]

- Solitary scalp lesions make up approximately 70% of all cases, although multiple lesions affecting the face, trunk, extremities, or any part of the body, can also be observed.
- The surface may present a variable presentation at birth including a granulation tissue, erosion, ulceration, membrane-covered defect, or scar, indicating intrauterine healing.

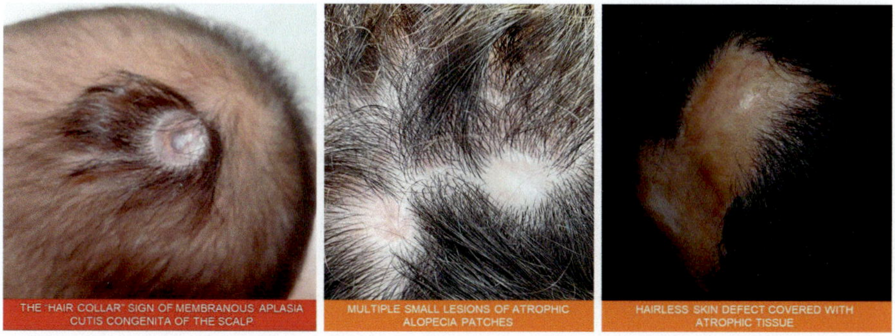

Fig. 9.7 Clinical photograph of patients with Aplasi Cutis Congenita (Courtesy of Dr. Luciana Rodino Lemes and Dr. Verena Florenço)

- Lesions vary in size from a few millimeters up to several centimeters. Large (>1 cm), irregular defects are often associated with defects of the underlying bone, dura, and intracranial vasculature. Underlying morphologic abnormalities occurs in approximately 37% of cases, including underlying bony defects, vascular anomalies, or neurologic malformations. Therefore, it is prudent for clinicians to assess disease involvement using appropriate imaging.
- The "hair collar" sign: Membranous aplasia cutis congenita of the scalp may have an abnormal surrounding circle of coarse, long hair. It is necessary to investigate an underlying neuroectodermal defect.
  - Small, scalp lesions are less likely associated with underlying defects and typically heal on their own within a couple of months; therefore, monitoring these lesions without further imaging is acceptable.
  - A midline vertex scalp lesion, hair collar sign, and vascular stains have all been shown to be strong indicators for cranial or central nervous system (CNS) involvement.
  - For larger, ulcerative lesions, ultrasound provides a relatively inexpensive evaluation while not putting the child through a great deal of discomfort. If there is any concern for underlying defects on ultrasound, further workup with MRI is warranted. MRI is more sensitive and specific for identifying underlying lesions according to a 2017 retrospective multicenter study; however, it is more costly than ultrasound and typically requires the child to be sedated for the duration of the procedure, limiting its utility as an initial screening investigation.
  - If the lesion is purulent or associated with surrounding erythema, laboratory evaluation—including complete blood count, blood cultures, and wound cultures— is recommended [10].

9.3.4 Trichoscopy (Fig. 9.8) [12]

- Translucency sign: shiny surface, with thin telangiectatic vessels.
- Absence of follicular openings on the alopecic area.
- Hair collar sign: hair follicles distributed around the edge of the plaque, and blue globules corresponding to horizontal hair bulbs (blue globules). In non bullous ACC, hair bulbs are arranged in a starburst pattern in the periphery of the patch. In bullous ACC, bulbs are arranged in a "golf club set" pattern, or a parallel pattern.

9.3.5 Histopathology [13]

- Histopathological findings in aplasia cutis are generally nonspecific, emphasizing the importance of clinical correlation. Histopathology may reveal a n discontinuity of the epidermis, granulation tissue at the lesional margin, and varying degrees of dermal fibrosis, ranging from scar-like to keloid-like pattern. These changes are consistent with cicatricial alopecia, characterized by a complete loss of hair follicles in the affected area.

9.3.6 Ultrasonography (Fig. 9.9) [14]

- Ultrasonography can identify the surface layers of the brain in cases of aplasia cutis congenita of the scalp.
- Ultrasonography precisely locates the sagittal sinus, reducing the risk of injury and potentially fatal complications.

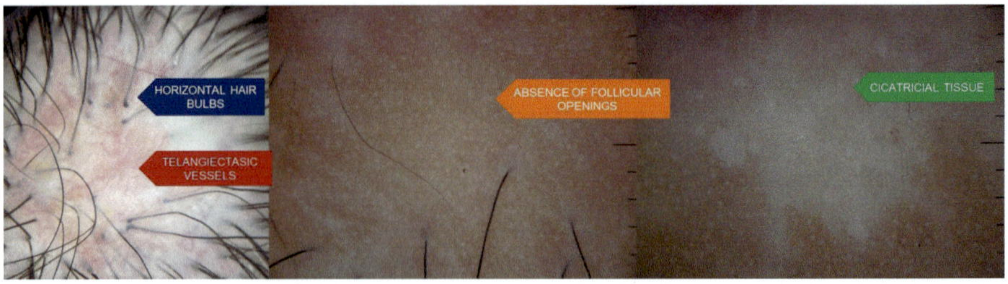

Fig. 9.8 Trichoscopy findings in aplasia cutis (x20) (Images courtesy from Dr. Verena Florenço)

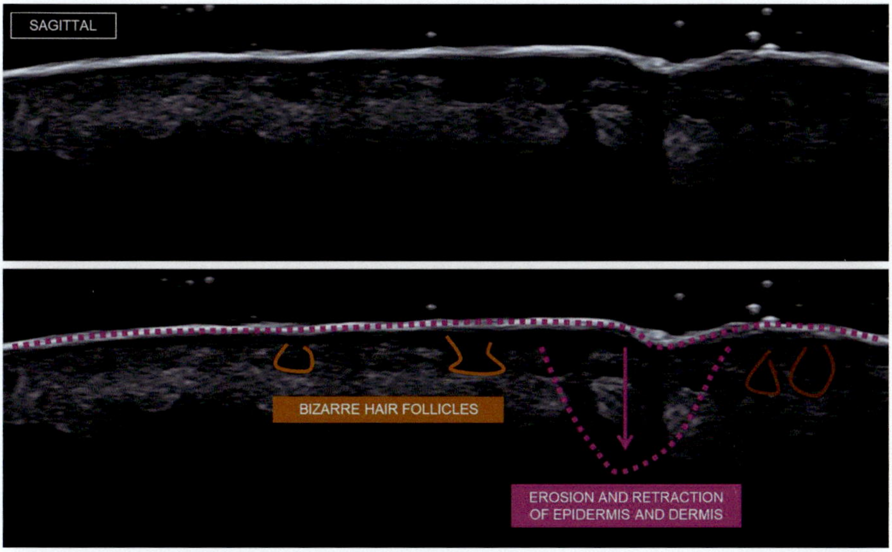

Fig. 9.9 Ultrasonographic findings of Aplasia Cutis Congenita of the scalp with a 24 MHz probe (Aplio i800, Canon Medical Systems)

- Visualization of the dura to evaluate dural defects, reducing risk of brain parenchyma damage and assessing potential brain herniation areas. Neural tube defects such as meningocele often manifesting as a midline lesion on the scalp covered by skin or a thin membrane. Ultrasonography is useful in confirming continuity with the central nervous system to support the diagnosis.
- Some membranous aplasia cutis congenita lesions may clinically resemble congenital dermoid cysts; however, they are typically more translucent. Ultrasonography can aid in confirming the diagnosis by demonstrating the characteristic cystic appearance and features of dermoid cysts, thus assisting in the differential diagnosis.

9.3.7 MRI [15]

- MRI reveals absence of the scalp layers.
- MRI may detect cutaneous ulceration of the scalp.
- Exact location and depth of the sagittal sinus can be determined.

9.4 Nevus Sebaceous of Jadassohn

9.4.1 Definition [16]

- Sebaceous nevus of Jadassohn, also known as nevus sebaceous, is a rare congenital malformation characterized as a non-hereditary hamartoma involving the adnexal structures of the skin.
- These structures include the epithelial, sebaceous, follicular, and apocrine elements. The condition results from hyperplasia of these skin components.
- The etiology of nevus sebaceous is not fully understood but is believed to involve post-zygotic mutations in the HRAS, NRAS, and KRAS genes.

9.4.2 Epidemiology [16]

- The incidence of sebaceous nevus in newborns ranges from 0.1% to 0.3%.
- The condition does not show any predilection for sex or ethnicity.
- Although familial cases have been reported, lesions typically appear sporadically.
- The common areas affected include the scalp (62.5%), cephalic segment (24.5%), trunk (4.7%), and cervical region (4.2%).
- Despite the benign nature of the condition, about 10% to 20% of cases may develop secondary neoplasms, with around 3% exhibiting malignancy, such as basal cell carcinoma and squamous cell carcinoma.

9.4.3 Clinical Findings (Fig. 9.10) [16]

- Nevus sebaceous manifests as plaques that can be alopecic and vary in color from skin-colored to yellowish-orange or brownish-black.

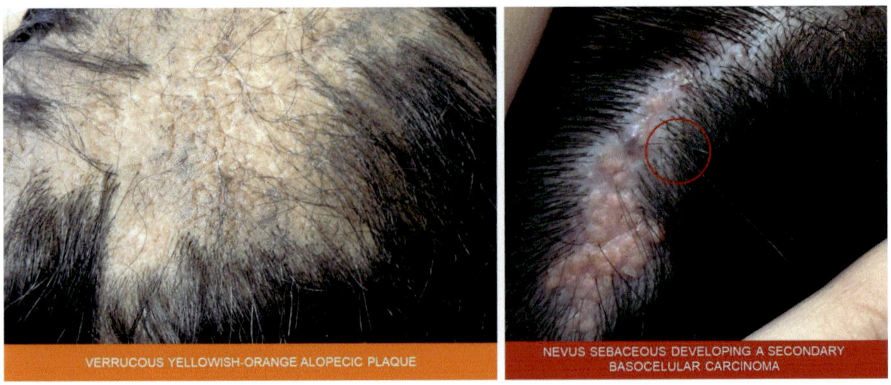

Fig. 9.10 Clinical photograph of a patient with a nevus sebaceous of Jadassohn

- The texture of these plaques can be smooth, nipple-like, or verrucous, depending on their stage of development.
- Commonly affected areas include the scalp, face, and neck, though lesions may also occur on the trunk and extremities, following Blaschko's lines.
- The clinical course of nevus sebaceous can be divided into three stages:
  - Infancy and childhood: Lesions appear as smooth, hairless patches or spots, typically pale or slightly yellowish.
  - Puberty: Hormonal influences cause hyperplasia of the sebaceous glands, leading to a verrucous appearance and more intense coloration due to hyperkeratosis, papillomatosis, and acanthosis.
  - Adulthood: There is an increased risk of secondary neoplasm development.
- Extracutaneous manifestations
  - When nevus sebaceous is associated with systemic abnormalities, it constitutes the linear nevus syndrome or Schimmelpenning-Feuerstein-Mims syndrome. This syndrome can involve a variety of organs and systems, leading to conditions such as hypophosphatemic rickets, intellectual disability, coloboma, strabismus, craniofacial defects, seizures, and various other neurological, ocular, cardiovascular, and genitourinary abnormalities.

9.4.4 Dermoscopy (Fig. 9.11) [16]

- The lesion often shows a homogenous yellow-orange background color, reflecting the sebaceous gland hyperplasia.
- Fine, linear, or branching blood vessels can be seen across the lesion, which is a common feature in sebaceous proliferations.

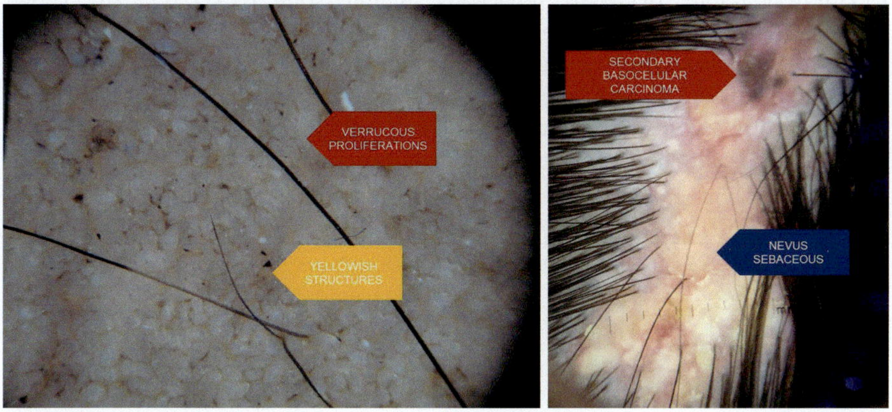

Fig. 9.11 Dermoscopy findings of a patient with a nevus sebaceous of Jadassohn (x20)

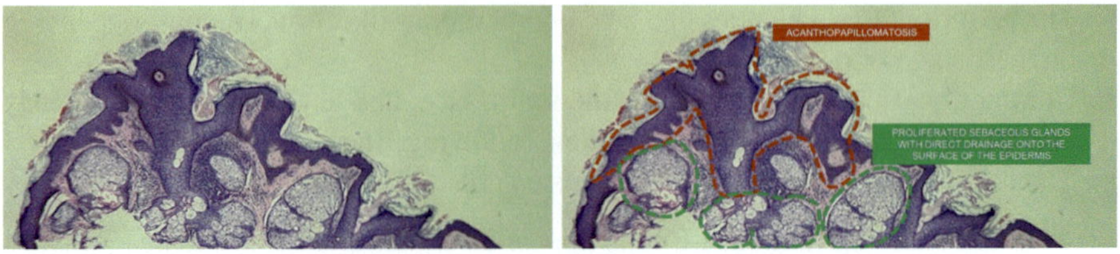

Fig. 9.12 Histological findings of nevus sebaceous of Jadassohn (H&E x4)

- In some cases, the lesion may present with a cerebriform pattern, which appears as brain-like convolutions on dermoscopy, especially in older lesions.
- Large, dilated follicular openings resembling comedones may also be observed.
- Unlike melanocytic lesions, nevus sebaceous lacks a typical pigment network, which helps in differentiating it from other pigmented lesions.

9.4.5 Histopathology (Fig. 9.12) [16]

- Nevus sebaceous exhibits hyperkeratosis, acanthosis, and papillomatosis, with hyperplasia of the sebaceous glands.
- The main concern in histopathological assessment is the potential for developing secondary neoplasms, which can range from benign tumors like trichoblastoma and syringocystadenoma papilliferum to malignant ones such as basal cell carcinoma and squamous cell carcinoma.

9.4.6 Ultrasonography (Figs. 9.13 and 9.14) [17]

- Ultrasonography of nevus sebaceous of Jadassohn (NSJ) typically shows hypoechoic lesions with hyperechoic spots.
- Correlation exists between ultrasonography features and histologic findings, including distorted and hypoechoic pilosebaceous units, presence of villus types of hair follicles, and areas with reduced hair follicles.
- Ultrasonography findings, such as thickening and mild undulation of the epidermis, correspond to histologic features like acanthosis and papillomatosis.

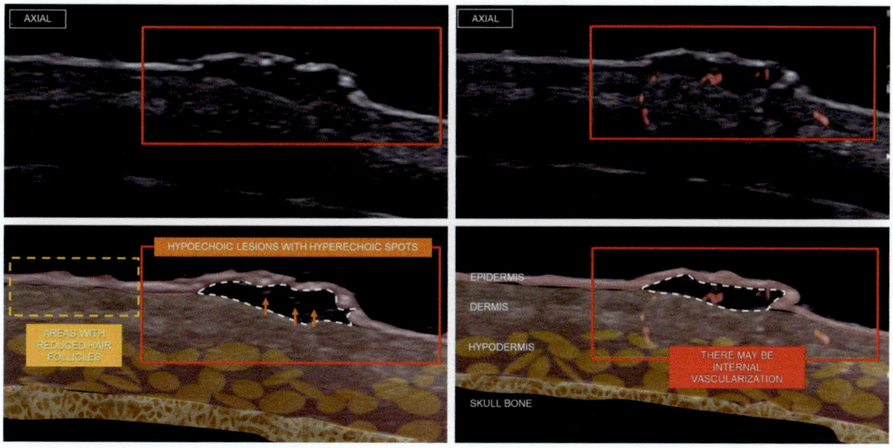

Fig. 9.13 Ultrasonographic findings of a nevus sebaceous of Jadassohn with a 24 MHz probe (Aplio i800, Canon Medical Systems)

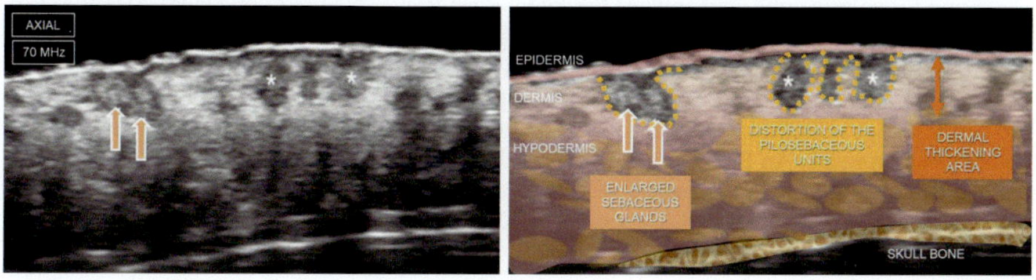

Fig. 9.14 Ultrasonographic findings of a nevus sebaceous of Jadassohn with a 70 MHz probe (Vevo MD Clinical High-Frequency Ultrasound, VisualSonics)

References

1. Shareef S, Horowitz D, Kaliyadan F. Cutis Verticis Gyrata. StatPearls; 2024. http://www.ncbi.nlm.nih.gov/pubmed/27294055.
2. Larsen F, Birchall N. Cutis verticis gyrata: three cases with different aetiologies that demonstrate the classification system. Australas J Dermatol. 2007;48:91–4.
3. Kolawole TM, Al Orainy IA, Patel PJ, Fathuddin S. Cutis verticis gyrata: its computed tomographic demonstration in acromegaly. Eur J Radiol. 1998;27:145–8.
4. Ortiz-Orellana G, Ferreira-Wortsman C, Wortsman X. Ultrasound pattern of cutis Verticis Gyrata. J Ultrasound Med. 2024;43:405–9.
5. Alorainy IA. Magnetic resonance imaging of cutis Verticis Gyrata. J Comput Assist Tomogr. 2008;32:119–23.

6. Yin Li V, Yesudian P. Congenital triangular alopecia. Int J Trichol. 2015;7:48. https://doi.org/10.4103/0974-7753.160089.
7. Guan Z, Shi W, Ren M, Bi T, Su H. Clinical and dermatoscopic features of temporal triangular alopecia in infants. Skin Res Technol. 2023;29:e13294.
8. Karadag Köse Ö, Güleç AT. Temporal triangular alopecia: significance of trichoscopy in differential diagnosis. J Eur Acad Dermatol Venereol. 2015;29:1621–5.
9. Coi A, Barisic I, Garne E, Pierini A, Addor M, Aizpurua Atxega A, et al. Epidemiology of aplasia cutis congenita: a population-based study in Europe. J Eur Acad Dermatol Venereol. 2023;37:581–9.
10. Bessis D, Bigorre M, Malissen N, Captier G, Chiaverini C, Abasq C, et al. The scalp hair collar and tuft signs: a retrospective multicenter study of 78 patients with a systematic review of the literature. J Am Acad Dermatol. 2017;76:478–87.
11. Chessa MA, Filippi F, Patrizi A, Vollono L, Sechi A, D'Ercole M, et al. Aplasia cutis: clinical, dermoscopic findings and management in 45 children. J Eur Acad Dermatol Venereol. 2020;34:e724.
12. Morgado-Carrasco D, Fustà-Novell X. Hallazgos dermatoscópicos en la aplasia cutis membranosa. Diagnóstico diferencial con otras formas de alopecia focal en lactantes. Actas Dermosifiliogr. 2021;112:275–7.
13. Gassenmaier M, Bösmüller H, Metzler G. Aplasia cutis congenita of the scalp: histopathologic features and clinicopathologic correlation in a case series. J Cutan Pathol. 2020;47:439–45.
14. Karakawa R, Yano T, Yoshimatsu H, Koto M, Nakao A, Ichi S. Use of ultra-high-frequency ultrasound for aplasia cutis congenita of the scalp. Plast Reconstr Surg Glob Open. 2021;9:e3876. https://doi.org/10.1097/GOX.0000000000003876.
15. Alexandros B, Dimitrios G, Elias A, Evangelos D, Andreas M, Sotirios P, et al. Aplasia cutis congenita: two case reports and discussion of the literature. Surg Neurol Int. 2017;8:273.
16. Neto MPS, Assis BR, Andrade GR. Sebaceous nevus of Jadassohn: review and clinical-surgical approach. An Bras Dermatol. 2022;97:628–36.
17. Wortsman X, Ferreira-Wortsman C, Corredoira Y. Ultrasound imaging of nevus sebaceous of Jadassohn. J Ultrasound Med. 2021;40:407–15. https://doi.org/10.1002/jum.15405.

Part III
Face, Ears and Nose

Chapter 10
Clinical, Imaging, and Histological Findings in Inflammatory Lesions of the Face, Ears, and Neck

Ana Luisa Sampaio, Viviane Maria Maiolini, Maria de Oliveira Buffara, Paula Figueiredo de Marsillac, Haizza Cristina de Almeida Cabral Monteiro, Daniel Cunha de Araujo, Renata Valente Lisboa, André da Silva Cartell, Carolina Ávila de Almeida, Priscilla Haui de Oliveira Galuzzi Fonseca, Laila Klotz de Almeida Balassiano, Felipe Aguinaga, Manuela Boleira Sieiro Guimarães, Veronica Rodrigues Bogado Leite, Roberto Souto, Simone Guarçoni, Mario Chaves, Heron Werner, Jéssica Gonçalves Povill, and Clarissa Canella Moraes do Carmo

In the realm of dermatology, accurately diagnosing inflammatory lesions of the face, ears, and neck requires a nuanced understanding of both clinical and imaging techniques. This chapter delves into the diagnostic imaging approaches used to evaluate these complex inflammatory conditions. Utilizing advanced imaging modalities such as high-frequency ultrasonography, magnetic resonance

---

Supplementary Information The online version contains supplementary material available at https://doi.org/10.1007/978-3-031-77987-9_10.

A. L. Sampaio · M. de Oliveira Buffara · P. F. de Marsillac · D. C. de Araujo · R. Souto
Department of Dermatology, Hospital Universitario Pedro Ernesto, Universidade Estadual do Rio de Janeiro—UERJ, Rio de Janeiro, Brazil

V. M. Maiolini
Faculty of Medicine, Cancer Institute of the State of São Paulo—ICESP, University of São Paulo—FMUSP, São Paulo, Brazil

H. C. de Almeida Cabral Monteiro
State University of Rio de Janeiro—UERJ, Pedro Ernesto Hospital—HUPE, Rio de Janeiro, RJ, Brazil

Department of Dermatology, Hospital Rio-Barra and Rede D'Or São Luiz, Rio de Janeiro, RJ, Brazil

R. V. Lisboa
Faculty of Medicine of Valença—Rio de Janeiro—UNIFAA, Valença, Brazil

A. da Silva Cartell
Adjunct Professor at Faculdade de Medicina da Universidade Federal do Rio Grande do Sul, Rio de Janeiro, Brazil

Dermatologist and Dermatopathologist in Private Practice, Rio de Janeiro, Brazil

© The Author(s), under exclusive license to Springer Nature Switzerland AG 2025

C. Canella Moraes do Carmo (ed.), *Atlas of Diagnostic Imaging in Dermatology*, https://doi.org/10.1007/978-3-031-77987-9_10

imaging with surface coil and computed tomography, clinicians can gain detailed insights into the depth, extent, and nature of inflammatory lesions. These imaging techniques complement clinical examination by revealing critical aspects of lesion morphology, tissue involvement, and potential complications that are not always visible on the surface. By integrating imaging findings with clinical assessments, this chapter aims to enhance the diagnostic accuracy and guide effective management strategies for inflammatory lesions in these challenging anatomical regions.

C. Á. de Almeida
Faculty of Medicine of Valença—UniFaa, Valença, Brazil

Federal University of Rio de Janeiro—UFRJ, Rio de Janeiro, Brazil

P. H. de Oliveira Galuzzi Fonseca
Clinica CDPI and ALTA—Rio de Janeiro, Barra da Tijuca, Rio de Janeiro, RJ, Brazil

L. K. de Almeida Balassiano
Sector of Dermatology and Post Graduate Course in Medical Clinics—UFRJ, University of Rio de Janeiro, Rio de Janeiro, RJ, Brazil

Medical Clinics—UFRJ, Federal University of Rio de Janeiro, Rio de Janeiro, Brazil

F. Aguinaga
Instituto de Dermatologia Professor Rubem David Azulay, Santa Casa da Misericórdia do Rio de Janeiro, Rio de Janeiro, RJ, Brazil

Department of Dermatology, Hospital Universitario Pedro Ernesto, Universidade Estadual do Rio de Janeiro—UERJ, Rio de Janeiro, Brazil

M. B. S. Guimarães
Dermatology Department, Policlinica geral do Rio de Janeiro, Castelo, RJ, Brazil

V. R. B. Leite
Hospital Universitario Antonio Pedro, Universidade Federal Fluminense—UFF, Niterói, Brazil

S. Guarçoni
Clinica ALTA—DASA—Rio de Janeiro, Rio de Janeiro, Brazil

M. Chaves
Department of Dermatology, Hospital Universitario Pedro Ernesto, Universidade Estadual do Rio de Janeiro—UERJ, Rio de Janeiro, Brazil

Dermatologic Surgery Outpatient Clinic at HCAP, Carlos Chagas Foundation, Rio de Janeiro, Brazil

H. Werner
Clinica ALTA—DASA—Rio de Janeiro, Rio de Janeiro, RJ, Brazil

Universidade Federal do Rio de Janeiro—UFRJ, Rio de Janeiro, RJ, Brazil

Biodesign Lab DASA—PUC—Rio de Janeiro, Rio de Janeiro, Brazil

J. G. Povill
Clinica de Diagnostico por Imagem, Dermatological Imaging at DASA, Barra da Tijuca, Rio de Janeiro, Brazil

C. Canella Moraes do Carmo (✉)
Fluminense Federal University—UFF, Rio de Janeiro, Brazil

Federal University of Rio de Janeiro—UFRJ, Rio de Janeiro, Brazil

Diagnóstico das Américas—DASA—RJ, Rio de Janeiro, Brazil

Biodesign Laboratory, DASA-PUC, Rio de Janeiro, Brazil

10.1 Acne

10.1.1 Nodulocystic Acne

10.1.1.1 Definition [1–3]

- Acne vulgaris is a chronic inflammatory disease affecting the pilosebaceous unit.
- The pathogenesis of acne involves a complex interplay of host factors:
  - Androgen-mediated stimulation of the sebaceous gland
  - Dysbiosis within the pilosebaceous follicle microbiome
  - Innate and cellular immune responses
- May be influenced by factors such as genetics and, possibly, diet.

10.1.1.2 Epidemiology [1, 3]

- Acne vulgaris is the eighth most common disease in the world, affecting more than 0.5 billion people.
- It occurs in more than 80% of adolescents.
- 50–60% of women aged 20–25 years.
- 12% of women over 25 years old.

10.1.1.3 Clinical Presentation (Fig. 10.1) [1, 3–5]

- Skin eruptions such as open and closed comedones, pustules, papules, and nodules.
- Deep, inflamed, erythematous, often painful papules or nodules (=1 cm).
- Although referred to as 'nodulocystic' acne, true cyst formation is rare.
- Characteristic distribution: face, chest, shoulders, back, or arms.
- Skin pigmentation may mask the erythema characteristic of inflamed lesions in patients with pigmented skin.

10.1.1.4 Dermoscopy [6]

- Comedosappear as dilated follicles filled with a white-yellow circle or a brown plug that represents oxidized keratin.
- Papules appear as erythematous roundish lesions, as a result of local inflammation.
- Pustules are centered by a white-yellowish area that corresponds to the collection of purulent material inside the cavity of the lesion.
- No peculiar vascular pattern was described.

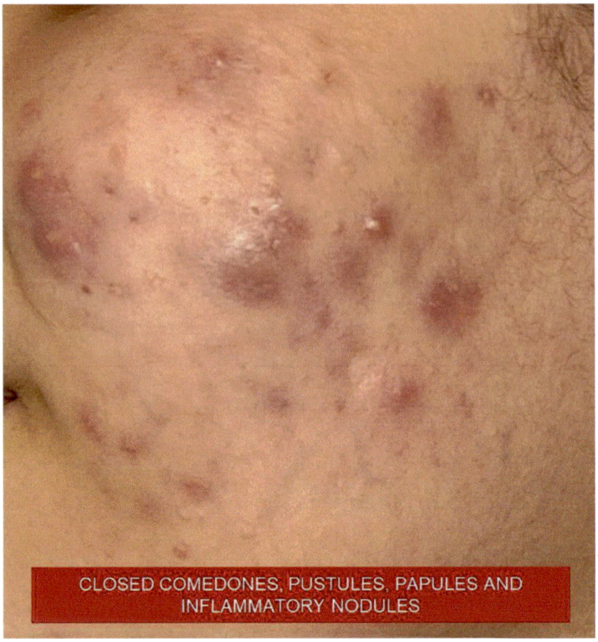

Fig. 10.1 Clinical photograph of patient with nodulocystic acne

10.1.1.5 Histopathology [2, 3, 7]

- Giant comedones, cysts, and nodules located in the cervical region and chest.
- Large, irregular fibrous scars and can cause inclusional epidermal cysts.
- Chronic suppurative and abscessed folliculitis with varying degrees of surrounding fibrosis and secondary cystification.

10.1.1.6 Ultrasonography (Fig. 10.2; Table 10.1) [8–10]

- Dilatation of pilosebaceous follicles.
- Thickening and decreased echogenicity of the dermis.
- Pseudocystic, oval, or round hypoechoic lesions of variable size in the dermis and hypodermis.
- Hypoechoic, elongated fistulous tracts in the dermis and hypodermis.
- Variable degrees of hypervascularity with slow flow vessels at power Doppler, along with increased vascularity in the periphery or within the alar nasal cartilages.
- There is an ultrasonographic scoring of the severity of acne named SOS-acne (sonographic scoring of acne) that counts the number of pseudocysts and fistulous tracts.

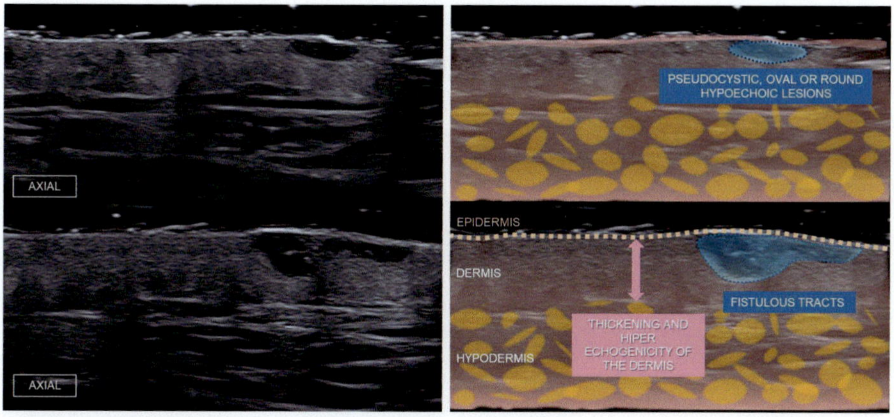

Fig. 10.2 Ultrasonographic findings of nodulocystic acne with a 24 MHz probe (Aplio i800, Canon Medical Systems)

Table 10.1 Sonographic scoring system acne severity classification

Acne Severity Classification	Number of Lesions
1. Mild	< 5 pseudocysts without fistulas
2. Moderate	5–9 pseudocysts without fistulas
3. Severe	= 10 pseudocysts with or without fistulas

10.1.1.7 MRI (Fig. 10.3)

- MRI with surface coil findings include dermal thickening with high signal intensity on STIR-weighted images.
- Dilatation of pilosebaceous follicles.
- Pseudocystic and fistulous tracts of variable size in the dermis and hypodermis on STIR images.
- Variable degrees of contrast enhancement of the peripheral of the lesions on T1 FS-weighted images.

10.1.1.8 3D Imaging (Fig. 10.4; Video 10.1)

- Most useful on deep and inflammatory lesions as pseudocystic and fistulous tracts.
- Allow the visualization of the extension of the lesion, enabling to assess the severity and relation with adjacent structures.
- Contribute to more precise surgical interventions, if applicable.
- Biomodels can be used and allows the creation of physical replicas of the affected area, offering representations that aid in surgical planning and patient education.

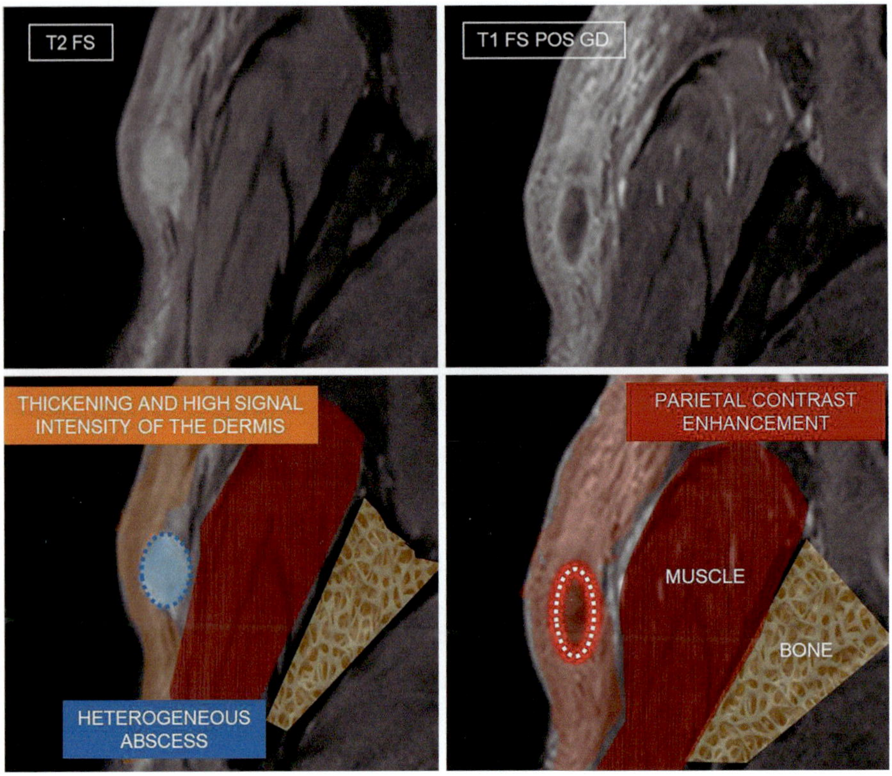

Fig. 10.3 MRI with surface coil findings of nodulocystic acne on T2 FS and T1 FS-weighted sequence after gadolinium administration (Magnetom Prisma 3T MRI, Siemens)

Fig. 10.4 3D virtual images of nodulocystic acne after segmentation of MRI isotropic images

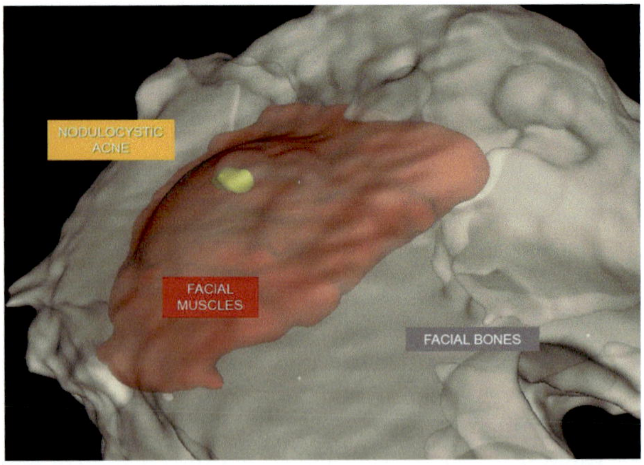

10.1.2 Scarring: Hypertrophic and Atrophic

10.1.2.1 Definition [3, 11]

- Scar is a skin lesion that results from the healing of wounds due to chemical, mechanical, or thermal injuries.
- Scarring acne can develop after skin inflammation as a complication due to the healing process of acne.
- Can be atrophic or hypertrophic.

10.1.2.2 Epidemiology [3, 11]

- Acne scars appear most often in people struggling with severe forms of acne.
- The underlying reasons why some patients develop distressing scars from acne while others do not are still not fully understood, although there is some evidence of genetic predisposition.

10.1.2.3 Clinical Presentation (Fig. 10.5) [3, 11]

- Inflammatory papules, pustules, nodules, subcutaneous cysts, and abscesses may develop into erosions and ulcerations, which may lead to atrophic, hypertrophic, and keloid scars.

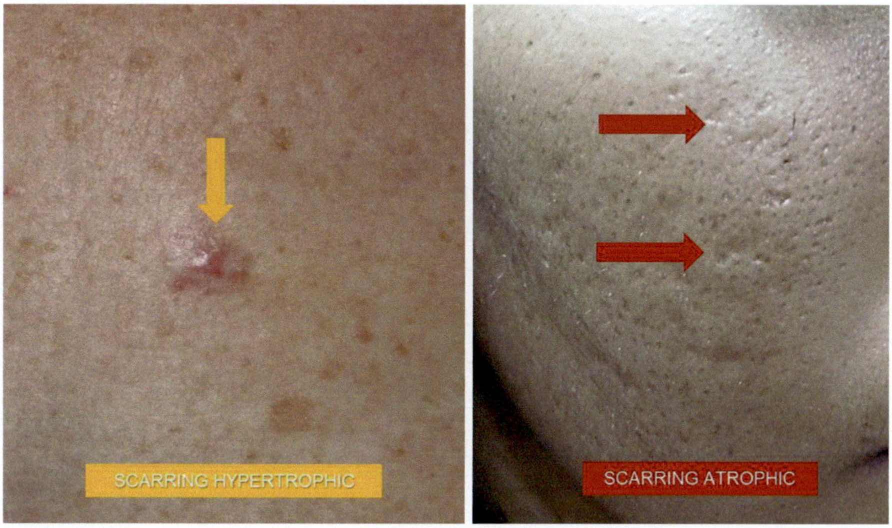

Fig. 10.5 Clinical photograph of patient with hypertrophic and atrophic scarring acne

- Atrophic (below the surface of the skin):
  - Icepick scars are deep, narrow, and can reach the border of the dermis with the subcutaneous tissue. They have sharp edges, a width of not more than 2 mm, and a V-shaped cross-section with a narrowing deep into the skin. Icepick scars account for 60% to 70% of atrophic scars.
  - Boxcar scars are oval or round but quite wide and flat and resemble the letter U or a square. Their edges are well marked and have a demarcated edge. They are usually 0.1–0.5 mm deep and 1.5–4 mm wide. They can combine to form clusters. Boxcar scars have the cross-section of the letter M and account for 15% to 20% of atrophic scars.
  - Rolling scars are the largest of all types and can reach a diameter of 5 mm. They comprise 15% to 25% of atrophic scars.
- Hypertrophic and keloids (above the skin surface):
  - Extend beyond the borders of original injury and fail to regress.
  - Keloids are elevated, firm bosselated papules and ill-defined plaques accompanied by variation in color, including erythematous, violaceous, or brown pigmentation.

10.1.2.4 Histopathology [7, 8]

- Uncharacteristic histology with fibrosis, which may be centered by a regressing sebaceous follicle.
- Fibrosis and keloidal pattern in some cases.
- Inclusional infundibular epidermal cysts.

10.1.2.5 Ultrasonography (Figs. 10.6 and 10.7) [8]

- Hypoechoic and elongated fistulous tracts in the dermis and hypodermis.
- Variable degrees of hypervascularity at power Doppler surrounding the lesions.
- Hypoechoic foci or hypoechoic bands with a fibrillar pattern in the dermis.
- Variable degrees of epidermal retraction.

10.1.2.6 MRI (Fig. 10.8)

- Pseudocystic and fistulous tracts of variable size in the dermis and hypodermis on STIR images.
- Variable degrees of contrast enhancement of the peripheral of the lesions on T1 FS-weighted images.
- Low signal intensity foci or bands with a fibrillar pattern in the dermis on T1 and STIR-weighted images.
- Variable degrees of epidermal retraction.

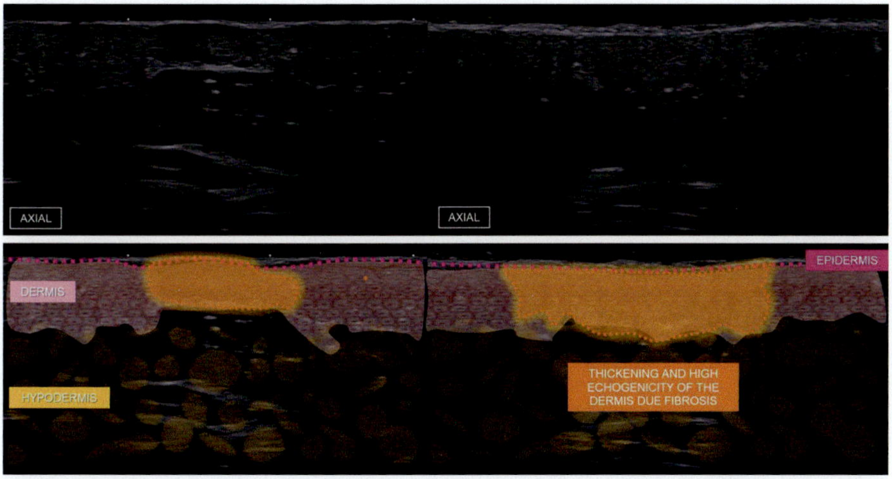

Fig. 10.6 Ultrasonographic findings of hypertrophic scarring acne with a 24 MHz probe (Aplio i800, Canon Medical Systems)

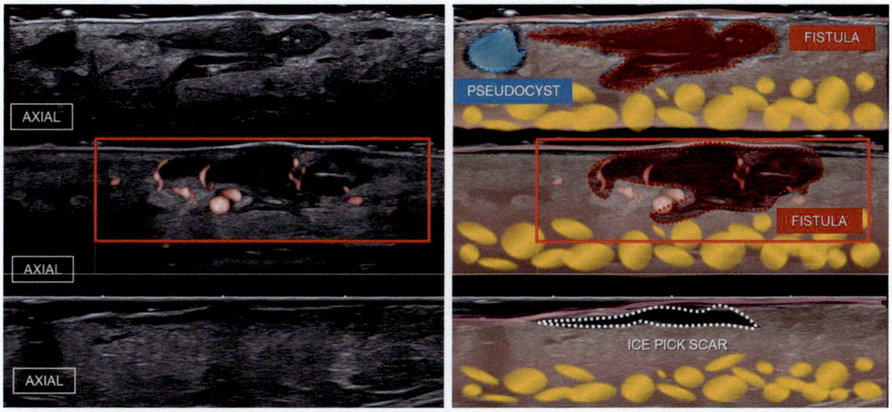

Fig. 10.7 Ultrasonographic findings of hypertrophic scarring acne with a 24 MHz probe (Aplio i800, Canon Medical Systems)

10.1.2.7 3D Imaging

- Most useful on deep and inflammatory lesions as pseudocystic and fistulous tracts.
- Allow the visualization of the extension of the lesion, enabling to assess the severity and relation with adjacent structures.
- Contribute to more precise surgical interventions, if applicable.
- Biomodels can be used and allows the creation of physical replicas of the affected area, offering representations that aid in surgical planning and patient education.

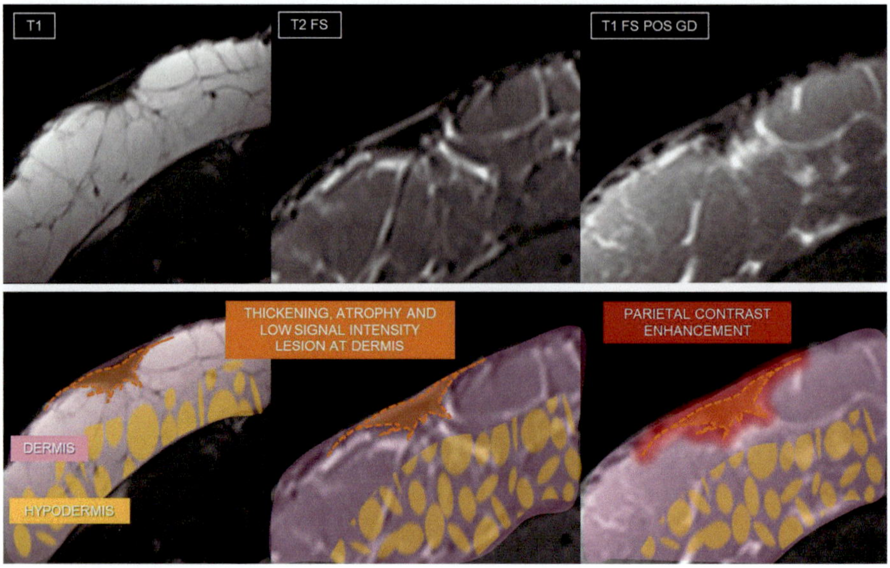

Fig. 10.8 MRI with surface coil findings of atrophic scarring acne on T2 FS, T1, and T1 FS-weighted sequence after gadolinium administration (Magnetom Prisma 3T MRI, Siemens)

10.2 Hidradenitis Suppurativa

10.2.1 Definition [12, 13]

- Chronic, inflammatory disease, characterized by follicular occlusion and rupture, which leads to recurrent nodules, comedones, abscesses, sinus tracts, and bridged scars.
- Usually present at flexural sites such as axillary, infra and intermammary, inguinal, perineal, perianal, and gluteal regions, which will be illustrated in Chap. 13.
- In addition to flexural sites, hidradenitis can also affect the facial region and will be illustrated in this chapter.

10.2.2 Epidemiology [12–14]

- Exact prevalence is unknown, but it is estimated to range from 0.03% to 4.1%.
- It is two to three times more common in women than in men.
- More prevalent in African Americans than Caucasians.
- Age of onset varies in literature but is more common between 18 and 44 years.

10.2.3 Clinical Presentation (Fig. 10.9) [14, 15]

- Nodules, abscesses, sinus tracts, bridged scars, comedones, and double-ended pseudo comedones are typical lesions.
- Most common at flexural sites as axillary, infra and intermammary, inguinal, perineal, perianal, and gluteal regions but can also be present in the face.
- Lesions are often accompanied by pain, pruritus, purulent, and malodorous discharge.

10.2.4 Dermoscopy [16]

- Double-ended pseudocomedones.
  - Under polarized dermoscopy are coupled cavities that deepen from the surface of the skin, in an oblique or parallel fashion, filled with superficial and deep-seated keratin accumulations.
  - The cavities are observed within a whitish cicatricial tissue and present large openings with irregular and undermined borders.
- Scars that on incident light dermoscopy are circinate and bridging scars with different depth levels and presenting hollows inside them.

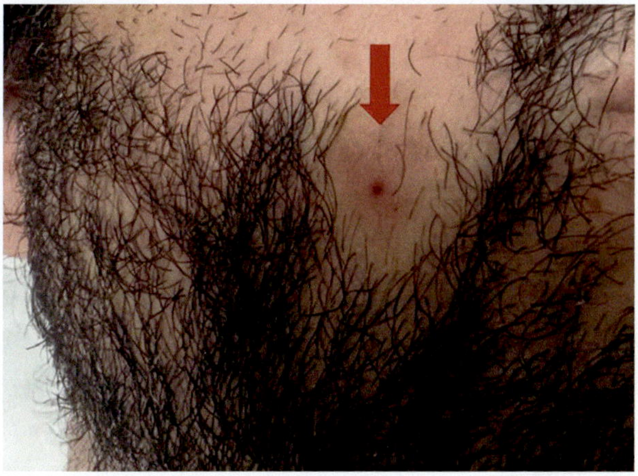

Fig. 10.9 Clinical photograph of patient with facial hidradenitis suppurativa

10.2.5 *Histopathology (Fig. 10.10) [13, 17, 18]*

- Early phase
  - Follicular plugging, acute suppurative folliculitis, and not always follicular rupture.
  - Follicular obstruction seems to be the initial event of hidradenitis suppurativa and is actually an abscessed folliculitis and not an apocrine lesion as the name suggests.
- Late phase (most frequently biopsied)
  - Chronic folliculitis with a mixed inflammatory pattern and extending from the lower half.
  - Abscesses and sinus tracts that may connect with the epidermis.
  - Marked fibrosis, destruction of hair follicles, eccrine, and apocrine glands secondarily.

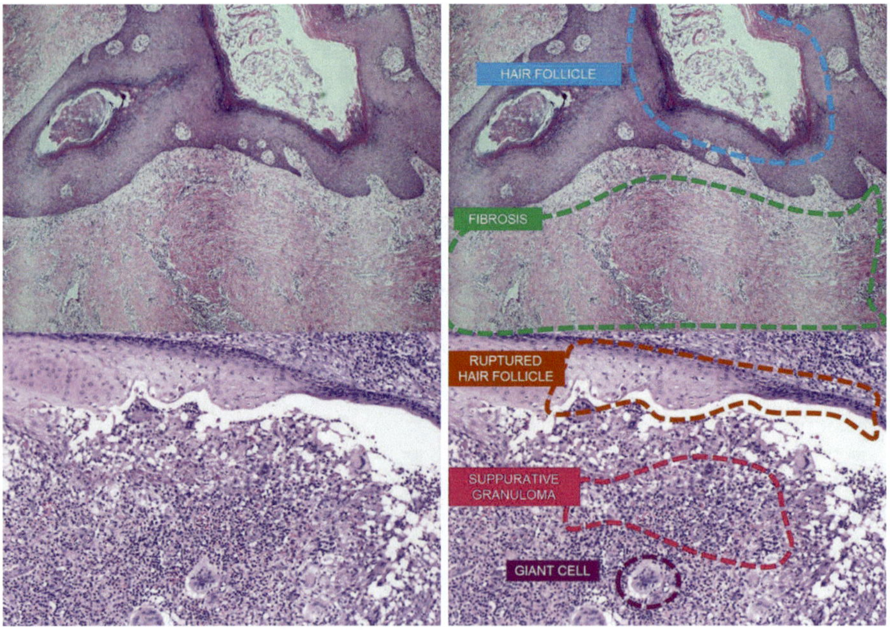

Fig. 10.10 Histological findings of facial hidradenitis suppurativa (H&E x10 and x20) (Image kindly provided by Dr. Gabbriella Giunta—Santa Catarina, Brazil)

10.2.6 Ultrasonography (Fig. 10.11) [16, 19–21]

- Ultrasonographic criteria of hidradenitis suppurativa.
  - Widening of the hair follicles.
  - Thickening or abnormal echogenicity of the dermis.
  - Dermal pseudocystic nodules (round or oval-shaped hypoechoic or anechoic nodular structures).
  - Fluid collections (anechoic or hypoechoic fluid deposits, in the dermis or hypodermis connected to the base of widened hair follicles).
  - Fistulous tracts (anechoic or hypoechoic band-like structures across skin layers in the dermis or hypodermis connected to the base of widened hair follicles).
- Ultrasonographic scoring for hidradenitis suppurativa (SOS-HS) criteria lesional features.
  - Stage I: Single fluid collection and dermal changes (hypoechoic or anechoic pseudocystic nodules, widening of the hair follicles, alterations in the dermal thickness or echogenicity) affecting a single body segment (e.g., axilla, groin, breast, buttock) (uni- or bilateral) without fistulous tracts.
  - Stage II: Two to four fluid collections or a single fistulous tract with dermal changes affecting up to two body segments (uni- or bilateral).

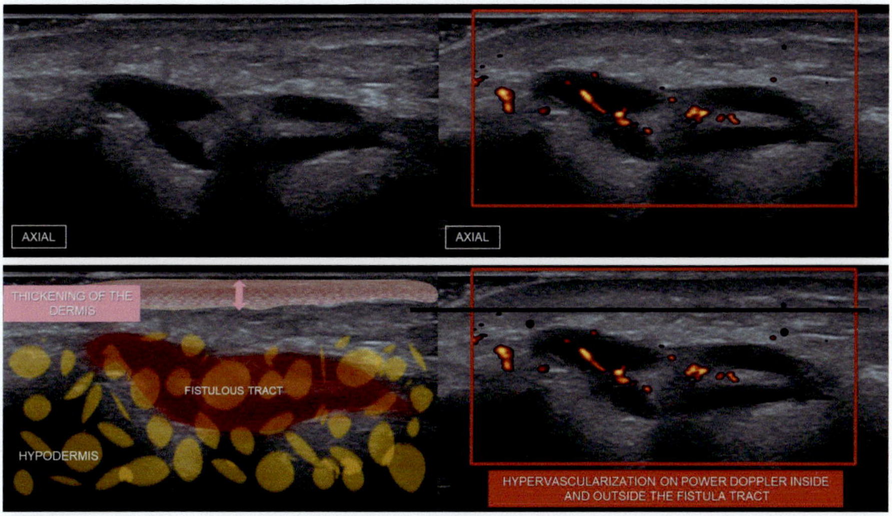

Fig. 10.11 Ultrasonographic findings of facial hidradenitis suppurativa with a 24 MHz probe (Aplio i800, Canon Medical Systems)

– Stage III: Five or more fluid collections or two or more fistulous tracts with dermal changes or involvement of three or more body segments (uni- or bilateral).

10.2.7 MRI (Fig. 10.12) [20, 22–25]

- Skin thickening, subcutaneous tissue induration, and abscess formation, with distinct signal characteristics on T1-weighted, T2-weighted, and STIR images.

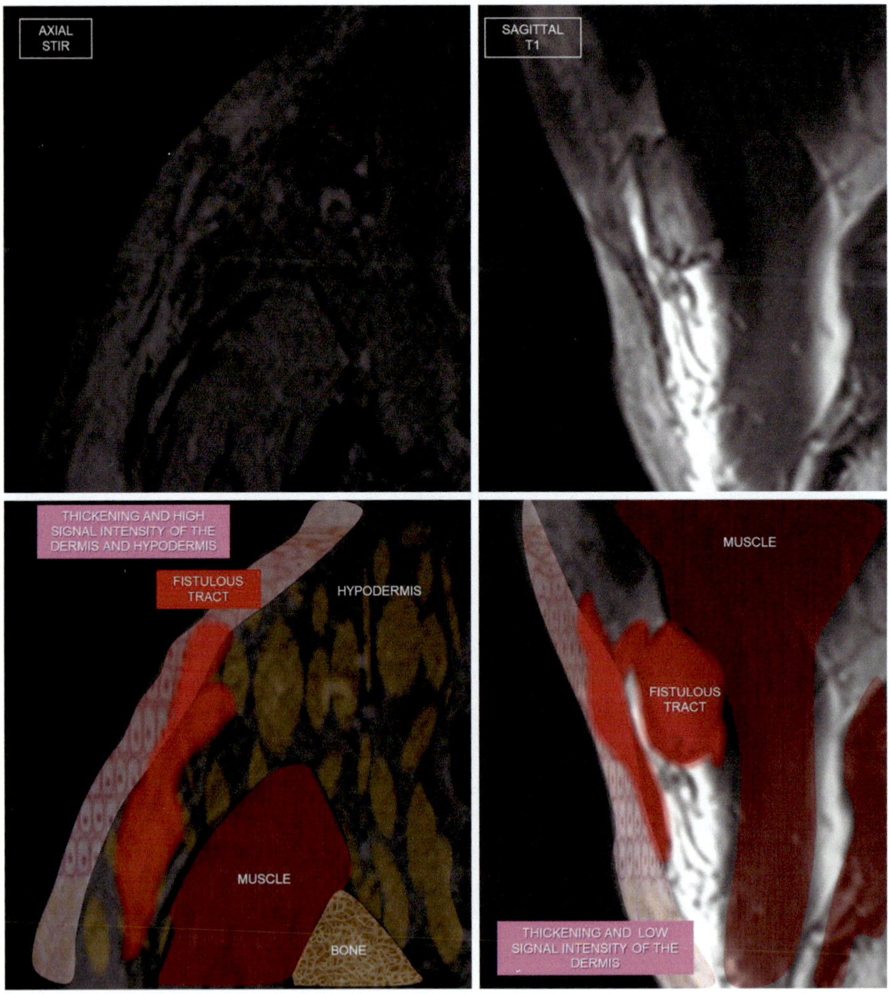

Fig. 10.12 MRI with surface coil findings of facial hidradenitis suppurativa on T1- weighted and STIR sequences (Magnetom Prisma 3T MRI, Siemens)

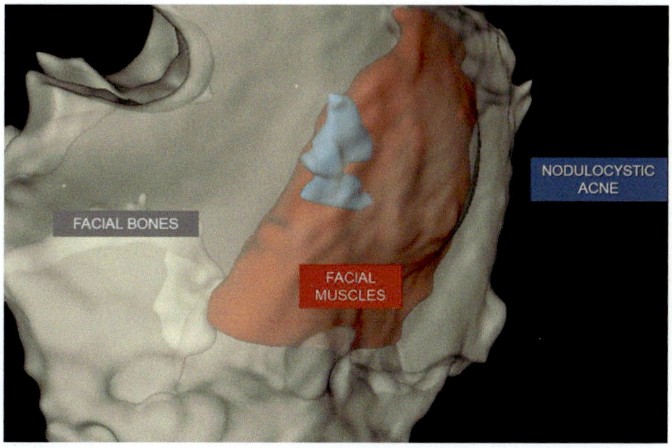

Fig. 10.13 3D virtual images of facial hidradenitis suppurativa after segmentation of MRI isotropic images

- Fistulous tracts (high signal band-like structures across skin layers in the dermis or hypodermis connected to the base of widened hair follicles.
- Exact extension of the inflammatory tissue surrounding the lesions.
- The high soft-tissue resolution of MRI can characterize the complex anatomy of the anal canal in great detail, providing particular utility of MRI for perianal HS cases, especially those with multiple tunnels.

10.2.8 3D Imaging (Fig. 10.13; Video 10.2)

- Allow the visualization of the extension of the abscess and fistula tracts, enabling to assess the severity and relation with adjacent structures in facial region.
- Contribute to more precise surgical interventions, if applicable, especially in the face.
- Biomodels can be used and allows the creation of physical replicas of the affected area, offering representations that aid in surgical planning and patient education.

10.3 Lupus Erythematosus

10.3.1 Definition [26, 27]

- Cutaneous lupus erythematosus primarily affects sun-exposed areas of the skin, including the face, scalp, ears, neck, and upper chest that will be illustrated in this chapter.
- In addition to sun-exposed areas, cutaneous lupus erythematosus can also affect other sites such as the arms, hands, and legs that will be illustrated in Chap. 13.
- Cutaneous lupus erythematosus comprises a wide range of manifestations of specific lesions erythematous lupus: acute, subacute, chronic, and intermittent.

- Acute and subacute are more inflammatory lesions that regress without scar.
- Intermittent lupus was previously called lupus tumidus.
- Chronic cutaneous lupus can leave atrophy if not treated effectively or quickly and are typified as
  - discoid lupus
  - lupus panniculitis
  - lupus profundus

10.3.2 Epidemiology [26–28]

- Female predominance of 4:1.
- More common between the ages of 20 and 40 years, with a mean age at onset of 43 years, varying according to the subtype.
- Discoid lupus erythematosus is by far the most common type of cutaneous lupus erythematosus, comprising 80% of all cases.
- Cutaneous lupus erythematosus is two to three times more frequent than systemic lupus erythematosus, with an annual incidence of 4.3 per 100,000.
- 70% to 80% of systemic lupus erythematosus patients have cutaneous involvement.
- 20% of patients diagnosed with cutaneous lupus erythematosus progress to systemic lupus erythematosus:
  - Acute cutaneous lupus erythematosus has the greatest chance of association with systemic lupus erythematosus (80% to 90% of cases).
  - Subacute cutaneous lupus erythematosus is associated to systemic lupus erythematosus in around 30%.
  - Generalized discoid lupus erythematosus is associated to systemic lupus erythematosus in 20%.
  - Localized discoid lupus erythematosus is associated to systemic lupus erythematosus in 5%.

10.3.3 Clinical Presentation (Fig. 10.14) [28]

- Acute lupus
  - Acute onset, with manifestations of malar rash, exanthematic (diffuse erythematous photodistributed) lesions and necrotic lesions (also called specific bullous lupus).
  - Acute lesions are more related to systemic lupus and ANA-positive antibodies.

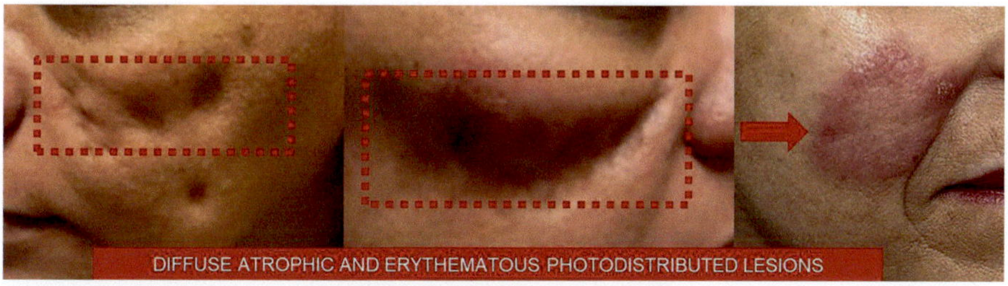

Fig. 10.14 Clinical photograph of patient with lupus erythematosus

- Subacute lupus is presented as
  - annular lesions
  - papulosquamous (or psoriasiform) lesions
  - Rowell's syndrome (target-like lesions that resembles erythema multiforme)
- Intermittent tumid lupus
  - Papules and plaques in sun-exposed localizations
  - Minimal epidermal involvement
- Chronic cutaneous lupus
  - Discoid lesions with hyperkeratotic, dyschromic, scarring plaques, and cicatricial alopecia in scalp lesions.
  - Can be presented as panniculitis with specific finding of lupus.

10.3.4 Dermoscopy (Fig. 10.15) [29]

- Acute cutaneous lupus erythematosus (ACLE)
  - Polymorphous vessels (linear, linear branched, linear curved, and, less frequently, dotted vessels) on a pink–red background.
  - There were also white or yellow scales of patchy distribution in 30% and 20% of the cases, respectively.
  - Red structureless (hemorrhagic) areas and dotted or globular structures were present in half of the cases.
- Subacute cutaneous lupus Erythematosus (SCLE)
  - Shows a pink–red background and polymorphous vessels (linear, linear branched, linear curved, and dotted vessels)
  - Scaling, peripheral pigmentation and red structureless (hemorrhagic)

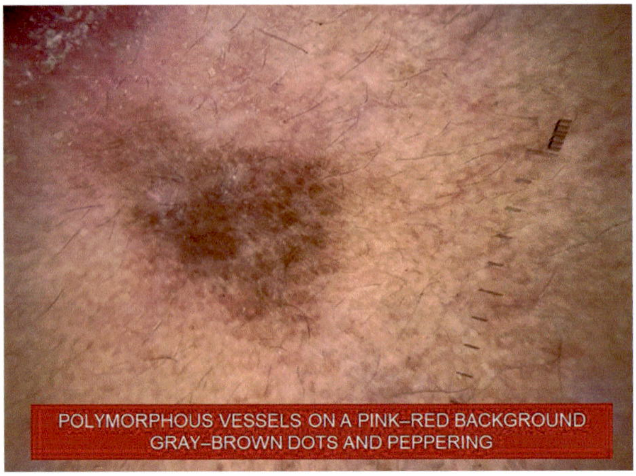

Fig. 10.15 Dermoscopic findings of patient with lupus erythematosus (X10)

- Intermittent cutaneous lupus erythematosus (ICLE):
  - Polymorphous vessels of unspecific distribution on a pink–red background.
  - This kind of cutaneous lupus erythematosus does not have scales, peripheral pigmentation, erosions, and crusting.
- Chronic cutaneous lupus erythematosus (CCLE)
  - Polymorphous vascular pattern (linear, linear curved, and linear branched vessels and less frequently dotted vessels)
  - White scaling and yellow scales (76.9% and 38.5%, respectively)
  - Follicular keratotic plug
  - Pink–red backgrounds
  - Perifollicular white halos
  - Dots or globules
  - Pink structureless areas
  - Red structureless (hemorrhagic) areas
  - White structureless areas
  - Follicular red dots
  - Gray–brown dots and peppering
  - Peripheral pigmentation, erosions, dilated follicles, and rosettes

10.3.5 Histopathology (Fig. 10.16) [29, 30]

- Chronic discoid lupus
  - Clinically and histologically, lupus erythematosus can present in different forms, varying depending on the stage of evolution of the biopsied lesion, inflammatory activity, and use of therapy. Therefore, a biopsy that includes a

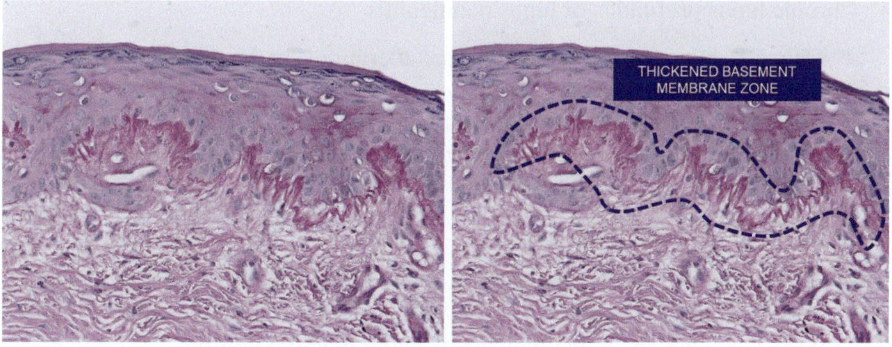

Fig. 10.16 Histological findings of lupus erythematosus (PAS x20)

hypodermis, punch 4 or greater or navet, informing the exact topography of the lesion and the biopsied area of the lesion, is essential.

- It usually presents as a vacuolar interface dermatitis with mononuclear inflammatory infiltrate, mainly lymphocytic, superficial, deep perivascular and/or periadnexal (adventitial); it is rarely lichenoid; the infiltrate may extend to the hypoderma or affect only the hypoderma (deep lupus); it can be variable and even quite discrete.
- There may be satellitosis.
- Hyaline thickening of the basement membrane zone (BMZ), positive magenta in SBP (Special Basement membrane Periodic acid-Schiff stain)and resistant diastasis; this thickening is irregular and may even fail and corresponds to the deposition of immunoglobulins (IgG and IgM) and complement with BMZ.
- Edema in the superficial dermis, more exuberant in the tumid forms.
- Epidermal atrophy at the expense of the spinous layer with compact hyperkeratosis; rarely exhibits irregular epithelial hyperplasia; parakeratosis may be present.
- Superficial venular ectasia; perivascular hyaline material corresponding to immunoglobulins and fibrin may be deposed; there may be extravasation of red blood cells. The association with hypersensitivity vasculitis (leukocytoclastic) or thrombotic vasculopathy related to antiphospholipid syndrome, seen in the same biopsy, is uncommon.
- Mucin deposition in the dermis reticularis, highlighted by PAS or alcian-blue, more common in the subacute and tumid forms.
- Conical follicular plugging, different from the lichen planus plug, where dilation is usually lower; sebaceous atrophy involving the vellus is the earliest adnexal alteration.
- Pigmentary incontinence.
- Direct immunofluorescence: granular deposits of IgM, IgG and complement in BZM in 50% to 90% of photo-exposed skin samples; it also marks apoptotic vessels and bodies; DIF is important for the differential diagnosis.

- Chronic lupus profundus or lupus panniculitis
  - Only 50% have dermal and epidermal alterations, in the other half, the alterations are restricted to hypoderm.
  - Lobular hypodermatitis with prominent lymphocytic infiltrate, lymphocytes with karyorexis (nuclear dust). Eventually, it may exhibit lymphoid follicles in 25% of cases.
- Intermittent lupus tumid
  - Absence of epidermal or junctional changes, presenting only dermal changes, including superficial and deep perivascular infiltrate and interstitial, papillary edema, and abundant mucin deposits in the reticular dermis.

10.3.6 Ultrasonography (Fig. 10.17) [10]

- Active cutaneous lupus
  - Thickening and hypoechogenicity of the upper hypodermis, typically seen on the face, particularly in the malar or cheek areas.
  - Power Doppler may show variable intralesional blood flow.
- Chronic cutaneous lupus
  - Cutaneous layer atrophy.
  - Hypovascularization on power Doppler, may lead to artery lumen narrowing and pearlization, causing Raynaud's phenomenon and vessel occlusion, commonly in digital arteries.

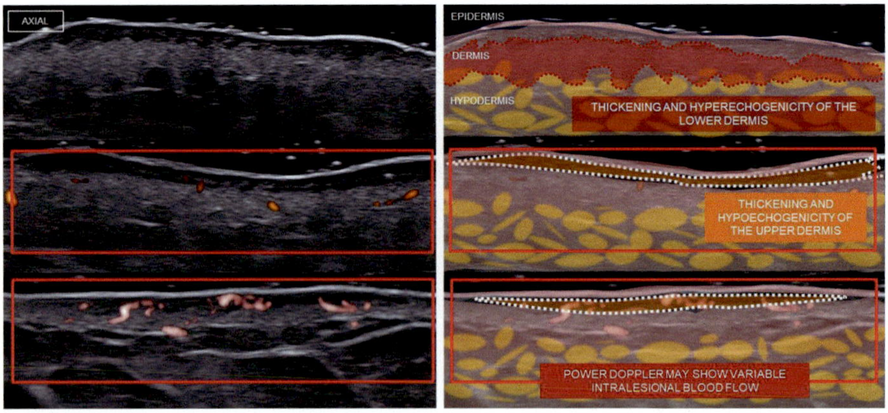

Fig. 10.17 Ultrasonographic findings of lupus erythematosus with a 24 MHz probe (Aplio i800, Canon Medical Systems)

- Lobular involvement seen on ultrasound as diffuse thickening and hyperechogenicity ("cloudy" pattern) or septal involvement with thickened hypoechogenic septa ("brick wall" pattern).

10.3.7 MRI (Fig. 10.18)

- Active cutaneous lupus
  - Thickening, high signal intensity on STIR images at upper hypodermis.
- Chronic cutaneous lupus
  - Lobular involvement similar to a panniculitis, seen as diffuse septal thickening and high signal intensity on STIR images.
  - Cutaneous layer atrophy.

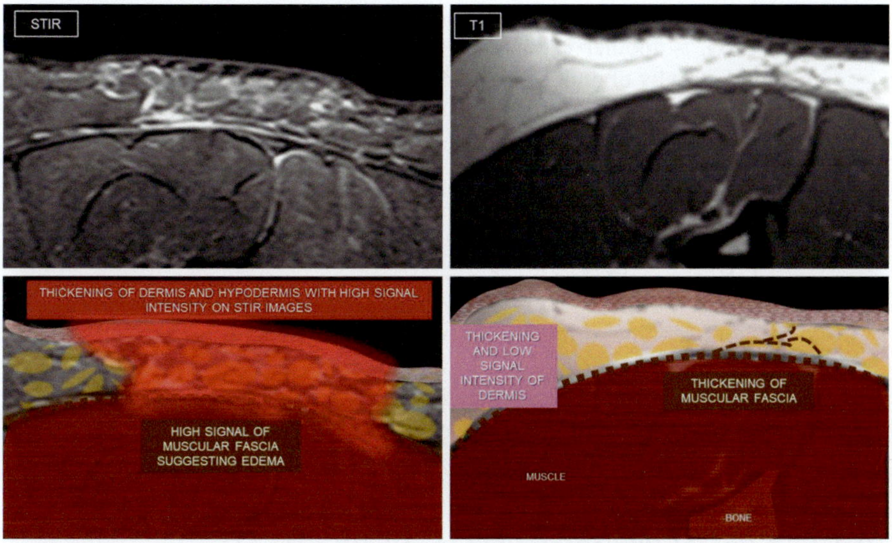

Fig. 10.18 MRI with surface coil with surface coil findings of lupus erythematosus on T1-weighted and STIR sequences (Magnetom Prisma 3T MRI, Siemens)

10.4 Scleroderma

10.4.1 Definition [31, 32]

- Chronic inflammatory connective tissue disorder, characterized by inflammation and fibrosis of the skin, with variable clinical presentations.
- Morphea, Pasini and Pierini atrophoderma, lichen sclerosus, eosinophilic fasciitis, and calcinosis are conditions associated with scleroderma, and will be described together in Chap. 13.
- Facial involvement in scleroderma presents in several ways, primarily characterized by linear scleroderma, which manifests as band-like localized lesions affecting the dermis, subcutaneous tissue, muscles, and underlying bones. This chapter will detail these manifestations:
  - Linear scleroderma en coup de sabre (LSCS) is a type of linear morphea that affects the head and neck.
  - Linear scleroderma that involves the forehead can affect the scalp, causing scarring alopecia, already described in Chap. 13.
  - Parry–Romberg syndrome (PRS), also known as progressive hemifacial atrophy (PHA), is another variant of linear morphea, which is characterized by unilateral atrophy of underlying soft tissue and bone with minimal overlaying cutaneous changes. It has been associated with various systemic manifestations, particularly neurologic, ophthalmologic, and maxillofacial.

10.4.2 Epidemiology [31, 32]

- Coup de sabre subtype of linear scleroderma affects about 6–7% of all cases of localized scleroderma.
- Parry–Romberg syndrome exact incidence is less well-defined but is generally considered to be even rarer than coup de sabre.

10.4.3 Clinical Presentation (Fig. 10.19) [31, 32]

- Coup de sabre
  - The lesion is usually unilateral.
  - Mixed hypopigmented and hyperpigmented skin overlying the frontoparietal area associated with a deep paramedian forehead scar separating atrophic from normal tissue.
  - Mostly affects the frontoparietal region or the paramedian forehead.

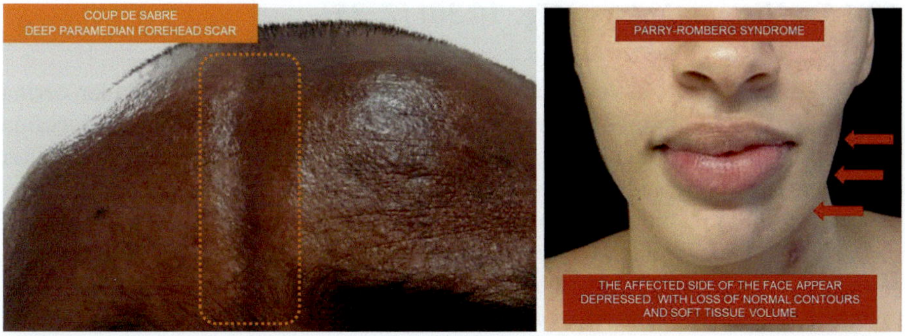

Fig. 10.19 Clinical photograph of patient with Parry–Romberg syndrome and coup de sabre lesion

- Parry–Romberg syndrome
  - Facial asymmetry characterized by progressive and often unilateral wasting of the skin, subcutaneous fat, and sometimes underlying muscle and bone. This asymmetry usually begins during childhood or adolescence and progresses slowly over time.
  - The affected side of the face may appear sunken or depressed, with loss of normal contours and soft tissue volume. The skin can become tight and atrophic, sometimes leading to a shiny appearance.
  - In some cases, there can be ocular manifestations such as enophthalmos (sunken eye), ptosis (drooping eyelid), and vision disturbances. Dental abnormalities, including malocclusion or teeth misalignment, may also be observed.
  - Neurological symptoms such as facial pain, migraine-like headaches, and sensory disturbances (such as numbness or tingling) may occasionally accompany the facial changes.

10.4.4 Dermoscopy [33, 34]

- Trichoscopic findings
  - Loss of follicular openings
  - Peripilar casts
  - Areas with short regrowing hairs
  - Pili torti and black dots or broken hair

10.4.5 Histopathology (Fig. 10.20) [7, 35]

- Deep dermal sclerosis; usually progresses from the superficial reticular derma toward the hypoderm. It is important to observe the location of the eccrine glands, as they are usually involved with obliteration of the perianexal adventitia leading to atrophy and disappearance of the cutaneous ducts and appendages.
- Thickening of the collagen fibers, with a tendency to homogenize and horizontalize the fibers in relation to the surface and loss of the interstitial space between the collagen fibers, making the collagen appear more compacted. In small magnification, scleroderma gives a square or rectangular appearance to the punch (square disease).
- There may be thickening of the vessel walls with narrowing of the lumen; superficial vascular ectasia leading to thromboangiitis obliterans.
- Elastic fibers preserved in the evaluation by orcein; it is an exception to the rule where fibrosis and elastosis are mutually exclusive phenomena.
- Thickening of the hypodermic septa in deep involvement.
- Deep perivascular lymphoplasmacytic infiltrate; more exuberant in the most recent phases.
- Usual or atrophic epidermis.
- Pigmentary incontinence may be present.

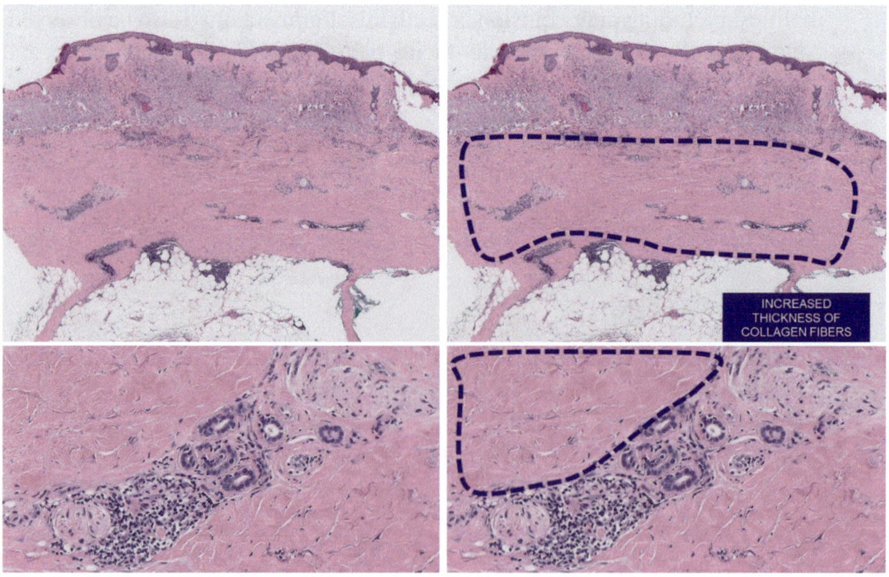

Fig. 10.20 Histological findings of scleroderma (H&E x4 and x20)

10.4.6 Ultrasonography (Figs. 10.21 and 10.22) [36, 37]

- Hemifacial atrophy demonstrated as unilateral wasting of the skin, subcutaneous fat, and sometimes underlying muscle.
- Areas of increased echogenicity in the hypodermis, with localized, scattered, or diffuse patterns.
- Increased dermal or hypodermal vascularization observed on power Doppler.

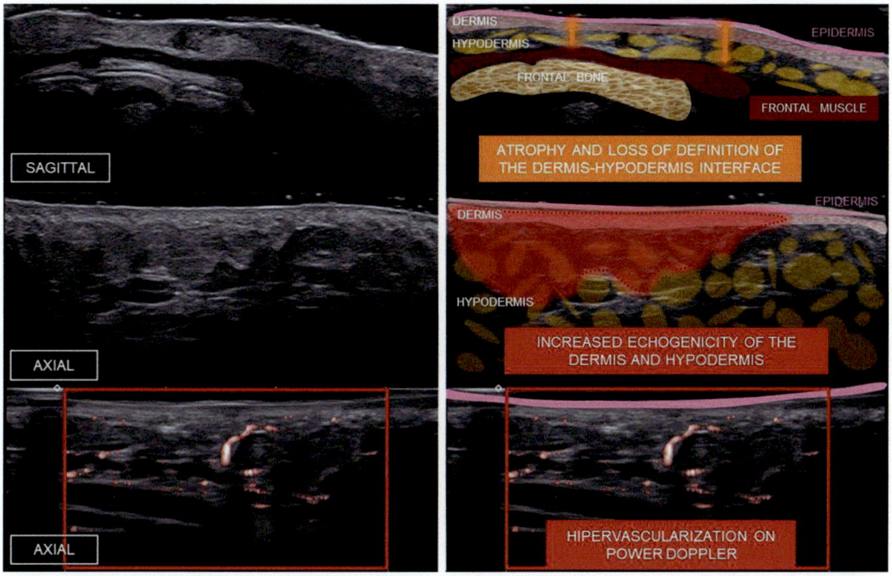

Fig. 10.21 Ultrasonographic findings of coup de sabre lesion with a 24 MHz probe (Aplio i800, Canon Medical Systems)

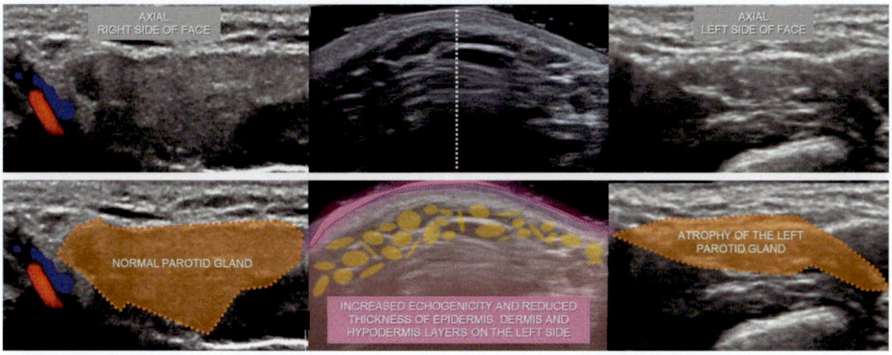

Fig. 10.22 Ultrasonographic findings of Parry–Romberg syndrome with a 24 MHz probe (Aplio i800, Canon Medical Systems)

- Thickening of the vessel walls, vascular ectasia with surrounding hyperechogenicity of hypodermis.
- Occasional detection of underlying muscular involvement, characterized by areas of increased echogenicity of the muscles and sometimes increased vascularization, suggesting a more severe form or mixed connective tissue disease.

10.4.7 MRI (Fig. 10.23) [38]

- Hemifacial atrophy demonstrated as unilateral wasting of the skin, subcutaneous fat, and sometimes underlying muscle. May extend to involve underlying facial bones, which can appear thinner and heterogeneous compared to the unaffected side.
- High signal intensity on STIR images of dermis or hypodermis, suggesting inflammatory lesions.
- Thickening on T1-weighted images of dermis or hypodermis on acute phases and atrophy on late stages.
- Underlying muscular involvement, characterized by areas of high signal intensity on STIR images.

10.4.8 3D Imaging

- Used to quantify and visualize the facial asymmetry, enabling to assess the severity precise involvement of muscles and bones.
- Facilitate more accurate surgical interventions, where appropriate.
- Biomodels can be used and allows the creation of physical replicas of the affected area, offering representations that aid in surgical planning and patient education.

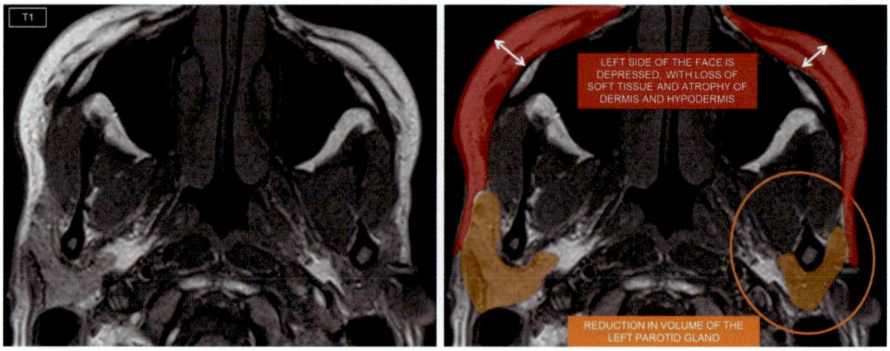

Fig. 10.23 MRI with surface coil findings of Parry–Romberg syndrome on T1-weighted sequence (Magnetom Prisma 3T MRI, Siemens)

10.5 Sarcoidosis

10.5.1 Definition [39, 40]

- The most common face dermatological lesion of sarcoidosis is lupus pernio (LP) characterized by violaceous or erythematous, indurated, infiltrative plaques that are primarily distributed on the central face.
- Has been associated with sarcoidosis of the upper respiratory tract, typically associated with pulmonary fibrosis, chronic uveitis, and bone cysts.

10.5.2 Epidemiology [39–41]

- The presence of lupus pernio appears to be associated with an increased risk for extracutaneous disease (particularly the respiratory tract).
- Prevalence ranging from
  - 1 to 5 per 100,000 in South Korea, Taiwan, Japan, and Spain
  - 140 to 160 per 100,000 in Sweden and Canada
- More common among some populations of African origin, women, and ages between 45 and 65.

10.5.3 Clinical Presentation (Fig. 10.24) [39–41]

- Chronic persistent violaceous skin lesion at nose, cheeks, and ears.
- Ranges from a few small button-like lesions or nodules under the tip of the nose to exuberant plaques covering the nose and spreading across the cheeks.
- Less commonly involves the dorsal hands, finger, and toes.

10.5.4 Dermoscopy (Fig. 10.25) [42]

- Well-defined red- or brownish-grayish areas.
- The lesions may exhibit a granular or mottled appearance, reflecting the underlying granulomatous inflammation.
- Small telangiectasias can sometimes be observed at the periphery of the lesions.
- Changes in pigmentation, including areas of hypopigmentation or hyperpigmentation, may be present within the lesions.
- In some cases, dermoscopy can reveal nodular or papular structures within the lesion, which correspond to the granulomas present in the skin.

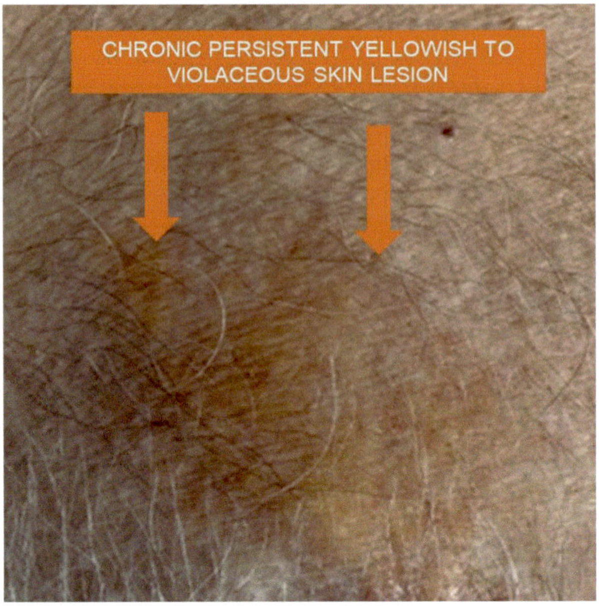

Fig. 10.24 Clinical photograph of patient with sarcoidosis

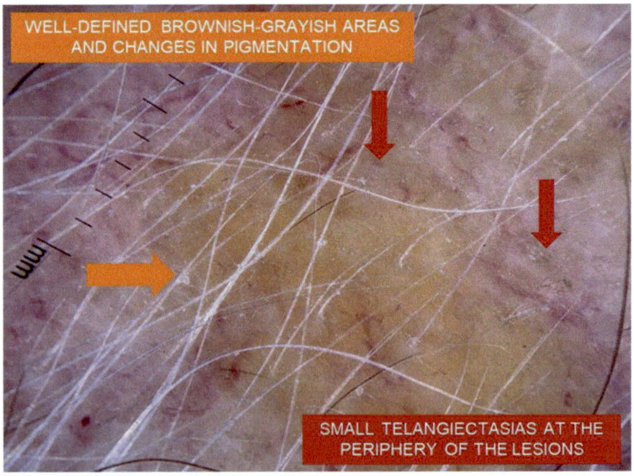

Fig. 10.25 Dermoscopic findings of patient with sarcoidosis (x10)

- Fine scaling or rough surface texture may be visible, particularly in cases with significant inflammatory involvement.
- The borders of the lesions might be well-defined and sometimes show a slight elevation compared to the surrounding skin.

10.5.5 Histopathology (Fig. 10.26) [7, 35]

- Atrophy, parakeratosis, or acanthosis of epidermis in 50% of cases.
- Non-caseifying granulomas (without central necrosis) of epithelioid cells with little or no lymphocyte crown at hypodermis, presenting histopathological pattern called naked or denuded granulomas, which are well demarcated and tend to have few gigantocytes.
- In the late phase, the granulomas present evident surrounding, responsible for the hardened consistency on palpation.
- Granulomas can have distinct locations: only superficial, diffuse, or subcutaneous in the Darier–Roussy sarcoid.
- Asteroid bodies: streliform eosinophilic inclusion with an apparent halo, caused by an antigen-antibody reaction.
- Schaumann bodies which are lamellar or concentric calcified inclusions within gigantocytes.

10.5.6 Radiography and Computed Tomography [41]

- Lytic and cystic bone lesions in the hands and feet can be present underlying lesions of lupus pernio.

10.5.7 Ultrasonography (Fig. 10.27) [43]

- Hypoechoic nodules or pseudonodules in dermal or hypodermal tissue, presenting peripheral hyperechoic halo.
- Panniculitis with mainly lobular pattern surrounding the nodules and septal involvement.
- Increased vascularity on power Doppler imaging.

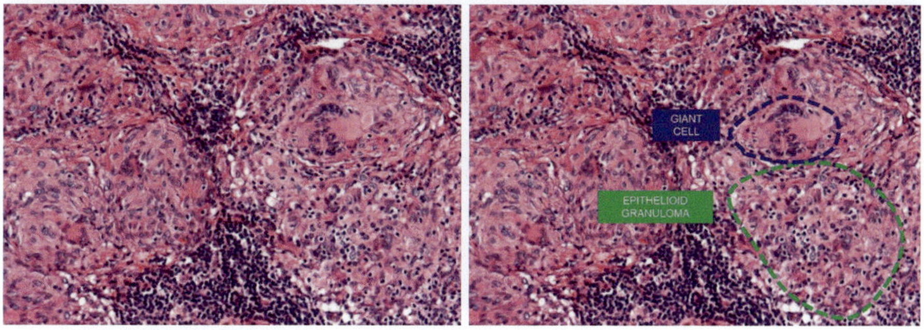

Fig. 10.26 Histological findings of sarcoidosis (H&E x20)

10.5.8 MRI (Fig. 10.28) [44]

- Nodules or pseudonodules in dermal or hypodermal tissue, presenting high signal intensity on T2 FS images and low signal intensity on T1-weighted image.
- Panniculitis with mainly lobular pattern and septal thickening associated with high signal intensity soft tissue edema.
- Increased vascularity on power Doppler imaging.
- Nodular enhancement observed on contrast-enhanced images.

10.5.9 3D imaging

- Used to quantify and visualize the extension of the nodule, enabling to assess the severity and relation with adjacent structures.

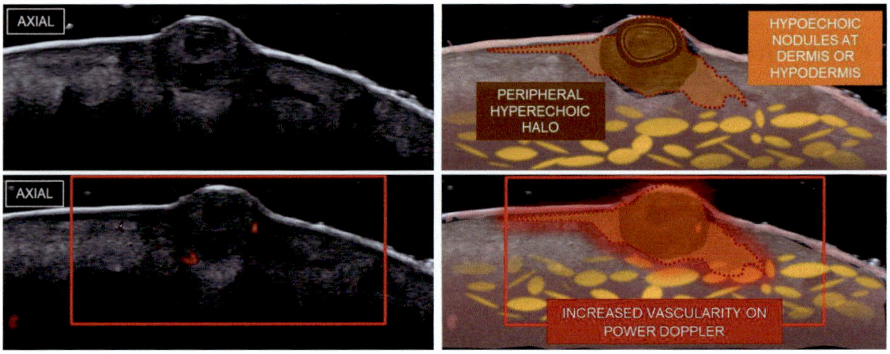

Fig. 10.27 Ultrasonographic findings of sarcoidosis with a 24 MHz probe (Aplio i800, Canon Medical Systems)

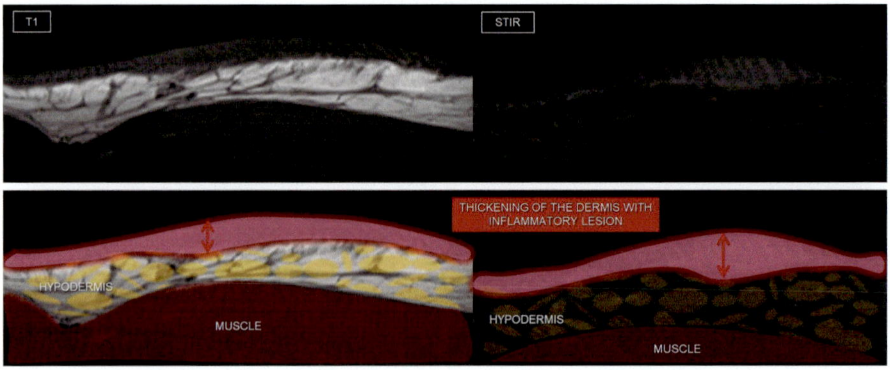

Fig. 10.28 MRI with surface coil findings of sarcoidosis on T1-weighted and STIR sequences (Magnetom Prisma 3T MRI, Siemens)

- Biomodels can be used and allows the creation of physical replicas of the affected area, offering representations that aid in surgical planning and patient education.

References

1. Kutlu Ö, Karadag AS, Wollina U. Adult acne versus adolescent acne: a narrative review with a focus on epidemiology to treatment. An Bras Dermatol. 2023;98:75–83.
2. McLaughlin J, Watterson S, Layton AM, Bjourson AJ, Barnard E, McDowell A. Propionibacterium acnes and acne vulgaris: new insights from the integration of population genetic, multi-Omic. Biochem Host-Microbe Stud Microorgan. 2019;7:128.
3. Sutaria AH, Masood S, Saleh HM, Schlessinger J. Acne vulgaris. StatPearls; 2024. http://www.ncbi.nlm.nih.gov/pubmed/30101990.
4. Mavranezouli I, Daly CH, Welton NJ, Deshpande S, Berg L, Bromham N, et al. A systematic review and network meta-analysis of topical pharmacological, oral pharmacological, physical and combined treatments for acne vulgaris. Br J Dermatol. 2022;187:639–49.
5. O'Neill AM, Gallo RL. Host-microbiome interactions and recent progress into understanding the biology of acne vulgaris. Microbiome. 2018;6:177.
6. Alma A, Sticchi A, Chello C, Guida S, Farnetani F, Chester J, et al. Dermoscopy, reflectance confocal microscopy and optical coherence tomography features of acne: a systematic review. J Clin Med. 2022;11:1783.
7. Hall BJ, Hall JC, Cockerell CJ, Affolter K, Alvarez P. Diagnostic pathology: nonneoplastic dermatopathology. Elsevier; 2017.
8. Lacarrubba F, Verzì AE, Tedeschi A, Catalfo P, Nasca MR, Micali G. Clinical and Ultrasonographic correlation of acne scars. Dermatologic Surg. 2013;39:1683–8.
9. Wortsman X. Role of color doppler ultrasound in cutaneous inflammatory conditions. Semin Ultrasound CT MR. 2024;45(3):264–86.
10. Wortsman X. Atlas of dermatologic ultrasound. Cham: Springer International Publishing; 2018. https://doi.org/10.1007/978-3-319-89614-4.
11. Chilicka K, Rusztowicz M, Szygula R, Nowicka D. Methods for the improvement of acne scars used in dermatology and cosmetology: a review. J Clin Med. 2022;11:2744.
12. Sabat R, Jemec GBE, Matusiak L, Kimball AB, Prens E, Wolk K. Hidradenitis suppurativa. Nat Rev Dis Primers. 2020;6:18.
13. Ballard K, Shuman VL. Hidradenitis Suppurativa. StatPearls; 2024. http://www.ncbi.nlm.nih.gov/pubmed/34057384.
14. Goldburg SR, Strober BE, Payette MJ. Hidradenitis suppurativa. J Am Acad Dermatol. 2020;82:1045–58.
15. Von Der Werth J, Williams H. The natural history of hidradenitis suppurativa. J Eur Acad Dermatol Venereol. 2000;14:389–92. https://doi.org/10.1046/j.1468-3083.2000.00087.x.
16. Lacarrubba F, Musumeci M, Nasca M, Verzì A, Fiorentini F, Micali G. Double-ended Pseudocomedones in hidradenitis Suppurativa: clinical, dermoscopic, and histopathological correlation. Acta Dermato Venereologica. 2017;97:763–4.
17. Napolitano M, Megna M, Timoshchuk E, Patruno C, Balato N, Fabbrocini G, et al. Hidradenitis suppurativa: from pathogenesis to diagnosis and treatment. Clin Cosmet Investig Dermatol. 2017;10:105–15.
18. Krajewski PK, Szepietowski JC, Martorell A. Tunnels in hidradenitis Suppurativa: active inflammatory entities with specific molecular and genetic profiles—a narrative review. Dermatology. 2023;239:323–7. https://doi.org/10.1159/000529848.
19. Wortsman X. Imaging of hidradenitis Suppurativa. Dermatol Clin. 2016;34:59–68.

20. Lopes AA, Moraes GN, Dias BMMDL, Souza GD, Souza LQ. Preoperative imaging assessment of hidradenitis suppurativa. Brazil J Plastic Surg. 2019;34:264–7. https://doi.org/10.5935/2177-1235.2019RBCP0143.
21. Der Sarkissian S, Frew JW. Ultrasound-guided de-roofing of epithelialised tunnels of hidradenitis suppurativa. Australas J Dermatol. 2021;62:360–3. https://doi.org/10.1111/ajd.13600.
22. Elkin K, Daveluy S, Avanaki K. Review of imaging technologies used in hidradenitis suppurativa. Skin Res Technol. 2020;26:3–10. https://doi.org/10.1111/srt.12772.
23. Srisajjakul S, Prapaisilp P, Bangchokdee S. Magnetic resonance imaging of hidradenitis suppurativa: a focus on the Anoperineal location. Korean J Radiol. 2022;23:785–93.
24. Kelly AM, Cronin P. MRI features of hidradenitis suppurativa and review of the literature. AJR Am J Roentgenol. 2005;185:1201–4.
25. Nazzaro G, Calzari P, Vaienti S, Passoni E, Marzano AV. The role of imaging technologies in the diagnosis of hidradenitis suppurativa. Clin Dermatol. 2023;41:611–21.
26. Maz MP, Michelle KJ. Cutaneous and systemic connections in lupus. Curr Opin Rheumatol. 2020;32:583–9.
27. Fijalkowska A, Kadziela M, Zebrowska A. The spectrum of cutaneous manifestations in lupus erythematosus: a comprehensive review. J Clin Med. 2024;13:2419.
28. Vale ECS, do, Garcia LC. Cutaneous lupus erythematosus: a review of etiopathogenic, clinical, diagnostic and therapeutic aspects. An Bras Dermatol. 2023;98:355–72.
29. Zychowska M, Reich A. Dermoscopic features of acute, subacute, chronic and intermittent subtypes of cutaneous lupus erythematosus in Caucasians. J Clin Med. 2022;11:4088.
30. Patel J, Borucki R, Werth VP. An update on the pathogenesis of cutaneous lupus erythematosus and its role in clinical practice. Curr Rheumatol Rep. 2020;22:69.
31. Papara C, De Luca DA, Bieber K, Vorobyev A, Ludwig RJ. Morphea: the 2023 update. Front Med (Lausanne). 2023;10:1108623.
32. Fett N, Werth VP. Update on morphea. J Am Acad Dermatol. 2011;64:217–28.
33. Saceda-Corralo D, Tosti A. Trichoscopic features of linear Morphea on the scalp. Skin Appendage Disord. 2018;4:31–3.
34. de Marsillac PF, Cortez de Almeida RF, Machado CJ, Piraccini BM, Starace M, Tosti A, et al. Clinical, epidemiological, trichoscopic and histopathological features of linear morphea on the scalp. J Eur Acad Dermatol Venereol. 2022;36:e892.
35. Patterson JW. Weedon's skin pathology. 6th ed. Elsevier; 2024.
36. Wortsman X, Vera-Kellet C. Ultrasound Morphea activity scoring (US-MAS: modified US-MAS). J Ultrasound Med. 2023;42:2447–50.
37. Wortsman X. Why, how, and when to use color Doppler ultrasound for improving precision in the diagnosis, assessment of severity and activity in morphea. J Scleroderma Relat Disord. 2019;4:28–34.
38. Khorasanizadeh F, Kalantari Y, Etesami I. Role of imaging in morphea assessment: a review of the literature. Skin Res Technol. 2023;29:e13410.
39. Ezeh N, Caplan A, Rosenbach M, Imadojemu S. Cutaneous sarcoidosis. Dermatol Clin. 2023;41:455–70.
40. Mañá J, Marcoval J. Skin manifestations of sarcoidosis. Presse Med. 2012;41:e355–74.
41. Hubail A, Belkharoeva R, Tepluk N, Belerosova T. Lupus pernio (Besnier-Tenneson syndrome): a rare form of sarcoidosis. Dermatol Rep. 2018;10:10.
42. Loo Lim AY, Tang PY, Oh CC. Dermoscopy in cutaneous sarcoidosis. Dermatol Online J. 2021;27 https://doi.org/10.5070/D327955144.
43. López-Llunell C, Romaní J, Roé E, Giavedoni P, Vidal D, Wortsman X. Ultrasonographic patterns of cutaneous sarcoidosis. J Ultrasound Med. 2021;40:2521–6.
44. Moore SL, Teirstein AE. Musculoskeletal sarcoidosis: spectrum of appearances at MR imaging. Radiographics. 2003;23:1389–99.

Chapter 11
Clinical, Imaging, and Histological Findings in Infectious Lesions of the Face, Ears, and Neck

Ana Luisa Sampaio, Paula Figueiredo de Marsillac, Jéssica Gonçalves Povill, Stacy Smith, André da Silva Cartell, Manuela Boleira Sieiro Guimarães, Flavia Martins Costa, Carolina Ávila de Almeida, and Clarissa Canella Moraes do Carmo

In the realm of dermatology and infectious disease, accurate diagnosis and effective management hinge on a thorough understanding of both clinical and imaging findings. This chapter explores the use of advanced imaging techniques—including

A. L. Sampaio
Department of Dermatology, Hospital Universitario Pedro Ernesto, Universidade Estadual do Rio de Janeiro—UERJ, Rio de Janeiro, RJ, Brazil

P. F. de Marsillac
State University of Rio de Janeiro—UERJ, Hospital Universitário Pedro Ernesto, Rio de Janeiro, RJ, Brazil

J. G. Povill
Clinica de Diagnostico por Imagem, Dermatological Imaging at DASA, Barra da Tijuca, Rio de Janeiro, Brazil

S. Smith
Division of Musculoskeletal Imaging and Intervention, Brigham and Women's Hospital, Harvard Medical School, Boston, MA, USA

A. da Silva Cartell
Adjunct Professor at Faculdade de Medicina da Universidade Federal do Rio Grande do Sul, Rio de Janeiro, Brazil

Dermatologist and Dermatopathologist in Private Practice, Rio de Janeiro, Brazil

M. B. S. Guimarães
Dermatology Department, Policlinica geral do Rio de Janeiro, Castelo, RJ, Brazil

F. M. Costa
Universidade Federal do Rio de Janeiro—UFRJ, Rio de Janeiro, Brazil

Department of Radiology, Diagnóstico das Americas—DASA, Rio de Janeiro, Brazil

C. Á. de Almeida
Faculty of Medicine of Valença—UniFaa, Valença, Brazil

Federal University of Rio de Janeiro—UFRJ, Rio de Janeiro, Valença, Brazil

© The Author(s), under exclusive license to Springer Nature Switzerland AG 2025

C. Canella Moraes do Carmo (ed.), *Atlas of Diagnostic Imaging in Dermatology*, https://doi.org/10.1007/978-3-031-77987-9_11

ultrasonography, magnetic resonance imaging (MRI), and 3D imaging—in conjunction with clinical assessments to distinguish between herpes simplex virus (HSV) infections, herpes zoster (shingles), and cellulitis. While HSV and herpes zoster present with distinct clinical features such as vesicular eruptions and dermatomal distributions, cellulitis is characterized by diffuse inflammation and swelling. Advanced imaging modalities offer enhanced visualization of these conditions, revealing subtle differences in tissue involvement, lesion morphology, and disease progression. Ultrasonography provides real-time, dynamic imaging of soft tissues and can detect inflammatory changes and fluid collections. MRI with surface coil offers detailed cross-sectional images, allowing for the assessment of deeper tissue involvement and potential complications. Meanwhile, 3D advanced imaging techniques provide comprehensive, three-dimensional views that aid in evaluating complex cases. This chapter aims to integrate these imaging modalities with clinical findings, offering a comprehensive approach to diagnosing and managing herpes simplex, herpes zoster, and cellulitis.

11.1 Herpes Simplex and Herpes Zoster

11.1.1 Definition [1–3]

- Herpes simplex virus and varicella-zoster virus are both human alpha-herpes viruses.
- They are capable of establishing latent infections in neural tissues.
- The primary way herpes simplex virus is acquired is through direct exposure of mucous membranes or broken skin to individuals with an active primary or recurrent infection.
- Herpes zoster is the result of reactivation of latent varicella-zoster virus and occurs more frequently in older adults and immunocompromised individuals.

11.1.2 Epidemiology [4, 5]

- An estimated 491 million people live with herpes simplex virus type 2 infection, 3583.5 million with oral herpes simplex virus type 1 infection, and around 155 million with genital herpes simplex virus type 1 infection, in those up to 49 years of age.
- An estimated 625 million people were genitally infected with either herpes simplex virus type 1 or 2.

C. Canella Moraes do Carmo (✉)
Fluminense Federal University—UFF, Rio de Janeiro, Brazil

Federal University of Rio de Janeiro—UFRJ, Rio de Janeiro, Brazil

Diagnóstico das Américas—DASA—RJ, Rio de Janeiro, Brazil

Biodesign Laboratory, DASA-PUC, Rio de Janeiro, Brazil

- The lifetime risk of herpes zoster in the general population ranges from 20% to 30%. However, the risk increases after 50 years of age, with the lifetime risk reaching 50% by age 85.

11.1.3 Clinical Presentation (Figs. 11.1 and 11.2) [1, 3, 5, 6]

- Herpes simplex virus
  - The clinical manifestations are variable and influenced by the portal of viral entry and degree of host immunity.
  - Herpetic primary infection is typically preceded by a sensation of burning at the site of inoculation, local lymphadenopathy associated with systemic symptoms. Few days later, numerous vesicles appear on oral mucosa and rapidly rupture to cause painful and superficial ulcerations.
  - Recurrence of herpes occurs within 24 h of the prodrome, multiple vesicles coalesce, and rupture to form tender superficial erosions which rapidly crust over.
  - Eczema herpeticum or Kaposi's varicelliform eruption has an acute onset of extensive vesicles and pustules coalesce into large superficial erosions which are susceptible to secondary bacterial infection.
- Varicella-zoster virus
  - Cutaneous rash preceded by neuropathic pain (tingling, burning, or severe pain), over the involved dermatome 1–5 days, even weeks before.
  - Cutaneous rash is initially maculopapular on an erythematous base, evolves into vesicular-pustular after 7–10 days.
  - Affects a unilateral dermatome and does not cross the midline.
  - Scarring and hypo- or hyperpigmentation may persist months to years after herpes zoster has resolved.

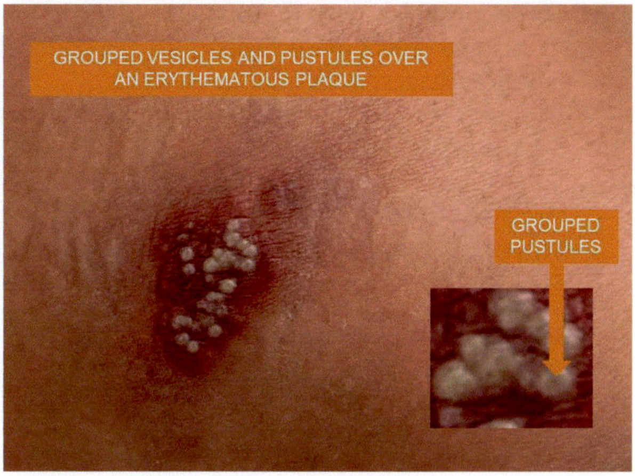

Fig. 11.1 Clinical photograph of a patient with herpes zoster

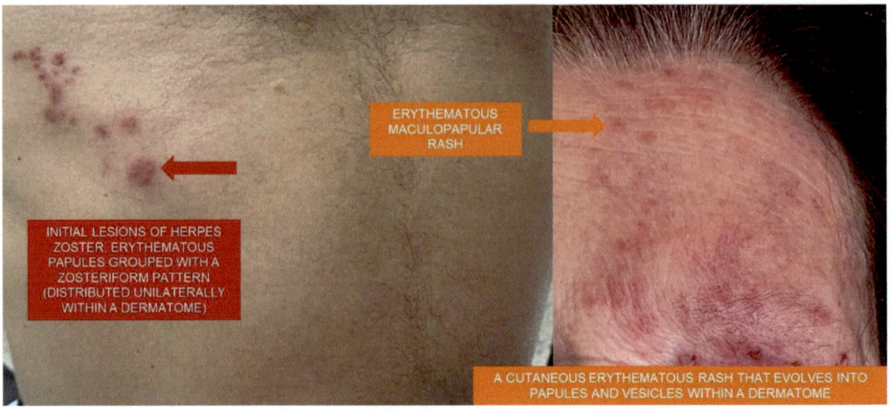

Fig. 11.2 Clinical photograph of a patient with herpes zoster

- The most commonly involved dermatomes are thoracic, followed by cranial (especially trigeminal), lumbar, and cervical. Simultaneous involvement of noncontiguous dermatomes rarely occurs in immunocompetent. Immunocompromised patients may have disseminated disease.
- The minority of the patients with herpes zoster develop systemic symptoms, such as fatigue, headache, fever, and malaise.

11.1.4 Dermoscopy (Fig. 11.3) [7]

- Herpes simplex
  - Dotted vessels: Small, red, dotted vessels may be seen in the affected area.
  - Scattered hemorrhages: Tiny bleeding spots that appear as red or dark blue dots.
  - Perilesional erythema: Redness around the lesion.
  - Crusts and ulceration: Irregular, uneven surfaces may be observed in more advanced stages.
  - Clustered vesicles: Early lesions may show grouped, translucent vesicles with a surrounding halo of redness.
- Early herpes zoster lesions
  - Poly-lobular gray and brown globules in a bright pink background.
  - Gray globules covered by grayish veil-like structure with gray rim.
- Late herpes zoster lesions
  - "Solar eclipse" pattern (poly-lobular gray and brown structures surrounded by erythematous zone).
  - "Crumpled fabric" patterns (folding of roof of flaccid bullae).

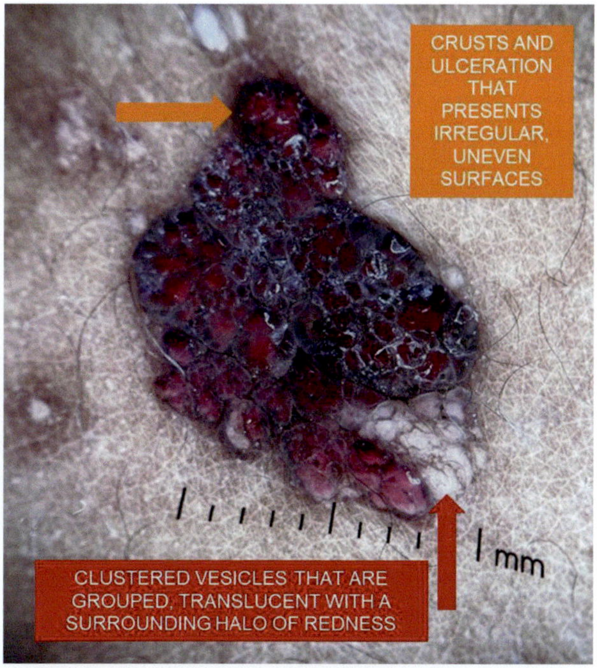

Fig. 11.3 Dermoscopy of a patient with herpes zoster (x10)

11.1.5 Histopathology (Fig. 11.4) [8, 9]

- Intraepidermal vesiculation in the early phase with epidermal necrosis and ballooning degeneration and necrotic bullae roof.
- Presence of acantholysis, perinuclear halos, and intracytoplasmic and intranuclear inclusion bodies containing multinucleated giant cells, chromatin margination, and central chromatolysis.
- Typical viral cytopathic changes are best seen at the borders of the vesicle or erosion.
- Multinucleation with central chromatolysis causes the phenomenon called shaped nuclei; herpes exhibits 3M: multinucleation, molding of nuclei, and margination of chromatin.
- Varicella-zoster has unique cytoplasmic or nuclear inclusions, usually basophilic, with retraction around the corpuscle (owl's eye), affecting epidermal cells. The blister pattern is not always distinct from herpes, especially in patients with altered immunity.

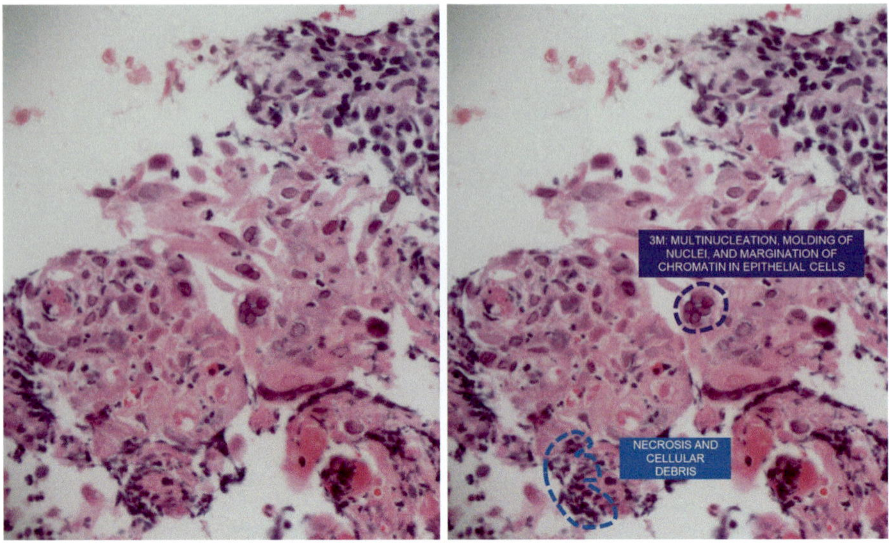

Fig. 11.4 Histological findings of herpes simplex (H&E x40)

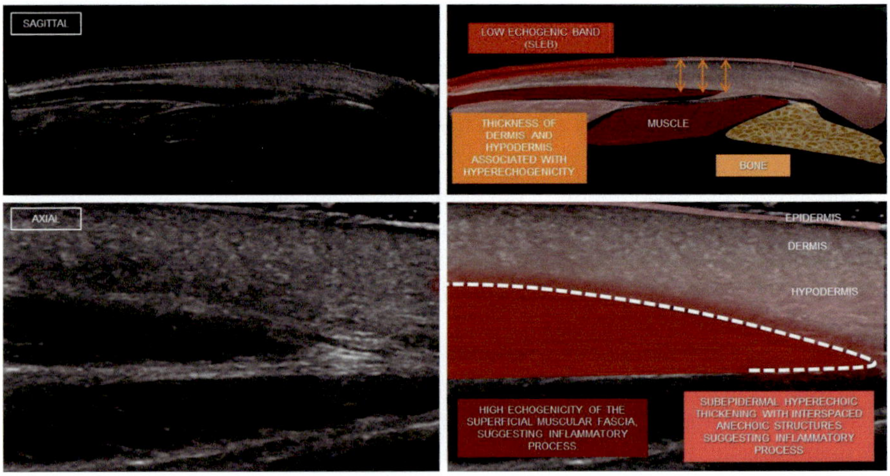

Fig. 11.5 Ultrasonographic findings of herpes with a 24 MHz probe (Aplio i800, Canon Medical Systems)

11.1.6 Ultrasonography (Fig. 11.5) [10]

- Ultrasonographic findings of herpes simples and herpes zoster are similar.
- Dermal hyperechogenicity and thickening with a prominent subepidermal low echogenic band (SLEB) indicating inflammatory origin.

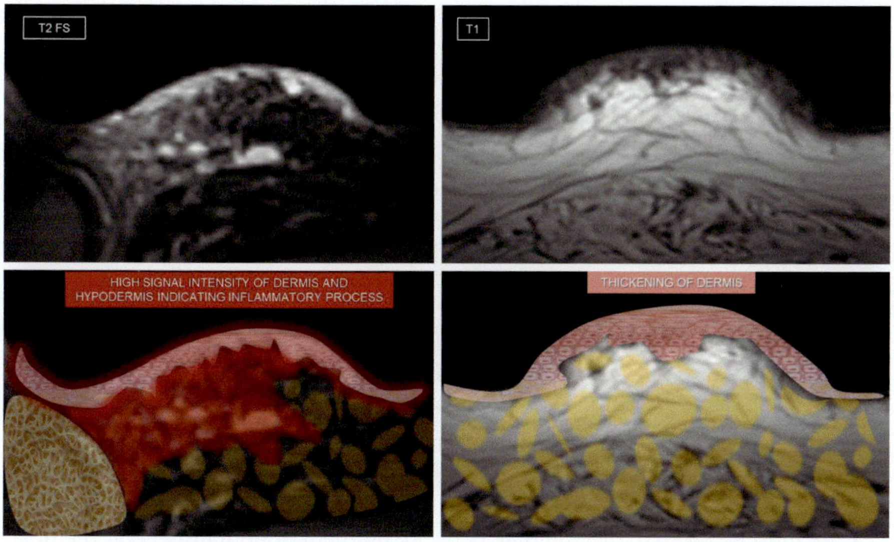

Fig. 11.6 MRI findings of herpes simplex on T1 and T2-weighted sequences with fat saturation using surface coil (Magnetom Avanto 1.5T MRI, Siemens)

- Subepidermal hypoechoic lesions associated with interspaced anechoic structures.
- Diffuse increase in vascularization on power Doppler imaging.

11.1.7 MRI (Fig. 11.6)

- MRI findings of herpes simples and herpes zoster are similar.
- Thickening of dermis and hypodermis with a high signal intensity on T2-weighted FS sequences indicating inflammatory origin.
- MRI is also important to detect extension of the inflammation to deep soft tissues and complications such myositis.

11.2 Cellulitis

11.2.1 Definition [11–13]

- Cellulitis is a bacterial infection involving skin and subcutaneous tissue
- May be classified as purulent or nonpurulent.
- Purulent cellulitis is defined as cellulitis associated with a pustule, abscess, or purulent drainage.

11.2.2 Epidemiology [14]

- Middle-aged and older adults.
- The most common diagnosis and accounted for an estimated 1.3% of all dermatology visits.
- Caused most commonly by beta-hemolytic streptococci from group A (*Streptococcus pyogenes*)
- *Staphylococcus aureus* is a significant, though less common, cause.

11.2.3 Clinical Presentation (Fig. 11.7) [12, 14, 15]

- Poorly demarcated erythema, edema, tenderness, and warmth of the affected skin.
- The lower extremities are the most common site of infection, but any area of skin can be involved.
- Care must be taken to differentiate between purulent or nonpurulent, as the treatment for nonpurulent cellulitis is antibiotic therapy without drainage. Typically, a purulent cellulitis will be fluctuant on examination.

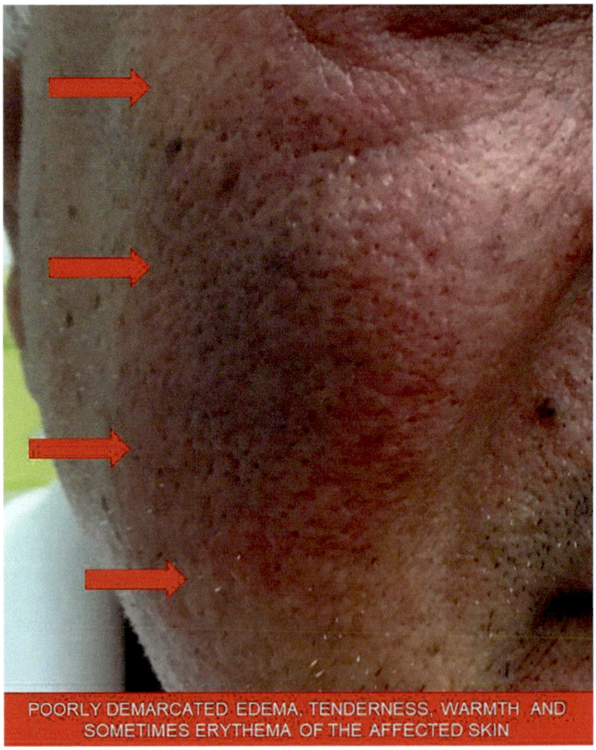

Fig. 11.7 Clinical photograph of a patient with cellulitis

11.2.4 Histopathology [9]

- Marked dermal and subcutaneous with venular and lymphatic ectasia.
- Initially, a perivascular neutrophilic inflammatory infiltrate is observed, which becomes more interstitial with the evolution of the lesion.
- Leukocytoclastic neutrophil cells may be present in the derma and hypodermis.
- The epidermis may present with secondary subepidermal cleavage blisters, usually associated with relevant dermal edema.
- Late lesions present granulation tissue fibrosis, predominance of mononuclear cells, including histiocytes and lymphocytes.
- Occasionally, hemorrhage, thrombotic vasculopathy or the presence of bacterial colonies may occur depending on the clinical situation.

11.2.5 Radiography and Computed Tomography (Fig. 11.8) [12, 14, 15]

- Radiography shows nonspecific diffuse soft tissue swelling and have the capability to detect radiopaque foreign bodies or soft tissue gas.
- Computed tomography provides a clearer view of cellulitis by showing the infiltration of subcutaneous adipose tissue and can also detect underlying abscesses, foreign bodies, or soft tissue gas.
- Abscesses on computed tomography are seen as fluid collection of low attenuation with surrounding irregular and thick rim-enhancement.

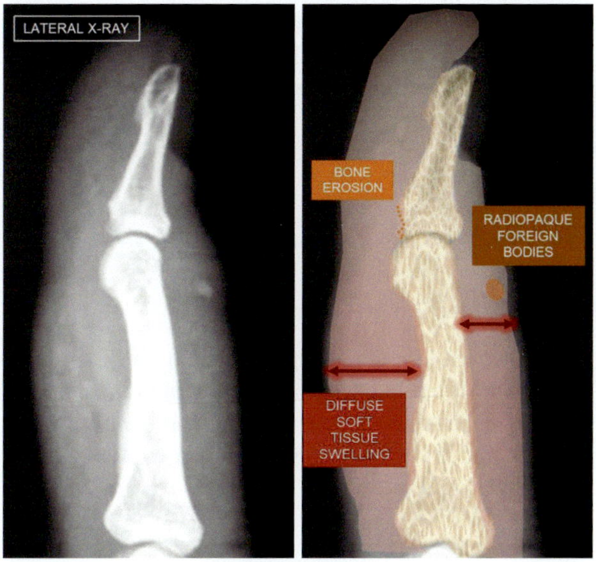

Fig. 11.8 Radiographic findings of cellulitis in a lateral X-ray (Philips Duo Diagnostic R&F Room Digital RF and Tomo System)

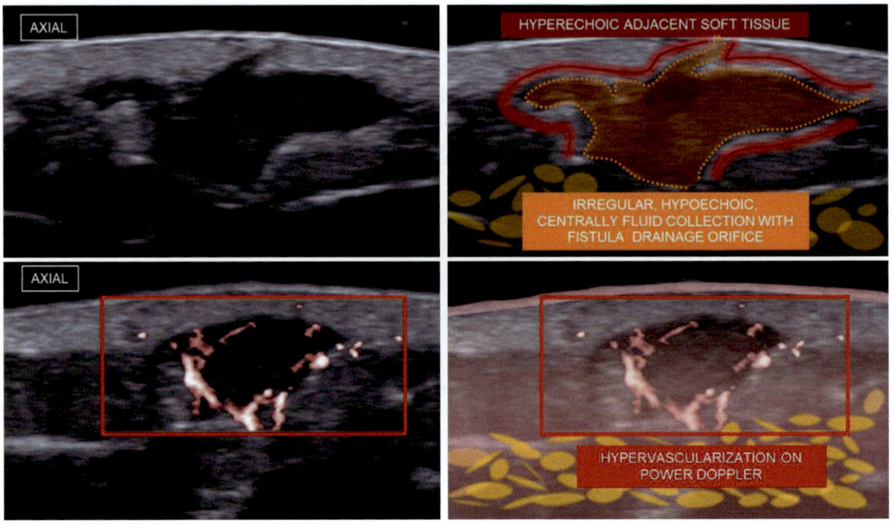

Fig. 11.9 Ultrasonographic findings of cellulitis and abscess with a 24 MHz probe (Aplio i800, Canon Medical Systems)

11.2.6 Ultrasonography (Fig. 11.9) [16–18]

- Irregular, hypoechoic, centrally avascular fluid collection on hypodermis surrounded by a hypervascular rim on power Doppler imaging.
- Fluid collections often show internal echos that may move with compression.
- Subcutaneous tissue edema with hypoechoic stranding amid echogenic fat lobules (cobblestone pattern).
- Surrounding dermal and hypodermal hyperechogenicity, thickening and increase in vascularization on power Doppler imaging with a prominent SLEB indicating inflammatory origin.

11.2.7 MRI (Fig. 11.10) [11, 19–21]

- Fluid collection presenting
  - low to intermediate signal intensity on T1-weighted images.
  - high signal intensity on T2-weighted images.
  - no enhancement after contrast administration
  - diffusion restriction on DWI images, that is hyperintense on high b-value and low signal on ADC.

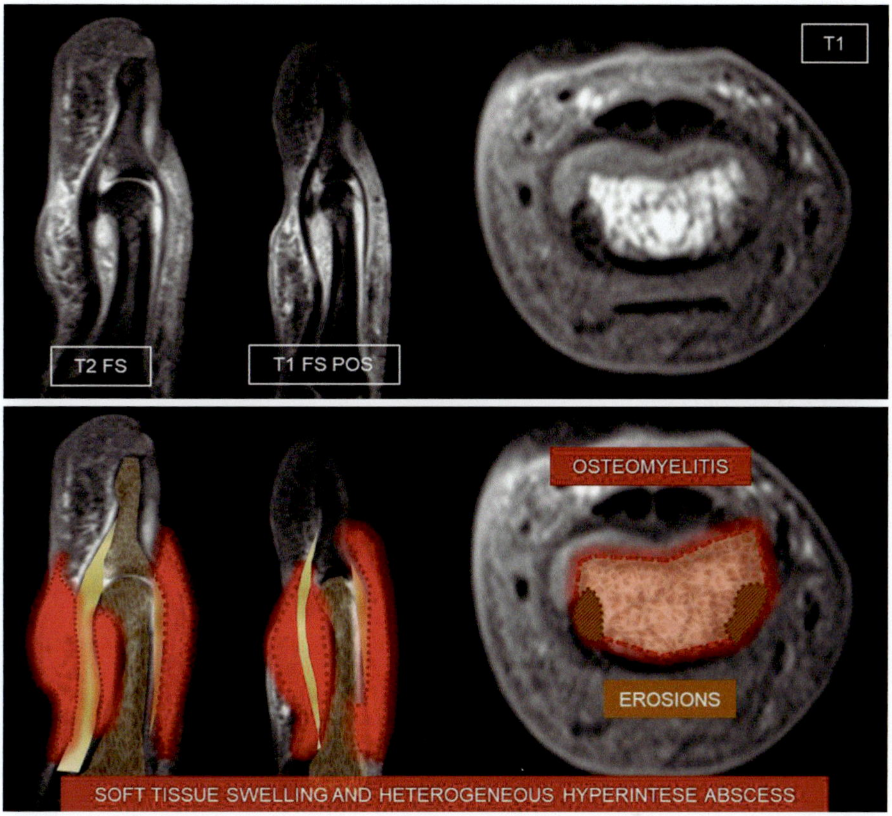

Fig. 11.10 MRI findings of cellulitis on T1 and T2-weighted sequences with fat saturation and T1 FS-weighted sequences after gadolinium administration using surface coil (Magnetom Avanto 1.5T MRI, Siemens)

- Capsular rim of the collection presenting
  - low signal intensity on T1-weighted images (high signal intensity of the penumbra sign is present on subacute abscesses, that represents a rim of vascularized granulation tissue surrounding the fluid collection).
  - low signal intensity on T2-weighted images.
  - marked enhancement after contrast administration.
- Diffuse linear or poorly defined thickening of surrounding soft tissue, presenting high signal intensity on T2-weighted images, low signal intensity on T1-weighted images, and diffuse enhancement post-contrast administration.
- MRI is also important to detect extension of the infection process to deep soft tissues and complications such as arthritis, osteomyelitis, and myositis.

References

1. Shah S, Singaraju S, Einstein A, Sharma A. Herpes zoster: a clinicocytopathological insight. J Oral Maxillofac Pathol. 2016;20:547.
2. Lautenschlager S. Herpes simplex und Varizella-Zoster-Virus-Infektionen. Ther Umsch. 2003;60:605–14.
3. Schmader K. Herpes zoster. Ann Intern Med. 2018;169:ITC17. https://doi.org/10.7326/AITC201808070.
4. James C, Harfouche M, Welton NJ, Turner KM, Abu-Raddad LJ, Gottlieb SL, et al. Herpes simplex virus: global infection prevalence and incidence estimates, 2016. Bull World Health Organ. 2020;98:315–29.
5. Fatahzadeh M, Schwartz RA. Human herpes simplex virus infections: epidemiology, pathogenesis, symptomatology, diagnosis, and management. J Am Acad Dermatol. 2007;57:737–63.
6. John AR, Canaday DH. Herpes zoster in the older adult. Infect Dis Clin N Am. 2017;31:811–26.
7. Ankad BS, Koti VR, Lallas A. Dermoscopic differentiation of blister beetle dermatitis and herpes zoster: an observational study. Dermatol Pract Concept. 2022;12:e2022180.
8. Hall BJ, Hall JC, Cockerell CJ, Affolter K, Alvarez P. Diagnostic pathology: nonneoplastic dermatopathology. Elsevier; 2017.
9. Patterson JW. Weedon's skin pathology. 6th ed. Elsevier; 2024.
10. Zattar L, Cerri GG. Ultrassonografia dermatológica. 1st ed. Manole; 2021.
11. Turecki MB, Taljanovic MS, Stubbs AY, Graham AR, Holden DA, Hunter TB, et al. Imaging of musculoskeletal soft tissue infections. Skeletal Radiol. 2010;39:957–71.
12. Altmayer S, Verma N, Dicks EA, Oliveira A. Imaging musculoskeletal soft tissue infections. Semin Ultrasound CT MRI. 2020;41:85–98.
13. de Almeida CÁ, Nakamura R, Leverone A, Costa F, Estrada BD, Haui P, et al. Imaging features for the evaluation of skin and nail infections. Skeletal Radiol. 2024;53:2051. https://doi.org/10.1007/s00256-023-04557-4.
14. Salastekar N, Su A, Rowe JS, Somasundaram A, Wong PK, Hanna TN. Imaging of soft tissue infections. Radiol Clin North Am. 2023;61:151–66.
15. Chin TY, Peh WC. Imaging update on musculoskeletal infections. J Clin Orthop Trauma. 2021;22:101600.
16. Cataldo-Cerda K, Wortsman X. Dissecting cellulitis of the scalp early diagnosed by color doppler ultrasound. Int J Trichol. 2017;9:147–8.
17. Wortsman X. Common applications of dermatologic sonography. J Ultrasound Med. 2012;31:97–111. https://doi.org/10.7863/jum.2012.31.1.97.
18. Wortsman X. Sonography of dermatologic emergencies. J Ultrasound Med. 2017;36:1905–14. https://doi.org/10.1002/jum.14211.
19. Weaver JS, Omar IM, Mar WA, Klauser AS, Winegar BA, Mlady G, et al. Magnetic resonance imaging of musculoskeletal infections. Pol J Radiol. 2022;87:141–62.
20. Hayeri MR, Ziai P, Shehata ML, Teytelboym OM, Huang BK. Soft-tissue infections and their imaging mimics: from cellulitis to necrotizing fasciitis. Radiographics. 2016;36:1888–910.
21. Pal D, Roy SG, Singh R, Hayeri MR. Imaging features of soft-tissue infections. Skeletal Radiol. 2024;53:2211.

Chapter 12
Clinical, Imaging, and Histological Findings in Tumoral Lesions of the Face, Ears, and Neck

Ana Luísa Sampaio, Viviane Maria Maiolini, Jéssica Gonçalves Povill, Maria de Oliveira Buffara, Camila Silveira Nobre, Haizza Cristina de Almeida Cabral Monteiro, Elisa de Oliveira Barcaui, Julia de Oliveira Barcaui, Marina Ramos Costa, Talita Caldas Oliveira, Rachel Marina Sá Rosado, Carolina Ávila de Almeida, André da Silva Cartell, Livia Guidoni, Curt Mafra Treu, Tatiana Fazecas, Laila Klotz de Almeida Balassiano, Fernada Miraldi, Marcos Decnop, Michele Azevedo Gomes, Thais Emanuelle Freire Barbosa, Julia Diva Zavariz, and Clarissa Canella Moraes do Carmo

Accurate imaging plays a crucial role in diagnosing and managing tumoral lesions of the face, ears, and neck, considering both medical and cosmetic implications. This chapter offers an in-depth examination of how advanced imaging technologies, such as ultrasonography, magnetic resonance imaging with surface coil, and 3D imaging,

Supplementary Information The online version contains supplementary material available at https://doi.org/10.1007/978-3-031-77987-9_12.

A. L. Sampaio
Department of Dermatology, Hospital Universitario Pedro Ernesto, Universidade Estadual do Rio de Janeiro—UERJ, Rio de Janeiro, Brazil

M. de Oliveira Buffara · C. S. Nobre
State University of Rio de Janeiro—UERJ, Pedro Ernesto Hospital—HUPE, Rio de Janeiro, RJ, Brazil

V. M. Maiolini
Faculty of Medicine, Cancer Institute of the State of São Paulo—ICESP, University of São Paulo—FMUSP, São Paulo, Brazil

J. G. Povill
Clinica de Diagnostico por Imagem, Dermatological Imaging at DASA, Barra da Tijuca, Rio de Janeiro, Brazil

H. C. de Almeida Cabral Monteiro
State University of Rio de Janeiro—UERJ, Pedro Ernesto Hospital—HUPE, Rio de Janeiro, RJ, Brazil

Department of Dermatology, Hospital Rio-Barra and Rede D'Or São Luiz, Rio de Janeiro, Brazil

© The Author(s), under exclusive license to Springer Nature Switzerland AG 2025

C. Canella Moraes do Carmo (ed.), *Atlas of Diagnostic Imaging in Dermatology*, https://doi.org/10.1007/978-3-031-77987-9_12

E. de Oliveira Barcaui
Ultrasonography, Clinica Dermatologica de Ipanema—CDI—Rio de Janeiro, Rio de Janeiro, RJ, Brazil

J. de Oliveira Barcaui
Souza Marques Faculty of Medicine, Rio de Janeiro, RJ, Brazil

M. R. Costa
State University of Rio de Janeiro—UERJ, Pedro Ernesto Hospital—HUPE, Rio de Janeiro, RJ, Brazil

Instituto de Dermatologia Professor Rubem David Azulay- Santa Casa da Misericórdia do Rio de Janeiro, Rio de Janeiro, Brazil

T. C. Oliveira
Department of Dermatology, Fluminense Federal University—UFF, Hospital Universitario Antonio Pedro—HUAP, Niterói, Brazil

R. M. Sá Rosado
State University of Rio de Janeiro—UERJ, Pedro Ernesto Hospital—HUPE, Rio de Janeiro, RJ, Brazil

Dermatologist and Rheumatologist in Private Practice, Rio de Janeiro, RJ, Brazil

C. Á. de Almeida
Faculty of Medicine of Valença—UniFaa, Valença, Brazil

Federal University of Rio de Janeiro—UFRJ, Rio de Janeiro, Brazil

A. da Silva Cartell
Adjunct Professor at Faculdade de Medicina da Universidade Federal do Rio Grande do Sul, Rio de Janeiro, Brazil

Dermatologist and Dermatopathologist in Private Practice, Rio de Janeiro, Brazil

L. Guidoni
Hospital Universitario Cassiano Antonio Moraes—UFES, Vitória, Brazil

C. M. Treu
Department of Dermatologic Surgery and Cutaneous Oncology, Policlinica Geral do Rio de Janeiro—PGRJ and Hospital Federal de Bonsucesso, Castelo, Brazil

T. Fazecas
Radiology Department, Hospital Municipal Jesus—HMJ and Diagnósticos da América—DASA, Rio de Janeiro, Brazil

L. K. de Almeida Balassiano
Sector of Dermatology and Post Graduate Course in Medical Clinics—UFRJ, University of Rio de Janeiro, Rio de Janeiro, RJ, Brazil

Medical Clinics—UFRJ, Federal University of Rio de Janeiro, Rio de Janeiro, Brazil

F. Miraldi
Fonte Imagem Medicina Diagnóstica, Casa de Saúde São José and Fleury Group, Rio de Janeiro, Brazil

M. Decnop
Department of Radiology, Instituto Nacional De Cancer—INCA, Centro, Rio de Janeiro, Brazil

M. A. Gomes
Head and Neck Oncological Surgery, National Institute of Cancer—INCA, Rio de Janeiro, Brazil

contribute to the assessment of these complex lesions. By highlighting the strengths and applications of each imaging technique, we aim to enhance understanding and clinical practice. From detailed visualization of tumoral structures to guiding surgical interventions and monitoring disease progression, these imaging modalities are indispensable tools in dermatological diagnostics and treatment planning. This chapter will provide dermatologists with the insights needed to effectively incorporate these technologies into their practice for improved patient outcomes.

12.1 Tumoral Lesions on the Face

12.1.1 Hemangiomas

12.1.1.1 Definition [1, 2]

- Hemangiomas are common benign tumors characterized by the abnormal proliferation of blood vessels.
- They can occur anywhere on the body but are most frequently found on the skin and internal organs.

12.1.1.2 Epidemiology [2, 3]

- Cutaneous hemangiomas are the most frequent benign tumors in infancy, affecting approximately 4–10% of infants.
- They are more prevalent in girls, premature infants, and Caucasian babies.
- Most cases are sporadic.

12.1.1.3 Clinical Presentation (Fig. 12.1) [2]

- Hemangiomas typically present as a bright red, raised lesion on the skin, often referred to as a "strawberry mark."

T. E. F. Barbosa
Marcilio Dias Naval Hospital, National Cancer Institute—INCA, Rio de Janeiro, Brazil

J. D. Zavariz
Radiology Institute of Clinical Hospital, São Paulo, Brazil

C. Canella Moraes do Carmo (✉)
Fluminense Federal University—UFF, Rio de Janeiro, Brazil

Federal University of Rio de Janeiro—UFRJ, Rio de Janeiro, Brazil

Diagnóstico das Américas—DASA—RJ, Rio de Janeiro, Brazil

Biodesign Laboratory, DASA-PUC, Rio de Janeiro, Brazil

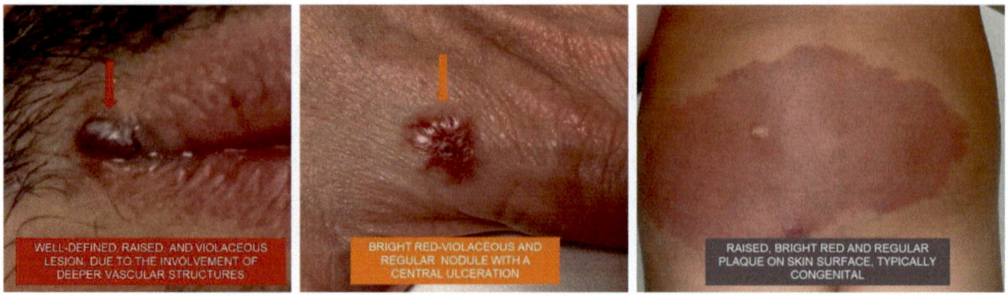

Fig. 12.1 Clinical photograph of patients with hemangioma

- They typically emerge within the first few weeks of life, undergo rapid growth in the initial months, and gradually regress over several years.
- They progress through three characteristic phases:
  - Proliferative phase: Lasts for the first 6 months, marked by rapid growth.
  - Stabilization phase: Occurs during the first year.
  - Involuting phase: Lasts until the child is 5 to 7 years old, during which the hemangioma gradually shrinks and fades.

12.1.1.4 Dermoscopy (Fig. 12.2) [4]

- Dermoscopy of infantile hemangioma
  - Infantile hemangiomas often display multiple lacunae (small, round, or oval spaces) with varying colors, typically red to blue, against a background that can also vary in color.
  - Visible isolated blood vessels may be present within the lesion.
  - In some cases, particularly when the hemangioma is thrombosed, there may be areas that appear jet-black due to the presence of clotted blood.
- Dermoscopy of cherry angioma:
  - Similar to infantile hemangiomas, cherry angiomas display multiple lacunae, typically exhibiting a more uniform red coloration.
  - Isolated vessels may also be seen within cherry angiomas.
  - While less common in cherry angiomas, thrombosed areas can present as jet-black regions.

12.1.1.5 Histopathology (Fig. 12.3) [5]

- Capillary hemangioma (cherry angioma): Small mature vessels lined with a single layer of flattened endothelial cells, tends to be superficial and forms small papules; epidermis usually normal or atrophic by compression.
- Cavernous hemangioma: large vessels, tendency to thrombosis, extends to the hypodermis or beyond.

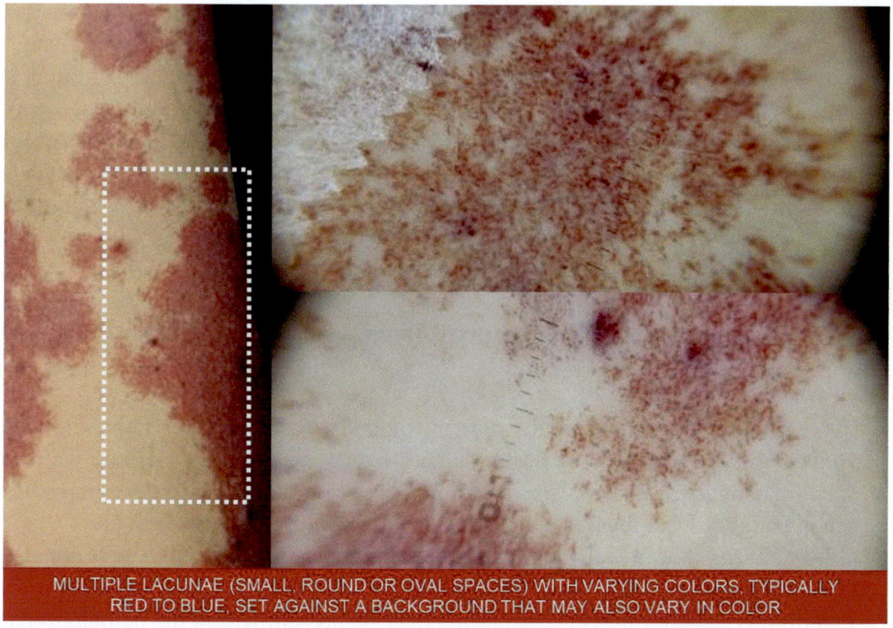

Fig. 12.2 Dermoscopic findings of patient with hemangioma (x10)

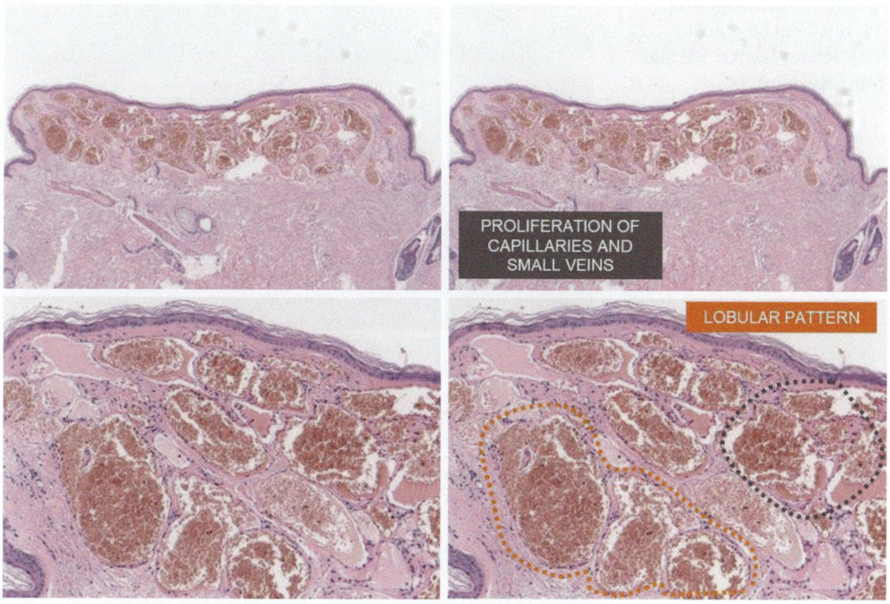

Fig. 12.3 Histological findings of hemangioma (H&E x4)

- Pyogenic granuloma or capillary lobular hemangioma: proliferation of capillaries and small veins in the derma or more deeply arranged in a lobular pattern, which may assume a polypoid profile with a characteristic collarette, often exhibiting a solution of epithelial continuity centrally; in the later phase of organization, it may present fibrosis, with fewer and dilated fused vessels, chronic inflammation, and hemosiderosis. It should be noted that in the initial phase the presence of ulceration, mitosis, inflammatory process and even endothelial atypia may occur and cause confusion with malignancy in small superficial biopsies.

12.1.1.6 Radiography and Computed Tomography (Figs. 12.4 and 12.5) [1, 3, 6]

- Typically, radiography is not the primary modality for evaluating hemangiomas. However, it may show soft tissue density overlying the affected area without specific bony involvement. In cases with deeper or more extensive lesions, radiographs might reveal displacement of adjacent structures and phebolytis.
- CT scans will show a well-defined, often lobulated, soft tissue mass with intense enhancement due to their vascular nature.
- Phleboliths (small round calcifications) may be present within the hemangioma.
- In some cases, specially with large or deep lesions, there may be evidence of bone remodeling or erosion adjacent to the hemangioma.

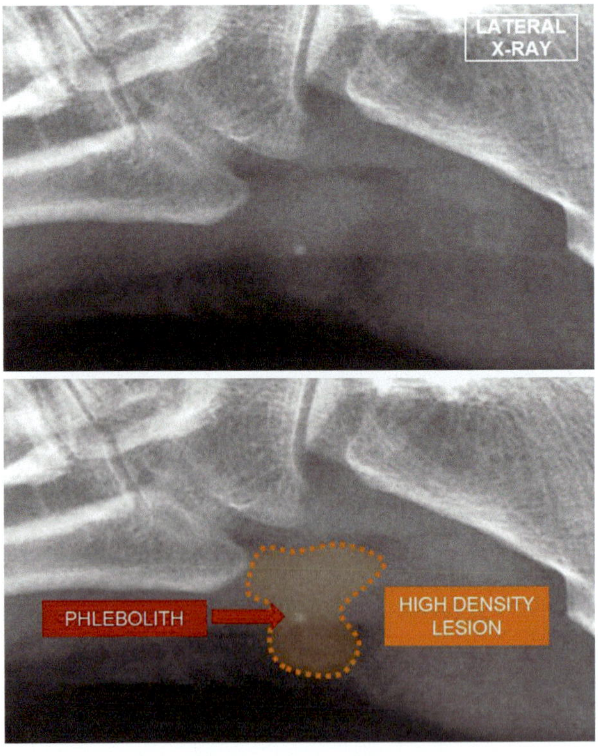

Fig. 12.4 Radiographic findings of hemangioma (Philips Duo Diagnost R&F Room Digital RF and Tomo System)

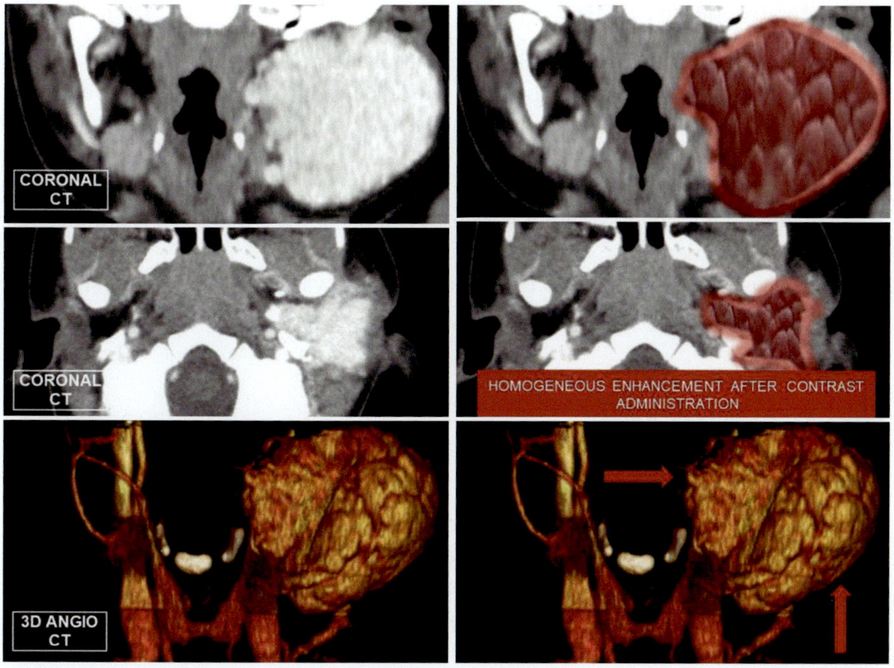

Fig. 12.5 Computed tomography findings of hemangioma (Philips Brilliance CT 64-slice)

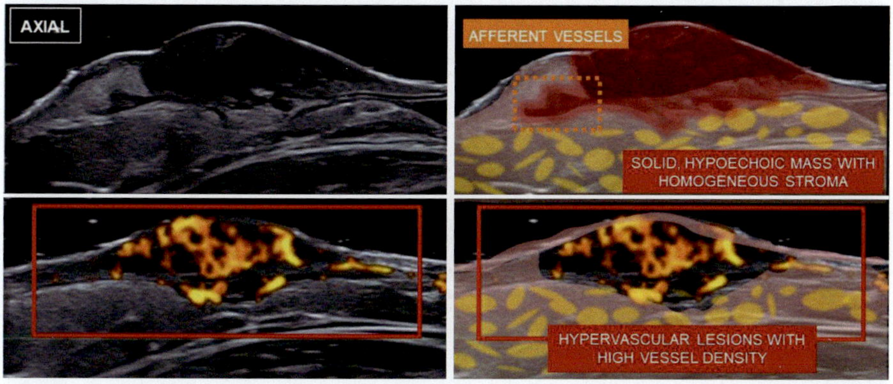

Fig. 12.6 Ultrasonographic findings of hemangioma with a 24 MHz probe (Aplio i800, Canon Medical Systems)

12.1.1.7 Ultrasonography (Fig. 12.6) [2, 7, 8]

- Ultrasonography is valuable in determining the depth and extent of hemangiomas.
- On ultrasonography, they commonly present as hypoechoic or mixed echogenic lesions with increased vascularization on Doppler imaging.

- Proliferative phase
  - Solid, hypoechoic tumor mass with homogeneous stroma.
  - Hypervascular lesions with high vessel density (>5 vessels/cm^2) and low resistive index on power Doppler imaging.
- Involuting phase
  - Increased echogenicity with a heterogeneous stroma due to fibroadipose tissue replacement.
  - Decreased power Doppler flow, though high systolic flow may persist compared to normal skin.

12.1.1.8 MRI (Fig. 12.7)

- Heterogeneous mass presenting:
  - Intermediate signal on T1-weighted sequences.
  - Hyperintense signal on T2-weighted images, although small areas of flow-voids, fibrous tissue, or calcification may be observed.
  - Homogeneous enhancement after gadolinium administration.

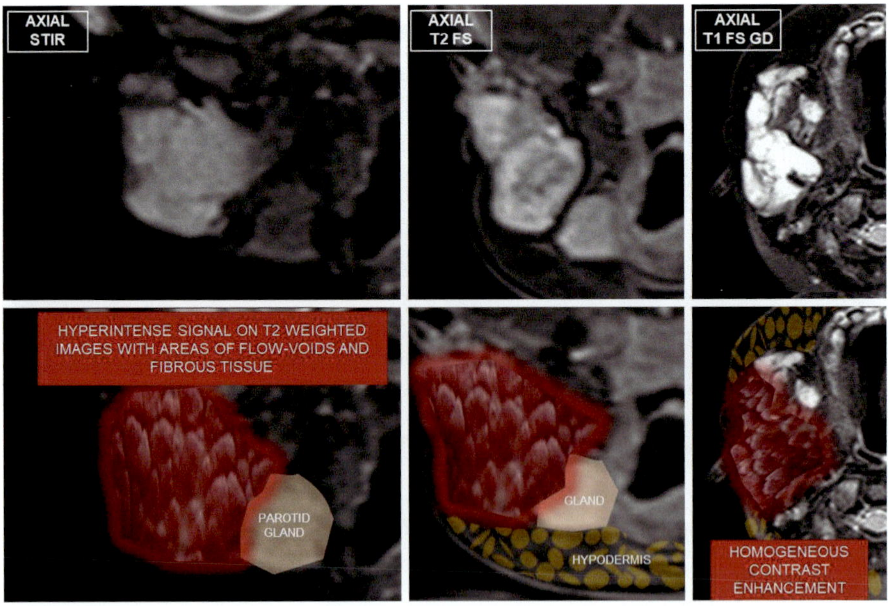

Fig. 12.7 MRI with surface coil findings of hemangioma on T2 FS, STIR, and T1 FS weighted sequences after gadolinium administration (Magnetom Prisma 3T MRI, Siemens)

12.1.2 Cylindroma

12.1.2.1 Definition [9]

- Cylindromas are rare adnexal neoplasms.
- Characterized by dual lineage cell proliferation within the dermis.
- Likely derived from apocrine cells in the hair follicle bulge.
- Exhibit a round, cylindrical morphology.
- Generally benign and slow-growing.
- Rare instances of malignant transformation and metastasis, especially in Brooke–Spiegler syndrome (autossomal dominant inherited disease with predisposition of multiple adnexal tumors, such as cilindromas and trichoepiteliomas).

12.1.2.2 Epidemiology [9]

- Rare, predominantly affecting females (9:1 ratio compared to males).
- More common in Caucasian populations.
- Sporadic forms typically present as solitary lesions in older patients.
- Familial forms present multiple lesions, often associated with syndromes like Brooke–Spiegler syndrome, and appear around puberty.
- Associated with other tumors, such as spiradenomas, trichoepitheliomas, and parotid tumors.

12.1.2.3 Clinical Presentation (Fig. 12.8) [9]

- Solitary lesions
  - Slow-growing, painless, round nodules.
  - Usually less than 1 cm in diameter.
  - Most often found on the scalp and face.
  - Pinkish or tan coloration with a smooth surface.
  - May feature small superficial blood vessels.
- Multiple lesions
  - Typically linked to familial syndromes.
  - Can grow larger, sometimes exceeding 20 cm.
  - May become painful and ulcerate.

12.1.2.4 Dermoscopy [9]

- Reveals round, well-defined nodules with a smooth surface.
- Vascular structures, such as small superficial blood vessels, may be visualized.
- Characteristic cylindrical shape supports diagnosis, especially on the scalp.
- Multiple lesions can merge to form larger masses in syndromic cases.

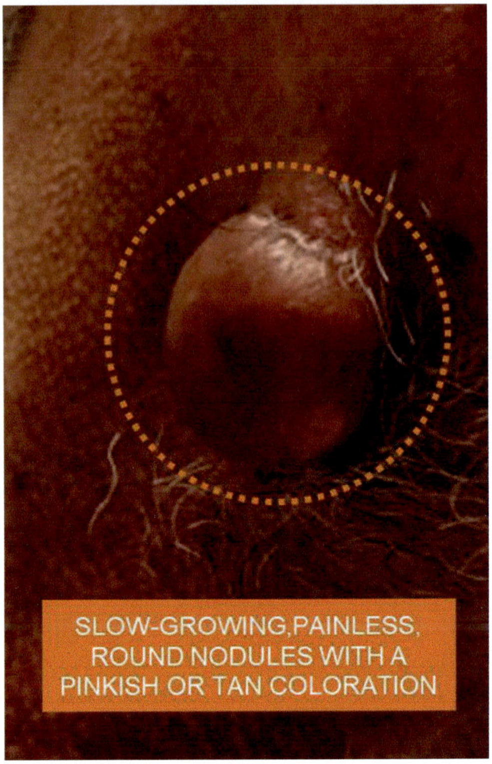

Fig. 12.8 Clinical photograph of patient with cylindroma

12.1.2.5 Histopathology [9]

- Characterized by variably sized rounded islands of basaloid cells.
- Arranged in a jigsaw puzzle-like pattern within the dermis, often extending into the subcutis.
- Islands do not connect to the overlying epidermis.
- Surrounded by an interconnecting hyalinized sheath.
- Cell populations
  - Peripheral lining of smaller, hyperchromatic cells.
  - Inner population of larger, paler cells with small duct-like structures.
  - Hyaline droplets (small round pink globules) are often interspersed within basaloid islands.

12.1.2.6 Ultrasonography (Fig. 12.9) [9]

- Well-defined, lobulated, heterogeneous mass in hypodermis, predominantly hypoechoic.

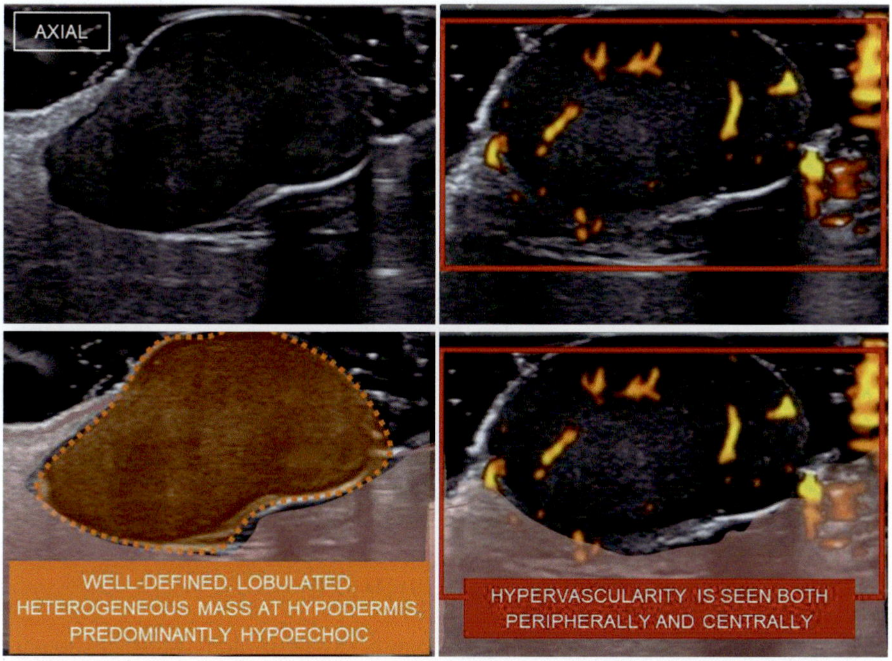

Fig. 12.9 Ultrasonographic findings of cylindroma with a 24 MHz probe (Aplio i800, Canon Medical Systems)

- Hypervascularity is seen both peripherally and centrally within the lesion on power Doppler imaging.
- Usually lack of invasion of adjacent structures.

12.1.2.7 MRI [9]

- Low signal intensity on T1-weighted images and intermediate to high signal intensity on T2-weighted images.
- Homogenous enhancement on contrast imaging.
- Giant lesions present high vascularity appearance and hemorrhagic features.

12.2 Tumoral Lesions on the Ears

12.2.1 Chondrodermatitis Nodularis Helicis

12.2.1.1 Definition [10, 11]

- Also called chondrodermatitis nodularis chronica helicis (CNH).

- Benign and painful inflammatory nodule or papule on the helix or antihelix of the ear.
- The exact etiology behind the development of CNH remains unclear.
- Chronic and excessive pressure on the pinna, autoimmune and connective tissue disorders, especially in young female patients, anatomical features, solar damage, and exposure to cold weather could be additional predisposing conditions.

12.2.1.2 Epidemiology [10, 11]

- CNH is infrequently documented in the literature. For this reason, the exact incidence of CNH remains unknown.
- Commonly affects men of middle age or later (70% to 90% of patients), when not associated with autoimmune processes.
- It is more frequent among fair-skinned people with a history of chronic sun exposure.

12.2.1.3 Clinical Presentation (Fig. 12.10) [10, 11]

- CNH is a painful, benign inflammatory nodule or papule on the helix or antihelix of the ear that is tender to touch or pressure.
- The nodule tends to be firm, tender, and usually fixed to the underlying auricular cartilage.
- Typical lesions are unilateral, 4 to 6 mm in size, and consist of an ulcerated nodule with a central crater. Crusting may or may not be present, and some lesions may have a cystic appearance.
- Bleeding and exudate accumulation after removal of the crust can be presented.

12.2.1.4 Dermoscopy [12]

- CNH presented dermoscopically with central keratin or an erosion surrounded by structureless white areas and ill-defined vessels.
- Dermoscopy did not allow the differentiation of CNH from squamous cell carcinoma. Histopathological examination is recommended.

12.2.1.5 Histopathology (Fig. 12.11) [13]

- Central erosion or ulceration, usually located at the apex of the helix, typically skin with relevant chronic photodamage, and may present with parakeratotic collarette or hemorrhagic scale-crust.
- Dermal edema in the acute phase.

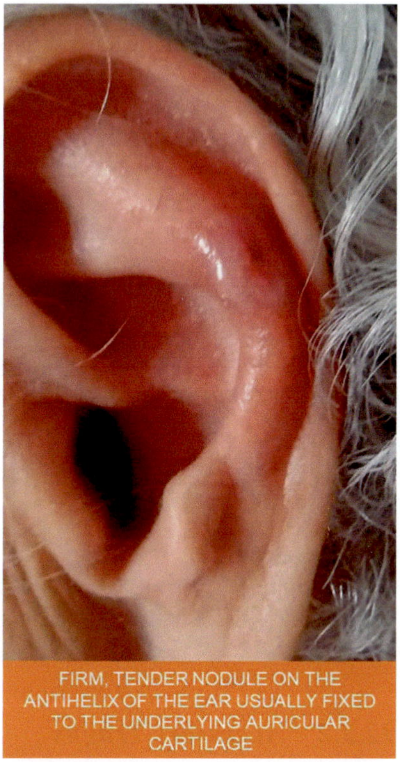

Fig. 12.10 Clinical photograph of patients with chondrodermatitis nodularis helicis

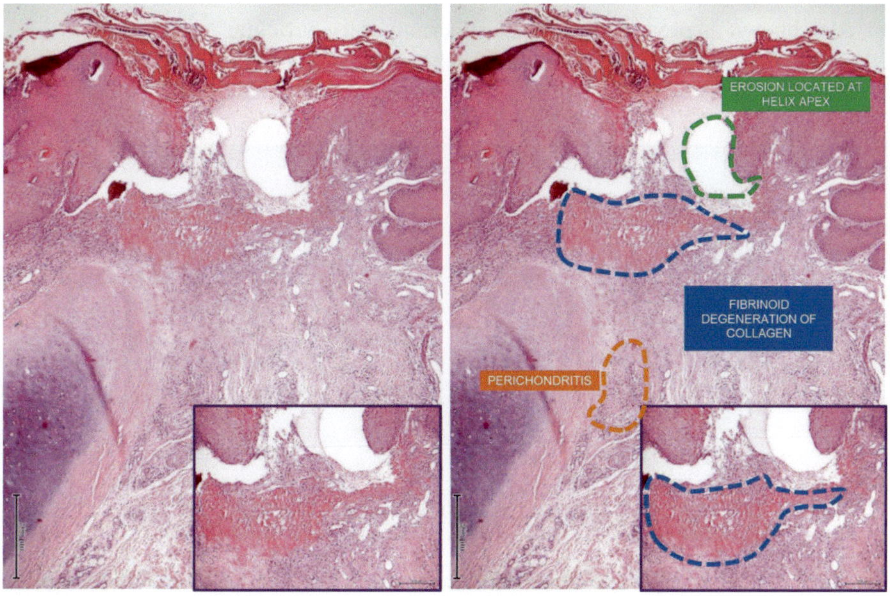

Fig. 12.11 Histological findings of chondrodermatitis nodularis helicis (H&E x4 and x10)

- Transepidermal elimination of degenerated collagen associated with granulation tissue and fibrinoid degeneration of collagen may be present; in the late stage it can organize as fibrosis.
- The presence of perichondritis or true focal chondritis, although rare, is usually associated with clinically disproportionate pain.

12.2.1.6 Ultrasonography (Fig. 12.12)

- Increased thickness and echogenicity reduction of auricular cartilage with ill-defined margins.
- Nodular lesions pattern and side asymmetry.
- Hypervascularity on power doppler imaging.

12.2.1.7 MRI

- Increased thickness of auricular cartilage with ill-defined edges presenting hyperintense signal on T2-weighted image.
- Nodular lesions pattern and side asymmetry.

12.2.2 *Accessory Tragus*

12.2.2.1 Definition [14]

- Also known as preauricular tag or supernumerary auricular appendage.
- Congenital anomaly characterized by the presence of extra skin or cartilage near the external ear.

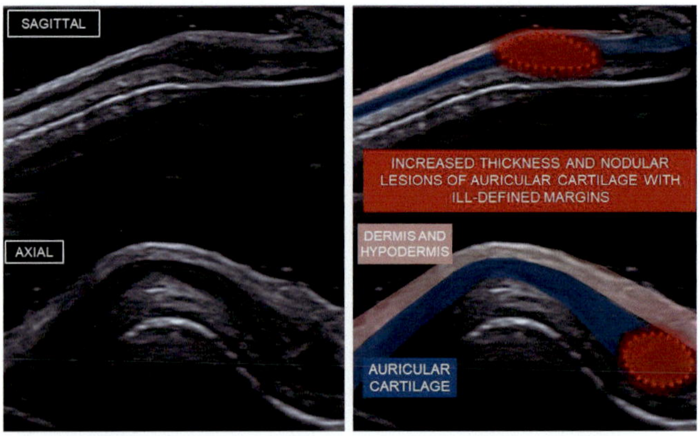

Fig. 12.12 Ultrasonographic findings of chondrodermatitis nodularis helicis with 24 MHz probe (Aplio i800, Canon Medical Systems)

- Often located in preauricular area, near the external ear canal, and can vary in size and shape.
- Accessory tragus is generally considered a benign and non-harmful condition. It does not typically cause pain or discomfort, and it is not associated with underlying health issues. While it is present from birth, it may become more noticeable over time as the child grows.

12.2.2.2 Epidemiology [14]

- The prevalence of accessory tragus is 1.7: 1000 and 9: 10,000–10: 10,000 for unilateral and bilateral lesions, respectively.
- A study in China reported a prevalence rate of 0.22% for this condition, whereas a more recent study indicated that there is 0.43% prevalence in Turkey.

12.2.2.3 Clinical Presentation (Fig. 12.13) [14]

- Skin-colored nodule or papule usually 3–10 mm in the preauricular region anterior to the tragus.
- Other less common locations are from the tragus down on an angle to the side of the mouth or anteriorly to the sternocleidomastoid muscle; and also on the cheek, lateral aspect of the neck, superior sternum, and glabella.
- Multiple lesions have also been rarely reported.

12.2.2.4 Histopathology [15, 16]

- Histological features of accessory tragus include a thin layer of stratum corneum with a rugated epidermis, presence of eccrine glands, and irregular spatial positioning of vellus hair follicles accompanied by sebaceous glands.

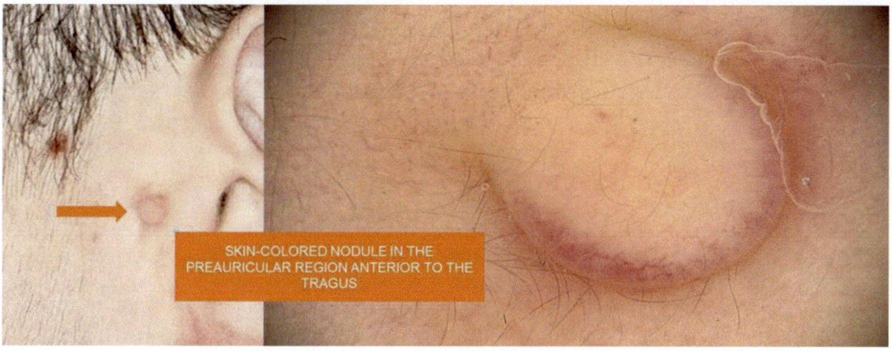

Fig. 12.13 Clinical photograph of patient with accessory tragus

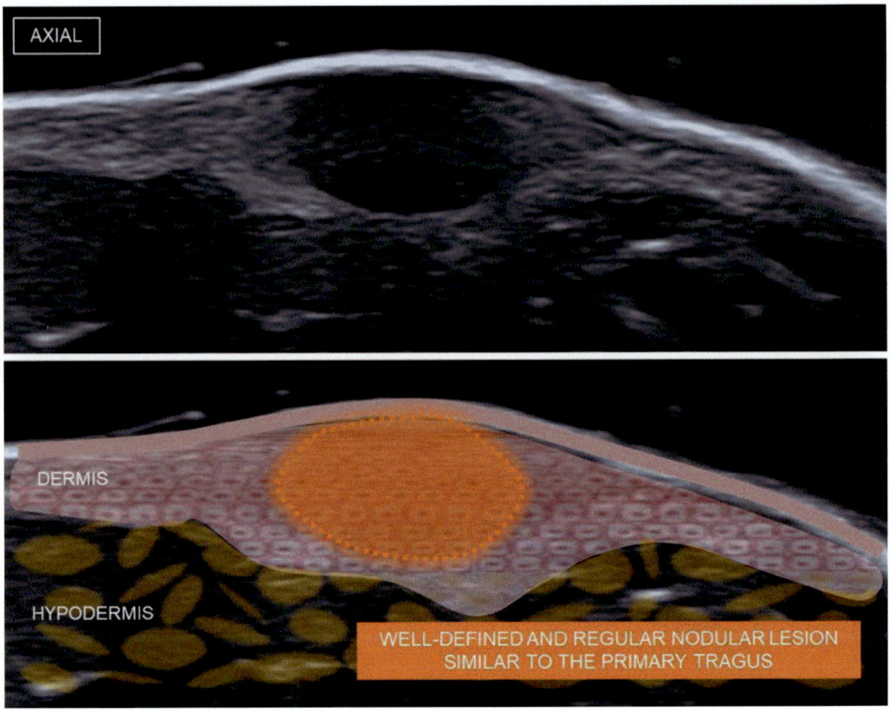

Fig. 12.14 Ultrasonographic findings of accessory tragus with a 24 MHz probe (Aplio i800, Canon Medical Systems)

- They are polypoid lesions with a loose fibrous stroma, which may or may not contain adipose tissue, the presence of vellus hairs with small sebaceous glands, and the characteristic central core consisting of cartilaginous tissue.

12.2.2.5 Ultrasonography (Fig. 12.14)

- Ultrasonography helps identify which layers compose the extra tissue.
- Nodular pattern with well-defined borders.
- Pattern and characteristics are similar to the primary tragus.

12.2.3 Keloid

12.2.3.1 Definition [17]

- Keloids result from abnormal wound healing in response to skin trauma or inflammation.
- Keloids can be formed by the trauma of earring or piercing.

12.2.3.2 Epidemiology [17]

- Dark-skinned individuals of African, Asian, and Hispanic descent have higher rates of keloid development compared to Caucasians.
- Incidence is notably higher during pregnancy and puberty.
- A positive family history increases the risk for keloid development.

12.2.3.3 Clinical Presentation (Fig. 12.15) [17]

- Keloids present as firm, rubbery nodules in an area of prior injury to the skin.
- Keloidal tissue extends beyond the initial site of trauma.
- Patients may experience pain, itching, or burning.

12.2.3.4 Histopathology (Fig. 12.16) [5]

- Most frequently, it occurs associated with a chronic healing process, which is better observed in the periphery and, centrally (place in another topic, on the line below), collagen fibers are replaced by irregular and branched strips of hyper

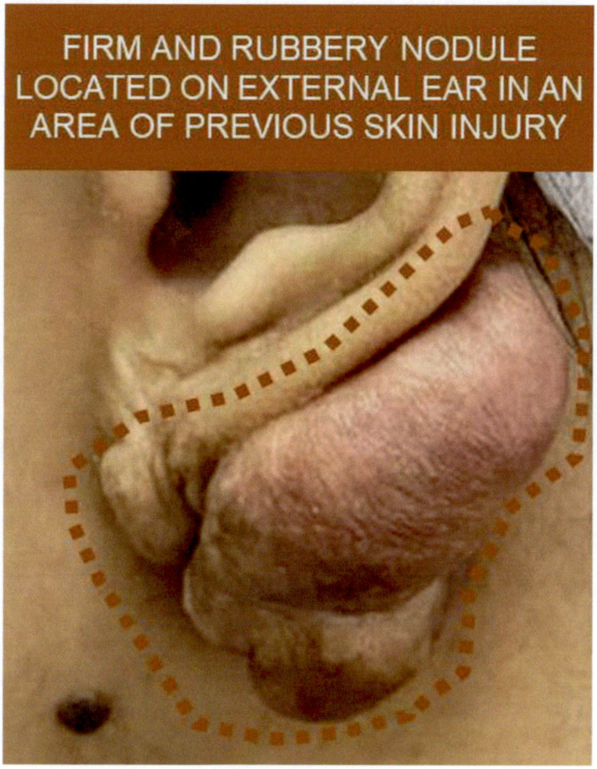

Fig. 12.15 Clinical photograph of patients with keloid tragus

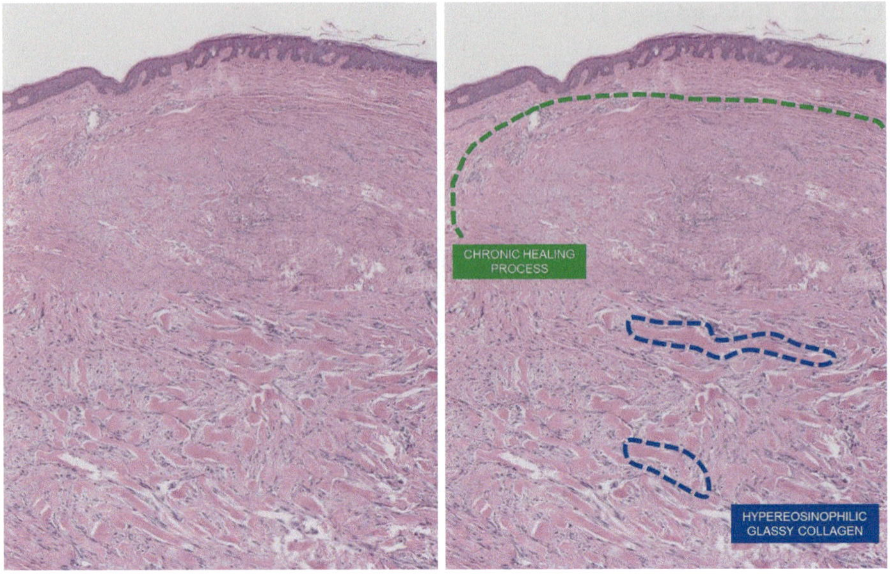

Fig. 12.16 Histological findings of keloid tragus (H&E x4)

eosinophilic collagen, glassy, of irregular length and width as well, presenting a decrease in the interfascicular space (place in another topic, on the line below), presence of fibroblasts with voluminous nuclei in the periphery (place in another topic, on the line below), absence of cutaneous appendages in the affected areas.

- There may be the presence of variable chronic inflammatory infiltrate in the periphery and even gigantocytes or granulomas due to a foreign body due to the causal agent.

12.2.3.5 Ultrasonography (Fig. 12.17) [18]

- Ultrasonography allows visualization of the internal structure of the keloid, providing information about its thickness, borders, and depth.
- Usually is a hypoechoic lesion in dermis that can demonstrates some calcifications.
- Increased vascularity on power Doppler may be indicative of active inflammation or growth.

12.2.3.6 MRI

- Low signal intensity on T1 and T2-weighted images.
- Mild to intense contrast can be observed after gadolinium administration depending on the phase of proliferation.
- Heterogenous or hypoenhancing areas can suggest necrosis.

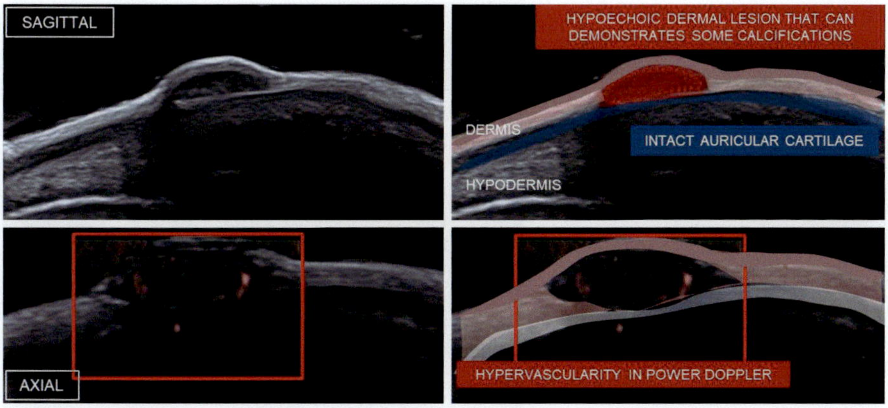

Fig. 12.17 Ultrasonographic findings of keloid tragus with a 24 MHz probe (Aplio i800, Canon Medical Systems)

12.2.4 Preauricular Sinus

12.2.4.1 Definition [19]

- Preauricular sinus is also known as preauricular pit or fistula.
- Common congenital anomaly characterized by a small pit or sinus located in front of the ear, typically along the ascending limb of the helix or other parts of the auricle.
- It arises due to incomplete fusion of the embryonic hillocks during development.

12.2.4.2 Epidemiology [19]

- Incidence ranges from 0.1% to 10%, with higher prevalence among Asian and African populations.
- It commonly presents unilaterally and sporadically, with a predisposition for the right side.
- Bilateral cases are often inherited in an autosomal dominant pattern with variable penetrance, linked to chromosome 8q11.1 to q13.3.
- May be associated with branchiogenic fistulas and other congenital anomalies like hearing loss and renal malformations.

12.2.4.3 Clinical Presentation (Fig. 12.18) [19]

- Small pit, hole, or sinus opening near the ear, most commonly along the ascending limb of the helix but can also appear in other areas such as the tragus or lobule.

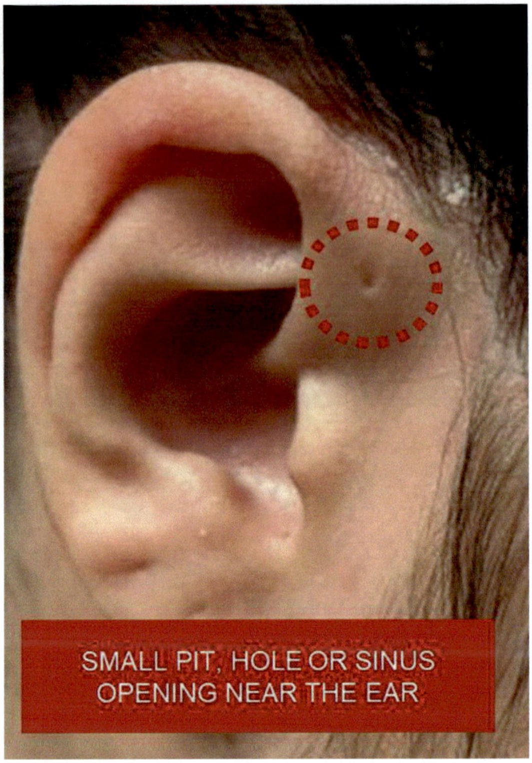

Fig. 12.18 Clinical photograph of patient with preauricular sinus

- In some cases, there is a variant type where the sinus opens posterior to a line drawn from the posterior aspect of the tragus to the ascending limb of the helix.
- This variant type may present with postauricular swelling, which can be mistaken for other conditions like lymphadenitis, cysts, or abscesses.

12.2.4.4 Histopathology [16]

- A preauricular sinus typically presents as a tiny pit or sinus near the external ear.
- Histologically, the pit or sinus is lined with squamous epithelium.
- Tiny follicles may open into the pit.

12.2.4.5 Ultrasonography (Figs. 12.19 and 12.20)

- Confirm the presence of a preauricular sinus. It helps visualize the structure, depth, and extent of the sinus tract and its direction.
- Evaluate complications by visualizing the presence of fluid collections, inflammatory changes, or other abnormalities in the surrounding tissues.

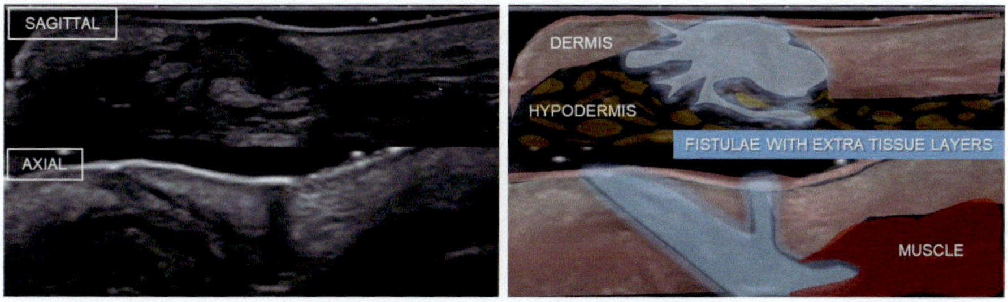

Fig. 12.19 Ultrasonographic findings of preauricular sinus with a 24 MHz probe (Aplio i800, Canon Medical Systems)

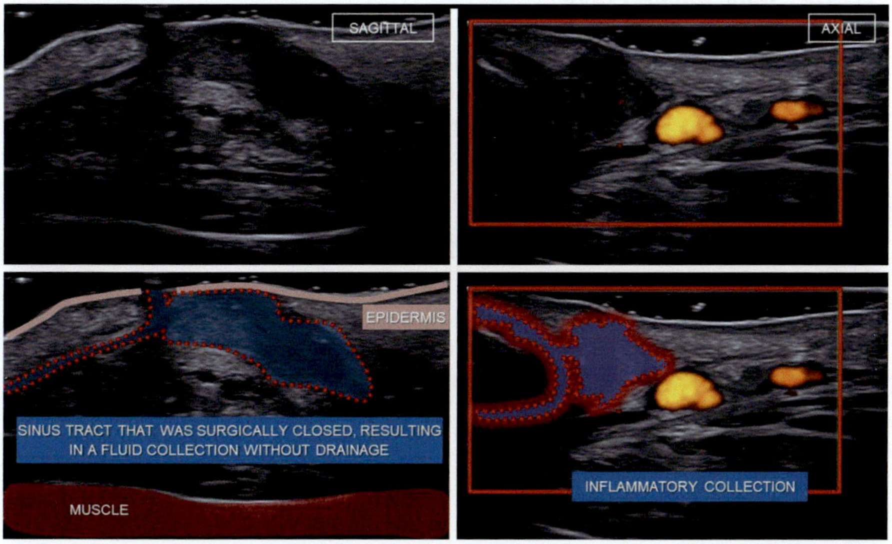

Fig. 12.20 Ultrasonographic findings of infected and complicated preauricular sinus with a 24 MHz probe (Aplio i800, Canon Medical Systems)

12.2.4.6 MRI

- Especially used to diagnose complications by visualizing the presence of fluid collections, fistulae, and inflammatory changes.
- Can help presurgical planning.

12.3 Tumoral Lesions on the Eyelids and Periorbital Region

12.3.1 Xantelasma

12.3.1.1 Definition [20]

- Also known as xanthelasma palpebrarum, is a type of yellowish deposit of fat or cholesterol that tends to form under the skin, usually on or around the eyelids.
- These lesions are typically soft and have a flat or slightly raised appearance.
- Xanthelasma is considered a subtype of xanthoma, which is a broader term used to describe cholesterol deposits in the skin.

12.3.1.2 Epidemiology [20]

- Xanthelasma palpebrarum affects approximately 1.1% of women and 0.3% of men. It is most commonly observed between the ages of 35 and 55.
- The condition is often associated with underlying lipid disorders, with about 50% of patients having abnormal lipid profiles.

12.3.1.3 Clinical Presentation (Fig. 12.21) [20]

- Symmetrical, yellowish papules or plaques on the medial aspect of the upper eyelid, followed by the lower eyelid and occasionally the lateral canthus
- These lesions are typically asymptomatic but can be a cosmetic concern due to their appearance.

12.3.1.4 Dermoscopy [20]

- Dermatoscopy of xanthelasma palpebrarum reveals yellowish-orange areas with a cobblestone-like surface pattern.
- Vascular structures may also be visible, and the lesions generally lack normal skin markings.

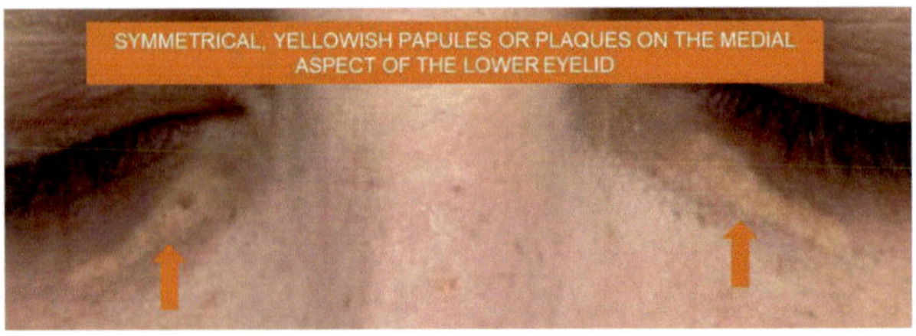

Fig. 12.21 Clinical photograph of patient with xanthelasma

12.3.1.5 Histopathology [16]

- Clusters of xanthomatous cells usually around a venule, an important clue for differential diagnosis with other xanthomatous cell infiltrates.

12.3.1.6 Ultrasonography (Fig. 12.22)

- Well-defined, homogeneous, and hyperechoic nodules in the dermis
- No vascularization on power Doppler imaging
- Note that ultrasonography of the periorbital region should be performed with the system's output power reduced to approximately 75–80%, given the anatomical proximity to the globe and the need to minimize acoustic energy exposure to ocular structures.

12.3.1.7 MRI

- Nodules of intermediate signal on T1 and T2 sequences, with higher T1 and T2 signal compared to the tendons.
- No enhancement after gadolinium administration.
- Striated appearance in sagittal sequences if the lesion is interposed between normal tendon fibers.

12.3.2 Hidrocystoma

12.3.2.1 Definition [21]

- Hidrocystomas are benign cystic tumors of apocrine or eccrine sweat glands.
- Apocrine hidrocystomas arises from cystic proliferation of the apocrine gland.
- Eccrine variant is caused by the retention of eccrine glands.

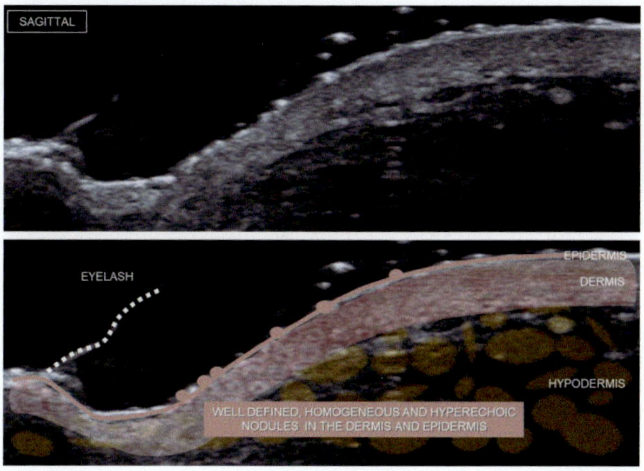

Fig. 12.22 Ultrasonographic findings of xanthelasma with a 33 MHz probe (Aplio i800, Canon Medical Systems)

12.3.2.2 Epidemiology [22]

- Eccrine hidrocystomas
  - Prevalent in adults between 30 and 70 years of age.
  - Solitary eccrine hidrocystomas are equally prevalent among males and females; however, the multiple eccrine hidrocystomas are mainly seen in female patients.
- Apocrine hidrocystomas
  - Same age groups as do eccrine hidrocystomas, single or multiple cystic lesions.
  - The multiple type is rare in the general population.
- Eyelid hidrocystomas are relatively common lesions which are among the top five benign eyelid lesions encountered in ophthalmic practice, accounting for 8% of benign eyelid lesions.

12.3.2.3 Clinical Presentation (Fig. 12.23) [21]

- Eccrine hidrocystomas: Solitary or multiple; typically dome-shaped, have an amber, brown, or bluish tint, and range from 1 to 6 mm in diameter; affect malar, periorbital, chest, axilla, or neck.
- Apocrine hidrocystomas: Primarily solitary, but occasionally manifesting as multiple lesions; ranges from dark-blue tint to black; affect face, ears, head, chest, or shoulders.

12.3.2.4 Dermoscopy [23]

- Dermoscopy is important to differentiate BCC from hidrocystomas.
- BCC showed eyelash destruction, in-focus arborizing telangiectasias and blotches and strands on dermoscopy. Induration, loss of lashes, a pearly appearance or pigmentation should raise suspicion of malignancy and warrant histological examination.
- Apocrine hidrocystomas can be clinically similar but on dermoscopy it had translucent homogenous areas, linear whitish structures, and no eyelash involvement.

12.3.2.5 Histopathology (Fig. 12.24) [24]

- Unilocular or multilocular dermal cyst, which may present apocrine or eccrine differentiation.

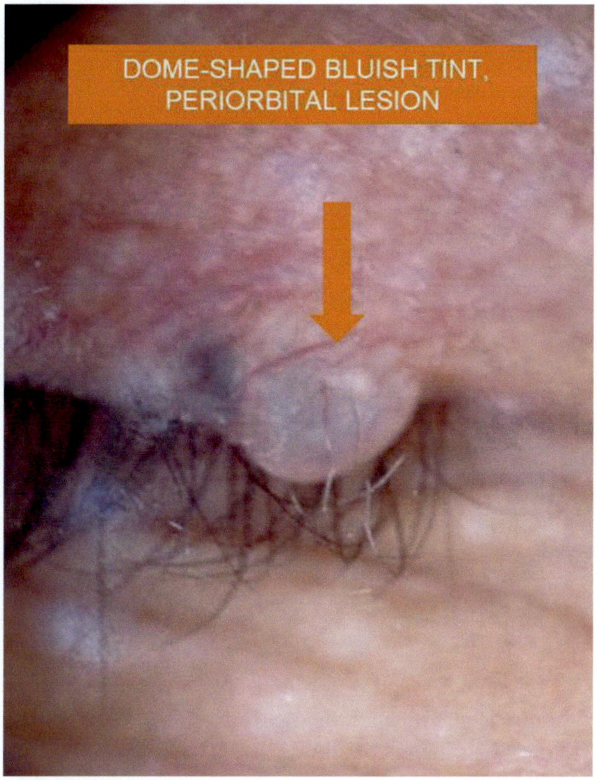

Fig. 12.23 Clinical photograph of patient with hidrocystoma

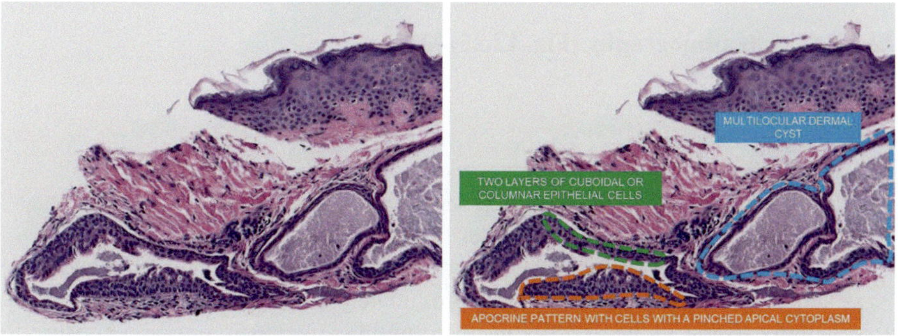

Fig. 12.24 Histological findings of hidrocystoma (H&E x10)

- Content of hyaline liquid that oozes during the macroscopic examination, so it appears empty on microscopy.
- The cyst is covered by one or two layers of cuboidal or columnar epithelial cells, often flattened with the evolution and increase of the cyst volume; there may be a clear apocrine pattern with cells with a pinched apical cytoplasm.

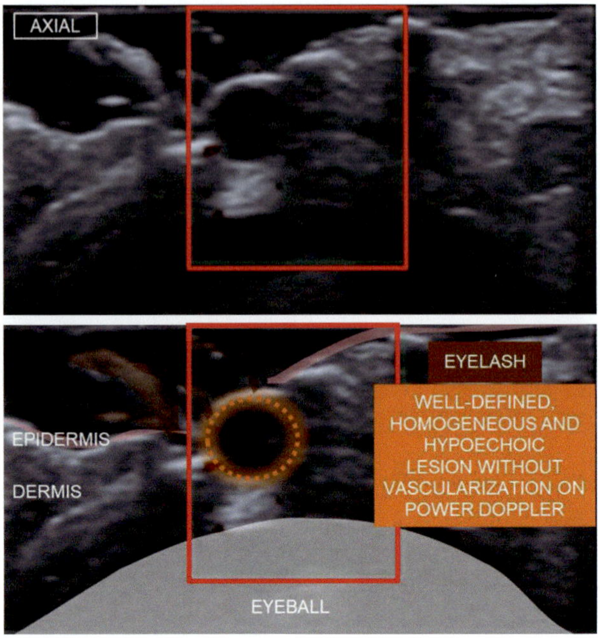

Fig. 12.25 Ultrasonographic findings of hidrocystoma with a 24 MHz probe (Aplio i800, Canon Medical Systems)

- The main clinical differential diagnosis is BCC, but in histopathology, the difficulty occurs in small or superficial biopsies in a cystic BCC that usually has more than one layer of lining cells and the presence of characteristic stroma-tumor clefts.

12.3.2.6 Ultrasonography (Fig. 12.25) [25]

- Well-defined lesion
- Homogeneous
- Hypoechoic
- No posterior enhancement or lateral acoustic shadow
- No vascularization on power Doppler
- Note that ultrasonography of the periorbital region should be performed with the system's output power reduced to approximately 75–80%, given the anatomical proximity to the globe and the need to minimize acoustic energy exposure to ocular structures.

12.3.2.7 MRI (Fig. 12.26)

- Well-defined lesion and homogeneous.
- Cystic appearance presenting low to intermediated signal on T1-weighted images and high signal intensity on T2-weighted images.
- No posterior enhancement after gadolinium administration.

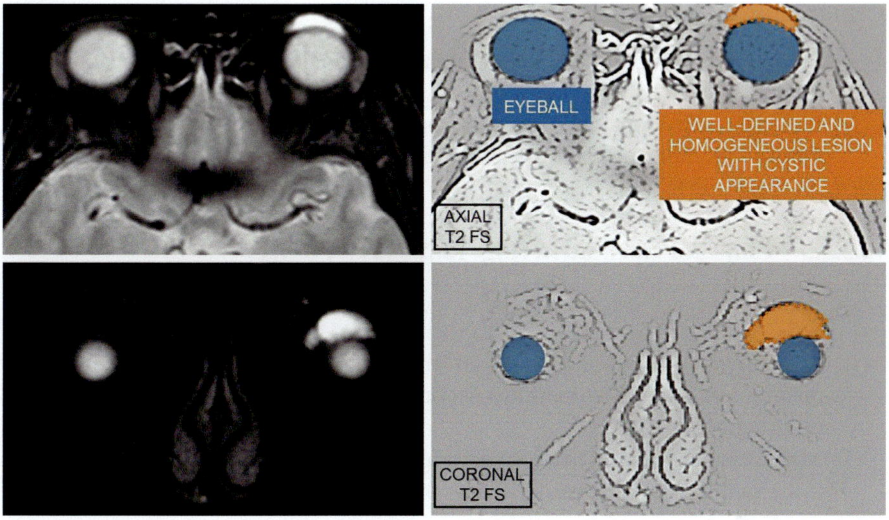

Fig. 12.26 MRI findings of hidrocystoma on T2 FS-weighted sequences (From Huang et al. [26]; with permission)

12.3.3 Lacrimal Glands Lesions

12.3.3.1 Definition [27]

- Lacrimal gland tumors and inflammatory lesions are abnormal growths or inflammatory processes affecting the lacrimal glands, which are responsible for tear production.
- Tumors can be benign or malignant, while inflammatory lesions can result from conditions like dacryoadenitis.

12.3.3.2 Epidemiology [27]

- Tumors
  - Lacrimal gland tumors are relatively rare, constituting a small percentage of orbital tumors.
  - Tumors can occur at any age, but certain types are more common in specific age groups (e.g., pleomorphic adenoma in middle-aged adults, lymphomas in older adults).
  - Some tumors have a slight gender predilection; for instance, pleomorphic adenomas are more common in females.

- Inflammatory lesions
  - Inflammatory conditions like dacryoadenitis are more common and can affect individuals of any age.
  - Includes infections (e.g., viral, bacterial), autoimmune diseases (e.g., Sjögren's syndrome), and systemic diseases.

12.3.3.3 Clinical Presentation (Fig. 12.27) [27]

- Tumors
  - Typically present as a painless or slowly growing mass in the upper outer quadrant of the eye, sometimes accompanied by eyelid swelling or proptosis (bulging of the eye).
  - May include palpable mass, eye discomfort, and occasionally vision changes if the tumor exerts pressure on the optic nerve.
- Inflammatory lesions
  - Often present with sudden onset of pain, redness, swelling, and tenderness over the lacrimal gland area.
  - Swelling of the eyelid, discharge, and possibly fever. Chronic cases may show more indolent symptoms with less acute inflammation.

12.3.3.4 Histopathology [16]

- Tumors
  - Pleomorphic adenoma: Characterized by a mix of epithelial and mesenchymal elements, with a well-circumscribed encapsulated lesion.
  - Lymphoma: Shows atypical lymphoid proliferation with varying degrees of cellularity.
  - Adenoid cystic carcinoma: Features perineural invasion and small, cribriform architectural patterns.

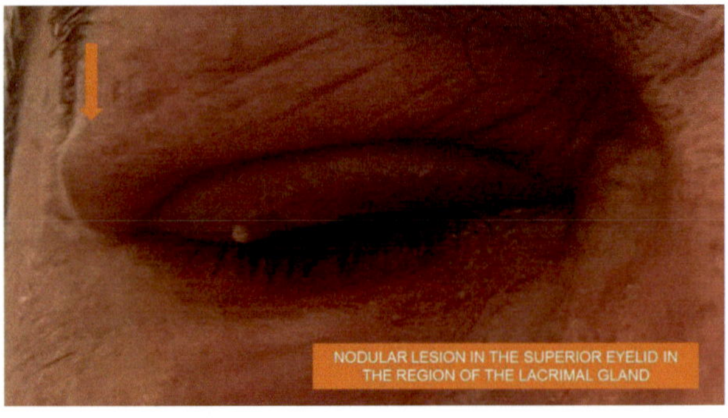

Fig. 12.27 Clinical photograph of patient with inflammatory lesion of the lacrimal gland

- Inflammatory lesions
  - Dacryoadenitis: Histology reveals inflammatory cell infiltration (lymphocytes, plasma cells, neutrophils) and possible granuloma formation in chronic cases.

12.3.3.5 Ultrasonography (Figs. 12.28, 12.29, and 12.30) [28]

- Note that ultrasonography of the periorbital region should be performed with the system's output power reduced to approximately 75–80%, given the anatomical proximity to the globe and the need to minimize acoustic energy exposure to ocular structures.

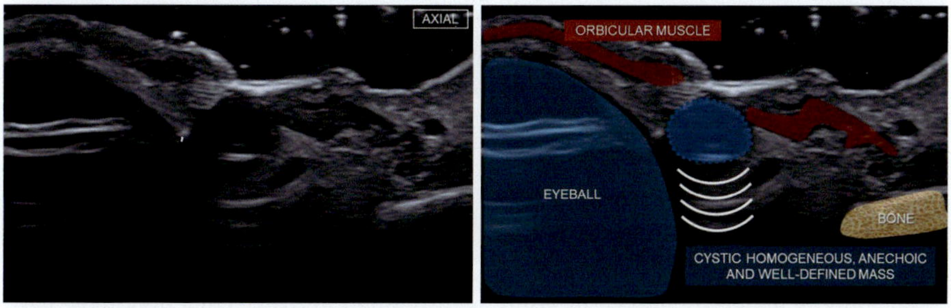

Fig. 12.28 Ultrasonographic findings of cystic lesion of the lacrimal gland with a 24 MHz probe (Aplio i800, Canon Medical Systems)

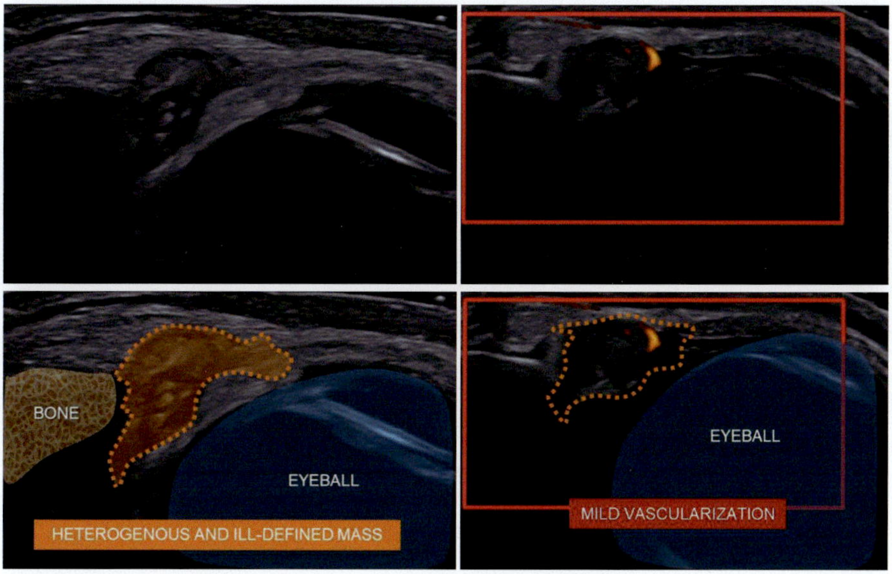

Fig. 12.29 Ultrasonographic findings of inflammatory lesion of the lacrimal gland with a 24 MHz probe (Aplio i800, Canon Medical Systems)

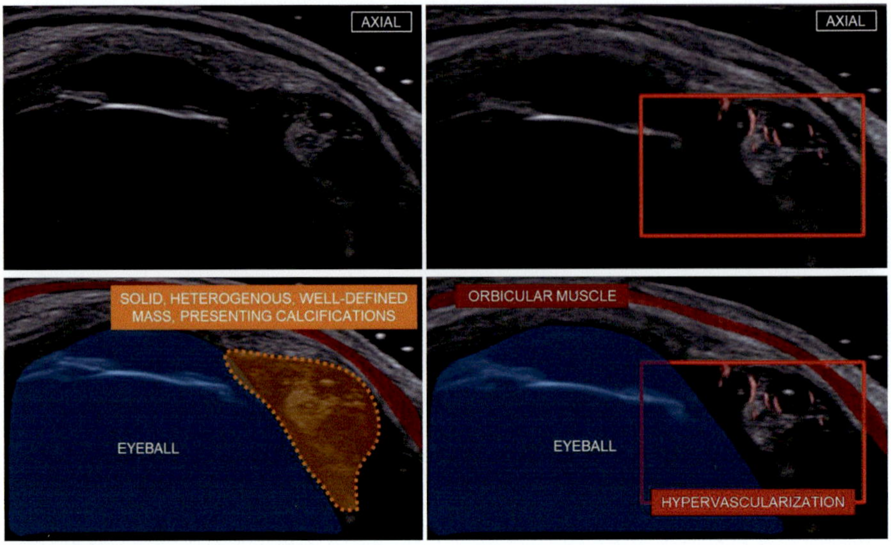

Fig. 12.30 Ultrasonographic findings of solid tumor lesion of the lacrimal gland with a 24 MHz probe (Aplio i800, Canon Medical Systems)

- Tumors
  - Tumors generally appear as solid, well-defined masses. They may have vari able echogenicity depending on their composition and can show internal cystic components or calcifications.
  - Increased blood flow may be seen within the tumor on Doppler imaging.
- Inflammatory lesions
  - Typically show diffuse hypoechoic areas in the lacrimal gland with possible focal areas of increased echogenicity due to edema or fibrosis.
  - Increased vascularity or hyperemia may be observed.

12.3.3.6 MRI [29]

- Tumors
  - Tumors often appear hypointense on T1-weighted images compared to surrounding tissues.
  - Tumors may appear hyperintense with variable signal intensities on T2-weighted images depending on their cellularity and composition.
  - Post-contrast images typically show enhancement patterns that can help in distinguishing between benign and malignant tumors.

- Inflammatory lesions
  - Edema and inflammation may appear hypointense on T1-weighted images.
  - Increased signal intensity due to edema and fluid accumulation on T2-weighted images.
  - Post-contrast images may show diffuse enhancement corresponding to inflammation and potential abscess formation if present.

12.3.4 Ocular and Extraocular Sebaceous Carcinoma

12.3.4.1 Definition [30]

- Sebaceous carcinoma is a rare malignant tumor originating from the sebaceous glands' adnexal epithelium.
- Can develop de novo or from benign sebaceous neoplasms.
- It is known for its aggressive behavior and varied clinical presentations.

12.3.4.2 Epidemiology [30]

- It occurs more frequently in regions with a higher concentration of sebaceous glands, such as the eyelids (ocular type) and the head and neck area (extraocular type).
- The majority of cases occur in the seventh and eighth decades of life.
- There is a slight female predominance in ocular sebaceous carcinoma, while extraocular sebaceous carcinoma affects both sexes equally.
- Sebaceous carcinoma is believed to have a higher incidence in Asian populations, but recent studies suggest no significant ethnic predominance.

12.3.4.3 Clinical Presentation (Fig. 12.31) [30]

- Painless and slowly enlarging subcutaneous nodule.
- Often appears as a yellow or pink nodule on the eyelid, frequently mistaken for a benign chalazion.
- Extraocular sebaceous carcinoma can present as pink, flesh-colored, red, brown, or yellow nodules or plaques, often resembling other neoplastic conditions.
- Bleeding can be associated with sebaceous carcinoma, particularly in extraocular lesions.

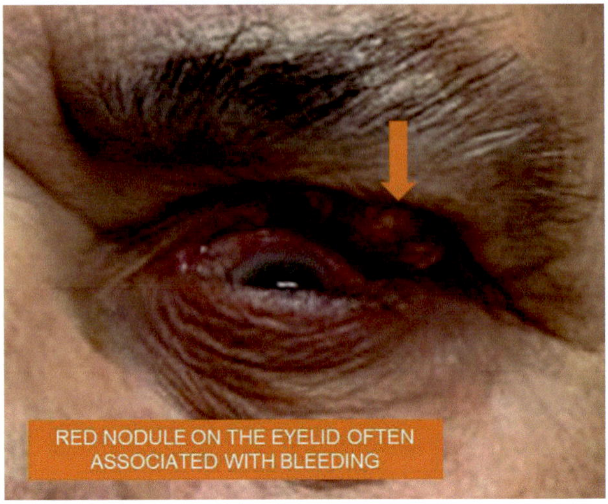

Fig. 12.31 Clinical photograph of patient with extraocular sebaceous carcinoma

12.3.4.4 Dermoscopy [31]

- Ocular sebaceous carcinoma
  - Yellowish areas
  - Polymorphous vessels (multiple types of vessels)
  - Vascular findings more brilliant due to thinner conjunctival epithelium and rich capillary site
- Extraocular sebaceous carcinoma
  - Yellowish areas
  - Polymorphous vessels
  - Similar patterns to ocular sebaceous carcinoma but less brilliant due to thicker cutaneous epithelium
- General dermoscopic features of sebaceous carcinoma`
  - Yellow color derived from foamy cells and mature sebocytes.
  - Homogeneous yellow patterns.
  - Polymorphous vessels indicating malignancy.
  - Co-occurrence of yellow areas and polymorphous vessels suggests sebaceous carcinoma and aids in early diagnosis.

12.3.4.5 Histopathology (Fig. 12.32) [24]

- Ocular and extraocular sebaceous carcinoma nodular dermal proliferation or in cords composed of different proportions of clear cells of sebaceous or basaloid pattern, with varying degrees of differentiation and atypia (place in another topic, on the line below), originating from the Meibomian gland.

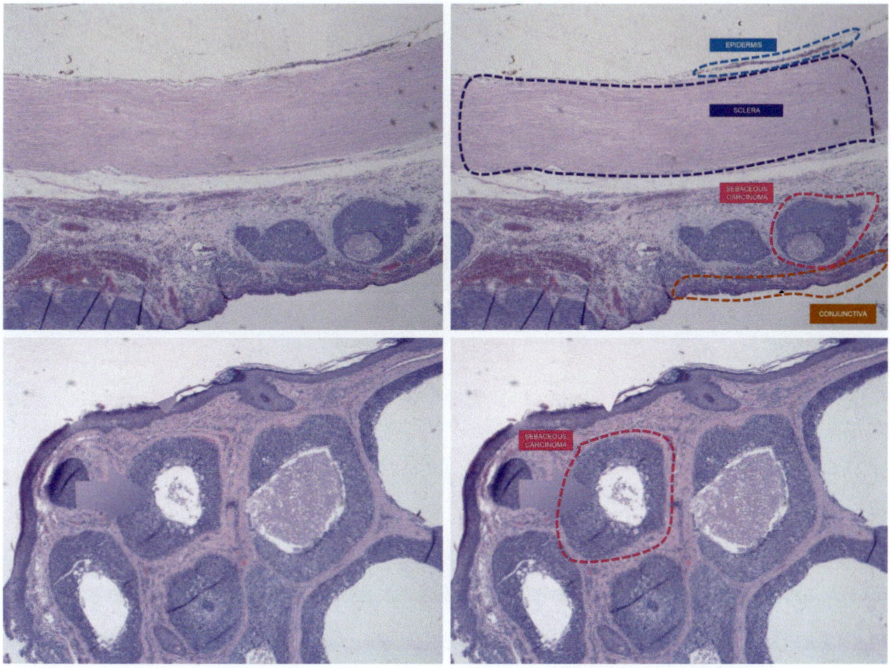

Fig. 12.32 Histological findings of extraocular sebaceous carcinoma (H&E x10)

- There may be mitosis and necrosis figures, and they may be graded as well, moderately and poorly differentiated (place in another topic, on the line below); may involve only the conjunctival epithelium.
- Occasionally, it may present epidermal or follicular connections (place in another topic, on the line below), it may present an intraepithelial component (in situ) with pagetoid dissemination occurring in about 30% of cases (place in another topic, on the line below); cells with characteristic sebaceous differentiation show clear cytoplasm with the nucleus showing several characteristic indentations, important for differentiating from other clear cell tumors, including metastasis from renal clear cell carcinoma.
- Angiolymphatic invasion is common.

12.3.4.6 Ultrasonography (Fig. 12.33)

- Ill-defined hypoechoic lesion at the glands' adnexal topography.
- Irregular and heterogeneous.
- Possible invasion of adjacent soft tissues.
- hypervascularity in power Doppler imaging.
- Note that ultrasonography of the periorbital region should be performed with the system's output power reduced to approximately 75–80%, given the anatomical

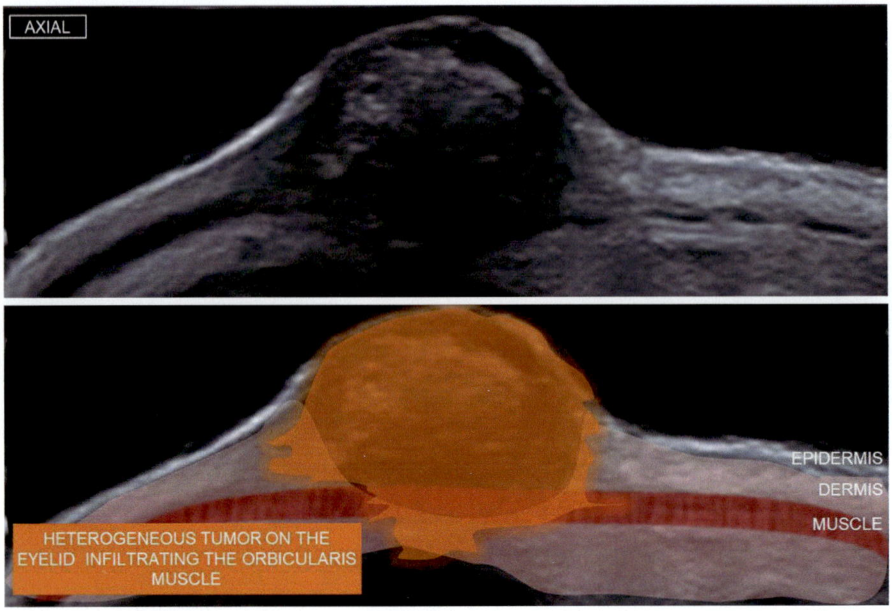

Fig. 12.33 Ultrasonographic findings of extraocular sebaceous carcinoma with a 33 MHz probe (Aplio i800, Canon Medical Systems)

proximity to the globe and the need to minimize acoustic energy exposure to ocular structures.

12.3.4.7 MRI

- Ill-defined and irregular lesion at the glands' adnexal topography presenting heterogeneous signal intensity on all sequences.
- Possible invasion of adjacent soft tissues.
- Enhancement after gadolinium administration.

12.4 Tumoral Lesions on the Lips

12.4.1 Mucocele and Ranula

12.4.1.1 Definition [32]

- Mucoceles and ranulas are the most common salivary gland disorders.
- Mucocele develops as a consequence of mechanical trauma to a minor salivary gland, with secondary saliva retention and accumulation inside the blocked and dilated excretory ducts of the gland.

- Ranula is similar to mucocele; however, it is caused by trauma to the excretory duct of the salivary glands located in the floor of the mouth.

12.4.1.2 Epidemiology [33]

- Mucocele
  - Prevalence of 2.4 cases per 1000 persons, primarily affecting individuals aged 3–20 years.
  - Frequently develop on the inner aspect of the lower lip due to trauma but can occur anywhere in the oral cavity.
- Ranula
  - Prevalence of 0.2 cases per 1000 persons, commonly occurring in teenagers and young adults.
  - Typically form on the floor of the mouth, with most arising from the sublingual glands and rarely from the submandibular gland.
- No racial or sexual predilection has been noted for these lesions.

12.4.1.3 Clinical Presentation (Fig. 12.34) [33]

- Mucocele: Presents as painless, fluctuant swellings that may suddenly enlarge. Superficial mucoceles have a bluish-translucent hue, while deeper lesions are pinkish. Common sites include the lower labial mucosa, floor of the mouth, ventral tongue, buccal mucosa, and palate.
- Oral ranula: Appears as a large, cystic, translucent to blue swelling in the floor of the mouth, resembling the belly of a frog. It can interfere with speech, swallowing, mastication, and respiration by displacing the tongue.
- Cervical ranula: Presents as an asymptomatic, mobile, fluctuant, enlarging mass in the neck. It typically occurs unilaterally but may cross the midline.

12.4.1.4 Histopathology [16]

- Mucocele (and ranula) is a mucous cyst usually present on the lower lip, usually presenting as a collection of mucus with surrounding chronic inflammation, due to rupture of the salivary duct.
- It is rarely seen in the cystic form. In the late stage, it organizes with fibrosis.

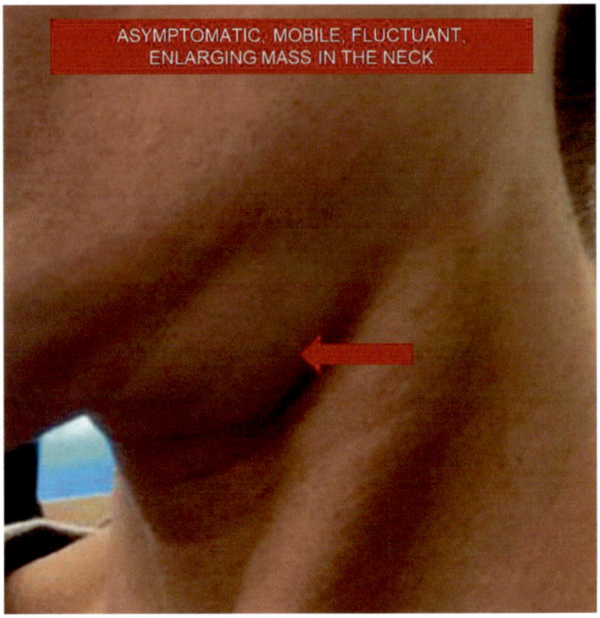

Fig. 12.34 Clinical photograph of patients with cervical ranula

12.4.1.5 Computed Tomography (Fig. 12.35) [34]

- Ranulas appear as thin-walled cystic lesions. Simple ranulas are confined to the sublingual space and closely mimic epidermoids of the floor of the mouth on CT scans.
- Mucoceles present as low-attenuation cystic lesions on CT scans.

12.4.1.6 Ultrasonography (Fig. 12.36) [35]

- Ranulas typically exhibit a hypoechoic to anechoic texture due to their composition of mucous saliva. Sludge-like echoes may be present, correlating with the thickness of mucous secretion.
- Often appear oval or round with regular contours. In larger or more complex ranulas, irregular contours may be observed.
- Ranulas are commonly found in the sublingual space. Plunging ranulas (PRs) can extend beyond the mylohyoid muscle, potentially into the submandibular or parapharyngeal spaces.
- Plunging patterns may exhibit plunging patterns through a hiatus in the mylohyoid muscle or beyond its posterior border.

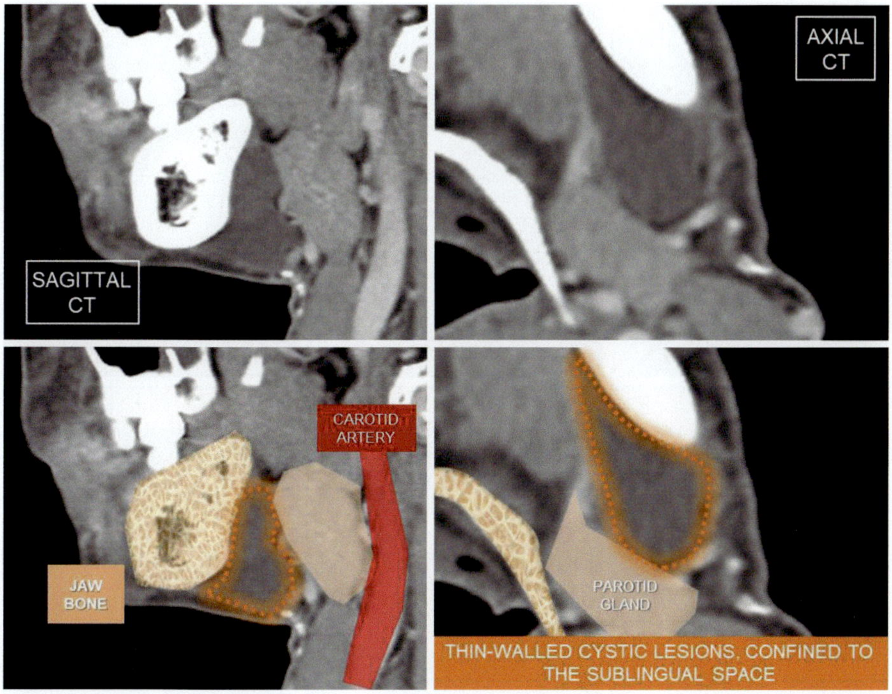

Fig. 12.35 Computed tomography findings of cervical ranula (Philips Brilliance CT 64-slice)

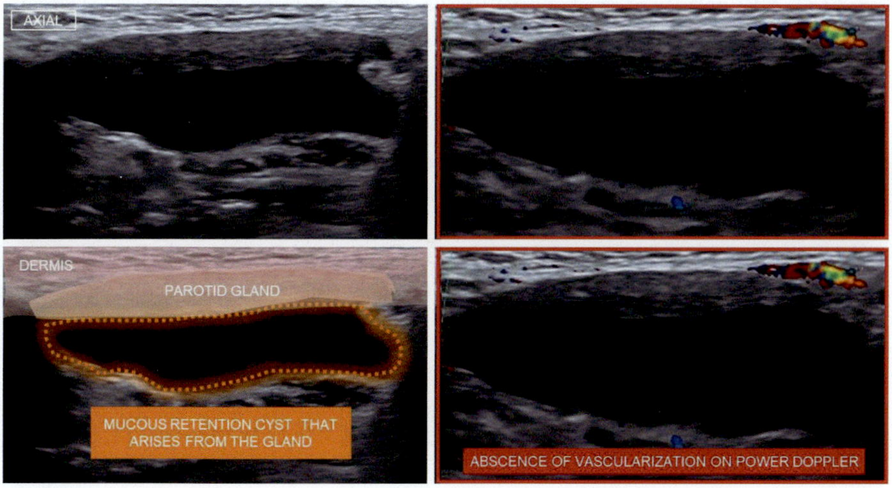

Fig. 12.36 Ultrasonographic findings of cervical ranula with a 24 MHz probe (Aplio 1800, Canon Medical Systems)

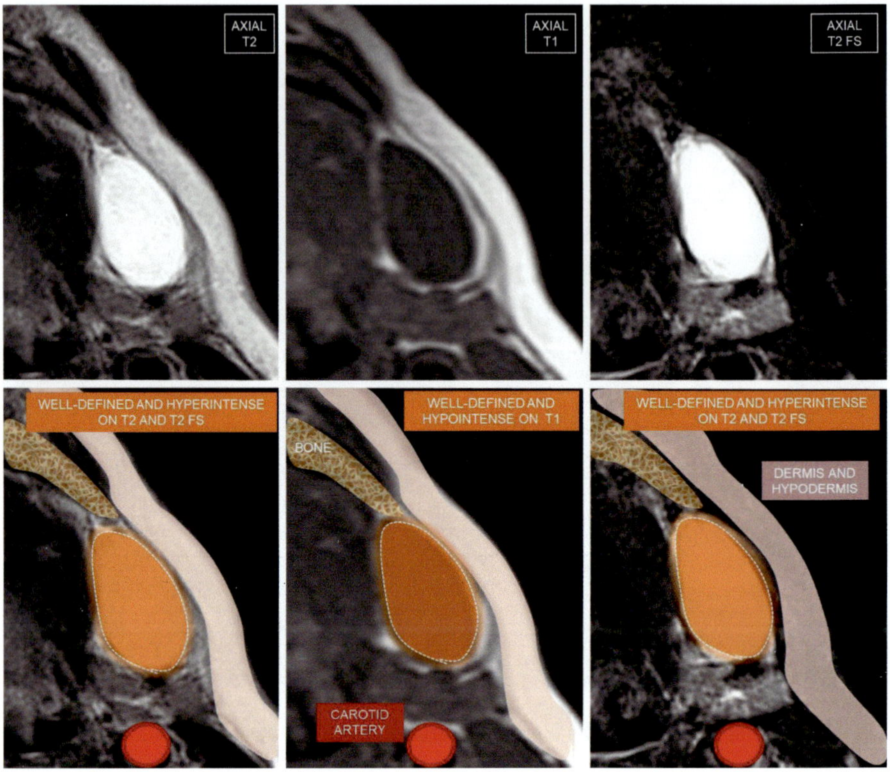

Fig. 12.37 MRI findings of ranula on T2 FS, T2, and T2 FS-weighted sequences (Magnetom Prisma 3T MRI, Siemens)

12.4.1.7 MRI (Fig. 12.37) [34]

- Simple ranulas are predominantly located in the sublingual space and resemble floor of mouth epidermoids on CT, but are distinguishable on MRI, which shows epidermoids with restricted diffusion.
- Mucoceles appear as hypointense lesion on T1-weighted and hyperintense on T2-weighted MRI scans. They show no signs of diffusion restriction, which distinguishes them from epidermoids.

12.4.2 Actinic Cheilitis and Squamous Cell Carcinoma (CEC)

12.4.2.1 Definition [36]

- Actinic cheilitis (AC) is the most common potentially malignant lesion affecting the lips. Defined by the clonal expansion of genomically unstable keratinocytes.

- Squamous cell carcinoma (SCC) is the most frequent oral malignancy, up to 95% of SCCs on the lip occur on preexisting ACs.

12.4.2.2 Epidemiology [36]

- Actinic cheilitis (AC) is a chronic condition that usually develops in patients with cumulative sun damage. It affects both men and women with men being at far greater risk compared with women. AC is frequently seen in elderly individuals.
- Squamous cell carcinoma (SCC) constitutes 90% of all cases of oral malignancy.

12.4.2.3 Clinical Presentation (Fig. 12.38) [36]

- Actinic cheilitis including pale, flaking, or scaly lips, chronic ulcerations and erosions, white plaques, blurring of the demarcation between the lip vermillion border and the skin and vermillion atrophy, areas of erythema, and potentially other lesions. Palpation of the lesional surface produces a fine, "sandpaper-like" feeling.
- Squamous cell carcinoma presents like a thickening and induration of the lips surface, nodularity, and rapid growth, and eventually one or more of them ulcerate, causing bleeding and pain.

12.4.2.4 Dermoscopy (Fig. 12.39) [36]

- Dermoscopic criteria for AC diagnosis include ill-demarcated lesion borders, white-colored projections, "island"-like structures and radially arranged vascular telangiectasia surrounding ulcerated areas.

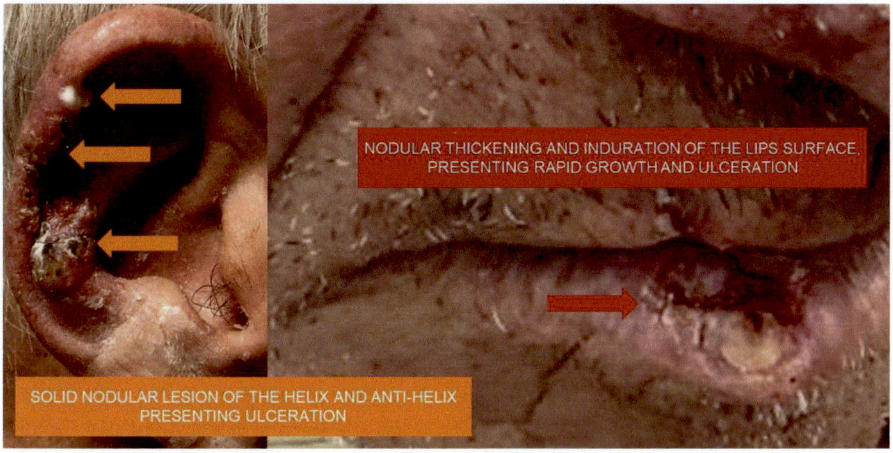

Fig. 12.38 Clinical photograph of patients with squamous cell carcinoma

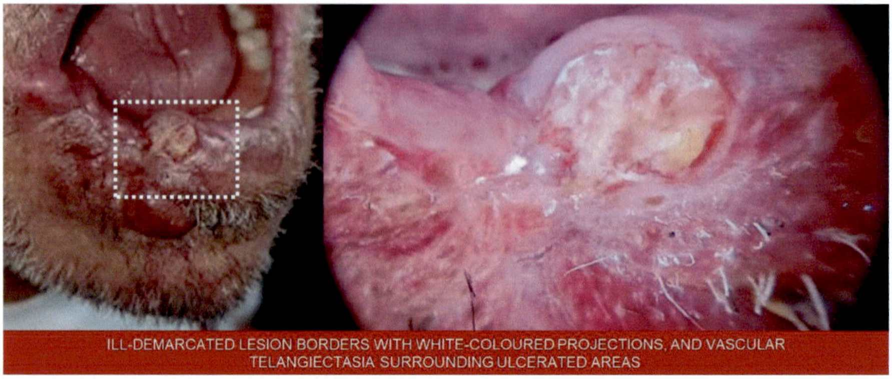

Fig. 12.39 Dermoscopic findings of patient with squamous cell carcinoma (x10)

- Classically described dermoscopic features of SCC are glomerular or dotted vessels against a red, scaly background. Vascular polymorphism: telangiectatic, branching, hairpin, serpiginous, linear, truncated, and dotted blood vessels is described. In addition to displaying white clods, white, structureless areas and ulceration are found in squamous cell carcinoma of the lip.

12.4.2.5 Histopathology (Fig. 12.40) [16]

- Actinic cheilitis
  - Typically occurs in the mucosal area of the lower lip vermilion (place in another topic, on the line below); the mucosa may be atrophic or proliferative and warty (place in another topic, on the line below); zonal parakeratosis—does not exhibit alternating parakeratosis because it does not have adnexal ostia, differentiating it from actinic keratosis (place in another topic, on the line below); increasing cellular atypia, similar to the grading of actinic keratosis (place in another topic, on the line below); may present inward endophytic buds (place in another topic, on the line below); submucosal tissue presents solar elastosis, telangiectasia, and variable lymphocytic infiltrate (place in another topic, on the line below); The presence of an accentuated lymphocytic infiltrate, up to the lichen planus-like pattern, may indicate focal invasion in a lesion of high dysplasia.
- Squamous cell carcinoma
  - SCC on the lip is like carcinomas of other sites, occurring in the mucocutaneous transition with clinically evident signs of chronic actinic damage, hence the predominance of the lower lip (place in another topic, on the line below). Lesions on the upper lip occur most often associated with previous diseases, especially lupus erythematosus (place in another topic, on the line below). Characteristically, it presents atypical and invasive keratinocytic proliferation with variable epithelial dysplasia, according to its gradation (Broders grades 1 to 4) from well to poorly differentiated and undifferentiated, forming nests,

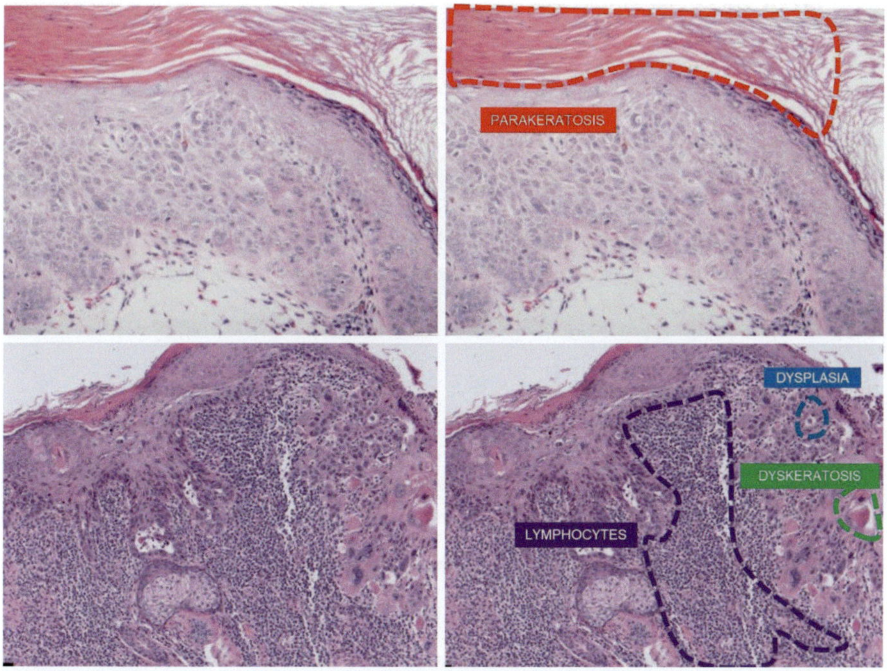

Fig. 12.40 Histological findings of squamous cell carcinoma (H&E x20)

cords and/or isolated cells, connected to the epidermis, most of the time, and may be associated with an intraepithelial component.

12.4.2.6 Computed Tomography [37]

- Lesions in the lip and oral cavity measuring less than 2 cm in size (T1 stage) may not be adequately visualized on either CT or MRI scans. In contrast, tumors larger than 2 cm (T2 and above) are more likely to infiltrate nearby anatomical regions and exhibit higher rates of cervical metastasis.
- Both MRI and CT are equally proficient in assessing cervical metastases.
- PET-CT serves as an imaging tool for evaluating both locoregional disease and distant metastases.

12.4.2.7 Ultrasonography (Figs. 12.41 and 12.42) [38]

- Ill-defined and irregular hypoechoic lesion at the dermis, usually affecting also the orbicularis muscle with invasive pattern.
- Power Doppler ultrasonography demonstrates strong vascularity.

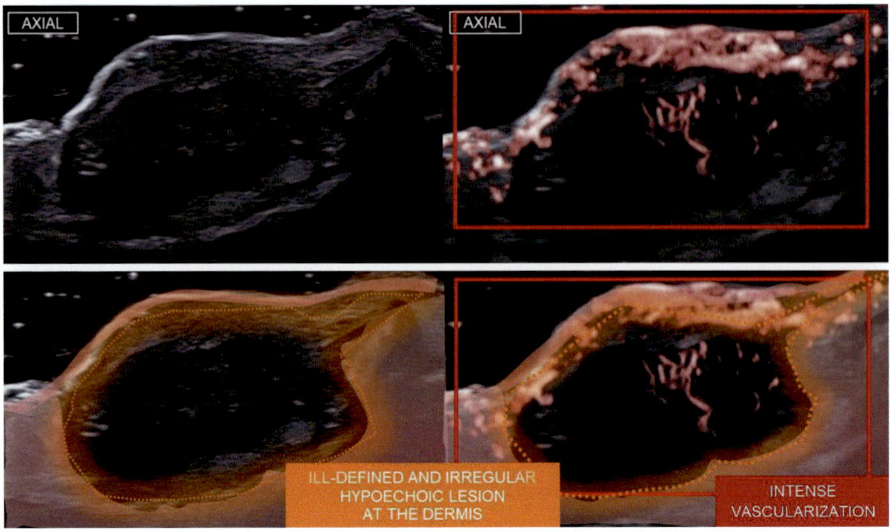

Fig. 12.41 Ultrasonographic findings of squamous cell carcinoma with a 24 MHz probe (Aplio i800, Canon Medical Systems)

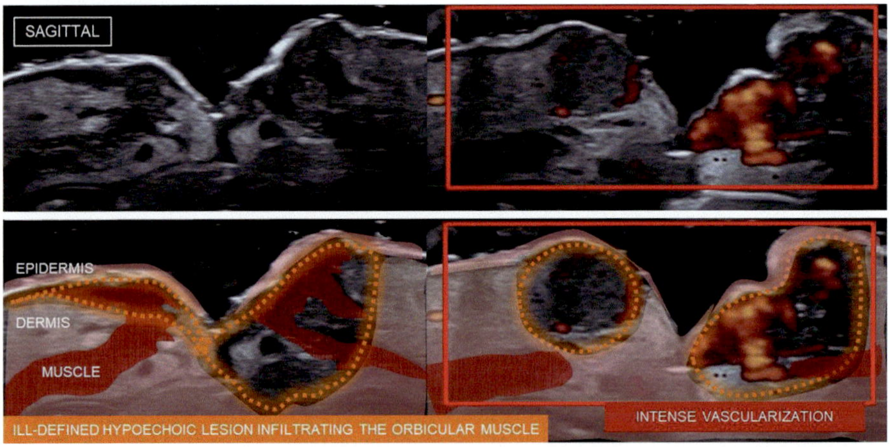

Fig. 12.42 Ultrasonographic findings of labial squamous cell carcinoma with a 24 MHz probe (Aplio i800, Canon Medical Systems)

12.4.2.8 MRI (Fig. 12.43) [37]

- Ill-defined and irregular lesion at the dermis, usually affecting also the orbicularis muscle, showing hypointense signal on T1-weighted images and hyper intense signal on T2-weighted images.
- Enhancement after gadolinium administration.

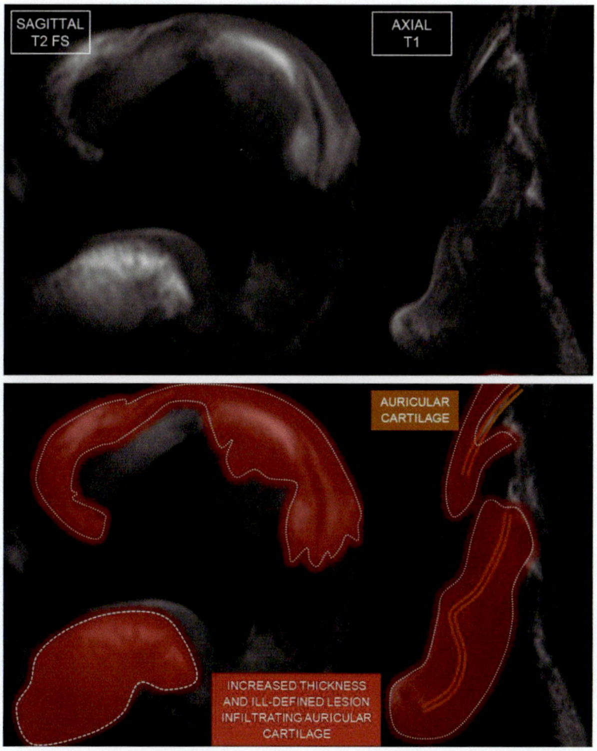

Fig. 12.43 MRI findings of squamous cell carcinoma on T2 FS and T1 FS-weighted sequences (Magnetom Prisma 3T MRI, Siemens)

- MRI excels in depicting details such as local soft tissue involvement, depth of invasion, perineural invasion, and bone marrow status.

12.4.2.9 3D Images (Fig. 12.44; Video 12.1)

- 3D images provide a detailed, accurate representation of the tumor and surrounding anatomy, allowing surgeons to better visualize the extent of the carcinoma. It also helps in clearly delineating the tumor boundaries, aiding in the precise determination of surgical margins.
- Surgeons can tailor the surgical plan to the patient's specific anatomy, improving outcomes by minimizing damage to healthy tissues and preserving critical structures like nerves and blood vessels.
- The 3D model allows for preoperative simulation of different surgical approaches, enabling the selection of the most effective and least invasive technique, leading to better aesthetic and functional outcomes.
- 3D models facilitate better communication among the surgical team and with the patient, ensuring everyone has a clear understanding of the planned procedure.

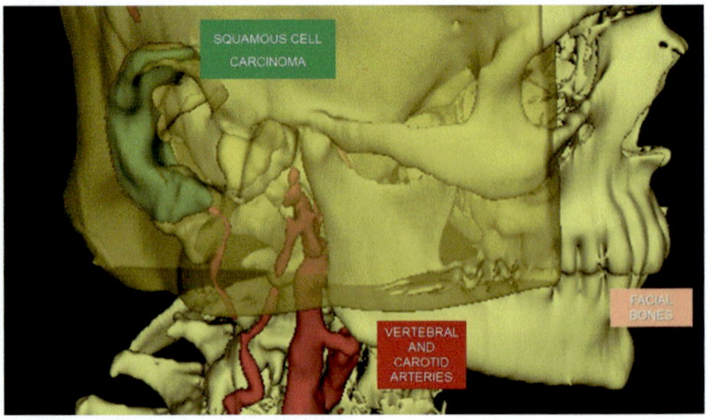

Fig. 12.44 3D images of squamous cell carcinoma after segmentation of MRI isotropic images used for surgical planning

12.4.3 Basal Cell Carcinoma

12.4.3.1 Definition [39, 40]

- Basal cell carcinoma (BCC) is a common form of skin cancer that originates from basal cells in the epidermis.
- Facial basal cell carcinoma specifically refers to BCCs located on the face, which is the most frequent site for this type of cancer.
- BCCs are usually slow-growing and have a low potential for metastasis but can cause local tissue damage and disfigurement.
- Basal cell carcinoma will also be covered in Chap. 15.

12.4.3.2 Epidemiology [39, 40]

- Basal cell carcinoma is the most common type of skin cancer, with facial lesions being particularly frequent.
- Primarily affects older adults, though it can occur in younger individuals, especially those with significant sun exposure.
- More common in males than females, possibly due to higher historical outdoor occupational exposures.
- Includes chronic sun exposure, fair skin, advanced age, and a history of skin cancer or genetic predispositions such as basal cell nevus syndrome.

12.4.3.3 Clinical Presentation (Fig. 12.45) [39, 40]

- BCCs often present as a persistent, nonhealing sore or lump. Patients may experience itching or tenderness in some cases.
- Nodular BCC: Appears as a pearly, waxy nodule with a central depression or ulceration. It may have telangiectasia (small blood vessels) on its surface.

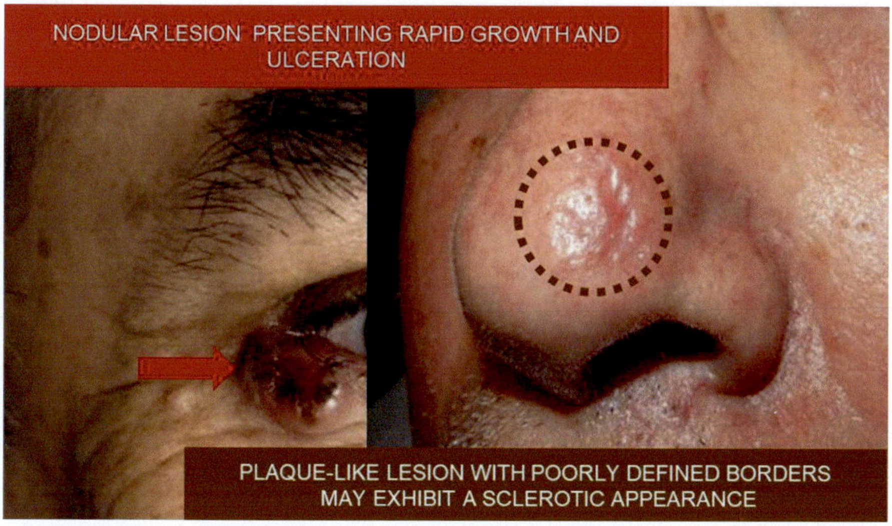

Fig. 12.45 Clinical photograph of patients with basal cell carcinoma

- Superficial BCC: Presents as a flat, scaly, reddish patch that may resemble eczema or psoriasis.
- Morpheaform (sclerosing) BCC: Appears as a scar-like area with a smooth, firm, and pale surface, often with indistinct borders.

12.4.3.4 Dermoscopy (Fig. 12.46) [41]

Nodular BCC

- Telangiectasia: Prominent, linear, or branching blood vessels on the surface of the lesion. These are often irregular and may be located at the edges of the lesion.
- Peripherally palisaded nests: Clusters of small, rounded structures often with a surrounding rim of palisaded nuclei, visible as white or light areas.
- Shiny, waxy appearance: A glossy or pearly surface due to the tumor's structure.
- Central ulceration or erosion may be seen, sometimes with crusting.

Superficial BCC

- Red or pink patches with a shiny surface and fine scaling.
- Blotch-like structure: Irregularly shaped, light-colored, or reddish blotches that may resemble eczema or psoriasis.
- Borders of the lesion are usually well-defined, with a slightly raised edge compared to the central area.

Morpheaform (sclerosing) BCC

- A firm, pale, and often smooth area resembling a scar or sclerotic plaque.

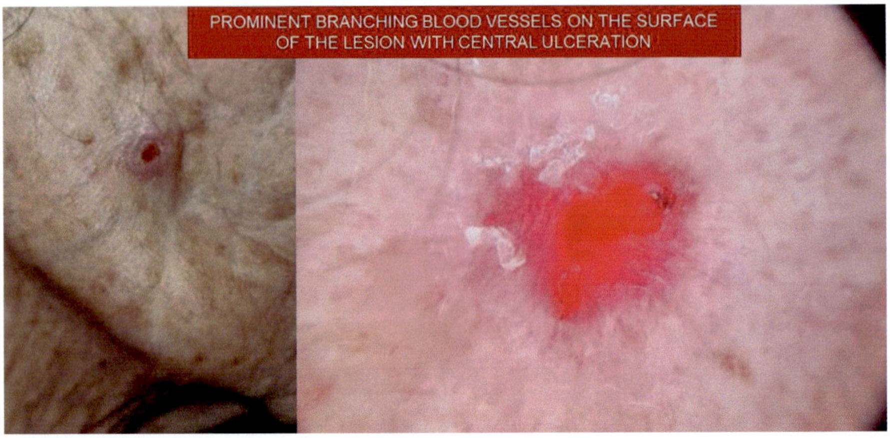

Fig. 12.46 Dermoscopic findings of patient with basal cell carcinoma (x10)

- Indistinct borders: The edges of the lesion are poorly defined, blending into the surrounding skin.
- Fine telangiectasia: Small, fine blood vessels may be visible, often less prominent than in nodular BCCs.

Pigmented BCC

- May present with varying degrees of pigmentation, ranging from brown to black. This can make the lesion appear similar to melanoma.
- Dark, comedo-like structures or black dots, representing pigment deposits.

12.4.3.5 Histopathology [16]

- Nodular BCC: Characterized by nests of basaloid cells in the dermis with peripheral palisading (aligning of nuclei at the edges of nests). The stroma between nests is often fibrous.
- Superficial BCC: Shows nests of basaloid cells in the superficial dermis with a less distinct peripheral palisading. The lesions may also have a somewhat infiltrative pattern.
- Morpheaform BCC: Exhibits small nests or strands of basaloid cells infiltrating the dermis, creating a sclerotic appearance with significant fibrous stroma.

12.4.3.6 Ultrasonography (Fig. 12.47) [42–44]

- BCCs typically appear as well-defined, hypoechoic nodules or masses on ultrasonography, with varying degrees of internal echogenicity depending on the amount of stroma and calcification.

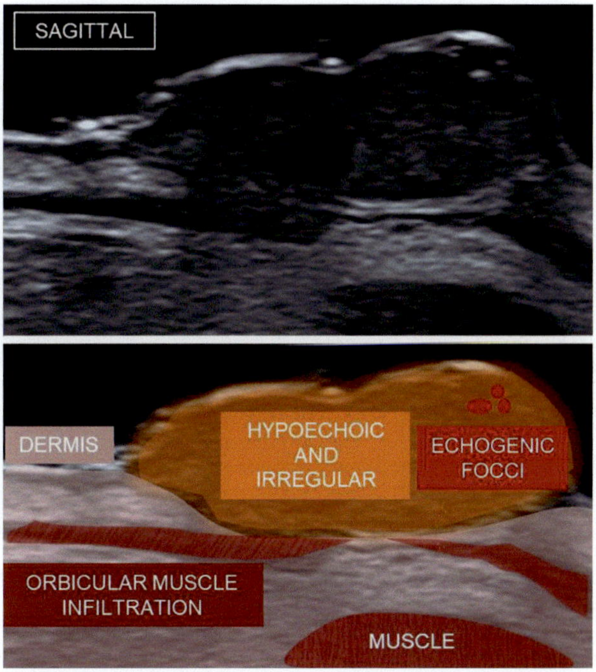

Fig. 12.47 Ultrasonographic findings of basal cell carcinoma with a 33 MHz probe (Aplio i800, Canon Medical Systems)

- Ultrasonography can help detect the depth of tumor infiltration into the dermis and subcutaneous tissue, which is important for surgical planning.
- Useful for assessing the extent of tumor invasion and guiding biopsy or excision.

12.4.3.7 MRI (Fig. 12.48) [45]

- BCCs often appear hypointense compared to surrounding tissues on T1-weighted images, due to their cellularity and fibrous stroma.
- Typically show hyperintense areas on T2-weighted images, reflecting the presence of fluid and increased cellularity.
- Post-contrast imaging usually shows variable enhancement, depending on the tumor's cellularity and vascularity. Morpheiform BCCs may exhibit less enhancement compared to nodular types due to their fibrous nature.
- MRI is valuable in assessing the depth of invasion and involvement of adjacent structures, which is crucial for surgical planning and evaluating the potential for local recurrence.

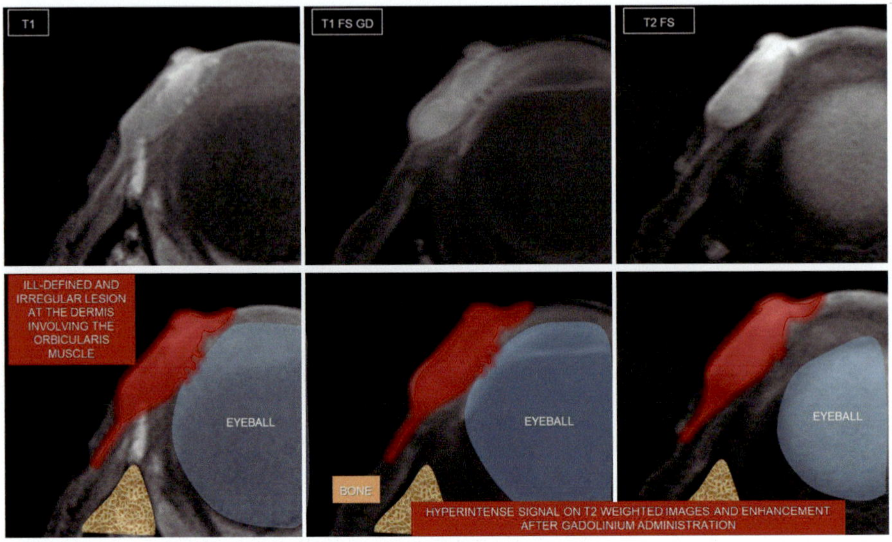

Fig. 12.48 MRI with surface coil findings of basal cell carcinoma on T2 FS and T1 FS-weighted sequences (Magnetom Prisma 3T MRI, Siemens)

12.4.3.8 3D Images (Fig. 12.49; Video 12.2)

- 3D imaging offers a precise and comprehensive view of the tumor and surrounding structures, enhancing the surgeon's ability to assess the full extent of the carcinoma. It also plays a crucial role in clearly defining the tumor boundaries, which is essential for accurately determining the surgical margins.
- By utilizing 3D images, surgeons can customize the surgical plan to match the patient's unique anatomy. This approach helps minimize damage to healthy tissues and safeguards vital structures such as nerves and blood vessels, ultimately improving surgical outcomes.
- The 3D model enables surgeons to simulate various surgical strategies before the operation, allowing them to choose the most effective and minimally invasive approach. This leads to improved aesthetic and functional results postsurgery.
- 3D models improve communication between the surgical team and the patient, ensuring that everyone involved has a clear and shared understanding of the surgical plan.

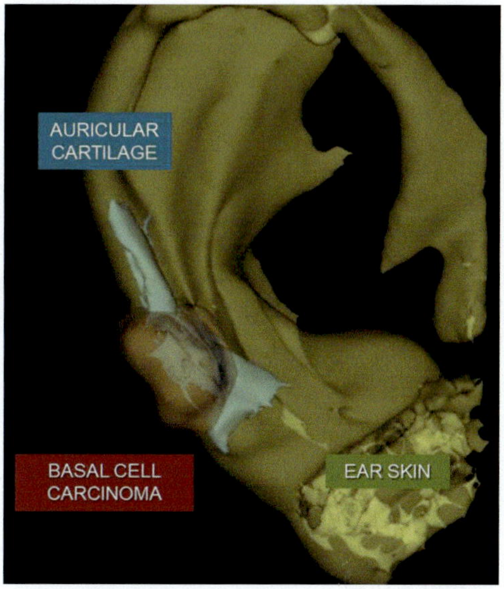

Fig. 12.49 3D images of basal cell carcinoma after segmentation of MRI isotropic images used for surgical planning

12.5 Tumoral Lesions on the Cervical Region

12.5.1 Thyroglossal Duct Cyst

12.5.1.1 Definition [46]

- Thyroglossal duct cysts are congenital anomalies that result from the persistence of the thyroglossal duct, a remnant of embryonic development.
- They form along the route of the thyroid gland's migration from the tongue base to the inferior neck.
- Thyroglossal duct cysts result from the failure of closure of the thyroglossal duct during embryonic development.
- In about 50% of people, the distal part of the duct differentiates into the pyramidal lobe of the thyroid gland.
- Normally, the thyroglossal duct involutes by the tenth week of gestation. However, if any portion persists, it can lead to cyst formation due to epithelial lining secretion.

12.5.1.2 Epidemiology [46]

- Thyroglossal duct cysts are found in approximately 7% of the global population.
- They occur equally in males and females.
- Although commonly seen in pediatric cases, they also present in adults with varying frequency.
- Their distribution includes approximately 20% to 25% at the suprahyoid level, 15% to 20% at the hyoid level, and 25% to 65% at the infrahyoid level.

12.5.1.3 Clinical Presentation (Fig. 12.50) [46]

- These cysts typically present as midline neck masses.
- They are closely associated with the hyoid bone.

12.5.1.4 Histopathology [16]

- A cyst lined with simple columnar or cuboidal epithelium or respiratory type with the presence of characteristic thyroid follicles in the periphery, containing mucinous material.

12.5.2 Computed Tomography [47, 48]

- Depicted as well-circumscribed lesions with mucoid attenuation, usually with thin walls.
- Enhanced CT shows mild to moderate enhancement of the cyst walls.
- Thick walls with rim enhancement may indicate current or past infection.
- Nodular enhancement within a thyroglossal duct cyst should prompt further workup for potential malignancy.

12.5.2.1 Ultrasonography [48]

- Simple, well-circumscribed anechoic cyst.
- Can have a pseudosolid appearance due to proteinaceous content.
- Histopathologic examination can confirm diagnosis by revealing cysts lined with squamous and respiratory epithelium.

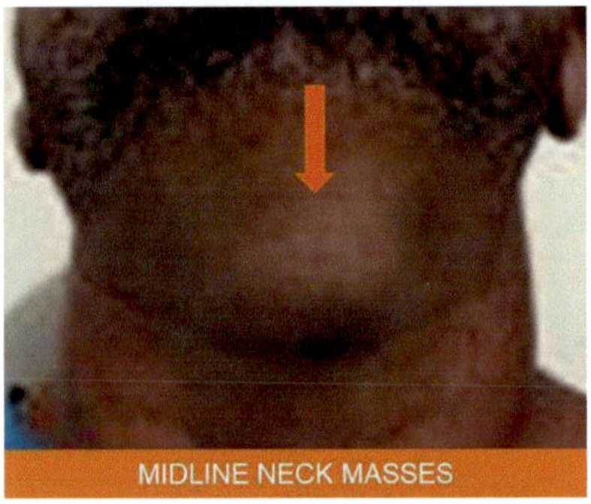

Fig. 12.50 Clinical photograph of patients with thyroglossal duct cyst

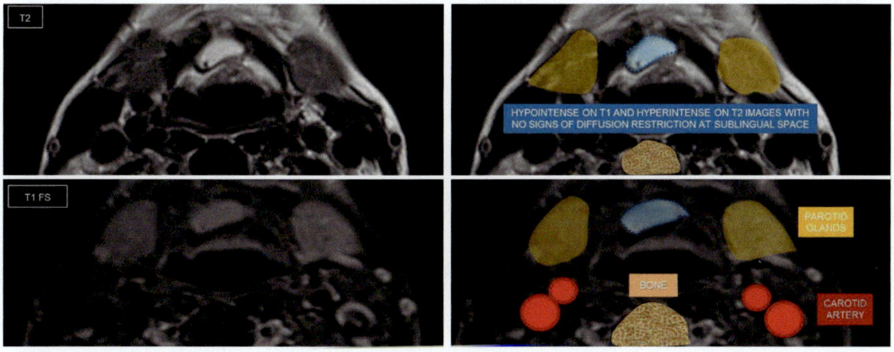

Fig. 12.51 MRI findings of thyroglossal duct cyst on T2 and T1 FS-weighted sequences (Magnetom Prisma 3T MRI, Siemens)

12.5.2.2 MRI (Fig. 12.51) [48]

- Demonstrates low signal intensity on T1-weighted sequences and high signal intensity on T2-weighted sequences.
- Non-enhancing in its cystic parts, unless there is an infection or complication, which causes rim enhancement.
- The cyst does not restrict diffusion, aiding in differentiation from other lesions.

12.5.3 Branchial Cleft Cyst

12.5.3.1 Definition [49]

- Branchial cleft cysts are congenital anomalies originating from the first through fourth pharyngeal clefts.
- The most common type arises from the second cleft, while anomalies from the first, third, and fourth clefts are rarer.
- These cysts are present at birth but may not be obvious or symptomatic until later.
- Childhood lesions often appear as visible puncta on the skin or neck masses, sometimes mistaken for abscesses.
- Branchial cleft anomalies can manifest as cysts, sinuses, or fistulae.
- Cysts have an epithelial lining without external openings and may be asymptomatic.
- Sinus tracts communicate externally with the skin or internally with the pharynx or larynx.
- Branchial cleft fistulae connect the pharynx or larynx to the external skin.

- First branchial cleft cysts
  - Make up approximately 5% to 25% of all branchial cleft anomalies.
  - Subclassified via the Work classification system.
  - Work Type I
    - Contain ectoderm only.
    - On physical exam, show preauricular masses or sinuses.
    - Track anterior and medial to the external auditory canal.
    - Typically present lateral to the facial nerve.
    - End within the external auditory canal or connect to the umbo of the middle ear (essentially a duplication of the external auditory canal).
  - Work Type II
    - More common.
    - Contain both ectoderm and mesoderm.
    - Classically present at the angle of the mandible or within the submandibular region.
    - Can course either lateral or medial to the facial nerve.
    - Pass superficially (57%), deeply (30%), or between (13%) branches of the facial nerve.
- Second branchial cleft cyst
  - Represents approximately 40–95% of branchial anomalies.
  - External punctum found anterior and medial to the sternocleidomastoid (SCM) on the neck skin.
  - Bilateral second branchial cleft cysts can be associated with branchio-oto-renal syndrome.
  - Course of a second branchial cleft sinus
    - External opening on the neck skin.
    - Fistula travels deep to platysma.
    - Passes between the internal and external carotids.
    - Courses superficially to both glossopharyngeal and hypoglossal nerves.
    - Connects to the tonsillar fossa.
    - Cysts or sinuses of the second branchial cleft can exist anywhere along this course.
- Third branchial cleft cyst
  - Represents an estimated 2–8% of all branchial cleft anomalies.
  - External skin opening is seen over the middle to lower third of the anterior sternocleidomastoid (SCM) muscle.
  - Course of the third branchial cleft sinus
    - From the skin opening described above, the tract courses deep to the platysma muscle.
    - It then courses posterior to the internal carotid artery.

    - The sinus passes between the glossopharyngeal and hypoglossal nerves.
    - It may be closely associated with the superior laryngeal nerve (often coursing superior to it).
    - Finally, it connects to the pyriform sinus in the larynx.

- Fourth branchial cleft cyst
  - Extremely rare, representing approximately 1% of all branchial cleft anomalies.
  - More commonly reported on the left side.
  - Skin opening near the medial lower border of the sternocleidomastoid (SCM) muscle.
  - Exact course not well characterized due to rarity.
  - Classically passes deep to the common carotid.
  - Can loop around either the aortic arch (left-sided anomaly) or the subclavian (right-sided anomaly).
  - Runs superficially to the recurrent laryngeal nerve and hypoglossal nerve.
  - Terminates in the apex of the pyriform sinus in the larynx.

12.5.3.2 Epidemiology [49]

- Exact incidence unknown due to presentation variations.
- No ethnic or gender predilection.
- Most common origin: Second branchial cleft (40–95% of cases).
- First, third, and fourth clefts are less frequent (5–25% combined).
- 10% of cases are bilateral.
- Typically present in the first decade of life, but presentation can be delayed.

12.5.3.3 Clinical Presentation (Fig. 12.52) [49]

- Often asymptomatic, but may become:
  - Tender
  - Enlarged
  - Inflamed
  - Infected (abscess formation)
  - Purulent drainage from a sinus tract (skin or pharynx) possible with infection
  - Dysphagia, dyspnea, and rare stridor due to airway compression
- Presentation varies based on cyst location
  - *First cleft cyst:* Smooth, non-tender, fluctuant mass between ear canal and submandibular area. May have a punctum with fluid expression.
  - *Second cleft cyst:* Skin pit or punctum at lower anterior sternocleidomastoid muscle. May connect to the tonsillar fossa. Tender with infection, possible airway compromise. Mucoid or purulent discharge possible.

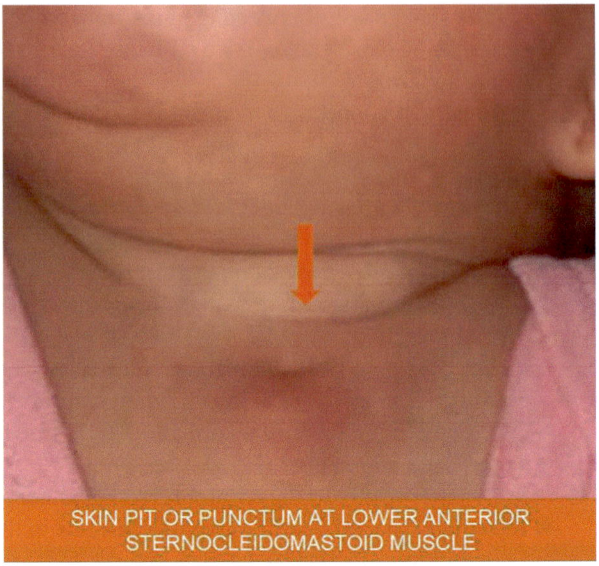

Fig. 12.52 Clinical photograph of patients with branchial cleft cyst

- *Third and fourth cleft cysts (rare):* Firm mass or infected cyst on left side of neck or near clavicle. May drain to the piriformis sinus or external neck skin. Often misdiagnosed and repeatedly drained.

12.5.3.4 Histopathology [49]

- Cyst lined by different types of epithelium, most of them (90%) by stratified squamous epithelium with marked lymphoid aggregates in the periphery and may contain keratinous debris inside the cyst.
- In some cases, the cyst wall is lined by ciliated columnar epithelium, resulting in more mucoid contents.
- Lymphoid tissue typically surrounds the epithelial lining.
- If infected or ruptured, inflammatory cells can be identified in the cavity or stroma.

12.5.3.5 Computed Tomography (Fig. 12.53) [50]

- *First branchial cleft cysts*
  - These cysts can be found along the course of the first branchial arch, extending from the submandibular triangle to the external auditory canal.
  - Type I: Usually present as cystic masses near the external auditory canal, composed entirely of ectodermal tissue.

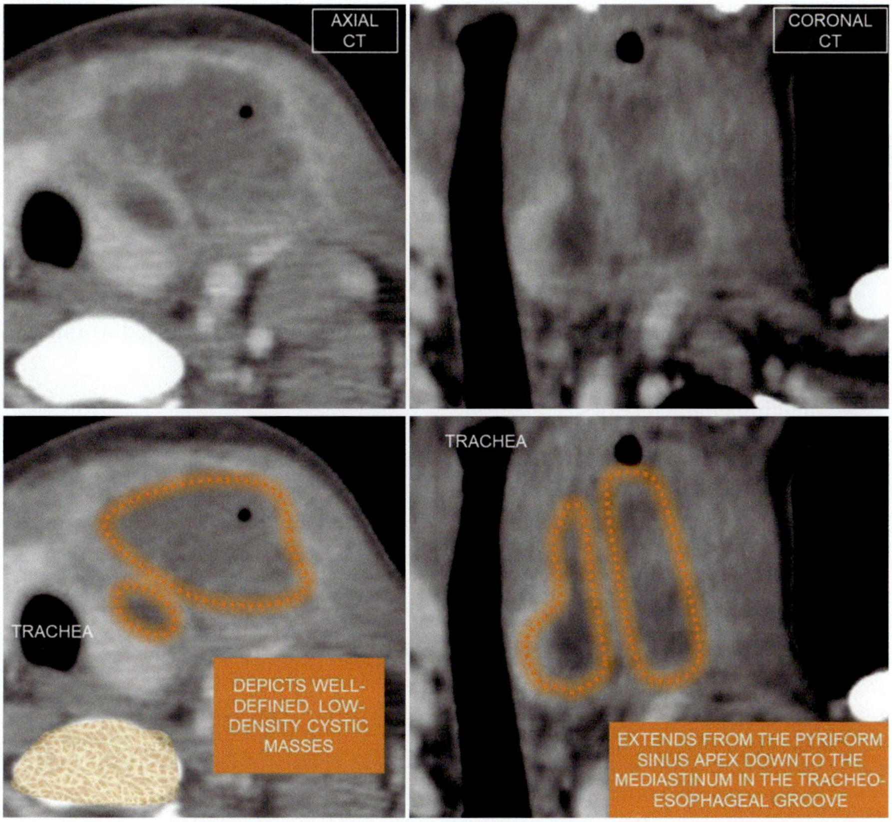

Fig. 12.53 Computed tomography findings of branchial cleft cyst (Philips Brilliance CT 64-slice)

- Type II: These can manifest as cysts, sinuses, or fistulae near the angle of the mandible and consist of both ectodermal and mesodermal tissues.
- CT san shows a cystic mass that can be superficial, within, or deep to the parotid salivary gland.

- *Second branchial cleft cysts*
  - Typically found within the submandibular space but can appear anywhere along the second branchial arch tract, from the supraclavicular fossa to the pharynx at the tonsillar fossa level.
  - Types:
    - Type I: Located superficially along the anterior surface of the sternocleidomastoid muscle, deep to the platysma.
    - Type II: Found anterior to the sternocleidomastoid muscle, posterior to the submandibular gland, and lateral to the carotid sheath.
    - Type III: Situated medially between the internal and external carotid arteries and lateral to the pharyngeal wall.

    - Type IV: Deep to the carotid sheath within the pharyngeal mucosal space, opening into the pharynx.
  - CT scans depict well-defined, low-density cystic masses with thin walls, which may thicken and enhance if infected.
- *Third and fourth branchial cleft cysts*
  - Location
    - Third: Found in the posterior cervical space, behind the sternocleidomastoid muscle.
    - Fourth: Extends from the pyriform sinus apex down to the mediastinum in the tracheoesophageal groove.
  - Imaging characteristics
    - Third branchial cleft cysts: Present as painless, fluctuant masses in the posterior cervical space that can become tender and enlarge if infected.
    - Fourth branchial cleft cysts: Often found on the left side, these may present as an abscess in the posterior triangle of the neck if infected.

12.5.3.6 Ultrasonography (Fig. 12.54) [50]

- *First branchial cleft cysts*
  - Displays a thick-walled cystic structure that is part of the sinus tract leading to the external auditory canal.
- *Second branchial cleft cysts*
  - Typically shows a well-defined, thin-walled, anechoic cyst with posterior acoustic enhancement, sometimes containing internal echoes.

12.5.3.7 MRI (Fig. 12.55) [50]

- *First branchial cleft cysts*
  - Thick-walled sinus tract extending to the external auditory canal, which might show signs of infection like purulent discharge.
- *Second branchial cleft cysts*
  - Usually hyperintense on T2-weighted images; wall thickening, and enhancement indicate inflammation.

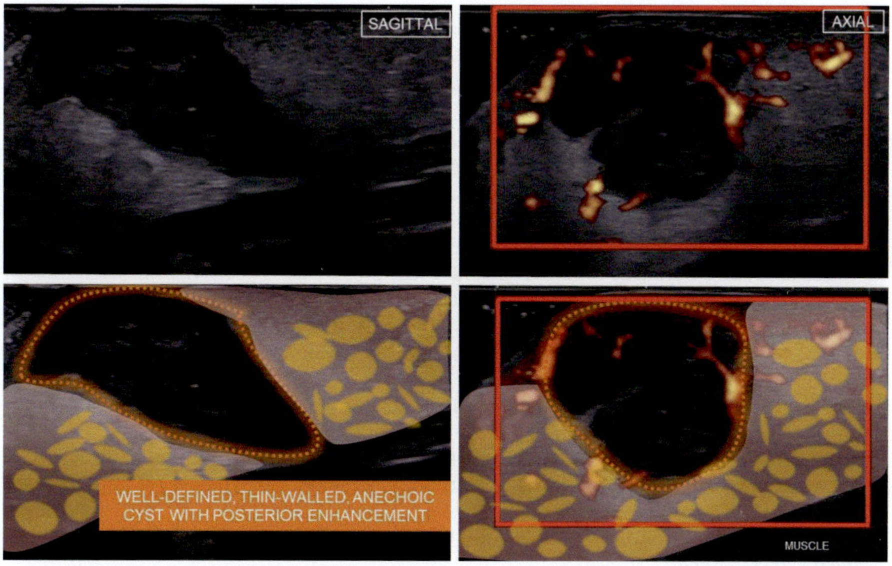

Fig. 12.54 Ultrasonographic findings of branchial cleft cyst with a 24 MHz probe (Aplio i800, Canon Medical Systems)

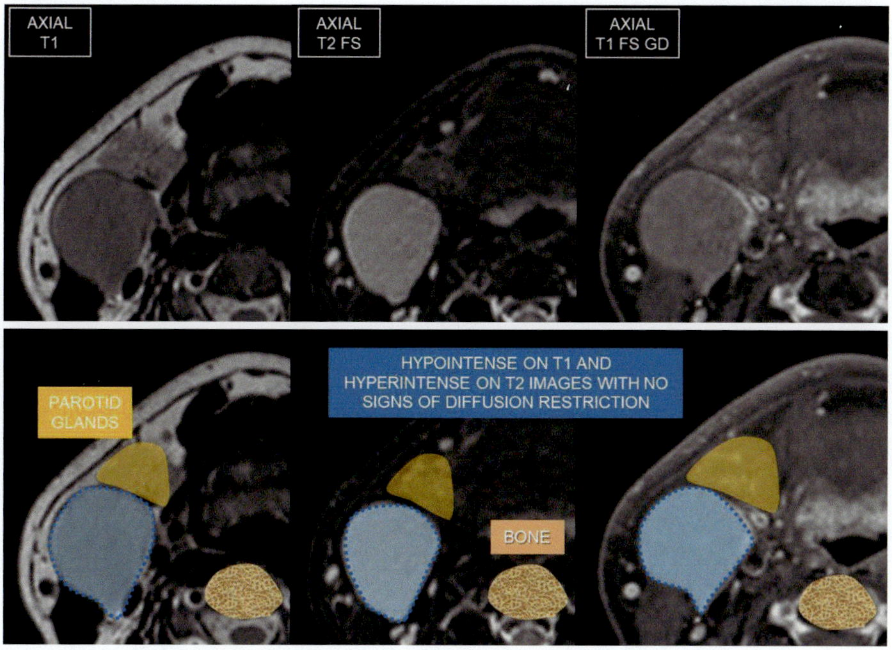

Fig. 12.55 MRI findings of branchial cleft cyst on T2 FS, T1, and T1 FS-weighted sequences after gadolinium administration (Magnetom Prisma 3T MRI, Siemens)

References

1. Shatzkes DR. Vascular anomalies: description, classification and nomenclature. Appl Radiol. 2018;18:4.
2. Alfageme Roldán F, Salgüero Fernández I, Zamanta Muñoz Garza F, Roustán Gullón G. Update on the use of ultrasound in vascular anomalies. Actas Dermo-Sifiliográficas. 2016;107:284–93.
3. Monsignore LM, Nakiri GS, Santos D, Giansante Abud T, Abud DG. Peripheral vascular malformations. Radiol Bras. 2010;43(3):185–94.
4. Piccolo V, Russo T, Moscarella E, Brancaccio G, Alfano R, Argenziano G. Dermatoscopy of vascular lesions. Dermatol Clin. 2018;36:389–95.
5. Calonje E, Lazar AJ, Luzar B. Diagnostic atlas of cutaneous mesenchymal neoplasia. Elsevier; 2020. https://linkinghub.elsevier.com/retrieve/pii/C20100684550.
6. Dzian A, Hamzík J. Intercostal hemangioma of the chest wall. Kardiochir Torakochirurgia Pol. 2016;1:58–60.
7. Bhatt K, Tambe S, Jerajani H, Dhurat R. Utility of high-frequency ultrasonography in the diagnosis of benign and malignant skin tumors. Indian J Dermatol Venereol Leprol. 2017;83:162.
8. Mittal A, Anand R, Gauba R, Choudhury SR, Abbey P. A step-by-step sonographic approach to vascular anomalies in the pediatric population: a pictorial essay. Indian J Radiol Imaging. 2021;31(1):157–71.
9. Myers DJ, Sathe NC, Fillman EP. Cylindroma. StatPearls; 2024. http://www.ncbi.nlm.nih.gov/pubmed/25354097.
10. So M, Edson RS. Chondrodermatitis nodularis helicis. Cleve Clin J Med. 2023;90:277–8.
11. Gupta G, Hohman MH, Kwan E. Chondrodermatitis nodularis helicis. StatPearls; 2024. http://www.ncbi.nlm.nih.gov/pubmed/21276202.
12. Morgado-Carasco D, Fustà-Novell X, Podlipnik S, Ferrandiz L. Dermoscopic features of chondrodermatitis nodularis chronica helicis: a case series. Dermatol Pract Concept. 2019;9:52–3.
13. Hall BJ, Hall JC, Cockerell CJ, Affolter K, Alvarez P. Diagnostic pathology: nonneoplastic dermatopathology. Elsevier; 2017. p. iii. https://linkinghub.elsevier.com/retrieve/pii/B9780323377133500017.
14. Bahrani B, Khachemoune A. Review of accessory tragus with highlights of its associated syndromes. Int J Dermatol. 2014;53:1442–6.
15. Patterson JW. Weedon's skin pathology. 6th ed. Elsevier; 2024.
16. Barnhill RL, Neil Crowson A, Magro CM, Piepkorn MW, Kutzner H, Desman GT. Barnhill's dermatopathology. 4th ed. McGraw Hill/Medical; 2019. https://dermatology.mhmedical.com/content.aspx?bookid=2802&sectionid=238125236.
17. McGinty S, Siddiqui WJ. Keloid. StatPearls; 2024. http://www.ncbi.nlm.nih.gov/pubmed/17276198.
18. Elrefaie AM, Salem RM, Faheem MH. High-resolution ultrasound for keloids and hypertrophic scar assessment. Lasers Med Sci. 2020;35:379–85.
19. Das C, Khaowas A. Pre-auricular sinus with post-auricular extension: an uncommon variant. Indian J Otolaryngol Head Neck Surg. 2019;71:1511–4.
20. Al Aboud AM, Shah SS, Blair K, Al Aboud DM. Xanthelasma Palpebrarum. StatPearls; 2024. http://www.ncbi.nlm.nih.gov/pubmed/29296091.
21. Koumaki D, Papadakis M, Lagoudaki E, Manios GA, Kassotakis D, Doxastaki A, et al. Apocrine and eccrine hidrocystomas: a clinicopathological study. Acta Dermatovenerol Alp Pannonica Adriat. 2021;30:53–6.
22. Jayaprakasam A, Rene C. A benign or malignant eyelid lump—can you tell? An unusual collision tumour highlighting the difficulty differentiating a hidrocystoma from a basal cell carcinoma. Case Rep. 2012;2012:bcr1220115307.
23. Ludzik J, Lee C, Mengden S, Nguyen H, Pleshakov D, Witkowski A. Dermoscopy and reflectance confocal microscopy of apocrine Hidrocystoma. Dermatol Pract Concept. 2023;13:e2023039.

24. Zhou C, Chai P, Xia W, Li J, Jia R, Fan X. Intraepithelial growth pattern for eyelid sebaceous carcinoma: a cohort of 214 patients from a single institution. Br J Ophthalmol. 2023;107:324–30.
25. Perez-Lopez I, Garrido-Colmenero C, Blasco-Morente G, Aneiros-Fernandez J, Arias-Santiago S. Utilidad de la ecografía cutánea en el diagnóstico diferencial de las lesiones azules, hidrocistoma. Dermatol Online J. 2015;21:13030/qt2mw2m8b0.
26. Huang V, Lee V, Briceño CA. Orbital apocrine hidrocystoma with ptosis. Am J Ophthalmol Case Rep. 2022;8(28):101747. https://doi.org/10.1016/j.ajoc.2022.101747.
27. von Holstein SL, Rasmussen PK, Heegaard S. Tumors of the lacrimal gland. Semin Diagn Pathol. 2016;33:156–63.
28. Kim SH, Min HK, Lee S-H, Lee K-A, Kim H-R. Ultrasonographic evaluation of lacrimal glands in patients with primary Sjögren's syndrome. Clin Exp Rheumatol. 2022;40:2283.
29. Nair JR, Syed R, Chan IYM, Gorelik N, Chankowsky J, del Carpio-O'Donovan R. The forgotten lacrimal gland and lacrimal drainage apparatus: pictorial review of CT and MRI findings and differential diagnosis. Br J Radiol. 2022;95:95.
30. Park S-K, Park J, Kim H-U, Yun S-K. Sebaceous carcinoma: clinicopathologic analysis of 29 cases in a tertiary Hospital in Korea. J Korean Med Sci. 2017;32:1351.
31. Satomura H, Ogata D, Arai E, Tsuchida T. Dermoscopic features of ocular and extraocular sebaceous carcinomas. J Dermatol. 2017;44:1313–6.
32. Horvat Aleksijevic L, Prpic J, Muhvic Urek M, Pezelj-Ribaric S, Ivancic-Jokic N, Peršic Bukmir R, et al. Oral mucosal lesions in childhood. Dent J (Basel). 2022;10:214.
33. Huzaifa M, Soni A. Mucocele and ranula. StatPearls; 2024. http://www.ncbi.nlm.nih.gov/pubmed/2193904.
34. Friedman E, Patiño MO, Udayasankar UK. Imaging of pediatric salivary glands. Neuroimaging Clin N Am. 2018;28:209–26.
35. Koch M, Mantsopoulos K, Leibl V, Müller S, Iro H, Sievert M. Ultrasound in the diagnosis and differential diagnosis of enoral and plunging ranula: a detailed and comparative analysis. J Ultrasound. 2022;26:487–95.
36. Lupu M, Caruntu A, Caruntu C, Boda D, Moraru L, Voiculescu V, et al. Non-invasive imaging of actinic cheilitis and squamous cell carcinoma of the lip. Mol Clin Oncol. 2018;8(5):640–6.
37. Howard A, Agrawal N, Gooi Z. Lip and oral cavity squamous cell carcinoma. Hematol Oncol Clin North Am. 2021;35:895–911.
38. Warszawik-Hendzel O, Olszewska M, Maj M, Rakowska A, Czuwara J, Rudnicka L. Non-invasive diagnostic techniques in the diagnosis of squamous cell carcinoma. J Dermatol Case Rep. 2015;9:9.
39. Heath MS, Bar A. Basal cell carcinoma. Dermatol Clin. 2023;41:13–21.
40. Kim DP, Kus KJB, Ruiz E. Basal cell carcinoma review. Hematol Oncol Clin North Am. 2019;33:13–24.
41. Álvarez-Salafranca M, Ara M, Zaballos P. Dermoscopy in basal cell carcinoma: an updated review. Actas Dermosifiliogr. 2021;112:330–8.
42. Khan R, Ahmed A, Khachemoune A. Ultrasound features of high-risk basal cell carcinoma: a systematic review. Arch Dermatol Res. 2024;316:210.
43. Barcaui EO, Valiante PMN, Carvalho ACP, Barcaui CB. High-frequency ultrasound associated with dermoscopy in pre-operative evaluation of basal cell carcinoma. An Bras Dermatol. 2014;89:828–31.
44. Laverde-Saad A, Simard A, Nassim D, Jfri A, Alajmi A, O'Brien E, et al. Performance of ultrasound for identifying morphological characteristics and thickness of cutaneous basal cell carcinoma: a systematic review. Dermatology. 2022;238:692–710.
45. Cipullo MB, Rahimian E, Tahsini M, Giavri Z, Bisdas S. Giant basal cell carcinoma of the scalp with intracranial invasion: MRI findings with tract visualisation. Case Rep Radiol. 2021;2021:1–5.
46. Amos J, Shermetaro C. Thyroglossal duct cyst. StatPearls; 2024. http://www.ncbi.nlm.nih.gov/pubmed/30194760.

47. Ahuja AT, Wong KT, King AD, Yuen EHY. Imaging for thyroglossal duct cyst: the bare essentials. Clin Radiol. 2005;60:141–8.
48. Zander DA, Smoker WRK. Imaging of ectopic thyroid tissue and Thyroglossal duct cysts. Radiographics. 2014;34:37–50.
49. Coste AH, Lofgren DH, Shermetaro C. Branchial cleft cyst. StatPearls; 2024. http://www.ncbi.nlm.nih.gov/pubmed/30725193.
50. Adams A, Mankad K, Offiah C, Childs L. Branchial cleft anomalies: a pictorial review of embryological development and spectrum of imaging findings. Insights Imaging. 2016;7:69–76.

Part IV
Trunk and Limbs

Chapter 13
Clinical, Imaging and Histological Findings in Inflammatory Lesions of the Trunk and Limbs

Ana Luisa Sampaio, Paula Figueiredo de Marsillac, Maria de Oliveira Buffara, Camila Silveira Nobre, Haizza Cristina de Almeida Cabral Monteiro, Priscilla Haui de Oliveira Galuzzi Fonseca, André da Silva Cartel, Thais Emanuelle Freire Barbosa, Gabriella di Giunta, Leonardo Rodrigues Campos, Izabela Machado Flores Pereira, Heron Werner, Ana Leticia Boff, André Francisco Gomes, Laila Klotz de Almeida Balassiano, Luna Azulay, Rodrigo Gaudio, Silvana Machado Mendonça, Ana Beatriz Vargas dos Santos, Mary Lane Alves Nemer, Felipe Mauricio Soeiro Sampaio, Carolina Ávila de Almeida, and Clarissa Canella Moraes do Carmo

In dermatology, precise imaging of inflammatory lesions is essential for accurate diagnosis and effective treatment. This chapter explores the application of ultrasonography and magnetic resonance imaging with surface coil in the assessment of inflammatory skin conditions affecting the trunk and limbs. By leveraging these

Supplementary Information The online version contains supplementary material available at https://doi.org/10.1007/978-3-031-77987-9_13.

A. L. Sampaio
Department of Dermatology, Hospital Universitario Pedro Ernesto, Universidade Estadual do Rio de Janeiro—UERJ, Rio de Janeiro, Brazil

P. F. de Marsillac · M. de Oliveira Buffara · C. S. Nobre
State University of Rio de Janeiro—UERJ, Pedro Ernesto Hospital—HUPE, Rio de Janeiro, RJ, Brazil

H. C. de Almeida Cabral Monteiro
State University of Rio de Janeiro—UERJ, Pedro Ernesto Hospital—HUPE, Rio de Janeiro, RJ, Brazil

Department of Dermatology, Hospital Rio-Barra and Rede D'Or São Luiz, Rio de Janeiro, RJ, Brazil

P. H. de Oliveira Galuzzi Fonseca
Clinica CDPI and ALTA—Rio de Janeiro, Barra da Tijuca, Rio de Janeiro, RJ, Brazil

© The Author(s), under exclusive license to Springer Nature Switzerland AG 2025

C. Canella Moraes do Carmo (ed.), *Atlas of Diagnostic Imaging in Dermatology*, https://doi.org/10.1007/978-3-031-77987-9_13

advanced imaging modalities, clinicians can achieve a detailed understanding of lesion characteristics, including their size, depth, and distribution. Ultrasonography provides real-time, dynamic views of the skin and underlying structures, while MRI with surface coil offers high-resolution, cross-sectional images that reveal deeper tissue involvement. Integrating these imaging techniques into clinical practice enhances diagnostic precision, guides therapeutic decisions, and improves overall patient management for complex inflammatory dermatologic conditions.

A. da Silva Cartel
Faculdade de Medicina da Universidade Federal do Rio Grande do Sul, Universidade Federal do Rio Grande do Sul, Porto Alegre, RS, Brazil

Dermatologist and Dermatopathologist in Private Practice, Porto Alegre, RS, Brazil

T. E. F. Barbosa
Marcilio Dias Naval Hospital and National Cancer Institute—INCA, Rio de Janeiro, RJ, Brazil

G. di Giunta
Federal University of Santa Catarina, Florianópolis, SC, Brazil

L. R. Campos
Department of Pediatric Rheumatology, Antônio Pedro University Hospital—UFF, Niterói, RJ, Brazil

I. M. F. Pereira
Felício Rocho Hospital—FELUMA, Belo Horizonte, Brazil

H. Werner
Clinica ALTA—DASA—Rio de Janeiro, Rio de Janeiro, RJ, Brazil

Universidade Federal do Rio de Janeiro—UFRJ, Rio de Janeiro, RJ, Brazil

Biodesign Lab DASA—PUC—Rio de Janeiro, Rio de Janeiro, RJ, Brazil

A. L. Boff
Santa Casa Hospital, Porto Alegre, RS, Brazil

Dermathopathologist Private Practice, Clinica Dermapat, Porto Alegre, RS, Brazil

A. F. Gomes
Clinica Diagnóstico Avançado por Imagem—DAPI—Curitiba, Curitiba, Brazil

L. K. de Almeida Balassiano
Sector of Dermatology and Post Graduate Course in Medical Clinics—UFRJ, Federal University of Rio de Janeiro, Rio de Janeiro, RJ, Brazil

Medical Clinics—UFRJ, Federal University of Rio de Janeiro, Rio de Janeiro, RJ, Brazil

L. Azulay
Professor Rubem David Azulay Institute of Dermatology—Santa Casa RJ, Rio de Janeiro, RJ, Brazil

State University of Rio de Janeiro—UERJ, Pedro Ernesto Hospital—HUPE, Rio de Janeiro, RJ, Brazil

R. Gaudio
Antônio Pedro University Hospital—UFF, Niterói, RJ, Brazil

Autoimmunity Center (NAI)—AMIL, Niterói, RJ, Brazil

13.1 Connective Tissue Diseases

13.1.1 Lupus Erythematosus

13.1.1.1 Definition [1–3]

- Cutaneous lupus erythematosus encompasses a wide range of manifestations, including acute, subacute, chronic, and intermittent forms.
- Acute and subacute forms are more inflammatory and tend to regress without scarring.
- Intermittent lupus was previously called lupus tumidus.
- Chronic cutaneous lupus can leave atrophy if not treated effectively or quickly and are typified as:
  - Discoid lupus.
  - Lupus panniculitis.
  - Lupus profundus.

S. M. Mendonça
Clinica de Diagnostico por Imagem, Clinica Cavallieri, Rio de Janeiro, RJ, Brazil

Dermatology and Musculoskeletal Imaging at Diagnóstico das Américas—DASA—RJ, Rio de Janeiro, RJ, Brazil

A. B. V. dos Santos
State University of Rio de Janeiro—UERJ, Pedro Ernesto Hospital—HUPE, Rio de Janeiro, RJ, Brazil

M. L. A. Nemer
Clinica DERMUS—Ultrassonografia Especializada, Vitória, Vitória, Brazil

F. M. S. Sampaio
Private Dermatology Practice, Rio de Janeiro, RJ, Brazil

C. Á. de Almeida
Faculty of Medicine of Valença—UniFaa, Valença, Brazil

Federal University of Rio de Janeiro—UFRJ, Rio de Janeiro, Brazil

C. Canella Moraes do Carmo (✉)
Fluminense Federal University—UFF, Rio de Janeiro, Brazil

Federal University of Rio de Janeiro—UFRJ, Rio de Janeiro, Brazil

Diagnóstico das Américas—DASA—RJ, Rio de Janeiro, Brazil

Biodesign Laboratory, DASA-PUC, Rio de Janeiro, Brazil

13.1.1.2 Epidemiology [1–3]

- There is a 4:1 female predominance.
- More common between the ages of 20 and 40 years, with a mean age at onset of 43 years, varying according to the subtype.
- Discoid lupus erythematosus is by far the most common type of cutaneous lupus erythematosus, comprising 80% of all cases.
- Cutaneous lupus erythematosus is two to three times more frequent than systemic lupus erythematosus, with an annual incidence of 4.3/100,000.
- 70% to 80% of systemic lupus erythematosus patients have cutaneous involvement.
- 20% of patients diagnosed with cutaneous lupus erythematosus progress to systemic lupus erythematosus:
  - Acute cutaneous lupus erythematosus has the greatest chance of association with systemic lupus erythematosus (80% to 90% of cases).
  - Subacute cutaneous lupus erythematosus is associated to systemic lupus erythematosus in around 30%.
  - Generalized discoid lupus erythematosus is associated to systemic lupus erythematosus in 20%.
  - Localized discoid lupus erythematosus is associated to systemic lupus erythematosus in 5%.

13.1.1.3 Clinical Presentation (Fig. 13.1) [2]

- Acute lupus.
  - Acute onset, with manifestations of malar rash, exanthematic (diffuse erythematous photodistributed) lesions and necrotic lesions (also called specific bullous lupus).
  - Acute lesions are more commonly associated with systemic lupus and ANA-positive antibodies.
- Subacute lupus is presented as:
  - Annular lesions.
  - Papulosquamous (or psoriasiform) lesions.
  - Rowell's syndrome (target-like lesions that resembles erythema multiforme).
- Intermittent tumid lupus.
  - Papules and plaques in sun-exposed localizations.
  - Minimal epidermal involvement.

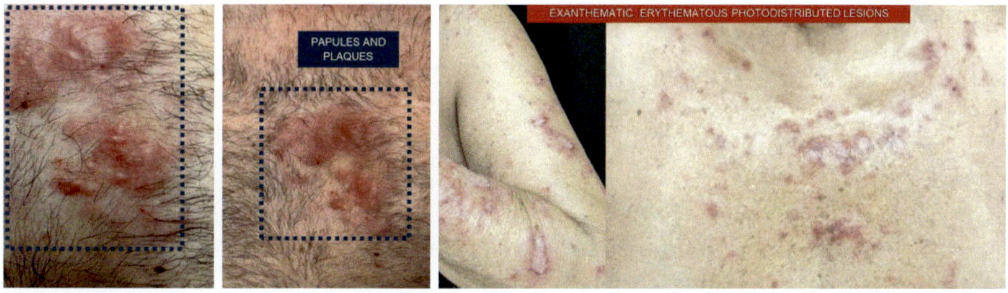

Fig. 13.1 Clinical photograph of patients with subacute and tumid cutaneous lupus erythematosus

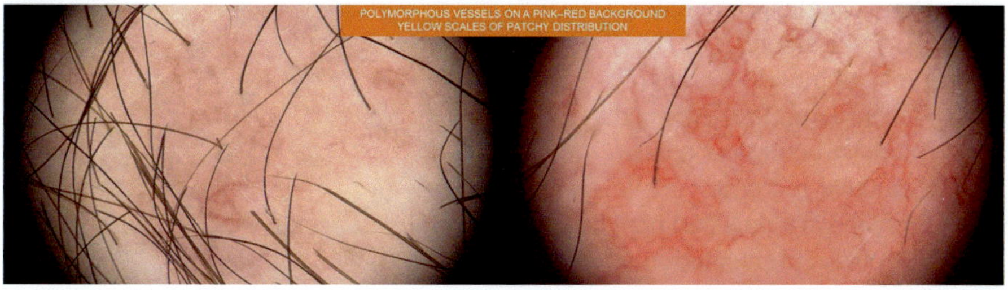

Fig. 13.2 Dermoscopic findings of patient with tumid cutaneous lupus erythematosus (x20)

- Chronic cutaneous lupus.
  - Discoid lesions with hyperkeratotic, dyschromic, scarring plaques, and cicatricial alopecia in scalp lesions.
  - Can be presented as panniculitis with specific finding of lupus.

13.1.1.4 Dermoscopy (Fig. 13.2) [4]

- Acute cutaneous lupus erythematosus (ACLE).
  - Polymorphous vessels (linear, linear branched, linear curved, and, less frequently, dotted vessels) on a pink–red background.
  - There were also white or yellow scales of patchy distribution in 30% and 20% of the cases, respectively.
  - Red structureless (hemorrhagic) areas and dotted/globular structures were present in half of the cases.
- Subacute cutaneous lupus erythematosus (SCLE):
  - Shows a pink–red background and polymorphous vessels (linear, linear branched, linear curved, and dotted vessels).
  - Scaling, peripheral pigmentation, and red structureless (hemorrhagic) areas.

- Intermittent cutaneous lupus erythematosus (ICLE).
  - Polymorphous vessels of unspecific distribution on a pink–red background.
  - This kind of cutaneous lupus erythematosus does not have scales, peripheral pigmentation, erosions, and crusting.
- Chronic cutaneous lupus erythematosus (CCLE).
  - Polymorphous vascular pattern (linear, linear curved and linear branched vessels and less frequently dotted vessels).
  - White scaling and yellow scales (76.9% and 38.5%, respectively).
  - Follicular keratotic plug.
  - Pink–red backgrounds.
  - Perifollicular white halos.
  - Dots or globules.
  - Pink structureless areas.
  - Red structureless (hemorrhagic) areas.
  - White structureless areas.
  - Follicular red dots.
  - Gray–brown dots and peppering.
  - Peripheral pigmentation, erosions, dilated follicles, and rosettes.

13.1.1.5 Histopathology (Fig. 13.3) [3, 5]

- Chronic discoid lupus.
  - Clinically and histologically, lupus erythematosus can present in different forms, varying depending on the stage of evolution of the biopsied lesion, inflammatory activity, and use of therapy. Therefore, a biopsy that includes a hypodermis, punch 4 or greater or navet, informing the exact topography of the lesion and the biopsied area of the lesion, is essential.

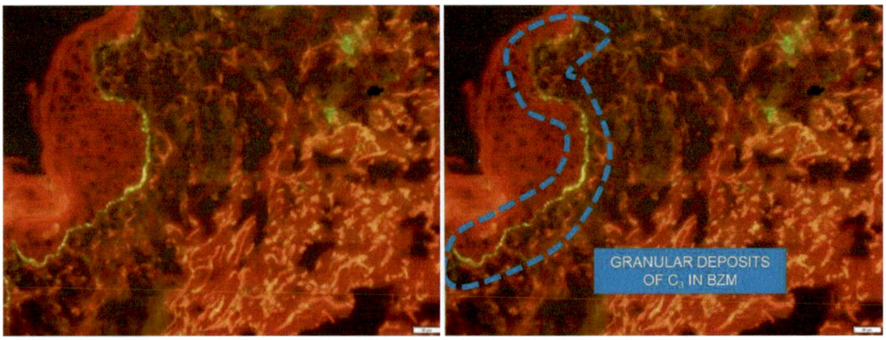

Fig. 13.3 Histological findings of cutaneous lupus erythematosus (Immunofluorescence or Polarized light microscopy)

- It usually presents as a vacuolar interface dermatitis with mononuclear inflammatory infiltrate, mainly lymphocytic, superficial, deep perivascular, and/or periadnexal (adventitial). It is rarely lichenoid. The infiltrate may extend to the hypoderma or affect only the hypoderma (deep lupus). It can be variable and even quite discrete.
- There may be satellitosis.
- Hyaline thickening of the basement membrane zone (BMZ) positive magenta in SBP (Special Basement Membrane Stains) and resistant diastasis. This thickening is irregular and may even fail and corresponds to the deposition of immunoglobulins (IgG and IgM) and complement with BMZ.
- Edema in the superficial dermis, more exuberant in the tumid forms.
- Epidermal atrophy at the expense of the spinous layer with compact hyperkeratosis; rarely exhibits irregular epithelial hyperplasia; parakeratosis may be present.
- Superficial venular ectasia; perivascular hyaline material corresponding to immunoglobulins and fibrin may be deposed. There may be extravasation of red blood cells. The association with hypersensitivity vasculitis (leukocytoclastic) or thrombotic vasculopathy related to antiphospholipid syndrome, seen in the same biopsy, is uncommon.
- Mucin deposition in the dermis reticularis, highlighted by PAS or alcian-blue, more common in the subacute and tumid forms.
- Conical follicular plugging, different from the lichen planus plug, where dilation is usually lower; sebaceous atrophy involving the vellus is the earliest adnexal alteration.
- Pigmentary incontinence.
- Direct immunofluorescence: granular deposits of IgM, IgG, and complement in BZM in 50% to 90% of photoexposed skin samples. It also marks apoptotic vessels and bodies. DIF is important for the differential diagnosis.

• Chronic lupus profundus or lupus panniculitis.

  - Only 50% have dermal and epidermal alterations, in the other half, the alterations are restricted to hypoderm.
  - Lobular hypodermatitis with prominent lymphocytic infiltrate, lymphocytes with karyorexis (nuclear dust). Eventually, it may exhibit lymphoid follicles in 25% of cases.

• Intermittent lupus tumid.

  - Absence of epidermal or junctional changes, presenting only dermal changes, including superficial and deep perivascular infiltrate and interstitial, papillary edema, and abundant mucin deposits in the reticular dermis.

13.1.1.6 Ultrasonography (Fig. 13.4) [6]

- Active cutaneous lupus.
  - Ultrasonography reveals thickening and hypoechogenicity of the upper hypodermis, typically seen on the face, particularly in the malar or cheek areas.
  - Power Doppler imaging may reveal variable intralesional vascularization.
- Chronic cutaneous lupus.
  - Cutaneous layer atrophy.
  - Hypovascularization on power Doppler, may lead to artery lumen narrowing and pearlization, causing Raynaud's phenomenon and vessel occlusion, commonly in digital arteries.
  - Lobular involvement seen on ultrasonography as diffuse thickening and hyperechogenicity ("cloudy" pattern) or septal involvement with thickened hypoechogenic septa ("brick wall" pattern).

13.1.1.7 MRI (Fig. 13.5)

- Active cutaneous lupus.
  - Thickening, high signal intensity on STIR images at upper hypodermis.

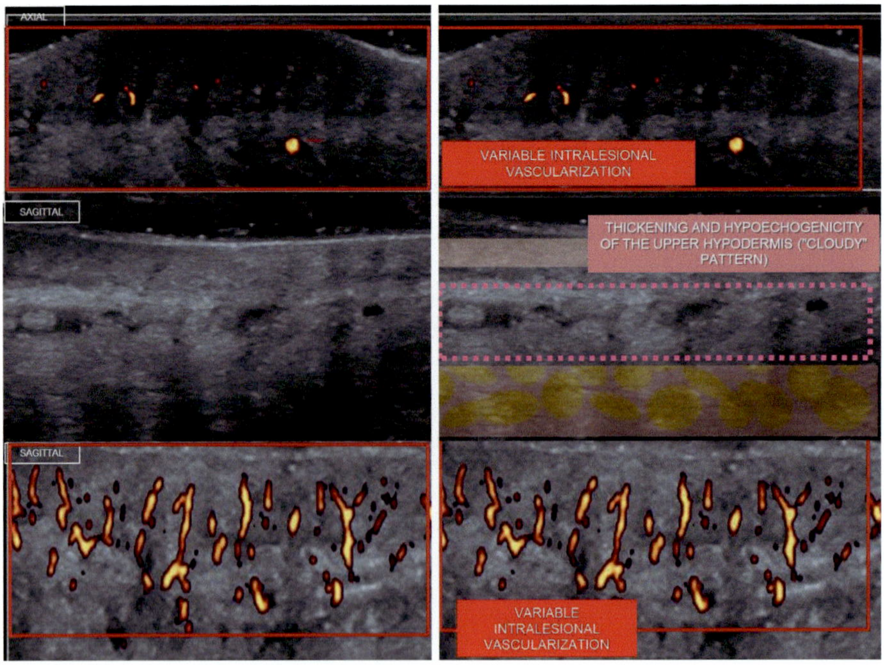

Fig. 13.4 Ultrasonographic findings of tumid cutaneous lupus erythematosus with a 24 MHz probe (Aplio i800, Canon Medical Systems)

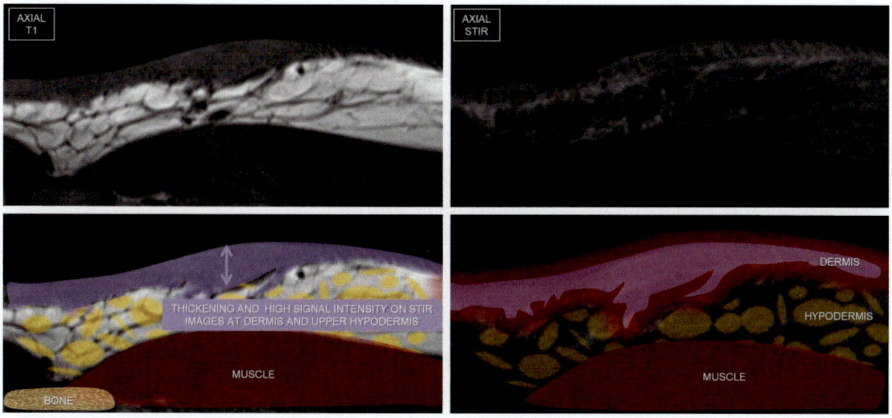

Fig. 13.5 MRI with surface coil findings of tumid cutaneous lupus erythematosus on T1-weighted and STIR sequences (Magnetom Prisma 3T MRI, Siemens)

- Chronic cutaneous lupus.
  - Lobular involvement similar to a panniculitis, seen as diffuse septal thickening and high signal intensity on STIR images.
  - Cutaneous layer atrophy.

13.1.2 Dermatomyositis

13.1.2.1 Definition [7–9]

- Dermatomyositis (DM) is an idiopathic inflammatory myopathy characterized by distinct skin lesions and systemic manifestations.
- Approximately 80% of patients with dermatomyositis have myopathy, that is, characterized by weakness of the proximal muscles over weeks to months.

13.1.2.2 Epidemiology [8, 9]

- The risk of developing malignancy is highest within a year of diagnosis of dermatomyositis and remains elevated for up to 5 years. The estimated prevalence of malignancy in adult patients is 20%.
- Prevalence has been estimated at 1–6 per 100,000 adults in the United States.
- Affects both genders with a 2:1 female: male ratio.

13.1.2.3 Clinical Presentation (Figs. 13.6, 13.7 and 13.8) [7, 8, 10]

- Cutaneous manifestations may be variable, including pathognomonic findings such as Gottron's papules and heliotrope eruption and non-specific cutaneous manifestations.
- Gottron's papules that represent erythematous violaceous papules covering the interphalangeal and metacarpophalangeal joints.
- Gottron's sign described as erythematous-violaceous macules over other joints, such as elbows or knees.
- Pink to violaceous erythema, with or without edema, involving the periorbital skin called heliotrope. The upper eyelid is the most affected site.
- Intense photosensitivity, with erythematous-violaceous lesions on the scalp, neck, shoulders, extensor surfaces of the upper extremities, upper chest region ("V-neck sign"), and upper back region ("shawl sign").
- Itchy and scale may be present on the scalp.
- Calcinosis of the skin, soft tissues, muscle, or bone is a challenging complication observed in patients with juvenile DM and occasionally develops in patients with adult DM.

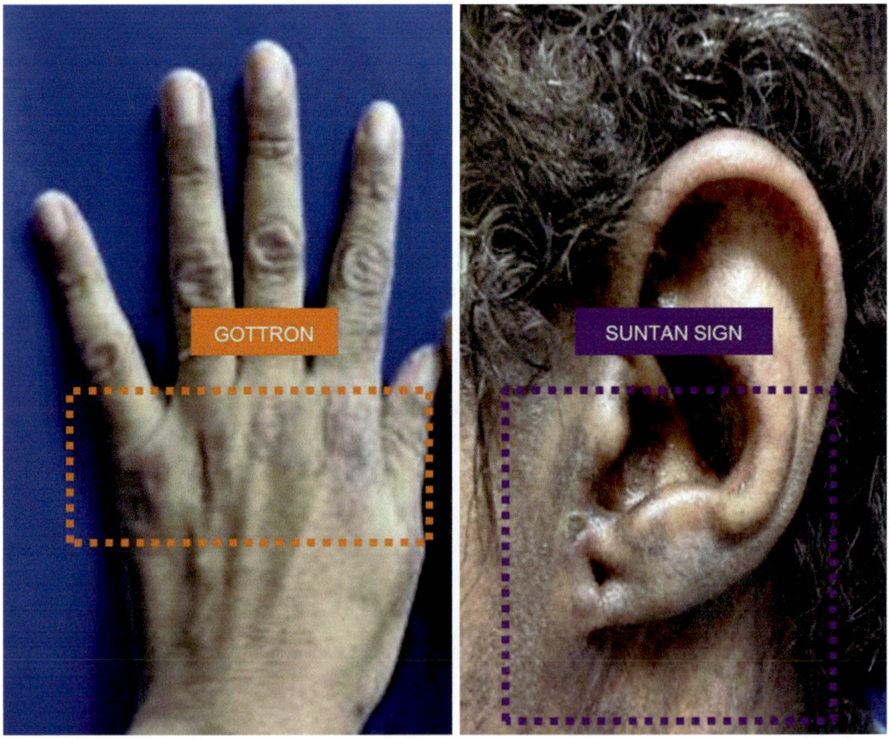

Fig. 13.6 Clinical photograph of patient with typical findings of dermatomyositis

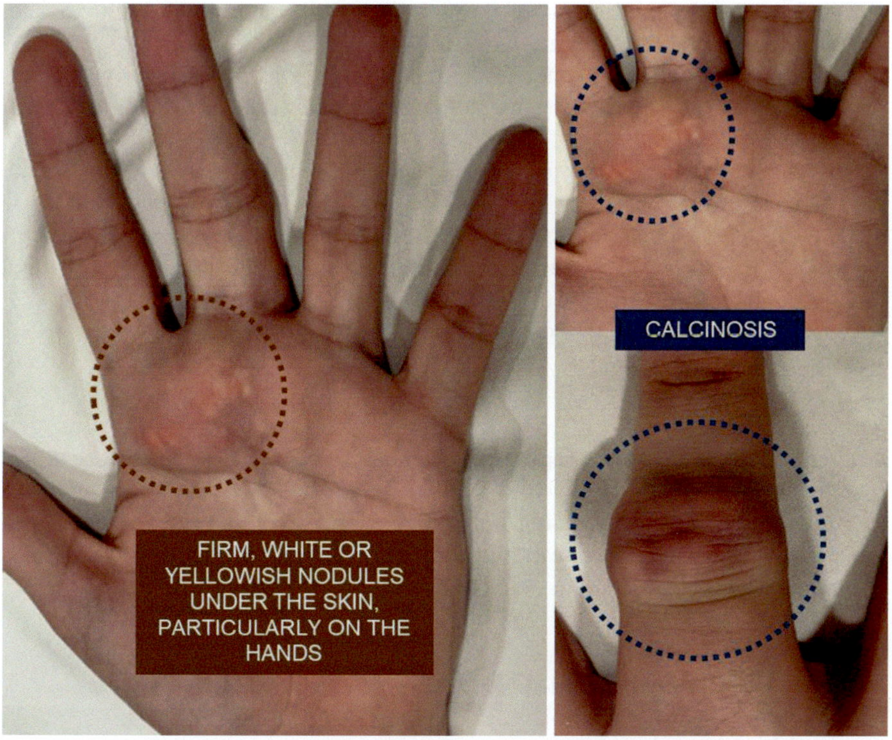

Fig. 13.7 Clinical photograph of patient with calcinosis due dermatomyositis

Fig. 13.8 Computed tomographic findings of calcinosis on sagittal reconstruction (Philips Brilliance CT 64-slice)

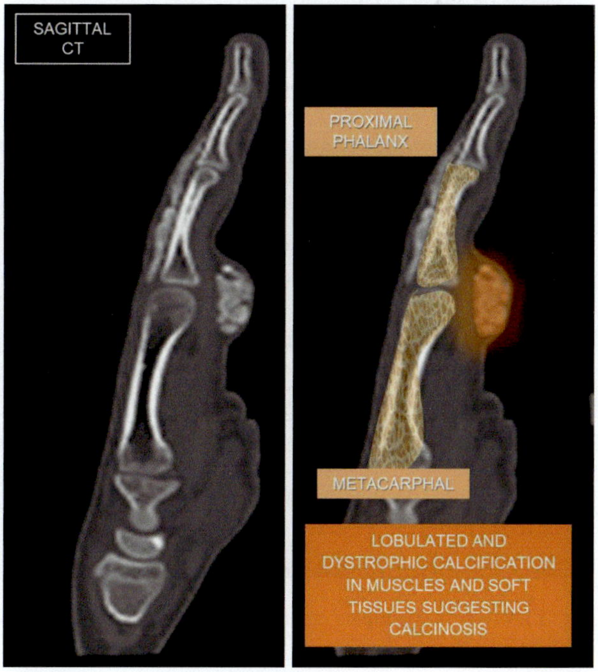

- The lateral and palmar areas of the fingers may become rough with cracked, "dirty" horizontal lines, resembling "mechanics' hands."
- Additional examples of cutaneous manifestations of DM include pruritus, hyperpigmentation, poikiloderma, panniculitis, periungual telangiectasias, and cuticular hypertrophy.
- The classic muscular manifestation is acute or subacute onset of symmetric, proximal muscle weakness.
- Dysphagia, dysphonia, and symptoms of aspiration indicate possible involvement of striated muscle of the pharynx and esophagus and are associated with a poor prognosis.

13.1.2.4 Dermoscopy [4, 11]

- Dermoscopy of Gottron's papule has been described as a lump of surface scales and dotted vessels.
- Polymorphic vessels, including linear, linear branched, and linear curved vessels, intermingled with white or pink structureless areas, are commonly observed under dermoscopy in various skin manifestations of DM.

13.1.2.5 Histopathology (Fig. 13.9) [8]

- Atrophic or normal epidermis.
- Damage to the basal layer.
- There may be thickening of the basement membrane (much more discrete compared to lupus erythematosus).
- Variable dermal edema.
- Alcian Blue positive dermal mucin may be present.
- Superficial perivascular infiltrate, lymphohistiocytic, sparse, and discrete.

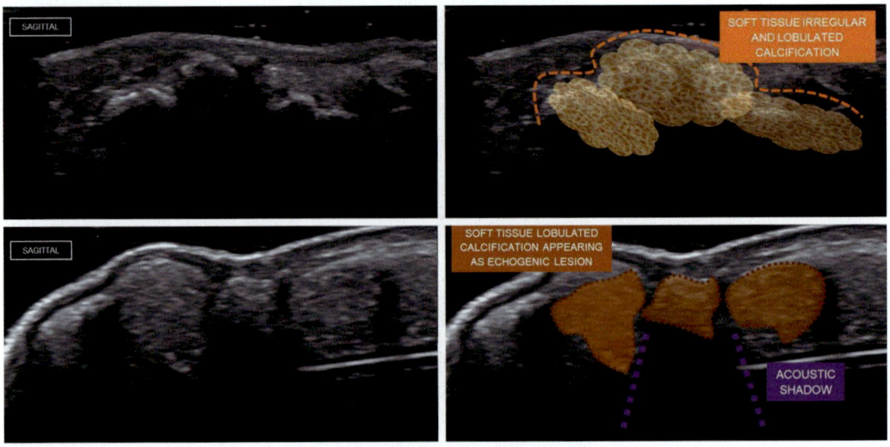

Fig. 13.9 Ultrasonographic findings of calcinosis with a 24 MHz probe (Aplio i800, Canon Medical Systems)

- There may be dystrophic dermal or hypodermic calcification, more intensely in children (resembles poikiloderma).
- Myositis presents variable lymphocytic infiltrate in the perimysium.

13.1.2.6 Radiography and Computed Tomography (Fig. 13.10) of Calcinosis

- Lobulated and dystrophic calcification in muscles and soft tissues suggesting calcinosis.

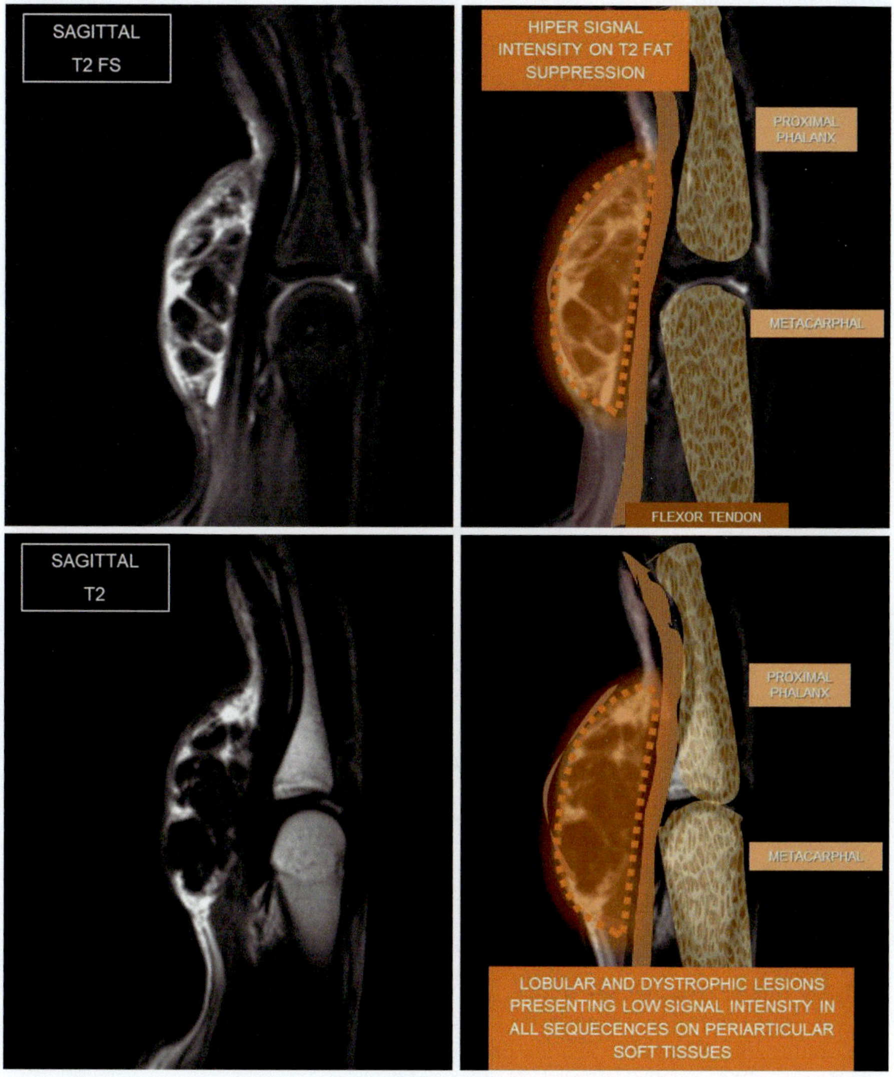

Fig. 13.10 MRI with surface coil findings of calcinosis on T1-weighted and STIR sequences (Magnetom Prisma 3T MRI, Siemens)

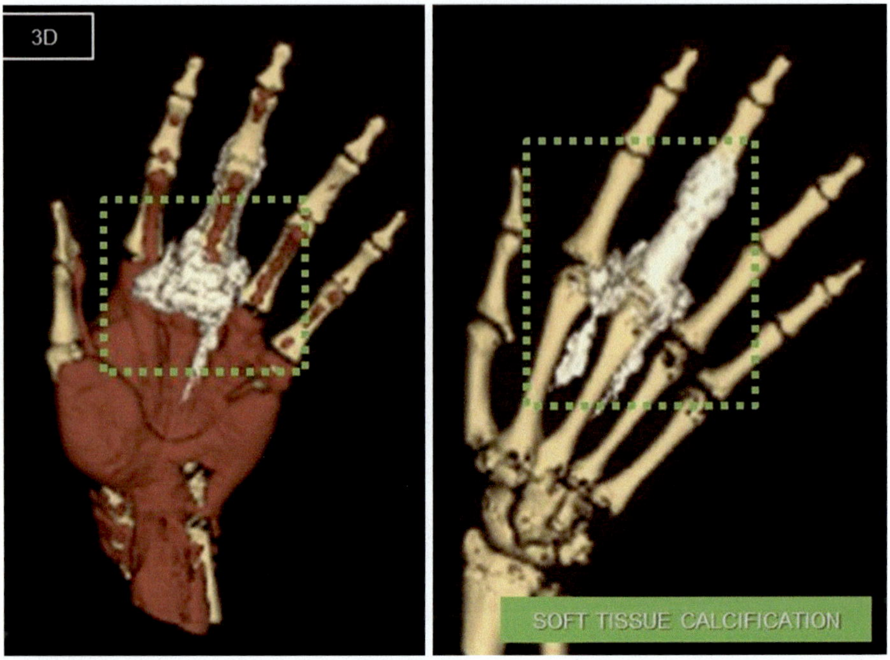

Fig. 13.11 3D images of calcinosis after segmentation of MRI isotropic images for monitoring disease

- Periarticular soft tissue thickening.
- Acro-osteolysis.

13.1.2.7 Ultrasonography (Figs. 13.11 and 13.12) [12]

- Lobulated and dystrophic echogenic calcification in muscles and soft tissues suggesting calcinosis.
- Periarticular hypoechoic soft tissue thickening corresponding to Gottron's papules.
- Inflammatory signs on hypodermis characterized by:
  - Loss of definition of the dermo-hypodermal transition.
  - Diffuse increased echogenicity in the hypodermis, with localized, scattered, or diffuse patterns.
  - Increased hypodermal vascularization observed on color Doppler.

13.1.2.8 MRI (Fig. 13.13)

- Lobular and dystrophic lesions presenting low signal intensity in all sequences on periarticular soft tissues suggesting calcinosis.

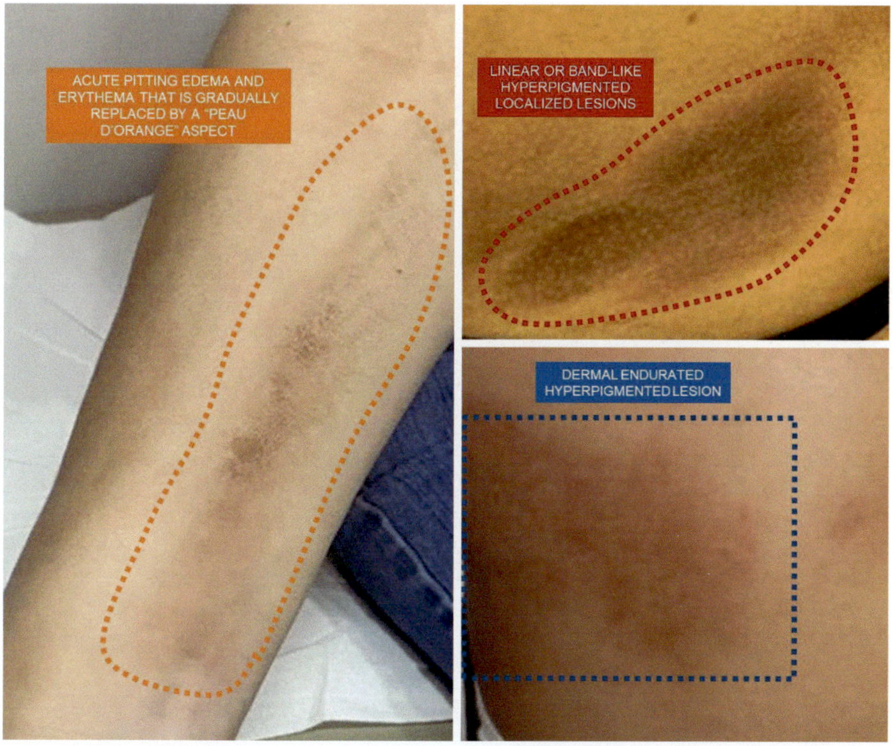

Fig. 13.12 Clinical photograph of patient with localized scleroderma

- Hyperintense signal intensity on T2 fat suppression and short-tau inversion recovery (STIR) suggesting edema on intermuscular septa, superficial muscular fascia, and hypodermis.
- Muscle edema on T2 FS and STIR images as high signal intensity. MRI STIR images are more sensitive (89–100%) but less specific (80–88%) than muscle biopsy (66% vs. 100%).
- T1 images show fatty infiltration as high signal intensity and volumetric muscle reduction, indicative of chronic injury.

13.1.2.9 3D Imaging (Fig. 13.14; Video 13.1)

- Used to quantify and visualize the extension of the soft tissue calcification, enabling to assess the severity and relation with adjacent structures.
- Contribute to precise surgical interventions, if applicable.
- Biomodels can be used and allows the creation of physical replicas of the affected area, aiding in surgical planning and patient education.

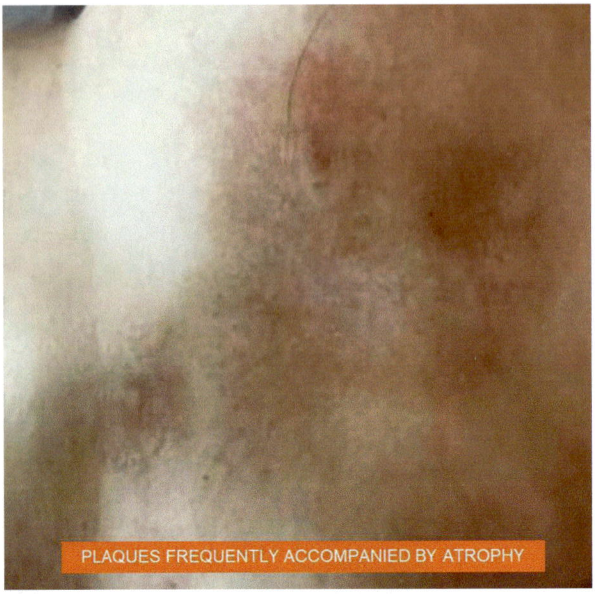

Fig. 13.13 Clinical photograph of patient with lichen sclerosus

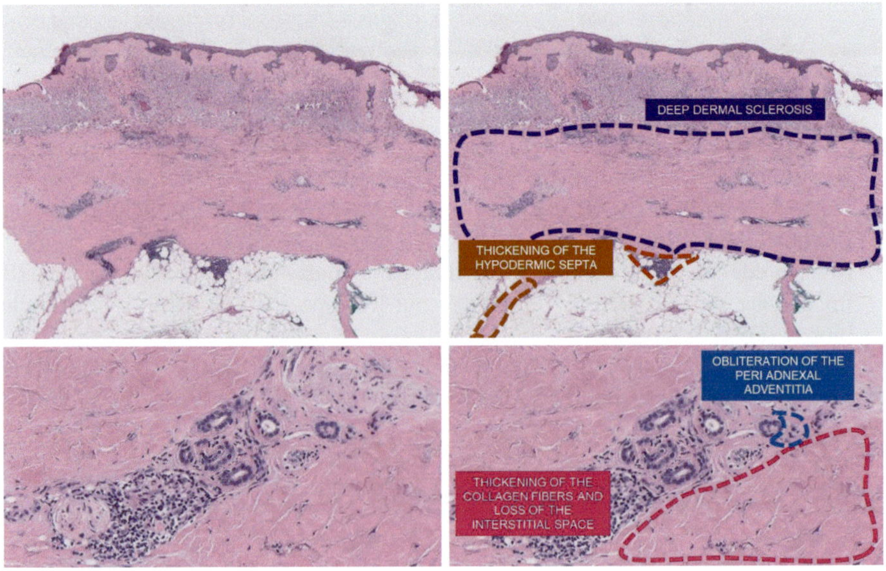

Fig. 13.14 Histological findings of morphea (H&E x4 and x20)

13.1.3 Scleroderma

13.1.3.1 Definition [13–16]

- Scleroderma, also known as systemic sclerosis, is a chronic autoimmune disease characterized by the hardening and tightening of the skin and connective tissues, due to an overproduction of collagen, leading to inflammation and fibrosis.
- Morphea, Pasini, and Pierini atrophoderma, lichen sclerosus, eosinophilic fasciitis, and calcinosis are conditions associated with scleroderma, and will be described together in this chapter due to their interconnected nature.
- Morphea.
  - Also known as localized scleroderma.
  - Linear scleroderma is reported as the most common subtype in children and is characterized by linear or band-like localized lesions that can affect the dermis, subcutaneous tissue, muscles as well as underlying bones.
  - Linear scleroderma en coup de sabre (which affects the head and neck), linear morphea that causes scarring alopecia, and Parry–Romberg syndrome (hemifacial unilateral atrophy of underlying soft tissue and bone) were already described previously in this book in Chap. 10.
- Pasini and Pierini atrophoderma.
  - Rare dermatologic disorder affecting dermal collagen and presenting with dermal atrophy lesions, which have no definitive pathogenesis or etiology.
- Lichen sclerosus.
  - Underdiagnosed inflammatory mucocutaneous condition affecting the anogenital areas, also presenting extragenital manifestations with a variety of clinical presentations.
  - Etiology is still unknown. Hormonal status, genetic predisposition, infection, frequent trauma and autoimmune diseases are well-known associations.
- Eosinophilic fasciitis.
  - Inflammatory disease that causes skin induration with an “orange peel” appearance.
  - Hypergammaglobulinemia, eosinophilia in the peripheral blood on laboratory tests.
  - Diffuse fasciitis on the histopathologic exam.
- Calcinosis.
  - Calcinosis in scleroderma might arise due to an active process where mesenchymal stem cells differentiate abnormally, creating a microenvironment conducive to bone formation.

13.1.3.2 Epidemiology [14–16]

- Morphea.
  - Morphea is a rare inflammatory connective tissue disease, with a total annual incidence ranging from 4 to 27 new cases per million people.
  - Female 3:1 male ratio.
  - Morphea can occur at any age, 50–65% develop the disease as adults.
- Pasini and Pierini atrophoderma.
  - Second and third decades of life.
  - Female 6:1 male ratio.
- Lichen Sclerosus.
  - Female-to-male ratio between 3:1 and 10:1.
  - Extragenital manifestations have been estimated between 15% and 20%, and are found mostly in females.
- Eosinophilic Fasciitis.
  - Predominantly affects patients in their fourth and fifth decade of life.
  - Manifests secondary to malignancy in a minority of patients (5–10%).
- Calcinosis.
  - Affect approximately 25–40% of patients with systemic sclerosis.
  - Prevalence can be higher in limited cutaneous systemic sclerosis (CREST syndrome).

13.1.3.3 Clinical Presentation (Fig. 13.15) [14–16]

- Morphea.
  - Usually unilateral.
  - Mixed hypopigmented and hyperpigmented skin overlying the frontoparietal area associated with a deep paramedian forehead scar separating atrophic from normal tissue.
  - Already described previously in this book in Chap. 10.
- Pasini and Pierini atrophoderma.
  - Single or multiple violaceous and hyperpigmented plaques with sharply demarcated areas of depression.
  - Generally symmetrical, they begin on the back and then progress to the trunk and arms, which may cause pruritus.
  - Unlike morphea, there is no induration or surrounding erythema.

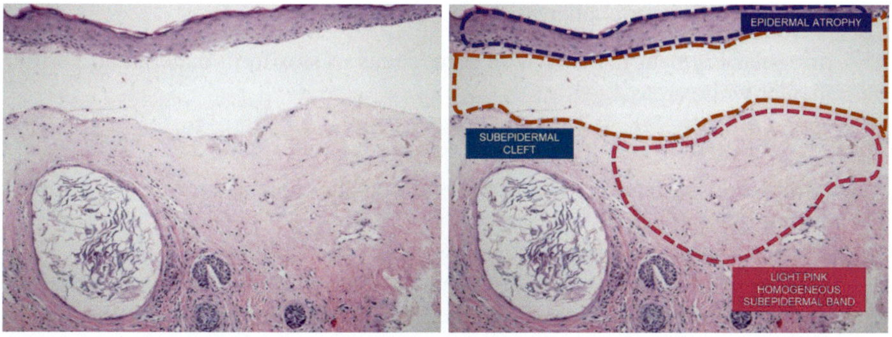

Fig. 13.15 Histological findings of lichen sclerosus (H&E x10)

- Lichen Sclerosus.
  - Genital lichen sclerosus occurs alone or can also overlie morphea.
  - Initial manifestations include itch, burning sensation. Later can be manifested with atrophy, fissures, erosions, vulvar, and perianal bruising.
  - Extragenital manifestations present as asymptomatic white opalescent papules, which cluster in plaques and progress over time in plaques frequently accompanied by atrophy and severe pruritus.
- Eosinophilic Fasciitis.
  - Usually, there is history of intense exercise few days to 2 weeks before.
  - Acute pitting edema and erythema. As the disease progresses, edema is gradually replaced by a "peau d'orange" aspect as deep sclerosis starts to develop.
  - In platelike hardness areas, only the blood vessels remain soft, which creates grooves (groove sign).
  - Commonly in extremities, trunk, and neck.
- Calcinosis.
  - Firm, white or yellowish nodules or plaques under the skin, particularly on the fingers, hands, elbows, and knees.
  - Can be painful and may cause inflammation or swelling in the surrounding tissues.

13.1.3.4 Dermoscopy [17–22]

- Morphea.
  - Trichoscopic findings.

    Loss of follicular openings.
    Peripilar casts.
    Areas with short regrowing hairs.
    Pili torti and black dots or broken hair.

- Pasini and Pierini atrophoderma.
  - Irregular pigment network with some areas of storiform pattern and perifollicular white areas.
- Lichen Sclerosus.
  - Structureless whitish or white-yellowish patches placed over a white atrophic background.
  - Early stages reveal irregular linear vessels and dotted vessels.
  - In later stages, most vessels disappear as dermal fibrosis may exceed the vascular, scattered gray-blue dots, the comedo-like openings and the scales. White chrysalis-like structures are not specific, but they have been documented.
- Eosinophilic Fasciitis.
  - One of the most characteristic dermoscopic features of eosinophilic fasciitis is a reticular or netlike pattern. This pattern reflects the fibrotic changes in the skin and underlying fascia and may appear as a network of fine lines or a grid-like appearance.

13.1.3.5 Histopathology (Fig. 13.16) [14, 15, 19, 23]

- Morphea.
  - Deep dermal sclerosis; usually progresses from the superficial reticular derma toward the hypoderm. It is important to observe the location of the eccrine glands, as they are usually involved with obliteration of the perianexal adventitia leading to atrophy and disappearance of the cutaneous ducts and appendages.
  - Thickening of the collagen fibers, with a tendency to homogenize and horizontalize the fibers in relation to the surface and loss of the interstitial space between the collagen fibers, making the collagen appear more compacted. In small magnification, scleroderma gives a square or rectangular appearance to the punch (square disease).
  - There may be thickening of the vessel walls with narrowing of the lumen; superficial vascular ectasia leading to thromboangiitis obliterans.
  - Elastic fibers preserved in the evaluation by orcein. It is an exception to the rule where fibrosis and elastosis are mutually exclusive phenomena.
  - Thickening of the hypodermic septa in deep involvement.
  - Deep perivascular lymphoplasmacytic infiltrate; more exuberant in the most recent phases.
  - Usual or atrophic epidermis.
  - Pigmentary incontinence may be present.
- Pasini and Pierini atrophoderma.
  - The histological changes are quite subtle, and may mimic normal skin or plaque scleroderma, and there is no fully characteristic lesion in histopathology.

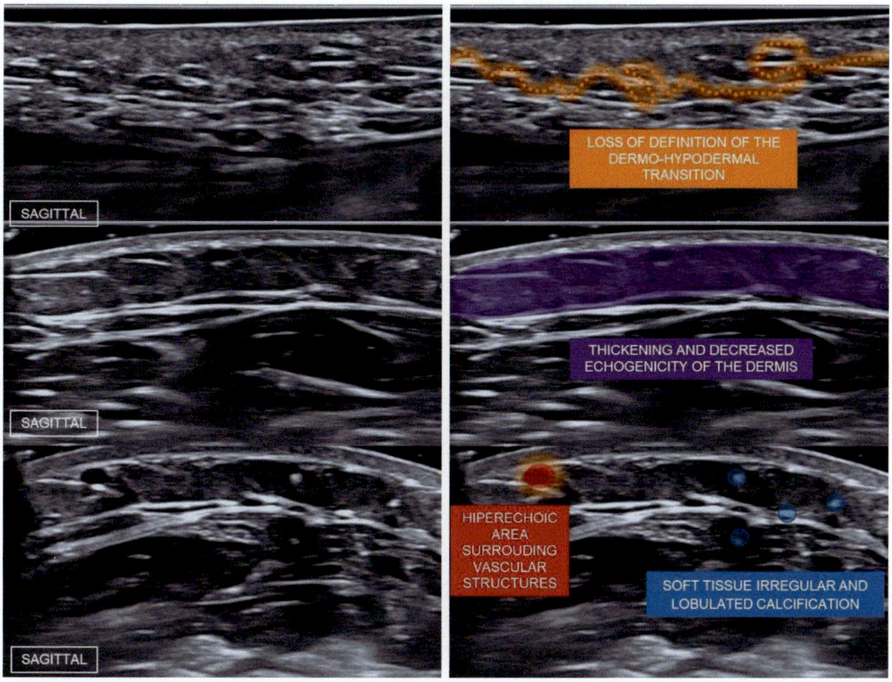

Fig. 13.16 Ultrasonographic findings of morphea with a 24 MHz probe (Aplio i800, Canon Medical Systems)

- Lichen Sclerosus.
  - Papillary dermis presenting as a light pink and homogeneous subepidermal band; there may be clefts, dermal edema, and superficial hyalinization.
  - ectasia and superficial vascular neoformation, more exuberant in the late phase.
  - Damage of the basal layer (focal and discrete vacuolization) and there may be pigmentary incontinence.
  - Sparse lymphoplasmacytic infiltrate in the papillary dermis in the initial phase, pushed down from the hyalinization area, eventually lichenoid.
  - Variable epidermal atrophy, and variable hyperkeratosis.
  - Destruction of elastic fibers.
- Eosinophilic Fasciitis.
  - Edema and thickening of the fascia due to the presence of marked and evident eosinophilic infiltration, with inflammatory cells including lymphocytes, histiocytes, and plasma cells.
  - The dermis and overlying adipose tissue may exhibit fibrous thickening and presence of eosinophils, as well as secondary atrophy of cutaneous appendages.
  - Eosinophilic infiltration may be present in the underlying skeletal muscle.

- Calcinosis.
  - Calcium phosphate deposits, often in the form of hydroxyapatite crystals, within the dermis and subcutaneous tissues.
  - Commonly surrounding the calcium deposits, there is granulomatous inflammatory response, with macrophages and multinucleated giant cells.

13.1.3.6 Radiography and Computed Tomography

- Soft tissue irregular and lobulated calcification in case of calcinosis.

13.1.3.7 Ultrasonography (Fig. 13.17) [6, 24]

- Morphea.
  - Employing the modified US-MAS (mUS-MAS) ultrasonography scoring system.
  - The ultrasonographic appearance of morphea will depend on the form of presentation and the phase of the lesions.
  - Signs of activity (inflammatory signs).

    Loss of definition of the dermo-hypodermal transition.
    Areas of increased echogenicity in the hypodermis, with localized, scattered, or diffuse patterns.
    Increased dermal or hypodermal vascularization observed on power Doppler.
    Thickening of the vessel walls, vascular ectasia with surrounding hyper echogenicity of hypodermis.

  - Other ultrasonographic signs of morphea.

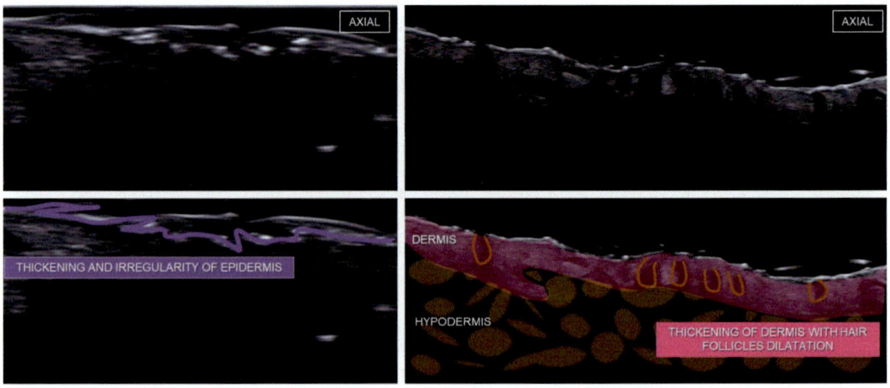

Fig. 13.17 Ultrasonographic findings of lichen sclerous with a 24 MHz probe (Aplio i800, Canon Medical Systems)

Thickening and decreased echogenicity of the dermis, which are generally not indicative of activity due to their nonspecific nature and possible association with other inflammatory dermal conditions.
In cases with prominent hypodermal involvement the ultrasonographic signs of panniculitis may range from predominantly lobular to predominantly septal in atrophic stages.
Thickening and increased echogenicity of the fascia, and occasional detection of underlying muscular involvement.
Soft tissue irregular and lobulated calcification.

- Pasini and Pierini atrophoderma.
  - Atrophic skin changes are characterized by decreased thickness and echogenicity.
  - Homogeneous skin texture and diminished layer distinction.
- Lichen Sclerosus.
  - Epidermal thickening and dermal echogenicity increase, with potential scarring and fibrosis presenting as echogenicity areas.
  - Decreased vascularization in power Doppler.
- Eosinophilic Fasciitis.
  - Fascial involvement may manifest as blurring or thickening with decreased echogenicity.
  - Increased echogenicity of the adjacent hypodermis.
  - Underlying muscular involvement, characterized by areas of increased echogenicity of the muscles.
  - Increased muscles vascularization on power Doppler.
- Calcinosis.
  - Soft tissue irregular and lobulated calcification appearing as echogenic lesion with acoustic shadow.

13.1.3.8 MRI (Figs. 13.18 and 13.19)

- Morphea.
  - High signal intensity on STIR images of dermis or hypodermis, suggesting inflammatory lesions.
  - Thickening on T1-weighted images of dermis or hypodermis on acute phases and atrophy on late stages.
  - Signs of panniculitis may range from predominantly lobular to septal involvement.

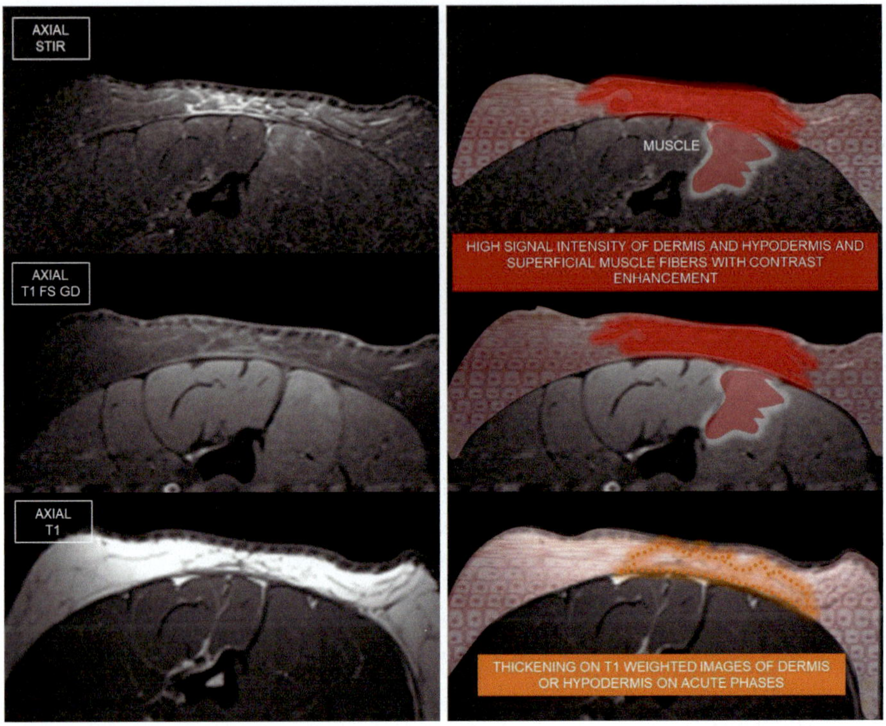

Fig. 13.18 MRI with surface coil findings of morphea on T1, STIR, and T1 FS-weighted sequences after gadolinium administration (Magnetom Prisma 3T MRI, Siemens)

- Pasini and Pierini atrophoderma.
  - Atrophic skin changes similar to the late stage of morphea.
- Lichen Sclerosus.
  - Similar findings comparable to morphea, occurs in the anogenital areas.
- Eosinophilic Fasciitis.
  - Thickening and high signal intensity on STIR images of the fascia, along with thinning hypodermic fat tissue.
  - Underlying muscular involvement, characterized by areas of high signal intensity on STIR images.
- Calcinosis.
  - Soft tissue irregular and lobulated calcification appearing as hyposignal intensity on all sequences.

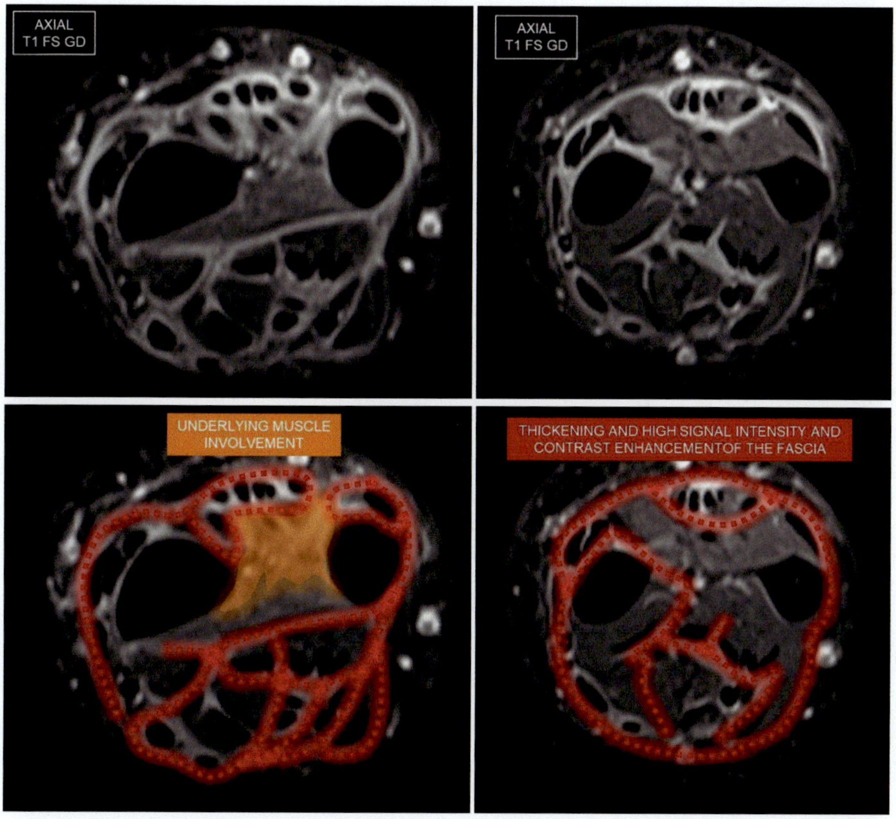

Fig. 13.19 MRI findings of eosinophilic fascitis on T1 FS-weighted sequences after gadolinium administration (Magnetom Prisma 3T MRI, Siemens)

13.1.3.9 3D Imaging

- Used to quantify and visualize the extension of calcinosis, enabling to assess the severity and relation with adjacent structures.
- Contribute to more precise surgical interventions, if applicable.
- Biomodels can be used and allows the creation of physical replicas of the affected area, offering representations that aid in surgical planning and patient education.

13.1.4 Psoriasis

13.1.4.1 Definition [25–27]

- Psoriasis is an immune-mediated, genetic disease manifesting in the skin, nails, and joints.

- Metabolic syndrome is the most frequent comorbidity in psoriasis and a risk factor for cardiovascular disease, a major cause of death among patients with psoriasis.

13.1.4.2 Epidemiology [25–27]

- The prevalence of psoriasis in adults ranged from 0.51% to 11.43%, and in children from 0% to 1.37%.
- Chronic plaque psoriasis is the most common form of the disease (90%).
- The prevalence of metabolic syndrome ranges from 20% to 50% and is the major cause of death among patients with psoriasis.

13.1.4.3 Clinical Presentation (Figs. 13.20 and 13.21) [25–27]

Five types of psoriasis have been reported:

- Plaque psoriasis (psoriasis vulgaris): monomorphic, sharply demarcated erythematous plaques covered by silvery lamellar scales. Lesions demonstrate symmetric distribution, and they are most frequently localized on knees, elbows, scalp, and sacral region.
- Guttate or eruptive psoriasis: Lesions onset suddenly with an appearance like small droplets, and less frequently as squamous psoriatic papules, generally manifesting after streptococcal infections.
- Inverse psoriasis (intertriginous or flexural): Psoriasis that is localized in skinfolds is termed flexural or inverse psoriasis.
- Pustular psoriasis: Is characterized by the onset of widespread 2- to 3-mm sterile pustules on erythematous skin or within psoriasiform plaques.
- Erythrodermic psoriasis: Corresponds to the generalized form of the disease, lesions affect nearly 80% of the body surface.

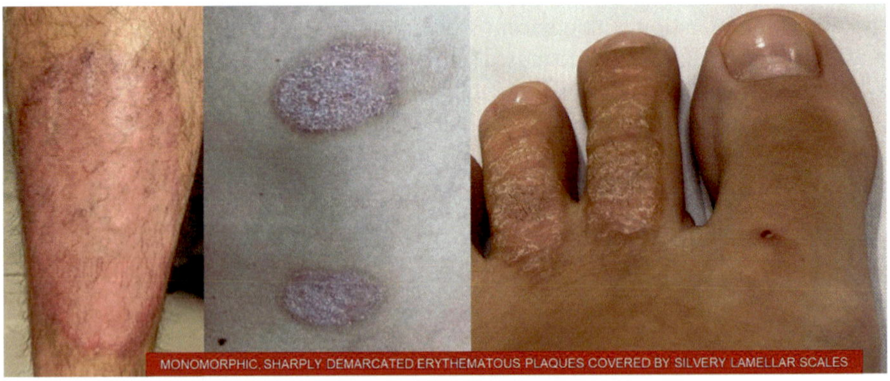

Fig. 13.20 Clinical photograph of patients with psoriasis vulgaris

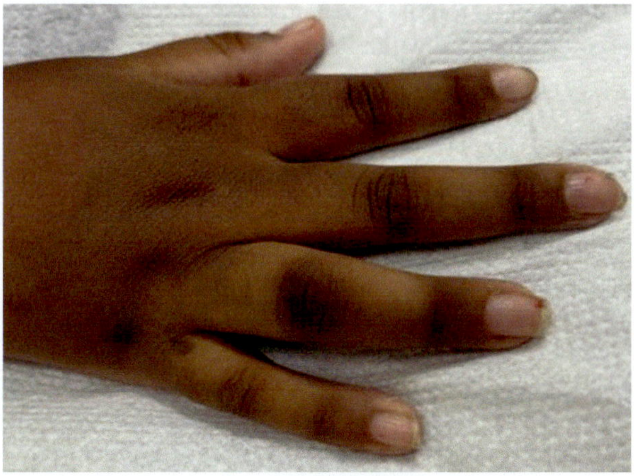

Fig. 13.21 Clinical photograph of patient with dactylitis of the fourth digit

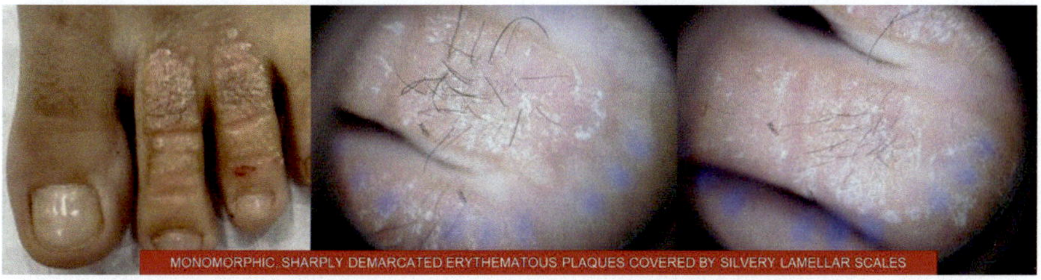

Fig. 13.22 Dermoscopic findings of patient with psoriasis vulgaris (x10)

13.1.4.4 Dermoscopy (Fig. 13.22) [26–28]

- Hemorrhagic dots are a common feature of psoriasis.
- Ringlike vessels hairpin-like vessels.
- Regular vessel distribution.

13.1.4.5 Histopathology (Fig. 13.23) [28]

- Focal or confluent parakeratosis; may alternate with lamellar hyperkeratosis.
- Focal or diffuse hypogranulosis or agranulosis; although psoriasis is a disease of the interadnexal epithelium, sparing the follicular ostia, in scalp psoriasis, parakeratosis can involve the edges of the hair infundibulum, mimicking seborrheic dermatitis.
- Regular acanthosis, characteristically without spongiosis.

- Viable neutrophils or not present at the top of the parakeratosis mounds, forming subcorneal collections called Munro's microabscesses. If they are in an intraepidermal location and associated with spongiosis, usually in the upper third of the epiderma, they are called Kogoj's spongiform pustules. Despite the predominance of neutrophils, lymphocytes may be present, especially in the early phase. Munro's microabscesses are more common in recent lesions.
- Extremely regular and downward growth of the interpapillary cones with bulbous due to the tendency of cones to melt with clubbing in the more developed lesions.
- Increase in the number of basal and suprabasal mitoses due to increased cell replication.
- Keratinocytes are more immature, with basaloid aspect, lower eosinophilia, and greater cellularity due to smaller cell diameter.
- Suprapapillary atrophy with upward elongation and narrowing of the dermal papillae; is the cause of Auspitz's sign, by the exposure of dilated vessels in the dermal papilla, which are ruptured during Brocq's methodical curettage. Suprapapillary atrophy greater than two-thirds of the thickness of the epidermis is characteristic of psoriasis. The papilla is elongated but usually retains its diameter, resembling the columns of the Parthenon.
- Dilation and tortuosity of the superficial dermal vessels, with the most important histopathological sign being the most precocious.
- Superficial mononuclear inflammatory infiltrate usually discrete.
- Focal hemorrhage in the derma papillary (nonspecific) especially in eruptive lesions, which may be mistaken for Gibert's pityriasis rosea.
- With the exception of the pustular form, spongiosis is absent or discrete, usually restricted to the lower third of the epiderma, unlike eczema.

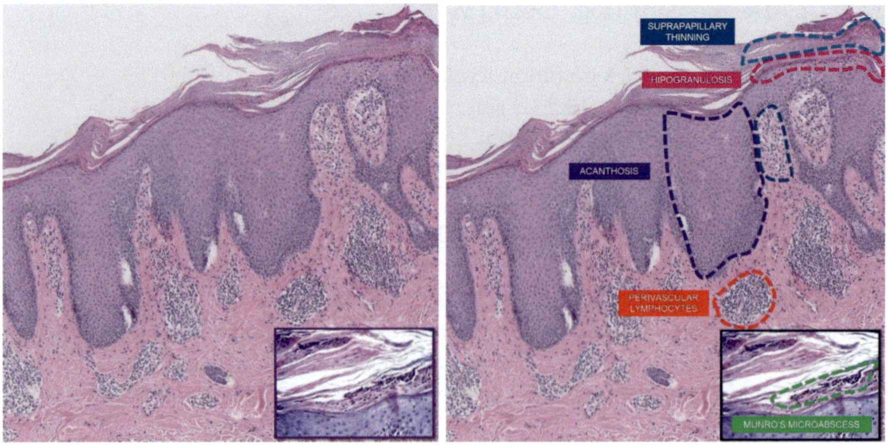

Fig. 13.23 Histological findings of psoriasis vulgaris (H&E x4)

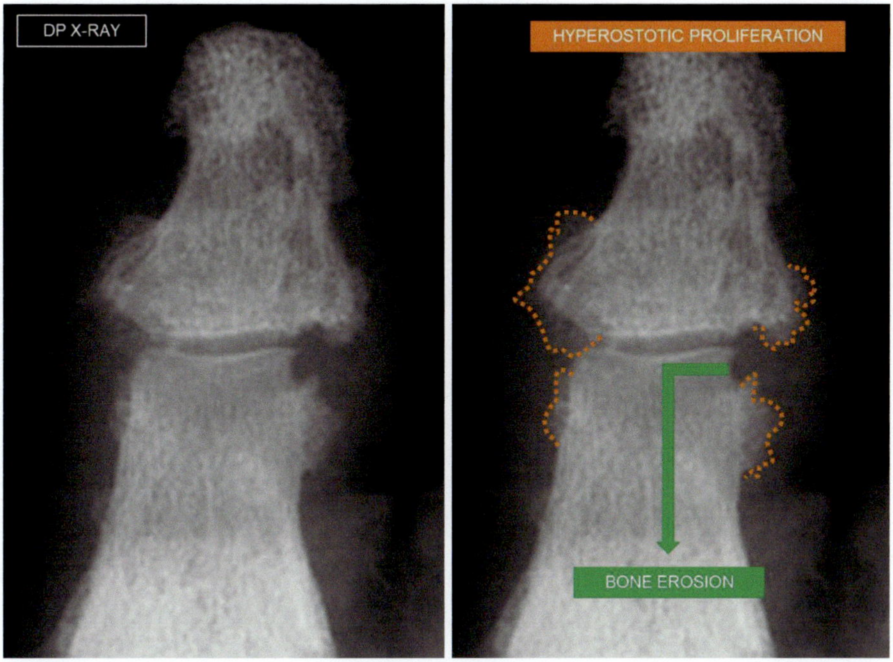

Fig. 13.24 Radiographic findings of psoriatic arthritis (Philips Duo Diagnost R&F Room Digital RF and Tomo System)

13.1.5 Radiography and Computed Tomography (Fig. 13.24)

- Unique cutaneous involvement by psoriasis cannot be detected through radiography or computed tomography.
- Only psoriatic arthritis is diagnosable by radiography, and this will be discussed in greater detail in Chap. 16.

13.1.5.1 Ultrasonography (Figs. 13.25, 13.26 and 13.27) [6, 29]

- Thickened epidermis due to acanthosis and increased echogenicity due to hyperkeratosis.
- Proeminent SLEB, indicating inflammatory condition.
- Hypoechoic areas in the dermis, indicating inflammatory infiltrates, with power Doppler hypervascularity.

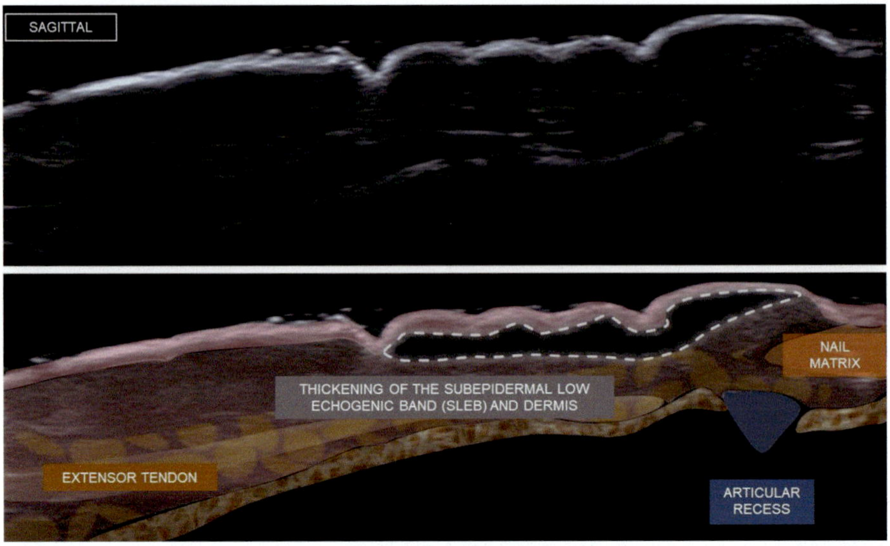

Fig. 13.25 Ultrasonographic findings of psoriasis vulgaris with a 24 MHz probe (Aplio i800, Canon Medical Systems)

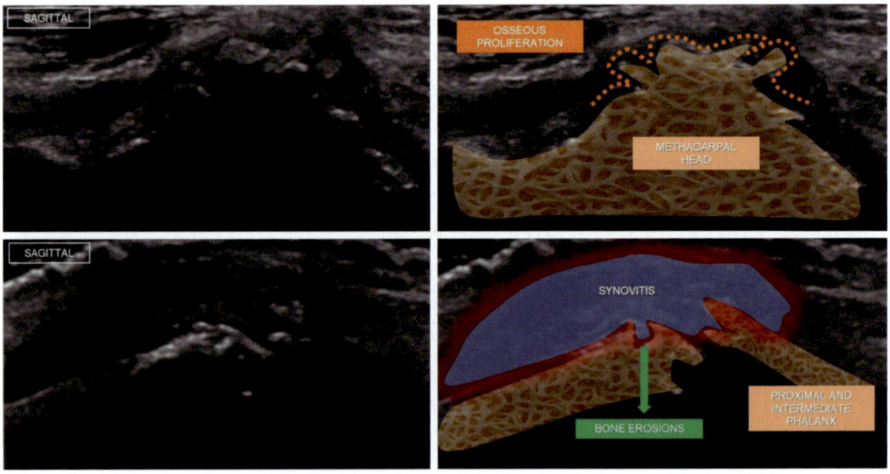

Fig. 13.26 Ultrasonographic findings of psoriatic arthritis with a 24 MHz probe (Aplio i800, Canon Medical Systems)

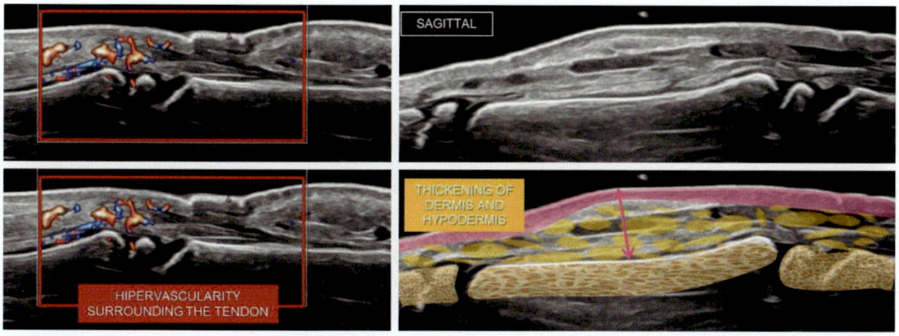

Fig. 13.27 Ultrasonographic findings of dactylitis with a 24 MHz probe (Aplio i800, Canon Medical Systems)

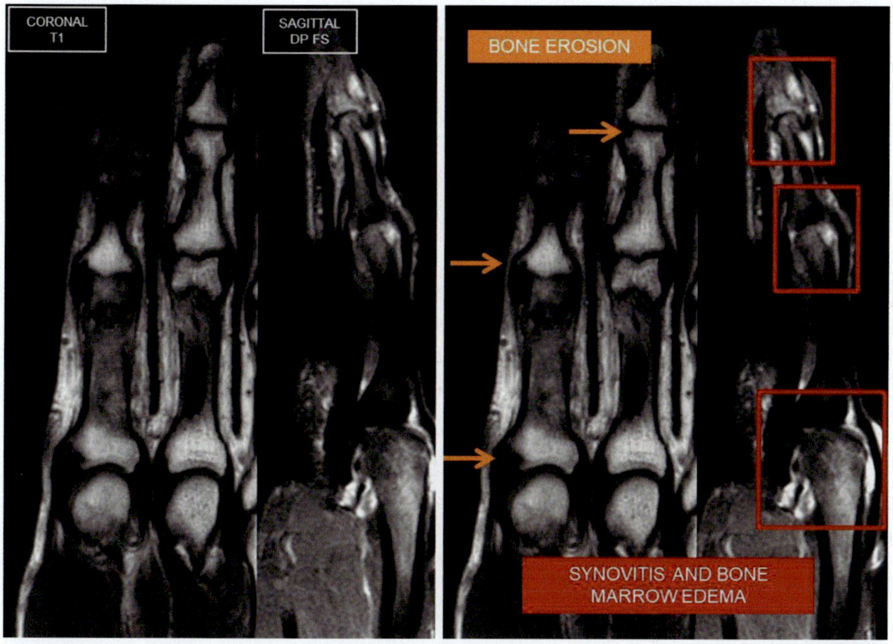

Fig. 13.28 MRI findings of psoriatic arthritis on T1 and DP FS-weighted sequences (Magnetom Avanto 1.5T MRI, Siemens)

13.1.5.2 MRI (Fig. 13.28)

- Thickening of the epidermis and dermis with increased signal intensity in the due to inflammation and hyperkeratosis on T1-weighted and T2-weighted images,
- Enhancement post-contrast administration, indicating increased vascularity within the plaques.

13.1.6 Pityriasis Rubra Pilaris

13.1.6.1 Definition [30]

- Inflammatory papulosquamous skin disease of unknown etiology.
- There are six different clinical subtypes. Well-demarcated plaques with reddish-orange color are found in all subtypes.

13.1.6.2 Epidemiology [30]

- Rare dermatosis that affects all ethnicities and both sexes.
- Bimodal age distribution, with incidence peaks in the first and fifth decades of life.
- Most cases are sporadic, but a small portion has a familial inheritance.

13.1.6.3 Clinical Presentation (Fig. 13.29) [30]

- Clinical findings to all subtypes include hyperkeratotic follicular papules, red-orange, well-demarcated plaques, and palmoplantar keratoderma.
- Classification:
  - Classical adult onset or type I: Affects 55% of patients with PRP. Plaques are sharply demarcated from healthy skin, producing the phenomenon called "islands of sparing." Yellow-orange, palmoplantar keratoderma associated with nail involvement arise within weeks or months.

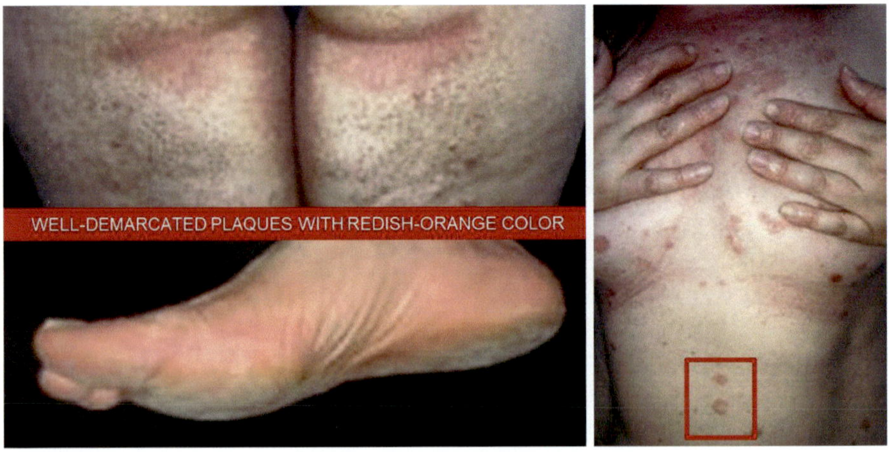

Fig. 13.29 Clinical photograph of patients with ptiriase rubra pilaris

- Atypical adult or type II: Affects 5% of patients. Ichthyosiform dermatitis, little hair on the scalp and thick palmoplantar keratoderma are the main clinical features.
- Classical juvenile or type III: represents 10% of all cases. Affects children and teenagers. It has the same sequence and clinical findings of type I PRP, with a better prognosis.
- Circumscribed juvenile or type IV: Affects 25% of patients. It is the only focal subtype. It presents grouped follicular papules on a sharply demarcated erythematous basis, localized on the knees and elbows. It is more common among prepubertal children.
- Atypical juvenile or type V: represents 5% of PRP cases. It is an inherited condition with early onset and chronic course. It presents as an ichthyosiform dermatitis and follicular hyperkeratosis.
- Type VI: It is a form associated with HIV infection, with poor prognosis and recalcitrant to therapy. Patients present nodulocystic and lichen-spinulosus-like lesions. Erythroderma is a common complication.

13.1.6.4 Dermoscopy [31]

- The most common findings of PRP under polarized dermoscopy are:
  - Perifollicular round and oval yellowish areas.
  - Keratotic follicular plugs.
  - Central hair.
- The majority of cases of PRP do not seem to have vessel structures.
- Erythrodermic PRP can present irregularly distributed dotted and linear vessels, besides the perifollicular yellow areas.

13.1.6.5 Histopathology (Fig. 13.30) [32]

- Alternating orthokeratosis with foci of parakeratosis horizontally and vertically, close to the follicular ostia, giving a pattern called "checkerboard pattern."
- Discrete irregular acanthosis with broad straight ridges and preserved granular layer or discrete hypergranulosis (in contrast with psoriasis).
- Parakeratotic follicular plugging near the follicular ostium; tending to be more exuberant in the hair follicles.
- Superficial and perifollicular perivascular lymphocytic infiltrate.

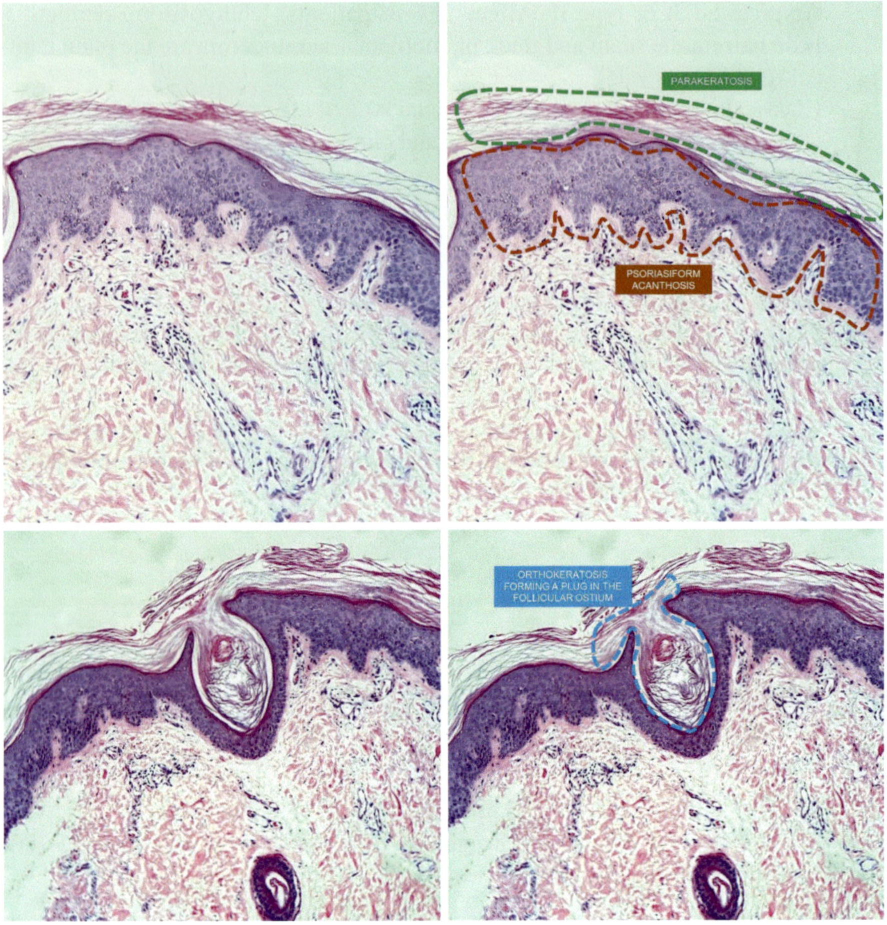

Fig. 13.30 Histological findings of ptiriase rubra pilaris (H&E x4)

13.1.6.6 Ultrasonography (Fig. 13.31)

- Thickened epidermis, which is consistent with the hyperkeratosis and acanthosis.
- Increased echogenicity of the dermis due to the accumulation of keratin and other structural changes in skin.
- Hypoechoic areas within the dermis that correspond to inflammatory infiltrates.
- In chronic cases, ultrasonography might show signs of dermal fibrosis. This appears as increased echogenicity in the dermal layer and reflects the fibrotic changes.
- Does not show significant changes in vascular patterns on ultrasonography.

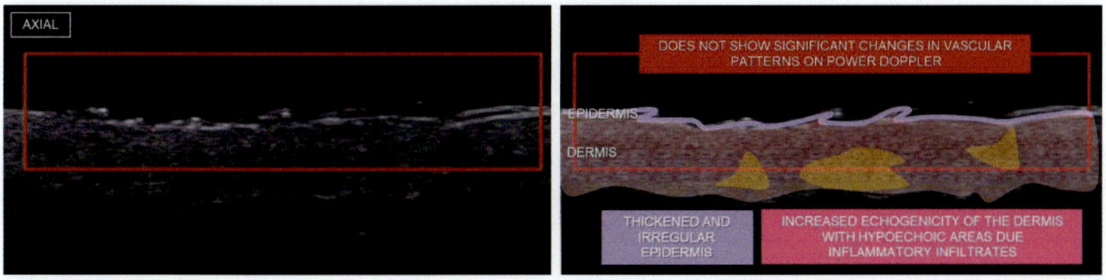

Fig. 13.31 Ultrasonographic findings of ptiriase rubra pilaris with a 33 MHz probe (H&E x4)

13.1.7 Darier's Disease

13.1.7.1 Definition [33]

- Also known as Darier–White disease.
- Rare genetic acantholytic disorder described by the French Dermatologist Ferdinand-Jean Darier in 1889.
- Skin lesions, nail abnormalities, and mucous membrane involvement.

13.1.7.2 Epidemiology [33]

- Darier's disease affects approximately 1 in 30,000–100,000 individuals worldwide.
- Autosomal dominant pattern.
- The associated gene is the ATP2A2, a key gene that regulates the calcium balance within the cells. Its mutation leads to impaired calcium signaling.
- Factors contributing to lesion development encompass environmental triggers and stressors, such as exposure to sunlight, heat, humidity, hormonal changes (as in pregnancy), and certain medications such as lithium and antiepileptic drugs.

13.1.7.3 Clinical Presentation (Fig. 13.32) [33]

- Skin lesions, the most common being the keratotic papules, described as small, firm papules, usually red or brown in color. These papules can occur in clusters. The most common sites are the chest, upper back, scalp, forehead, temples, and groin area. The lesions may vary in severity, and can become crusted, scaly, or greasy.
- Nail abnormalities may also occur, such as ungueal pitting, ridges, red or white streaks.
- Mucous membrane involvement could particularly affect the mouth, throat, and genital áreas. It usually presents as white or grayish patches, painful sores, or inflammation.

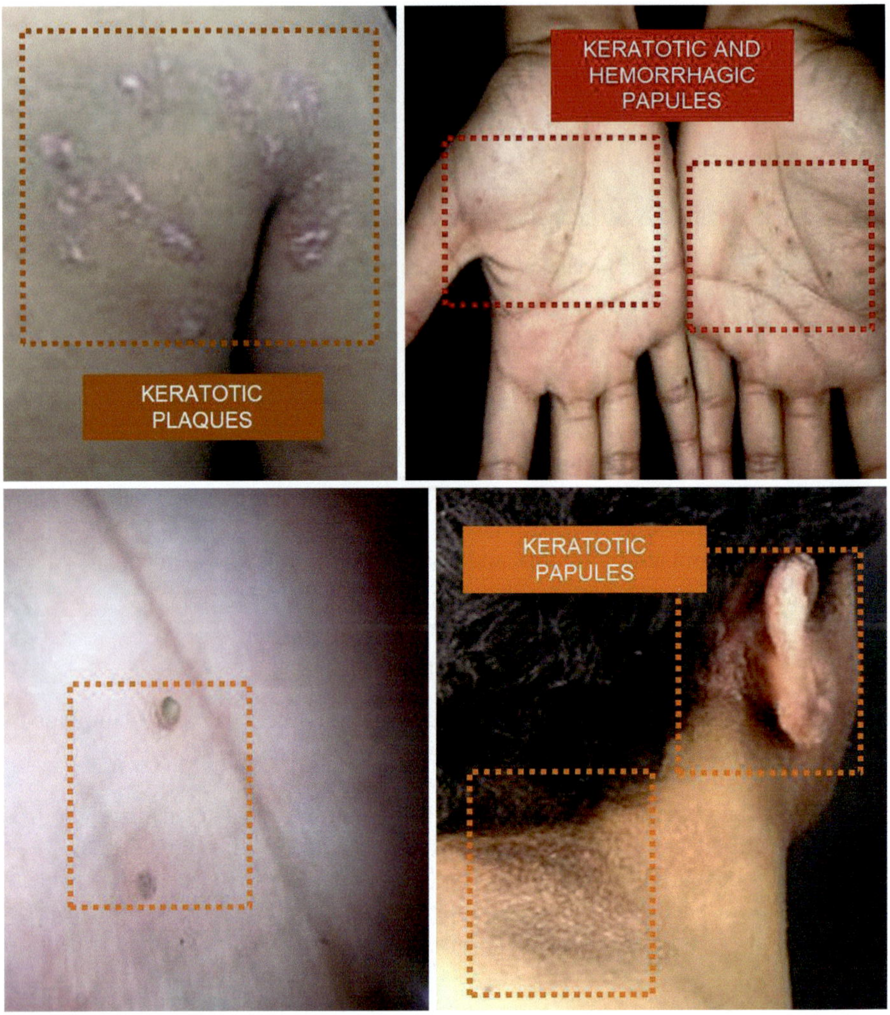

Fig. 13.32 Clinical photograph of patients with Darier's disease

13.1.7.4 Dermoscopy [33–35]

- The characteristic finding is "dirt-like" or "dried mud" appearance.
- Brownish to grayish scales and crusts, often arranged in a reticular or cobblestone pattern.

13.1.7.5 Histopathology (Fig. 13.33) [34, 36]

- Acantholysis (separation of epidermal cells).
- Dyskeratosis (abnormal keratinization).
- Corps rounds (rounded eosinophilic cells) and grains (small dark basophilic bodies) in the epidermis.

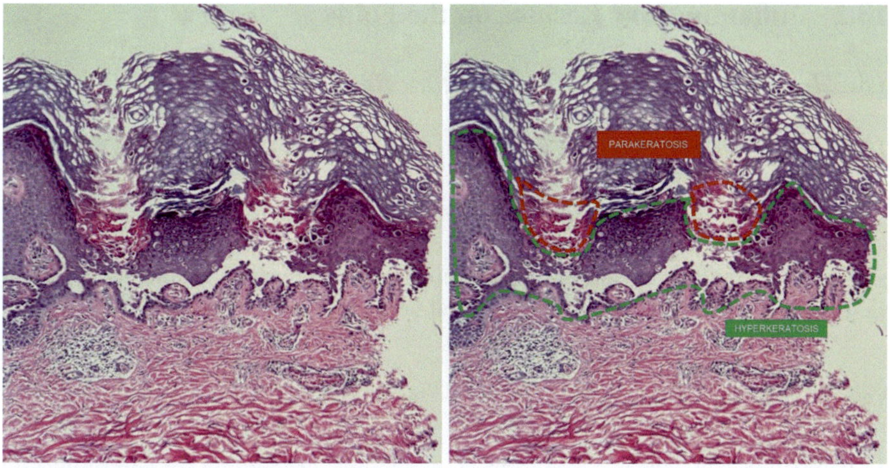

Fig. 13.33 Histological findings of Darier's disease (H&E x4)

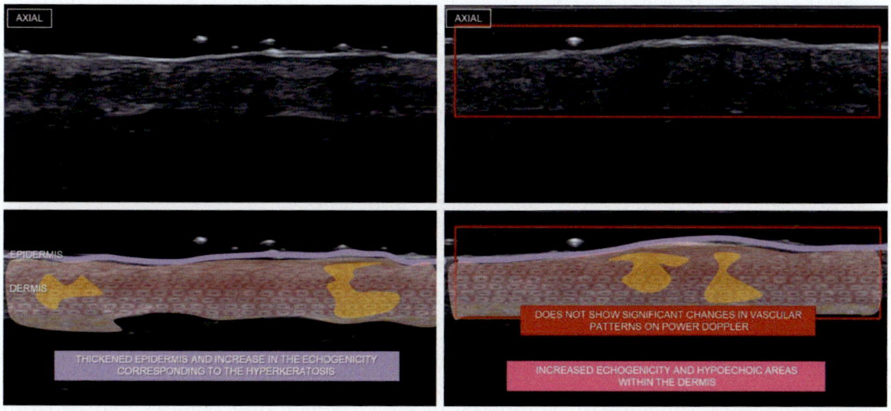

Fig. 13.34 Ultrasonographic findings of Darier's disease with a 33 MHz probe (Aplio i800, Canon Medical Systems)

13.1.7.6 Ultrasonography (Fig. 13.34)

- Thickened epidermis and increase in the echogenicity corresponding to the hyperkeratosis and accumulation of keratin and abnormal keratinocyte proliferation.
- Increased echogenicity reflecting the dense, scale-like plaques and the thickened stratum corneum.
- Irregular dermal thickness.
- Absence of prominent vascular changes on power Doppler.

13.2 Inflammatory Lesions on the Folds

13.2.1 Pemphigus Vegetans (Neumann's Disease)

13.2.1.1 Definition [37–39]

- Pephigus vegetans is a variant of pemphigus that is an autoimmune blistering disorder.
- Characterized by vegetating plaques, pustules, or verrucous lesions.
- Typically affects the axillae, groins, and other skin folds.

13.2.1.2 Epidemiology [37–39]

- Pemphigus vegetans is a rare form of pemphigus, accounting for approximately 1–3% of all pemphigus cases.
- Most commonly seen in adults, although it may affect individuals of any age.
- Slight predilection for females.

13.2.1.3 Clinical Presentation (Fig. 13.35) [37–39]

- Initially the lesion is small, flaccid blisters that rapidly evolve into vegetating or warty plaques with a typical "snail-track" appearance.
- The plaques are often reddish-brown in color and have a moist or greasy surface. May be accompanied by or evolve to erosions crusts, and pustules.
- Affect sites are flexural areas, like axillae, groin, perianal region, and inframammary folds.
- Two clinical distinct variants are described:
  - Pemphigus vegetans of Neumann, in which vegetating plaques evolve from classic pemphigus vulgaris lesions.
  - Pemphigus vegetans of Hallopeau, a milder form, in which the vegetating plaques are not preceded by bullae.
- The oral cavity may be involved, with the development of erosions, blisters or vegetating plaques on the lips, tongue, buccal mucosa, and gingiva.

13.2.1.4 Dermoscopy [37–39]

- White lines or dots may be seen on the surface of the skin lesions, typically irregular, with a reticular pattern.
- Yellow crusts may be appreciated under dermoscopy.

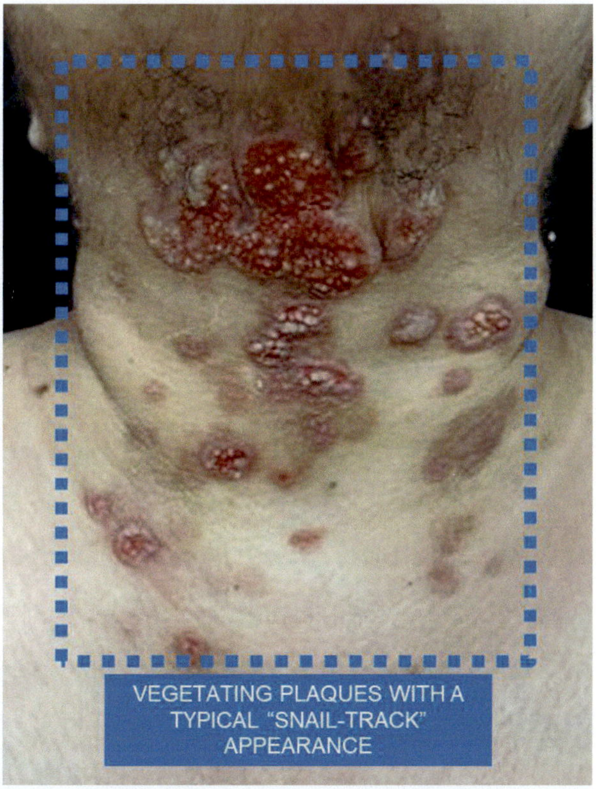

Fig. 13.35 Clinical photograph of patients with penfigo vegetans

13.2.1.5 Histopathology (Fig. 13.36) [28, 37, 38]

- Acantholysis that represents the loss of cohesion between the skin cells (keratinocytes) in the epidermis.
- Pemphigus vegetans typically shows suprabasal clefting, which means that the separation of cells occurs above the basal layer of the epidermis.
- Intraepidermal neutrophilic collections may also be appreciated.

13.2.1.6 Ultrasonography (Fig. 13.37) [40]

- Blister formation in epidermis.
- Thickening and decreased echogenicity of the epidermis and dermis, along with blister formation.
- Hypervascularization on power Doppler imaging suggesting inflammatory process.

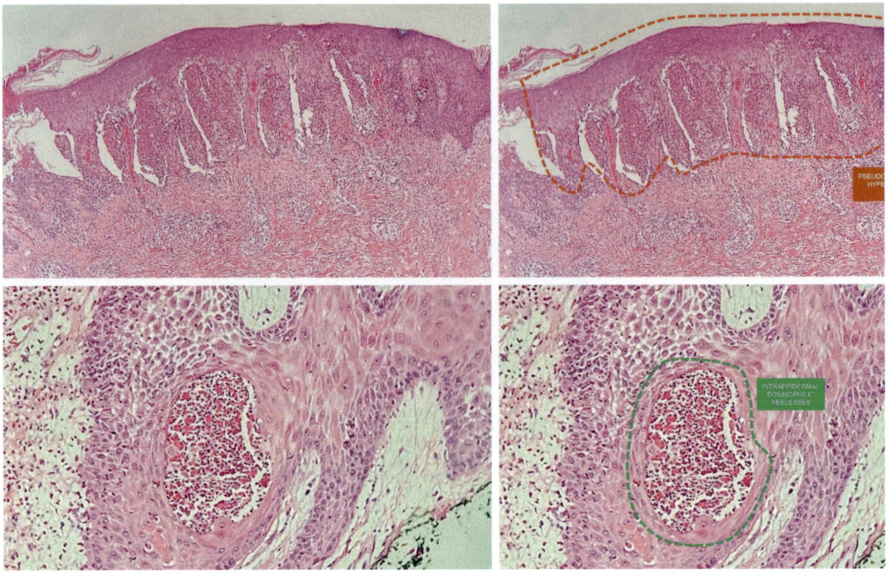

Fig. 13.36 Histological findings of penfigo vegetans (H&E x4 and x10)

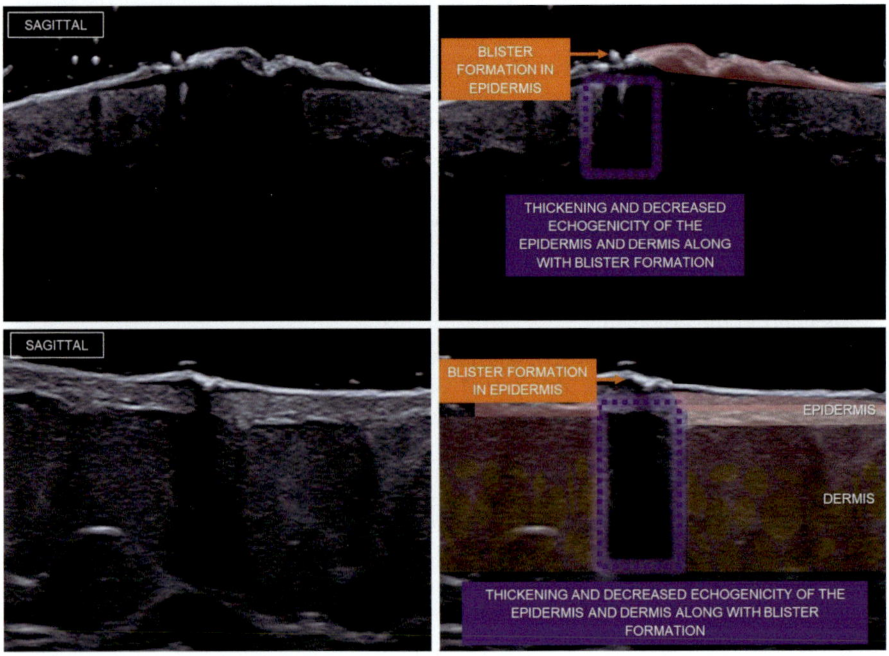

Fig. 13.37 Ultrasonographic findings of penfigo vegetans with a 33 MHz probe (Aplio i800, Canon Medical Systems)

13.2.2 Hailey-Hailey Disease

13.2.2.1 Definition [33, 41]

- Also known as familial benign chronic pemphigus.
- Autosomal dominant genetic disorder characterized by recurrent painful blisters, mainly in skin folds, secondary to intraepidermal acantholysis.
- It was first described by Hugh Edward Hailey and William Howard Hailey in 1939.

13.2.2.2 Epidemiology [33, 41]

- Rare disorder with an estimated prevalence of 1 in 50,000 to 100,000 individuals.
- Affects both males and females equally.
- Third or fourth decade of life. There are cases described earlier, in adolescence, and late in the eighth decade.
- Caused by mutations in the ATP2C1 gene, which encodes a protein responsible for cellular calcium homeostasis.

13.2.2.3 Clinical Presentation (Fig. 13.38) [33, 41]

- Primarily affects areas of friction and moisture on the body, such as the neck, axillae, groin, and under the breasts.
- Recurrent, painful, blistering, reddish rash and plaques that can become erosive and crusted. It typically assumes a symmetrical pattern.
- The most common clinical presentation is "intertriginous dermatitis." The affected areas may exhibit an unpleasant odor due to secondary bacterial or fungal infections.
- Some factors may trigger or worsen the symptoms, such as heat, sweating, friction, sunlight exposure, and skin trauma.

13.2.2.4 Dermoscopy [33, 41]

- Dermoscopy findings are nonspecific.
- May include erythema, erosions, and scales.

13.2.2.5 Histopathology (Fig. 13.39) [33, 41]

- Suprabasal acantholysis.
- Characteristic pattern of "dilapidated brick wall" appearance, where the individual keratinocytes remain attached at the basal layer, but detached from each other above it.

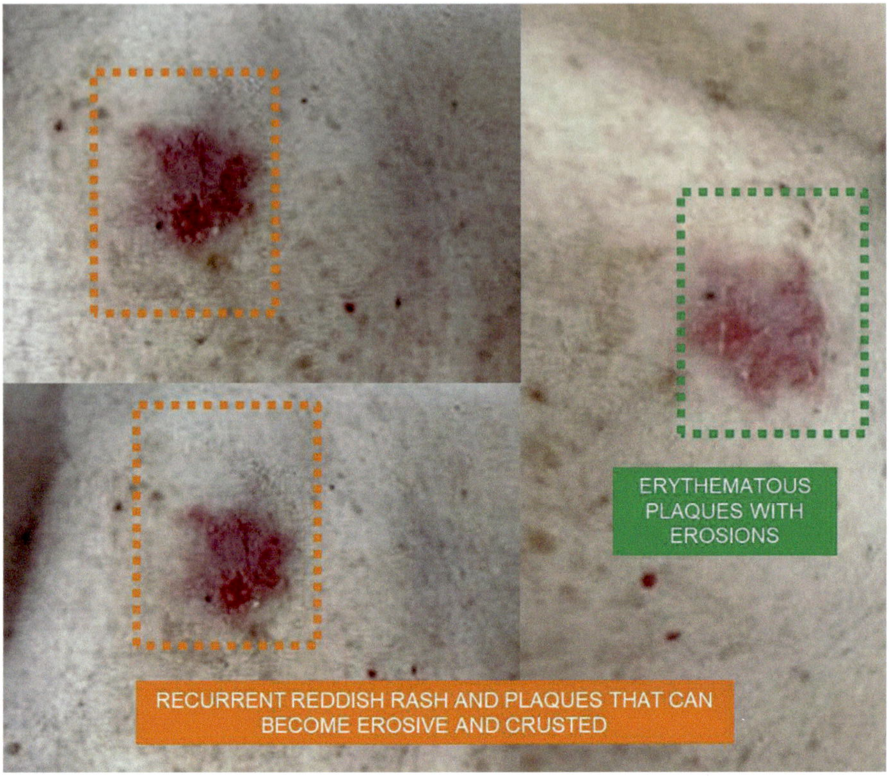

Fig. 13.38 Clinical photograph of patients with Hailey Hailey disease

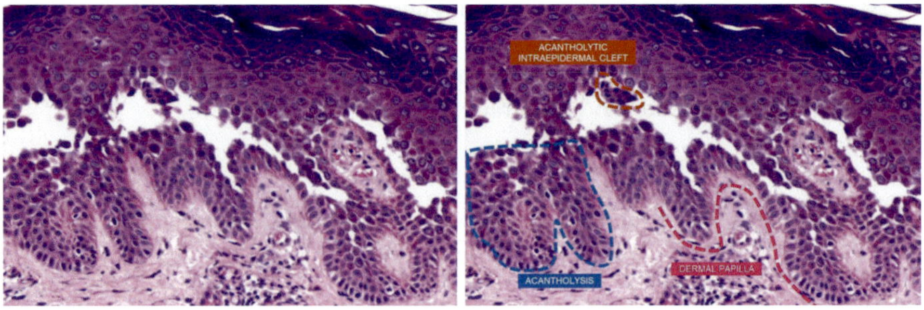

Fig. 13.39 Histological findings of Hailey Hailey disease (H&E x4) (Image kindly provided by Dr. Gabbriella de Giunta)

13.2.2.6 Ultrasonography (Fig. 13.40) [42]

- Blister formation in epidermis.
- Thickening and decreased echogenicity of the epidermis and dermis, along with blister formation.
- Hypervascularization on power Doppler imaging suggesting inflammatory process.

13.2.3 Hidradenitis Suppurativa

13.2.3.1 Definition [43, 44]

- Chronic, inflammatory disease, characterized by follicular occlusion and rupture, that leads to recurrent nodules, comedones, abscesses, sinus tracts, and bridged scars.
- It has a significant impact on patients' quality of life and is associated with multiple comorbidities.

13.2.3.2 Epidemiology [44–46]

- Exact prevalence is unknown, but it is estimated to range from 0,03% to 4,1%.
- It is two to three times more common in women than in men.
- More prevalent in African Americans than Caucasians.
- Age of onset varies in literature but is more common between 18 and 44 years.

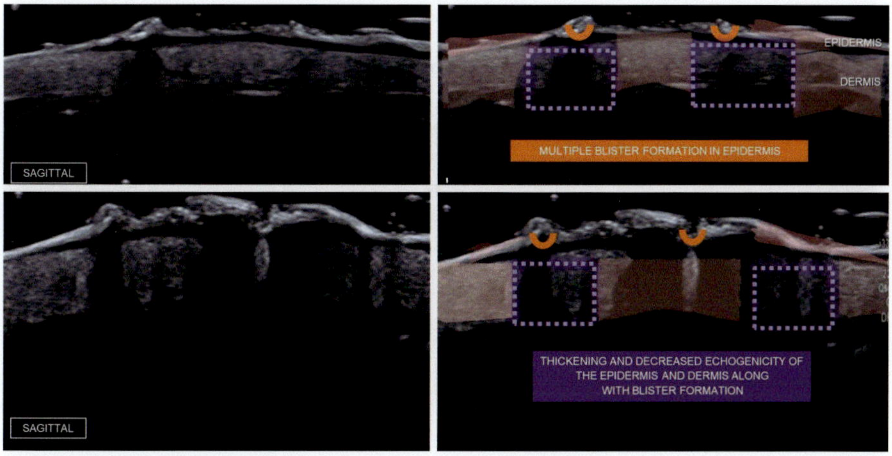

Fig. 13.40 Ultrasonographic findings of Hailey Hailey disease with a 33 MHz probe (Aplio i800, Canon Medical Systems)

13.2.3.3 Clinical Presentation (Figs. 13.41 and 13.42; Table 13.1) [43–46]

- Diagnosis is defined by typical lesions, predilection for flexural sites, and recurrence.
  - Typical lesions: Nodules, abscesses, sinus tracts, bridged scars, comedones, and double-ended pseudo comedones.
  - Flexural sites: Axillary, infra and intermammary, inguinal, perineal, perianal, and gluteal regions.
  - Recurrence: Two or more episodes of painful or suppurating lesions in 6 months.
- Lesions are often accompanied by pain, pruritus, purulent, and malodorous discharge.

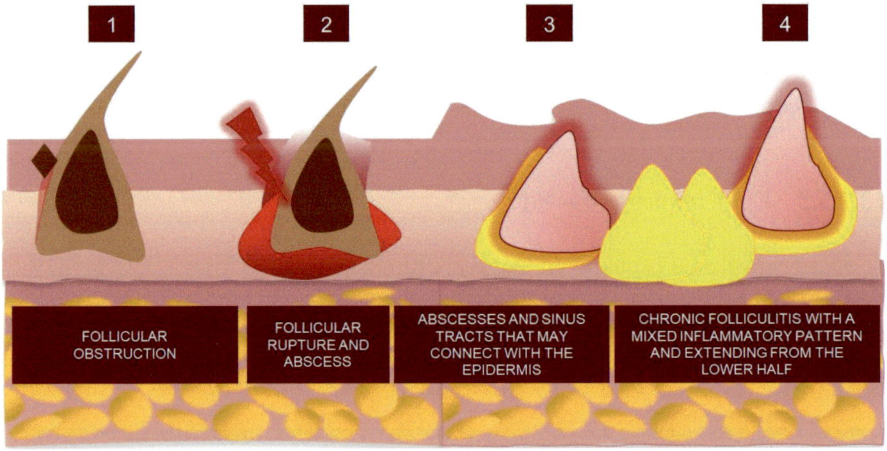

Fig. 13.41 Drawing schema pathophysiology of hidradenitis suppurativa

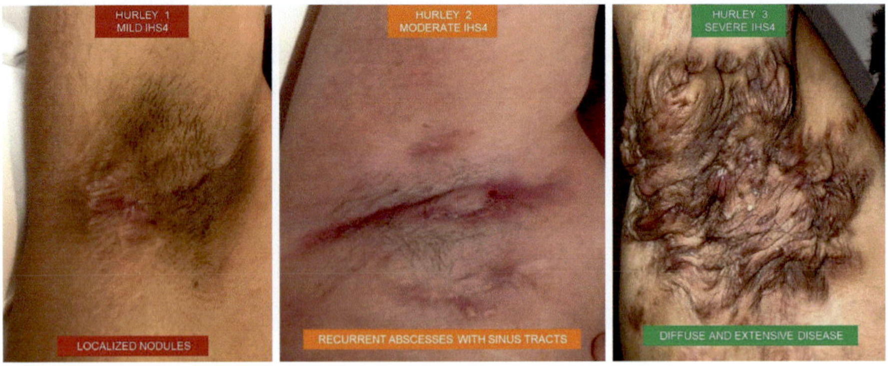

Fig. 13.42 Clinical photograph of patients with hidradenitis suppurativa

Table 13.1 International Hidradenitis Suppurativa Severity Score System (IHS4)

Aspect	Weight	Scoring description
Nodules, *n*	1	Count of nodules[a] present in affected areas
Abscesses, *n*	2	Count of abscesses[b] observed
Draining tunnels, *n*	4	Counting of draining tunnels[c] (fistulae or sinuses) detected

Severity classification	
Score range	Interpretation
0–3	Mild HS
4–10	Moderate HS
11 or higher	Severe HS

(From Sabat et al. [43]; with permission)

[a]Nodule: Elevated lesions or bumps beneath the skin surface, often painful and indicative of inflammatory activity

[b]Abscess: Pus-filled pockets or localized infections within the skin, typically manifesting as swollen, tender area

[c]Draining tunnels: Nodule: Tracts or channels connecting abscesses or nodules beneath the skin, often accompanied by discharge or drainage

- The Hurley staging system is used to classify the severity of hidradenitis suppurativa:
  - Stage I: Localized nodules.

    This stage is characterized by the presence of single or multiple abscesses or nodules, often with sinus tracts that may occasionally form.
  - Stage II: Recurrent abscesses with sinus tracts.

    In this stage, patients experience recurrent abscesses and nodules in one or more areas. There are multiple sinus tracts and scars.
  - Stage III: Diffuse and extensive disease.

    This stage involves diffuse, widespread involvement with multiple, interconnected abscesses and extensive sinus tracts. The area affected by the disease is larger, with significant scarring and the development of numerous sinus tracts.

13.2.3.4 Dermoscopy [28, 44]

- Double-ended pseudocomedones.
  - Under polarized dermoscopy are coupled cavities that deepen from the surface of the skin, in an oblique or parallel fashion, filled with superficial and deep-seated keratin accumulations.

  - The cavities are observed within a whitish cicatricial tissue and present large openings with irregular and undermined borders.
- Scars that on incident light dermoscopy are circinate and bridging scars with different depth levels and presenting hollows inside them.

13.2.3.5 Histopathology (Fig. 13.43) [43, 44, 46]

- Early phase.
  - Follicular plugging, acute suppurative folliculitis, and not always follicular rupture.
  - Follicular obstruction seems to be the initial event of hidradenitis suppurativa and is actually an abscessed folliculitis and not an apocrine lesion as the name suggests.
- Late phase (most frequently biopsied).
  - Chronic folliculitis with a mixed inflammatory pattern and extending from the lower half.
  - Abscesses and sinus tracts that may connect with the epidermis.
  - Marked fibrosis, destruction of hair follicles, eccrine, and apocrine glands secondarily.

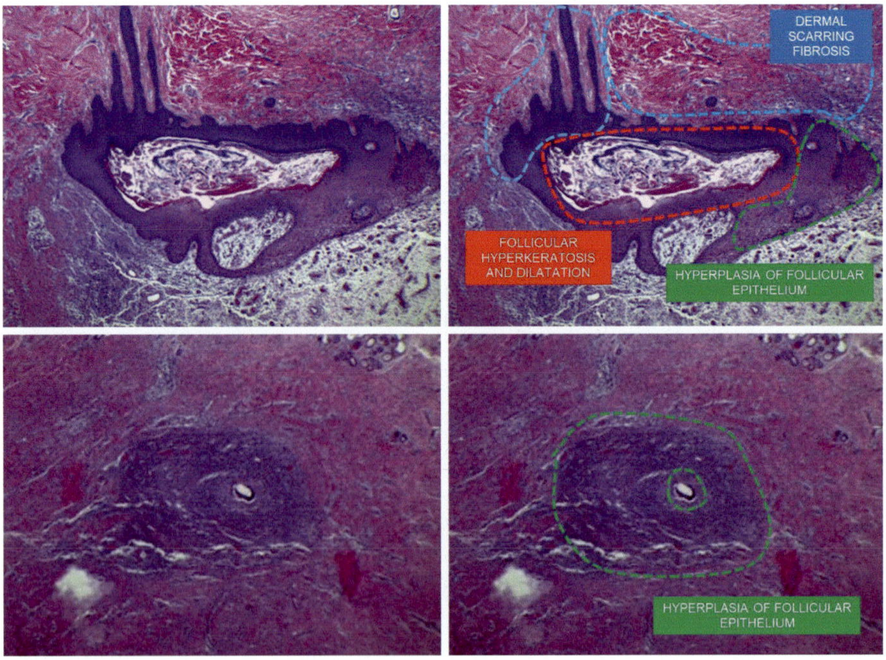

Fig. 13.43 Histological findings of hidradenitis suppurativa (Masson's trichrome stain X10 and H&E x40)

13.2.3.6 Radiography and Computed Tomography [47–52]

- Low-attenuation collections with thick walls in subcutaneous tissues.
- Abnormally enhanced infiltration of adjacent soft tissue, indicating a pronounced inflammatory response.
- Thickening of the overlying skin.
- Reactive lymph nodes.

13.2.3.7 Ultrasonography (Fig. 13.44; Tables 13.2 and 13.3) [9–12]

- These ultrasonographic findings assist in diagnosing, staging, and monitoring hidradenitis suppurativa. The protocols of study of HS recommend the power Doppler ultrasonography examination of all the affected regions bilaterally.
- Ultrasonographic criteria of hidradenitis suppurativa.
  - Widening of the hair follicles.
  - Thickening or abnormal echogenicity of the dermis.
  - Dermal pseudocystic nodules (round or oval-shaped hypoechoic or anechoic nodular structures).
  - Fluid collections (anechoic or hypoechoic fluid deposits, in the dermis or hypodermis connected to the base of widened hair follicles).

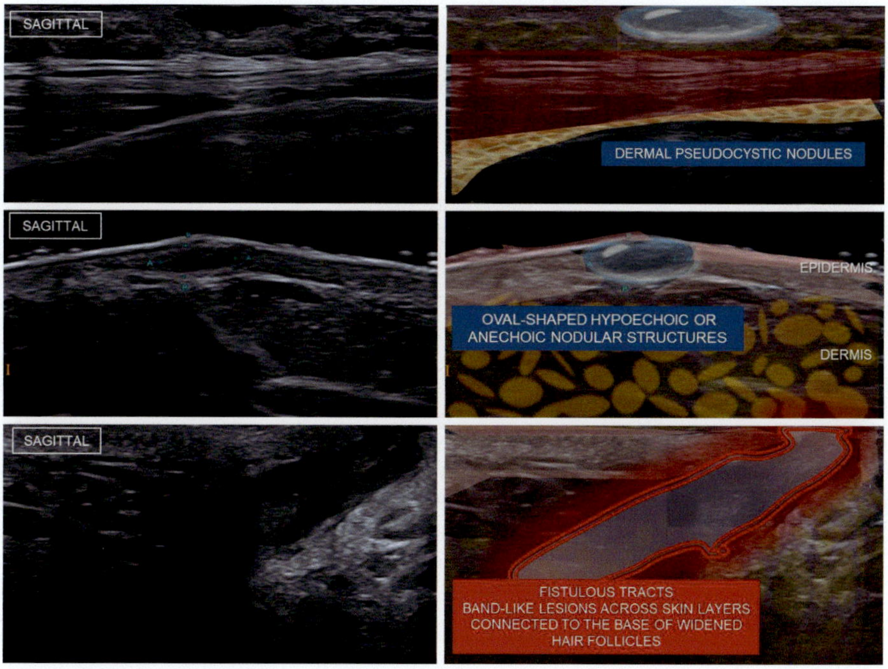

Fig. 13.44 Ultrasonographic findings of hidradenitis suppurativa with a 24 MHz probe (Aplio i800, Canon Medical Systems)

Table 13.2 Ultrasonography Hidradenitis Suppurativa Activity Score (US-HSA)

Variable	Score
Increased subcutaneous echogenicity	0 = Negative +2 = Positive
Dermal and/or subcutaneous vascularity	0 = Negative +2 = Positive
Type of flow	0 = No increase +1 = Venous or arterial <2 cm/s +2 = Arterial >2 cm/s
Corporal extension	+1 = Fewer than two corporal segments affected +2 = Two or more corporal segments affected +3 = Five or more corporal segments affected
Subregions within corporal region's extension	+1 = Fewer than two subregions affected within a corporal region +2 = Two subregions affected within a corporal region +3 = Three or more subregions affected within a corporal region
Variables added in examination control (compared with the previous examination)[a]	
Increase in size of key lesions or abnormalities	0 = Negative +1 = Increase in size or abnormalities in one previously affected subregion +2 = Increase in size or abnormalities in two to four previously affected subregions +2 = Extension in size or abnormalities in five or more of previously affected subregions
Appearance of new affected subregions	0 = Negative +2 = Positive (less than new subregions or one new corporal segment) +3 = Positive (two to four new subregions or two new corporal segments) +4 = Positive (five or more new subregions or three or more new corporal segments)
Decrease in maximum size of key lesions or abnormalities (grayscale abnormalities)	0 = Negative -1 = Partially -2 = Completely
Decrease of vascularity in periphery or within key lesions (color Doppler number or thickness [mm] of vessels in the lesional areas)	0 = Negative -1 = Partially -2 = Completely
Maximum scoring	18 points

(From Wortsman [95]; with permission)

[a]These additional variables in the control examination (compared with the previous examination) provide insights into changes in lesion characteristics and vascularity over time, contributing to a comprehensive assessment of HS activity

Table 13.3 Modified Sonographic Scoring System for Hidradenitis Suppurtiva (mSOS-HS)

Stage	Description
Stage I	A single fluid collection along with dermal changes, such as pseudocystic nodules, widened hair follicles, or alterations in dermal thickness or echogenicity, either unilaterally or bilaterally
Stage II	Two or four fluid collections or a single tunnel (fistulous tract) accompanied by dermal changes, either unilaterally or bilaterally
Stage III	
Stage IIIa	Five or more fluid collections or two to four noncommunicated tunnels or up to two communicated tunnels, either unilaterally or bilaterally
Stage IIIb	Five or more noncommunicated tunnels or three or more communicated tunnels, either unilaterally or bilaterally

(From Wortsman [95]; with permission)

  - Fistulous tracts (anechoic or hypoechoic band-like structures across skin layers in the dermis or hypodermis connected to the base of widened hair follicles).

- Ultrasonographic scoring for hidradenitis suppurativa (SOS-HS) criteria lesional features:
  - Stage I: Single fluid collection and dermal changes (hypoechoic or anechoic pseudocystic nodules, widening of the hair follicles, alterations in the dermal thickness or echogenicity) affecting a single body segment (axilla, groin, breast, buttock) (uni or bilateral) without fistulous tracts.
  - Stage II: Two to four fluid collections or a single fistulous tract with dermal changes affecting up to two body segments (uni or bilateral).
  - Stage III: Five or more fluid collections or two or more fistulous tracts with dermal changes or involvement of three or more body segments (uni or bilateral).
- Early signs of hidradenitis suppurativa (HS) linked with increased severity using ultrasonography:
  - Sword sign (hyperechoic linear structure suggestive of extruded hair shaft fragment through a ballooned hair follicle.
  - Bridge sign (hypoechoic band connecting the base of 2 or more dilated hair follicles).
  - Thick cylindrical fragments of hypoechoic keratin retained in the dermis or within the lesions.

13.2.3.8 MRI (Fig. 13.45) [53, 54]

- Skin thickening, subcutaneous tissue induration, and abscess formation, with distinct signal characteristics on T1-weighted, T2-weighted, and STIR images.

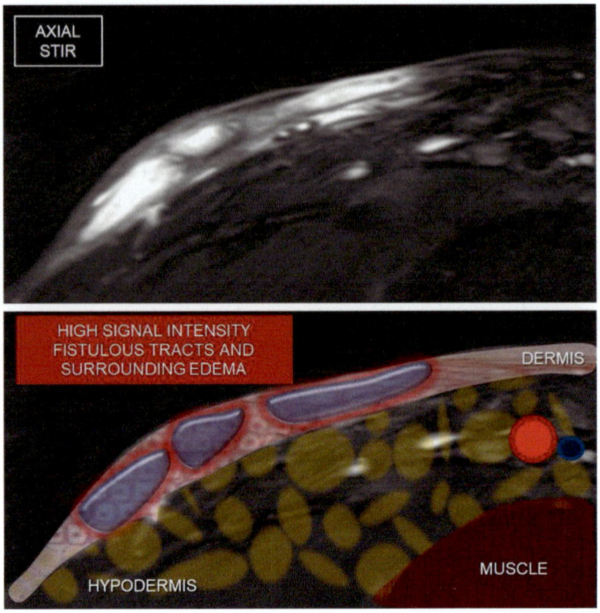

Fig. 13.45 MRI with surface coil findings of hidradenitis suppurativa on STIR sequence (Magnetom Prisma 3T MRI, Siemens)

- Fistulous tracts (high signal band-like structures across skin layers in the dermis or hypodermis connected to the base of widened hair follicles.
- Exact extension of the inflammatory tissue surrounding the lesions.
- The high soft-tissue resolution of MRI with surface coil can characterize the complex anatomy of the anal canal in great detail, providing particular utility of MRI for perianal HS cases, especially those with multiple tunnels.

13.2.3.9 3D Imaging (Fig. 13.46; Video 13.2)

- Allow the visualization of the extension of the abscess and fistula tracts, enabling to assess the severity and relation with adjacent structures.
- Contribute to more precise surgical interventions, if applicable.
- Biomodels can be used and allows the creation of physical replicas of the affected area, offering representations that aid in surgical planning and patient education.

13.2.4 Pilonidal Cyst

13.2.4.1 Definition [55–57]

- Dermis and hypodermis infections occurring at the upper part of the gluteal cleft of the buttocks.

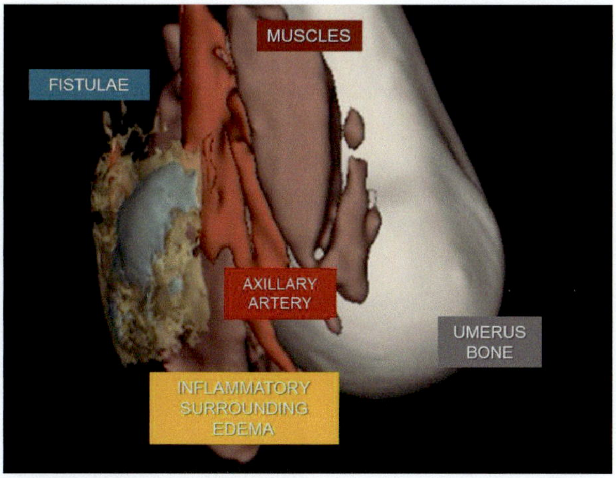

Fig. 13.46 3D image of hidradenitis suppurativa after segmentation of MRI isotropic images used for surgical planning

- Actually described as an acquired disease, which results from the suction of hair from surrounding skin, leading to a foreign body reaction and granuloma.

13.2.4.2 Epidemiology [57]

- Incidence of pilonidal disease is around 26 per 100,000 people.
- Occur at any age (less common in children and patients older than 45 years old).
- Incidence males 4:1 females.
- Risk factors.
  - Sedentary occupations and lifestyle.
  - Hirsutism.
  - Deep natal cleft.

13.2.4.3 Clinical Presentation (Fig. 13.47) [55, 56]

- Midline pits in the superior gluteal cleft.
- May be associated with cephalad or lateral tracking sinuses.

13.2.4.4 Histopathology [57]

- Hair within the pilonidal cysts originates from the overlying surrounding skin and microscopically had a hook architecture and suggested unidirectional hair migration.
- The walls of pilonidal cysts are composed of vascular pyogenic granulation tissue.

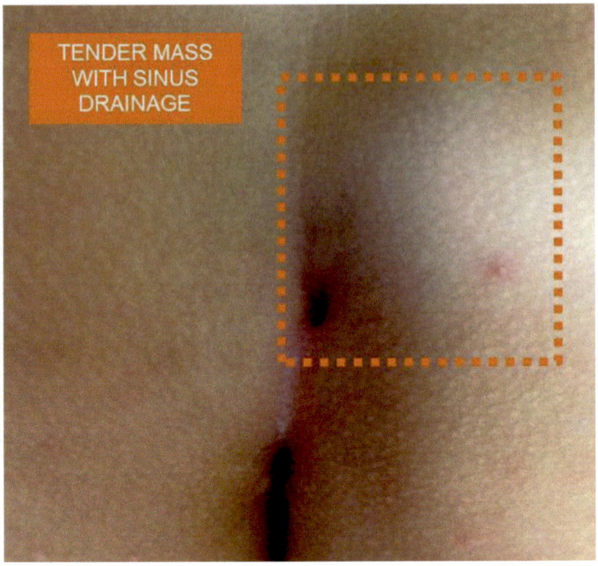

Fig. 13.47 Clinical photograph of patients with pilonidal cyst

13.2.4.5 Radiography and Computed Tomography

- CT may show the fistulous tract with parietal contrast-enhancement.
- Bone erosions and destruction may be present if the infectious tissue extend to sacral bone.

13.2.4.6 Ultrasonography (Fig. 13.48)

- Demonstrates fistulous tract associated with collection with parietal thickening and surrounding hypoechoic tissue.
- Hypervascularization on power Doppler imaging.
- Bone erosions can be identified if infectious tissue extend to sacral bone.

13.2.4.7 MRI (Fig. 13.49) [55]

- Demonstrates fistulous tract and the collection with high signal intensity on T2-weighted and STIR images associated with inflammatory surrounding edema.
- Thick and irregular parietal enhancement after gadolinium administration.
- Bone erosions and edema can be identified.
- Allows better visualization of fistulous tract anatomy and extension.

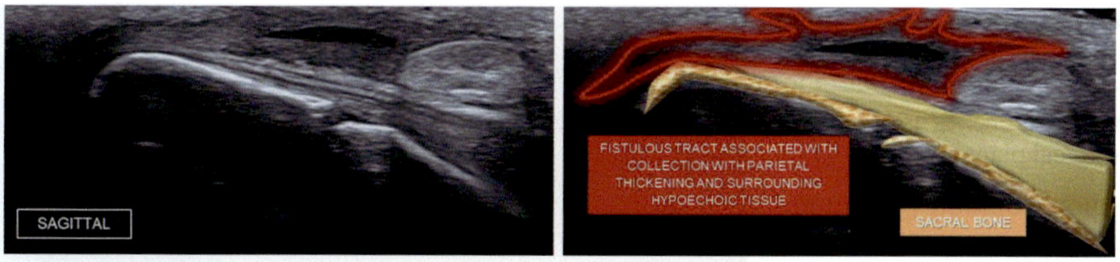

Fig. 13.48 Ultrasonographic findings of pilonidal cyst with a 24 MHz probe (Aplio i800, Canon Medical Systems)

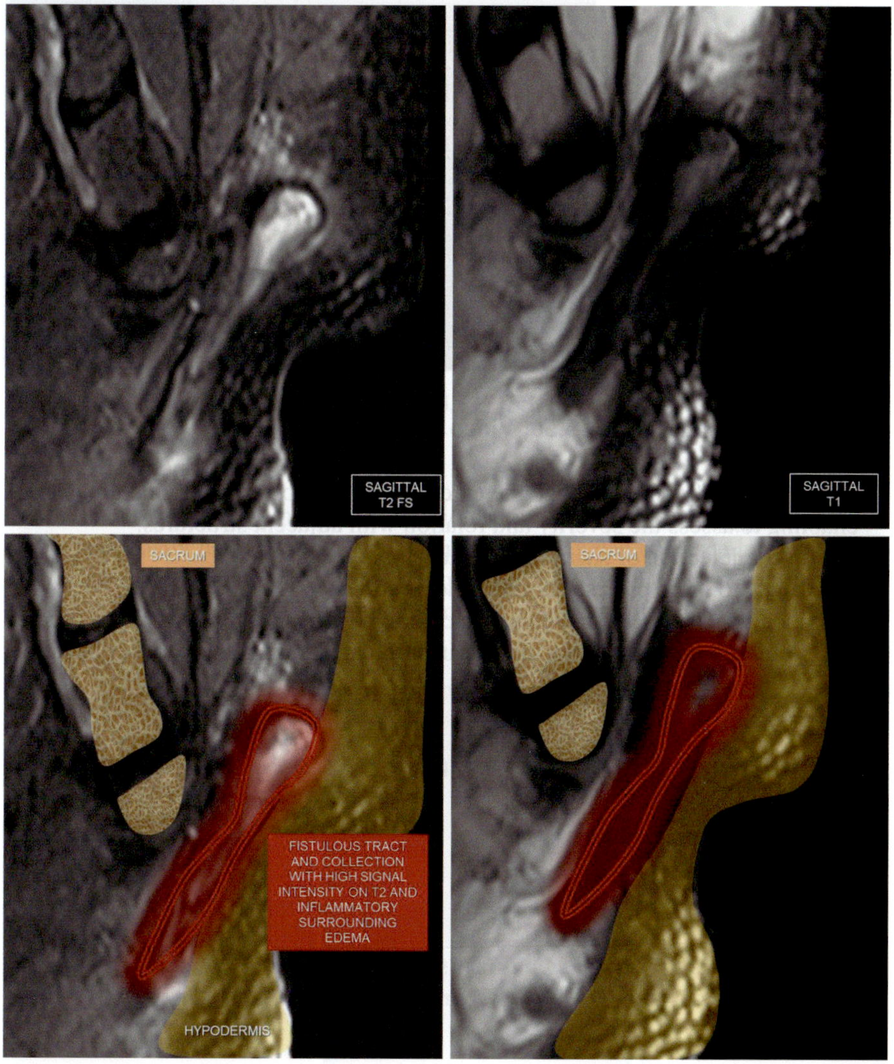

Fig. 13.49 MRI with surface coil findings of pilonidal cyst on T2 FS and T1-weighted sequences (Magnetom Prisma 3T MRI, Siemens)

- Nodular vasculitis.
  - Violaceous nodules or plaques on the posterior and anterolateral areas of the legs. Feet, thighs, arms, and face are rarely affected. Different from the lesions of erythema nodosum, nodular vasculitis' nodules are cold, not painful and tend to ulcerate.
  - Skin surface usually show desquamation and crusts over the ulcers. Most lesions resolve spontaneously and leave atrophic pigmented scars.

13.3.1.4 Histopathology [58, 59]

- Erythema nodosum.
  - Acute phase presents septal edema with mixed inflammatory infiltrate and vascular neoformation in the periphery of the septum, extending around the adipose lobe; there may be formation of Miescher's nodules, corresponding to aggregates of macrophages and neutrophils around the blood vessel, presence of fibrin, hemorrhage, endothelial edema, and lymphocytic infiltrate.
  - Chronic phase, there is septal thickening due to fibrosis and the presence of lipid-laden macrophages, neutrophils disappear, the presence of gigantocytes, and a decrease in the inflammatory process may occur. Adipose necrosis is uncommon.
- Nodular vasculitis.
  - Focal or diffuse lobular panniculitis occurs, usually associated with neutrophilic vasculitis of a small to medium-sized septal artery, and may present with fibrinous thrombus, lymphocytes, macrophages, and fibrosis as it progresses.
  - Vasculitis is not always present in biopsies, especially if small or shallow.
  - Adipose tissue may present a granulomatous inflammatory pattern with central foci of necrosis, mimicking mycobacteriosis, and it is important to perform AFB by Fite-Faraco staining.

13.3.1.5 Ultrasonography (Fig. 13.52)

- The ultrasonographic findings are identical for both erythema nodosum and nodular vasculitis.
- The most common finding is septal panniculitis.
- Prominent hyperechoic fatty lobules and hypoechoic, thick septa in the hypodermis.
- Dermis above this site appears to have decreased echogenicity.
- Power Doppler ultrasonography further reveals dermal and hypodermal hypervascularity in affected areas.

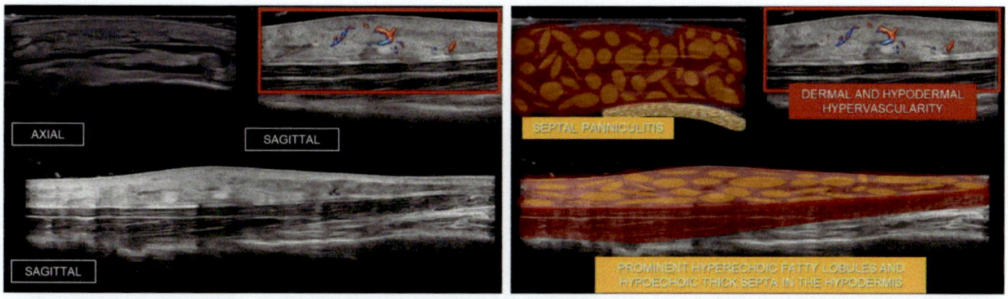

Fig. 13.52 Ultrasonographic findings of erythema nodosu with a 24 MHz probe (Aplio i800, Canon Medical Systems)

13.3.1.6 MRI

- The MRI findings are identical for both erythema nodosum and nodular vasculitis.
- Soft tissue inflammation showed as increased signal intensity on T2-weighted images in subcutaneous fat tissue with contrast enhancement.
- Prominent fatty lobules with thick septa in the hypodermis.

13.3.2 Sclerosing Panniculitis

13.3.2.1 Definition [60–62]

- Chronic venous insufficiency may lead to degenerative changes in the subcutaneous fatty tissue following lobular panniculitis (sclerosing panniculitis) and subsequent septal fibrosis associated with vascular proliferation, a condition known as Lipodermatosclerosis. The appearance of the chronic phase, referred to as lipodermatosclerosis, is characterized by induration and hyperpigmentation of the skin, particularly affecting the lower legs in a distinctive 'inverted champagne bottle' shape.

13.3.2.2 Epidemiology [60–62]

- Associated with venous insufficiency.
- Most common in middle aged women.
- Lipodermatosclerosis is frequently chronic and recurrent, emphasizing the need for ongoing management.

13.3.2.3 Clinical Presentation (Fig. 13.53) [60–62]

- Acute form may be painful and is frequently misdiagnosed as cellulitis.

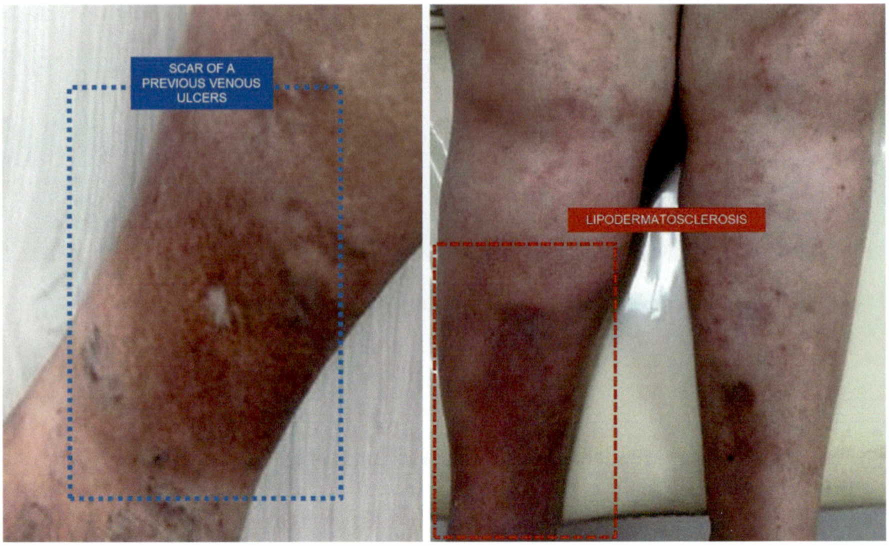

Fig. 13.53 Clinical photograph of patients with lipodermatosclerosis

- The hyperpigmentation, induration, and depression of lipodermatosclerosis are usually restricted to the medial leg but can be widespread.
- Can progress to venous ulcers and chronic pain is a common symptom.

13.3.2.4 Histopathology [60–62]

- Acute phase:
  - Lymphocytic infiltration of the septa surrounding fat lobules.
  - Cystic fat necrosis.
  - Capillary hemorrhage accompanied by hemosiderin deposition.
- Chronic phase:
  - Lobular panniculitis with a mixed cellular infiltrate.
  - Breakdown of adipocytes.
  - Lipomembranous change leading to the formation of "pseudocysts" within the subcutaneous tissue, that is defined by deteriorating adipocytes with thick and eosinophilic borders.
  - Septal fibrosis and hyaline sclerosis.

13.3.2.5 Radiography and Computed Tomography

- Thickening and dense soft tissue of the legs.

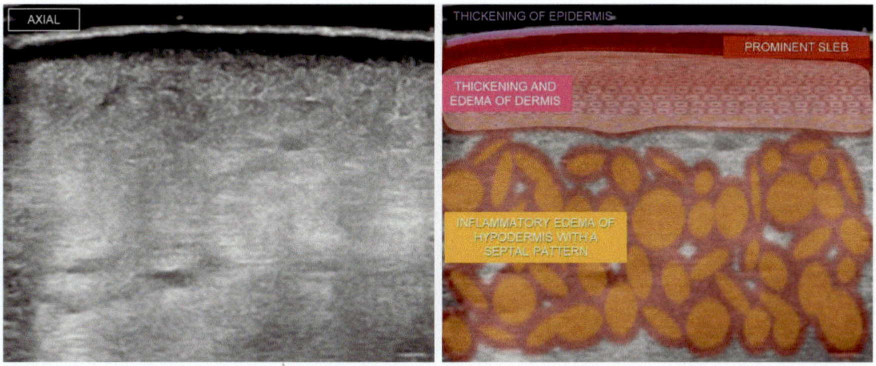

Fig. 13.54 Ultrasonographic findings of lipodermatosclerosis with a 24 MHz probe (Aplio i800, Canon Medical Systems)

13.3.2.6 Ultrasonography (Fig. 13.54)

- Acute stage:
  - Panniculitis.
  - Thickening and hypoechogenicity of the dermis and hypodermis.
  - Power Doppler may show high blood flow.
- Chronic stage:
  - Increased echogenicity of the subcutaneous tissue due to fibrosis.
  - Thickening of the dermis with loss of the dermal-hypodermal differentiation.
  - Areas of septa fibrosis.

13.3.2.7 MRI (Fig. 13.55)

- Acute stage:
  - Thickening, high signal intensity on STIR images at dermis and hypodermis suggesting panniculitis.
  - Thickening of the dermis and hypodermis.
  - Enhancement after gadolinium administration.
- Chronic stage:
  - Cutaneous layer atrophy.
  - Low signal intensity in the subcutaneous tissue due to fibrosis.
  - Thickening of the dermis and hypodermis.
  - Areas of septa fibrosis.

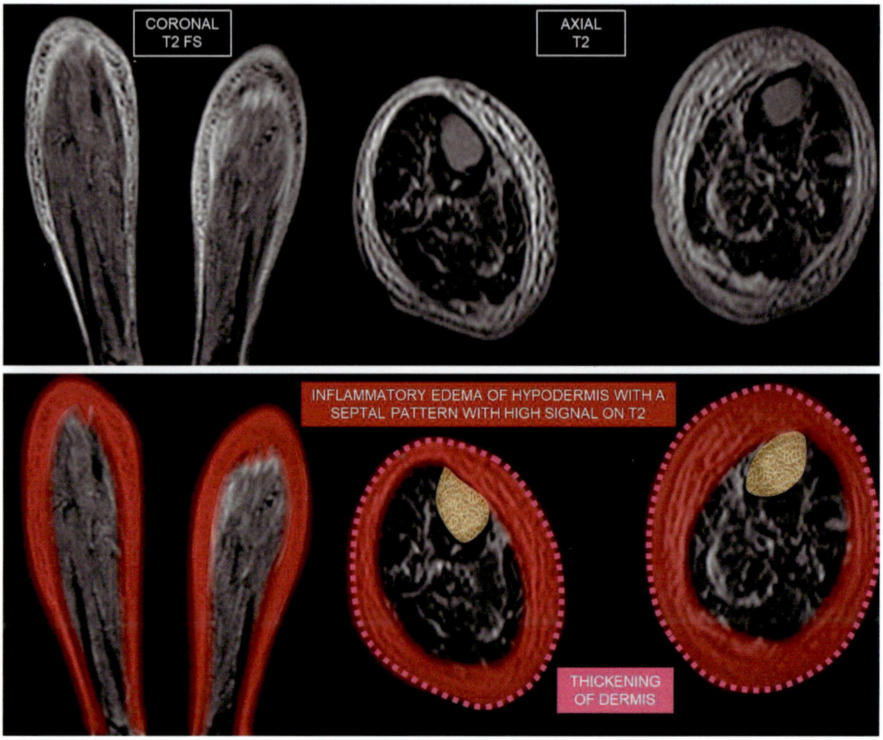

Fig. 13.55 MRI findings of lipodermatosclerosis on T2 and T2 FS-weighted sequences (Image reproduced from the article. From Chan et al. [94]; with permission)

13.3.3 Semicircular Lipoatrophy

13.3.3.1 Definition [63, 64]

- Benign, reversible, and rare disease, characterized by tissue atrophy subcutaneous adipose, without muscle or skin involvement.
- Areas of the skin of the extremities with contact with the furniture, mainly in the thigh.
- Etiology is unknown, multiple associated factors:
  - Contact of the affected area with furniture.
  - Presence of electromagnetic radiation.
  - Presence of electrostatic discharge.
  - Low relative humidity.

13.3.3.2 Epidemiology [63, 64]

- More common in women than in men.
- Repeated and prolonged microtrauma on the thighs, such as continued support on the edge of the work table, the pressure of the chair and the use of clothing compressive.
- Electrostatic charges and electromagnetic fields would produce the activation of macrophages, which would secondarily activate the secretion of factor.
- alpha tumor necrosis, resulting in adipocytes damaged by phagocytosis.

13.3.3.3 Clinical Presentation (Fig. 13.56) [63, 64]

- Depressed semicircular bands.
- Unilateral or bilateral.
- Symmetrical.
- Frequently located in the anterior and lateral region of the thigh (approximate height of 72 cm from the ground).

13.3.3.4 Histopathology (Fig. 13.57) [63, 64]

- Microscopic changes in semicircular lipoatrophy are uncharacteristic and rarely biopsied.
- The major characteristic is the subtotal or total loss of subcutaneous adipose tissue.

13.3.3.5 Ultrasonography (Fig. 13.58)

- Increased echogenicity of the subcutaneous tissue due to fibrosis.
- Atrophy of subcutaneous tissue comparing with the normal skin.
- May present thickening of the skin with areas of denser fibrosis.

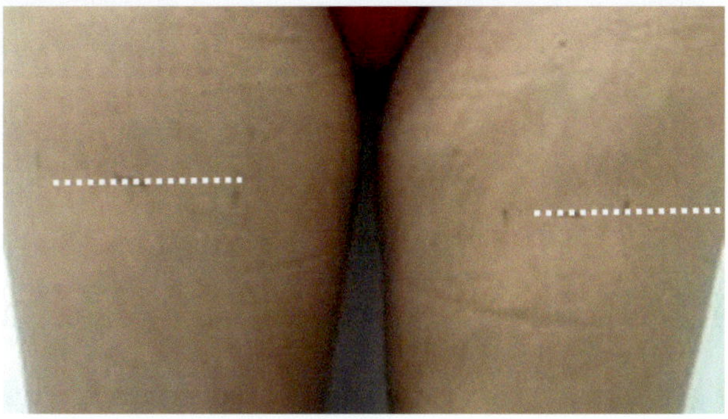

Fig. 13.56 Clinical photograph of patient with semicircular lipoatrophy

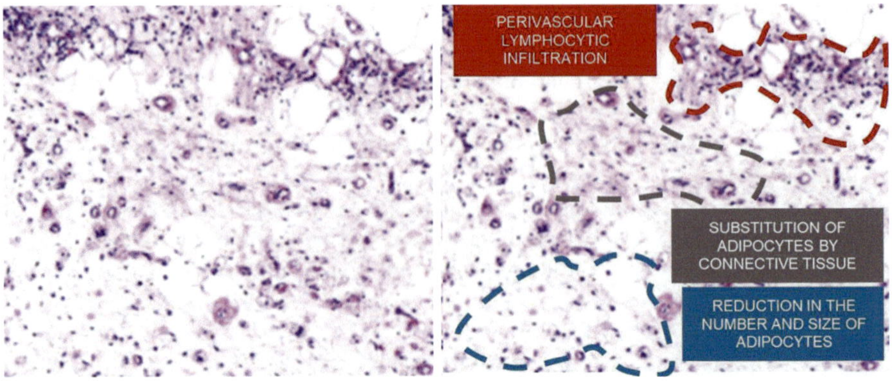

Fig. 13.57 Histological findings of semicircular lipoatrophy (H&E x2)

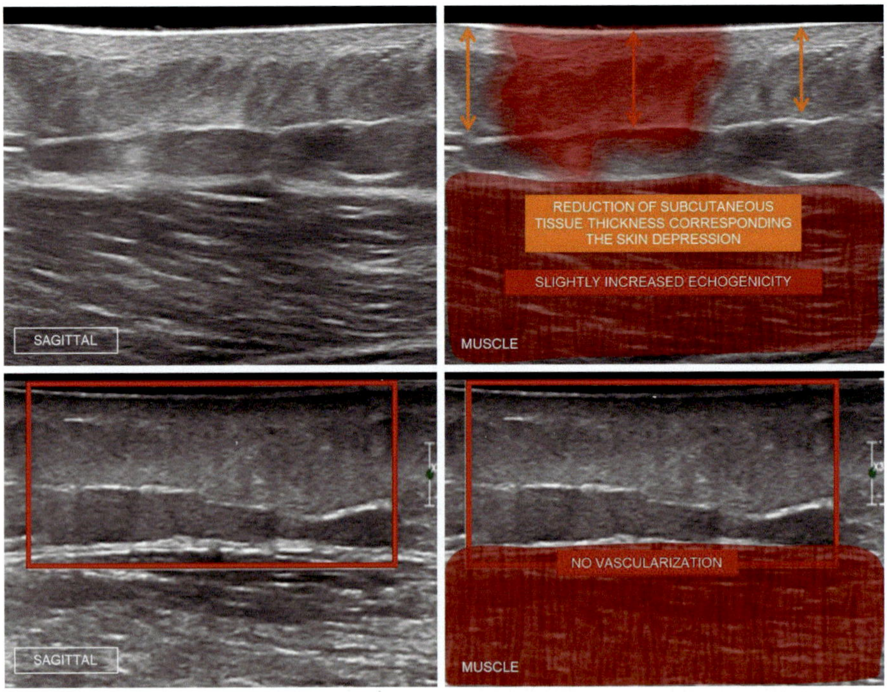

Fig. 13.58 Ultrasonographic findings of semicircular lipoatrophy with a 24 MHz probe (Aplio i800, Canon Medical Systems)

13.3.3.6 MRI [65]

- Loss of superficial subcutaneous adipose tissues T1 and T2-weighted images, showing atrophy.
- No alteration of the thickness of subcutaneous septa.
- Fat lobules were normal in size and shape.

13.3.4 Flebitis

13.3.4.1 Definition [66, 67]

- Flebitis, or phlebitis, is the inflammation of a vein, typically occurring in the superficial veins of the arms or legs.
- Characterized by pain, swelling, and redness along the affected vein, and can be caused by factors such as injury, infection, or irritation from intravenous catheterization.

13.3.4.2 Epidemiology [66, 67]

- Flebitis is relatively common and can occur in both hospitalized patients and those receiving intravenous therapy. It is especially prevalent in individuals with prolonged or repeated venous access.
- Includes the use of intravenous catheters, particularly in patients receiving long-term or frequent infusions, recent surgery, trauma, and conditions affecting blood flow or vessel integrity.
- Can affect individuals of all ages, though it is more common in older adults due to increased likelihood of venous catheter use and comorbid conditions.

13.3.4.3 Clinical Presentation (Fig. 13.59) [66, 67]

- Pain, tenderness, redness, and swelling along the course of the affected vein. The area may feel warm to the touch, and there may be visible redness along the vein.
- A palpable, hardened cord-like structure may be felt along the vein. In more severe cases, there may be associated fever or systemic symptoms if an infection is present.

13.3.4.4 Histopathology [66, 67]

- Acute phlebitis: Neutrophil infiltration and edema in the vessel wall and surrounding tissue.
- Chronic phlebitis: Lymphocytic infiltration, fibrosis, and possible formation of granulation tissue.
- Thrombus formation: Often associated with phlebitis, with evidence of clotting within the vein and inflammatory changes in the vessel wall.

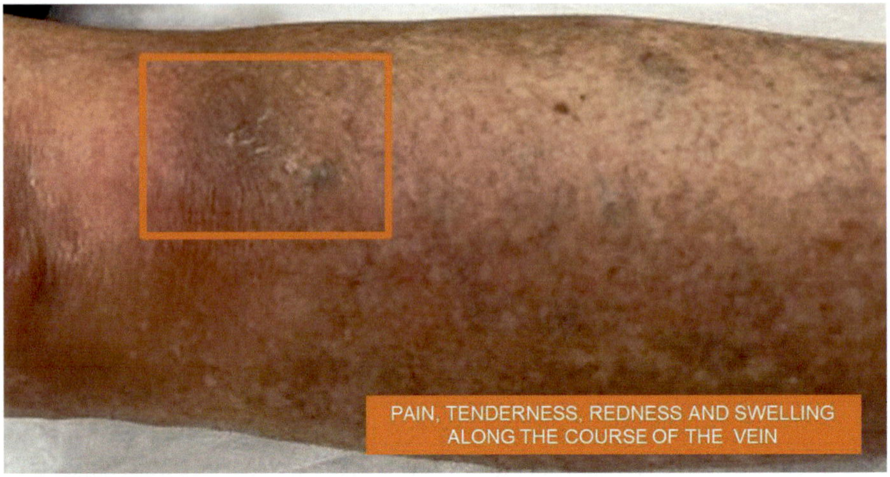

Fig. 13.59 Clinical photograph of patient with flebitis

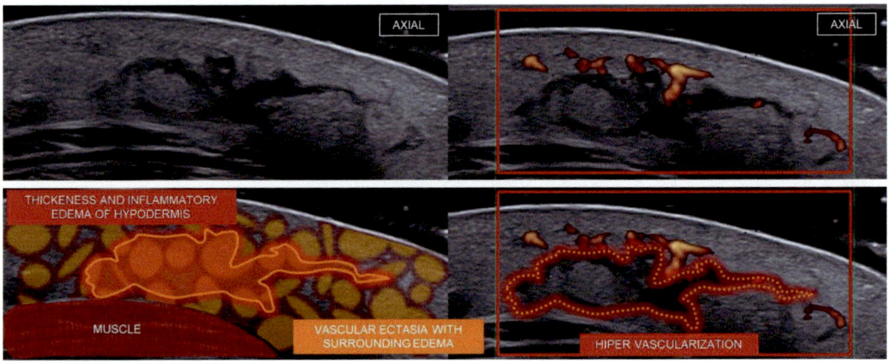

Fig. 13.60 Ultrasonographic findings of flebitis with a 24 MHz probe (Aplio i800, Canon Medical Systems)

13.3.4.5 Ultrasonography (Fig. 13.60)

- Increased blood flow in the affected vein as shown by power Doppler imaging.
- Hypoechoic areas around the vein indicating inflammation.
- he presence of an echogenic thrombus within the vein may be visible, sometimes accompanied by decreased venous compressibility.
- Ultrasonography can detect secondary complications such as abscess formation in the surrounding tissues.

13.3.4.6 MRI (Fig. 13.61)

- T2-weighted images often show increased signal intensity in the affected vein and surrounding tissue due to edema and inflammation.
- Hyperintense signal in the affected vein on T1-weighted images may indicate the presence of a thrombus.
- Thickening of the venous wall and surrounding soft tissue can be visualized.
- MRI can detect complications such as abscess formation or deeper tissue involvement, which may not be as easily seen with other imaging modalities.

13.3.5 Small and Medium Vessel Vasculitis

13.3.5.1 Definition [66, 68, 69]

- Small vessel vasculitis is a group of inflammatory conditions that affect the small blood vessels of the body, leading to a variety of symptoms and clinical features.
- Some of well-known types of small vessel vasculitis include:
  - the ANCA-related group,

    Granulomatosis with polyangiitis (GPA), former known as Wegener's granulomatosis.
    Microscopic polyangiitis (MPA).
    Eosinophilic granulomatosis with polyangiitis (EGPA), formerly known as Churg-Strauss syndrome.

  - IgA vasculitis (the former Henoch-Schönlein Purpura - HSP).
  - Cryoglobulinemic vasculitis.

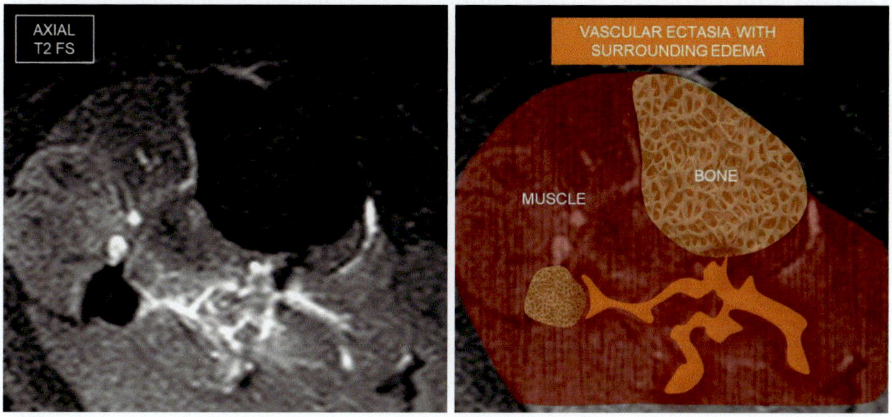

Fig. 13.61 MRI findings of flebitis on T2 FS-weighted sequence (Magnetom Avanto 1.5T MRI, Siemens)

- Cutaneous small vessel vasculitis or IgM/IgG vasculitis.
- Medium vessel vasculitis: - Poliarteritis Nodosa (PAN).

13.3.5.2 Epidemiology [66, 68, 69]

- Variable prevalence rates are reported, ranging from 10 to 30 cases per 100.000 individuals.
- The incidence and prevalence of small vessel vasculitis can vary geographically. GPA is more common in northern European populations, while MPA is more prevalent in Asian populations.
- It may occur at any age, depending on the specific condition.
  - IgA vasculitis (Henoch-Schönlein Purpura) occurs mainly in children.
  - GPA and MPA predominantly affects adults between 40 and 60 years old.
- Cutaneous small vessel vasculitis is more prevalent in female, while GPA has a slightly male predominance.

13.3.5.3 Clinical Presentation (Fig. 13.62) [68, 69]

- Cutaneous manifestations usually are identified as livedo reticularis, subcutaneous nodules and ulcers.
- Cutaneous small vessel vasculitis (leukocytoclastic angiitis) primarily affects the skin. Usually presents with palpable purpura, which are small red or purple spots on the skin caused by extravasation of red cells. These spots may be assymptomatic or accompanied by pain or itching.
- GPA is characterized by inflammation of the respiratory tract (upper and lower) and kidneys. Dermatological involvement includes palpable purpura, nodules, ulcers, and livedo reticularis (a purplish, mottled discoloration of the skin).
- EGPA primarily affects the respiratory tract and kidneys, with asthma and eosinophilia as usual hallmarks. Skin involvement in EGPA includes purpura, papules, and nodules.
- IgA vasculitis typically presents as palpable purpura, usually symmetrical reddish-purple spots on the skin, on the lower extremities, buttocks and sometimes arms and trunks. The lesions can evolve to vesicles or ulcers, in severe cases. Renal involvement is not uncommon and can have a poor prognosis. The purpura may be preceded by joint pain and gastrointestinal symptoms.
- PAN is the prototypical medium-sized vessel vasculitis, predominantly arteries. Skin involvement presents as livedo reticularis, with a classic lace-like mottled pattern, usually on lower extremities. Nodules, which are tender, raised, more palpable than visible lesions, may develop, particularly on the legs. Ulcers may also be the manifestation of a compromised deep vessel.

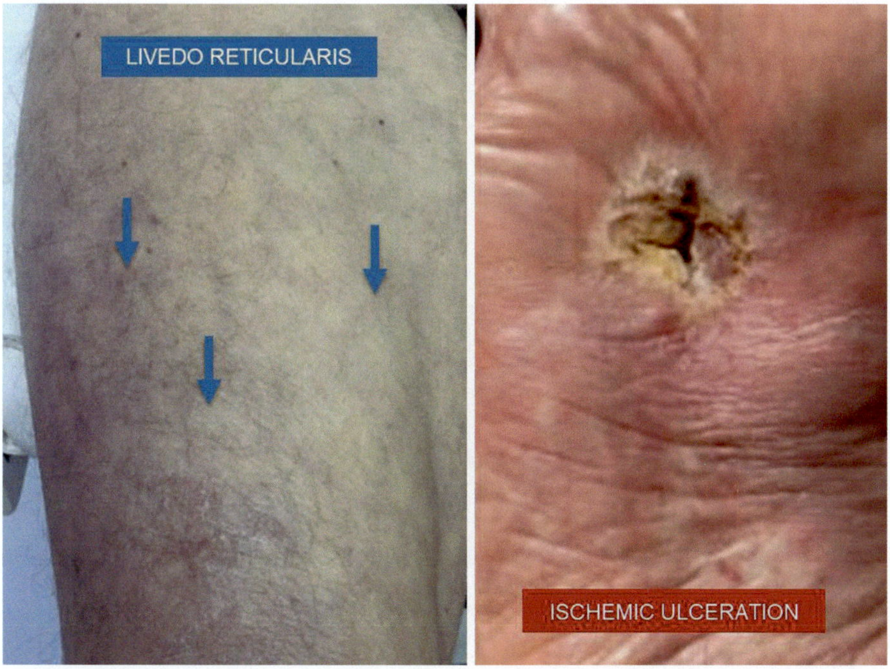

Fig. 13.62 Clinical photograph of patient with ulceration and livedo reticularis due small vessel vasculitis (Images kindly provided by Dr. Luiza Kassunga—Rio de Janeiro, Brazil)

13.3.5.4 Histopathology (Fig. 13.63) [68, 69]

- Leukocytoclastic vasculitis is a neutrophilic vasculitis of small venules presenting with fibrinoid necrosis or damage of the vessel wall, endothelial edema and hyperplasia, perivascular neutrophilic infiltrate with leukocytoclasia or karyorrhexis (nuclear dust), hemorrhage or hemosiderosis; there may be peripheral edema, vascular thrombosis, epithelial changes secondary to ischemia, fibrosis, histiocytes or eosinophils.
- Livedo reticularis or livedoid vasculopathy: absence of neutrophilic vasculitis; perivascular lymphocytic infiltrate is present without damage to the vessel wall, as in leukocytoclastic vasculitis. Occasionally, fibrinous thrombosis may occur with the presence of secondary ischemic skin changes.

13.3.5.5 Radiography and Computed Tomography

- Nodules.
  - Heterogeneous soft tissue high density in the affected area.
  - Sometimes dystrophic calcification can be identified.

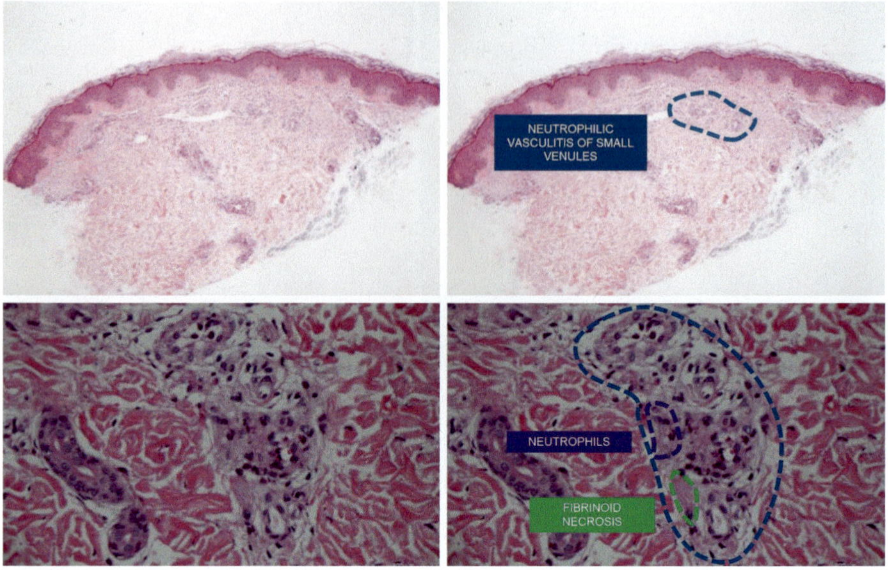

Fig. 13.63 Histological findings of small vessel vasculitis (H&E x4 and x20)

- Ulcers.
  - Loss of soft tissue density in the affected area, with irregular margins and increased soft tissue density surrounding the ulcer may indicate edema or inflammation.
  - If the ulcer is chronic or infected, there might be a bone erosions and periosteal reaction in adjacent bones, appearing as new bone formation along the periosteum.
  - In cases of infected ulcers, there might be evidence of localized fluid collections or abscesses.

13.3.5.6 Ultrasonography (Fig. 13.64)

- Nodules.
  - Ultrasonography imaging may show hypoechoic lesions and thickness of the skin and subcutaneous tissue in affected areas.
  - There may be evidence of increased or altered blood flow in the underlying vessels, especially in active cases of vasculitis.
- Ulcers.
  - Irregular soft tissue defects, with hypoechoic areas on the skin surface, often with a disruption of the normal soft tissue layers, May be surrounded by inflammation with a "panniculitis appearance".

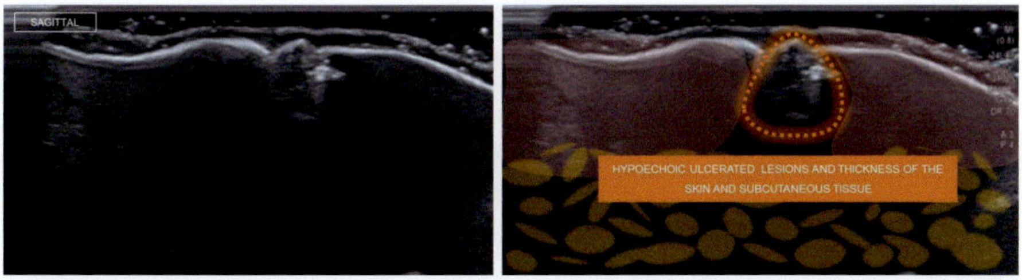

Fig. 13.64 Ultrasonographic findings of ulceration due small vessel vasculitis with a 24 MHz probe (Aplio i800, Canon Medical Systems)

- Ulcers, particularly if infected, may have associated fluid collections or abscesses, which appear as anechoic or hypoechoic areas with possible internal debris and septations.
- Power Doppler ultrasonography may show increased vascularity around the ulcer, suggesting active inflammation.
- In severe cases, cortical disruption of underlying bone and periosteal reaction can be identified if the ulcer extends deeply.

13.3.5.7 MRI (Fig. 13.65)

- Nodules.
  - Low to intermediate signal intensity nodules on T1-Weighted images and high signal intensity on T2-Weighted images due to the presence of fluid or necrotic material within the nodule.
  - After administration of gadolinium contrast, often enhance, indicating active inflammation or vascularity within the nodules.
- Ulcers.
  - Soft tissue defects with irregular margins showing abnormal signal intensity on both T1 and T2-weighted images, with edema and inflammation of the surrounding tissue.
  - Fluid collections can be observed as areas of high signal intensity on T2-weighted images with possible internal debris and septations presenting parietal restricted diffusion on DWI.
  - Cortical disruption, erosions and periosteal reaction of underlying bone can also be detected if the ulcer extends deep enough.

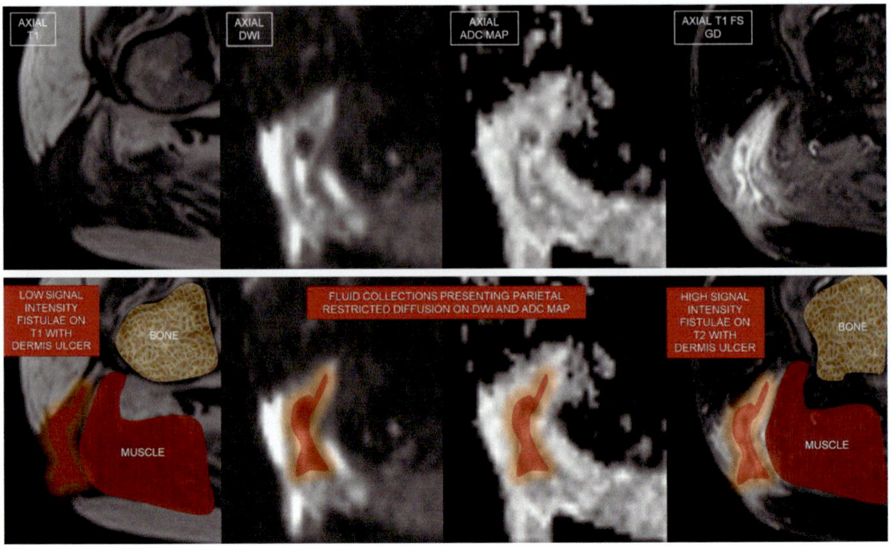

Fig. 13.65 MRI findings of ulceration due small vessel vasculitis on T1, T2 FS, DWI, and T1 FS-weighted sequences after gadolinium administration (Magnetom Avanto 1.5T MRI, Siemens)

13.3.6 Pretibial Myxedema

13.3.6.1 Definition [70, 71]

- Cutaneous manifestation of Graves' disease (autoimmune hyperthyroidism), characterized by the accumulation of glycosaminoglycans in the dermis.

13.3.6.2 Epidemiology [70]

- In patients with Graves' disease, the estimated prevalence of pretibial myxedema ranges from 0.5 to 4%.
- It is more common in those with serious ophthalmopathy and four times more common in women than men.

13.3.6.3 Clinical Presentation (Fig. 13.66) [70]

- Diffuse, non-depressible edema, with "peau d'orange" appearance.
- Lesions can also have nodular or plaque-like shape and usually vary in color.
- Few cases are pruritic or painful, but it is usually asymptomatic.
- Lymphedema and elephantiasis are possible complications that can arise from severe lymphatic obstruction.

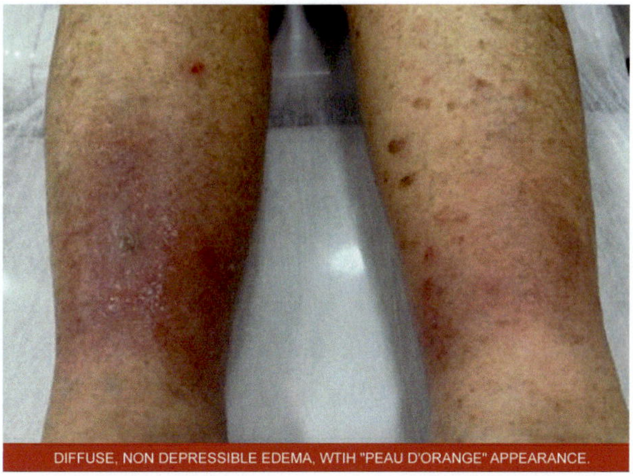

Fig. 13.66 Clinical photograph of patient with pretibial myxedema

13.3.6.4 Dermastocopy [70]

- Scale and white clouds.
- Shiny white lines on pink or brownish background.

13.3.6.5 Histopathology [70]

- Diffuse dermal mucinosis, usually pronounced, different from other localized mucinosis that are usually discrete, present throughout the dermis reticularis, positive by the staining of Alcian Blue.
- There may be variable hyperkeratosis and acanthosis and the presence of fibrosis in the chronic phase.
- Because it is a clinically characteristic lesion, it is rarely biopsied.

13.3.6.6 Ultrasonography (Fig. 13.67)

- Increase in skin thickness.
- Increase in the echogenicity of the dermis and hypodermis, with possible appearance of panniculitis.

13.3.6.7 MRI

- Thickening and high signal intensity on STIR images at dermis and hypodermis suggesting panniculitis.
- Thickening of the dermis and hypodermis.
- Enhancement after gadolinium administration.

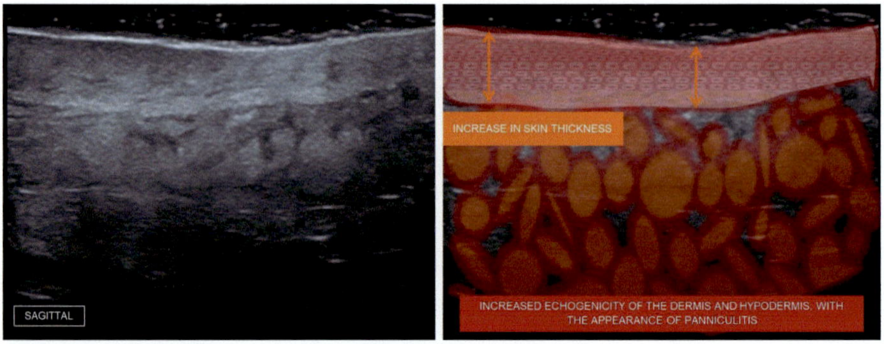

Fig. 13.67 Ultrasonographic findings of pretibial myxedema with a 24 MHz probe (Aplio i800, Canon Medical Systems)

13.3.7 Granuloma Annulare

13.3.7.1 Definition [72]

- Chronic, inflammatory, benign granulomatous cutaneous condition.
- Presents 4 types of appearance: localized, generalized or disseminated, subcutaneous and perforating.

13.3.7.2 Epidemiology [72]

- It is two times more common in women than men, when the lesion is localized.
- Usually starts before the age of 30.
- Subcutaneous subtype affects more children under the age of 5 and perforating GA, which is a rare presentation, affects more people under 30 years old.

13.3.7.3 Clinical Presentation (Fig. 13.68) [72]

- Localized: most common subtype, characterized by erythematous or skin-coloured papules grouped in a ring-like pattern. Rings grow centrifugally and are usually localized on dorsal hands and feet.
- Generalized or disseminated: ten or more lesions, involving any part of the body, especially the scalp, neck and trunk.
- Subcutaneous: deep, mobile, asymptomatic nodules that grow slowly and present spontaneous resolution.
- Perforating: rare subtype that presents millimetric, umbilicated papules, with central crust; pustules and scars. It is usually localized on the palms of the hands.

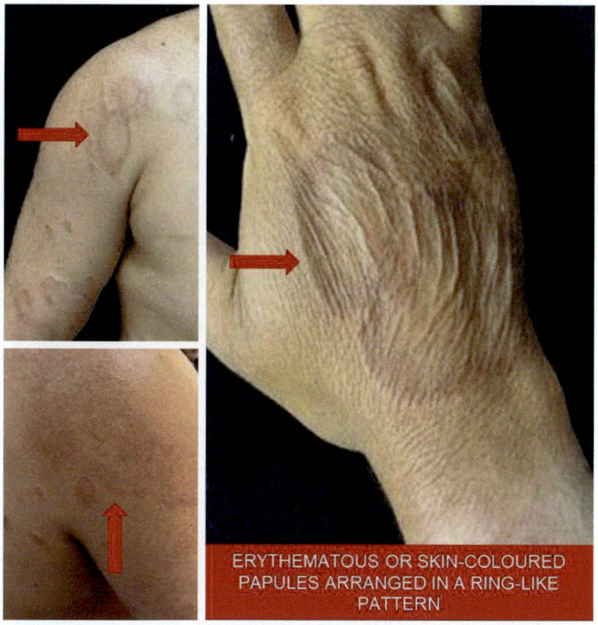

Fig. 13.68 Clinical photograph of patient with granuloma annulare

13.3.7.4 Dermoscopy [73, 74]

- Whitish areas and yellowish-orange structureless areas seem to be the most common non-vascular finding. Other findings include rosettes, crystalline structures and whitish scaling.
- Unfocused vessels, over a pinkish background, with different morphologies: dotted, linear or branching. Sparsely distributed dotted ones are the most frequent.

13.3.7.5 Histopathology (Fig. 13.69) [75]

- Begins as superficial perivascular dermatitis, predominantly lymphocytic, with foci of interstitial infiltration by histiocytes in the initial lesions.
- Evolution, there is degeneration of the fibers or necrobiosis with interstitial deposition of alcian blue mucin at pH 2.5 and positive colloidal iron. The area of collagen degeneration has a hypereosinophilic aspect in the HE compared to the unaltered collagen fibers.
- It forms several round or multifocal ovals, in the middle and upper dermis.
- There is a non-granulomatous interstitial form, with histiocytes squeezed between the collagen bands, with a busy dermis pattern, minimal necrobiosis, and minimal mucin.
- There may be eosinophils, sometimes with intense infiltrate, variable presence of gigantocytes in the periphery.
- In actinic gigantocellular forms occur the presence of elastophagocytosis.

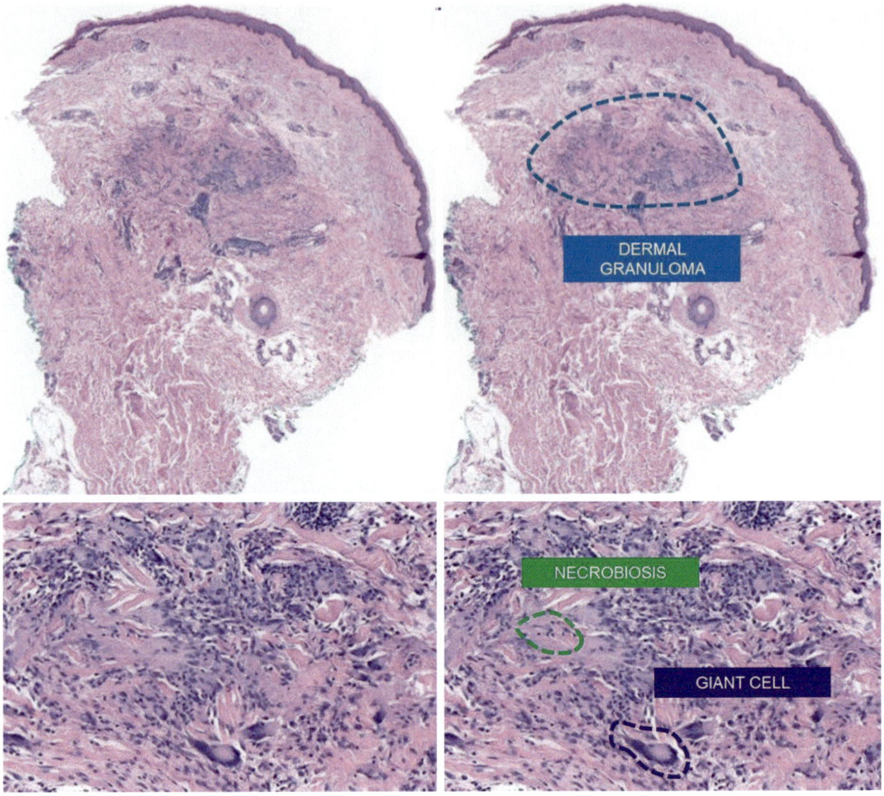

Fig. 13.69 Histological findings of granuloma annulare (H&E x4 and x20)

13.3.7.6 Ultrasonography (Fig. 13.70) [72, 76]

- Three distinct sonographic patterns were identified depending on the clinical variant of granuloma annulare:
  - Dermal pattern: poorly defined hypoechoic band or a double oval-shaped hypoechoic bands in the superficial dermis. Some cases show prominent hyperechogenic dots on the surface of the lesion.
  - Hypodermis pattern: irregularly shaped hypoechoic hypodermal lumps also located in reticular dermis.
  - Mixed pattern: ill-defined hypoechoic dermal and subcutaneous lesions.
- Some cases showed hypervascularity on power Doppler.

13.3.7.7 MRI (Fig. 13.71)

- Subcutaneous ill-defined lesions with isointense or slightly hyperintense to muscle on T1-weighted images and heterogeneous signal intensity on T2-weighted images.

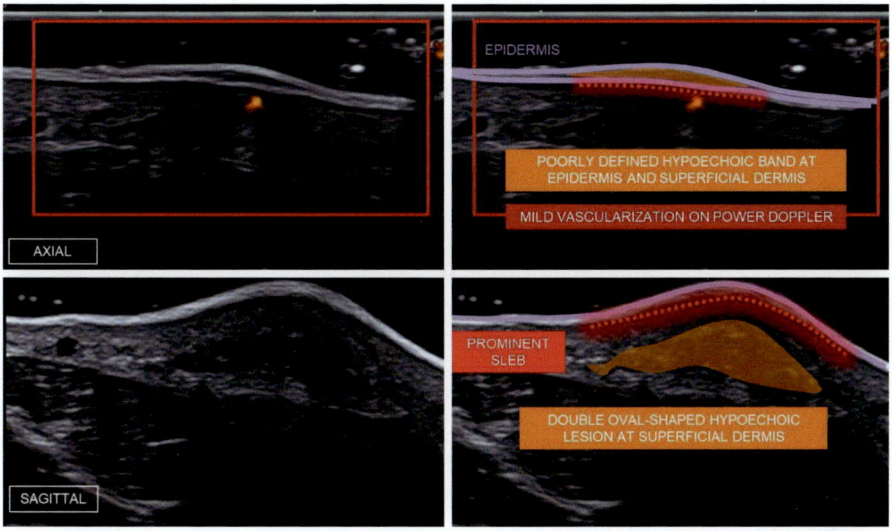

Fig. 13.70 Ultrasonographic findings of granuloma annulare with a 24 MHz probe (Aplio i800, Canon Medical Systems)

Fig. 13.71 MRI findings of granuloma annulare on T1 and PD FS-weighted sequences (Magnetom Avanto 1.5T MRI, Siemens)

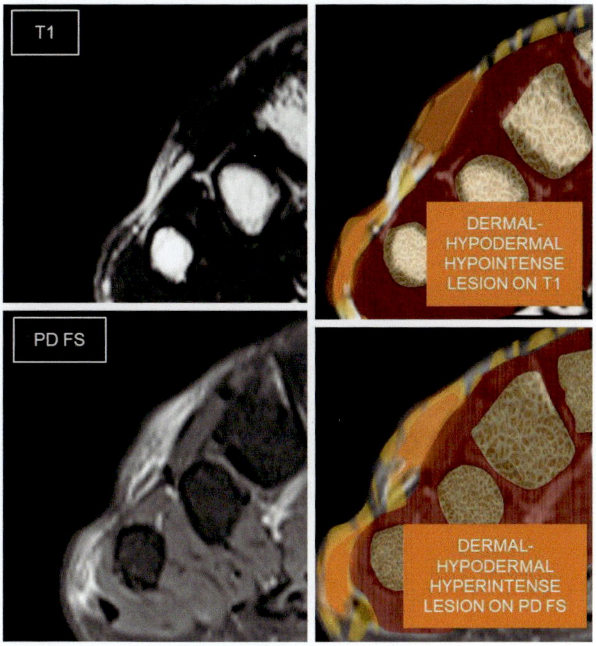

- Homogeneously contrast enhanced after gadolinium administrationT1: ill-defined subcutaneous mass, isointense to muscle.

13.3.8 *Pachydermodactyly*

13.3.8.1 Definition [77]

- Pachydermodactyly is a rare dermatological condition characterized by thickening and hypertrophy of the skin and soft tissues of the fingers.
- It is often associated with a distinct appearance of the fingers, resembling a "pachyderm" or thick-skinned animal.

13.3.8.2 Epidemiology [78]

- Pachydermodactyly is extremely rare, with only a few documented cases in medical literature.
- The condition can be congenital or acquired, with possible associations to systemic disorders, trauma, or genetic factors. It is not well-understood and lacks broad epidemiological data.
- Affects individuals across various ages, but cases are more frequently reported in adults. No significant gender predilection has been noted.

13.3.8.3 Clinical Presentation (Fig. 13.72) [78]

- Patients typically present with thickened, swollen, and hypertrophied skin on the fingers. This can cause discomfort and functional impairment.
- The affected fingers may exhibit a "pachydermatous" appearance with increased skin thickness and possible nodular formations. There may be associated changes in skin texture and color, and the condition can lead to decreased dexterity or range of motion in severe cases.

13.3.8.4 Histopathology (Fig. 13.73) [78]

- Hyperkeratosis characterized by thickened stratum corneum.
- Thickening of the epidermis called acanthosis.
- Dermal fibrosis observed as increased collagen deposition in the dermis.
- Mild inflammatory infiltrates may be present, depending on the underlying cause.

13.3.8.5 Ultrasonography (Fig. 13.74)

- Hypoechoic areas indicating thickened skin and subcutaneous tissue.
- Increased echogenicity in the dermal layer may reflect fibrosis or increased collagen deposition.
- Presence of well-defined nodules or masses in the subcutaneous tissue.

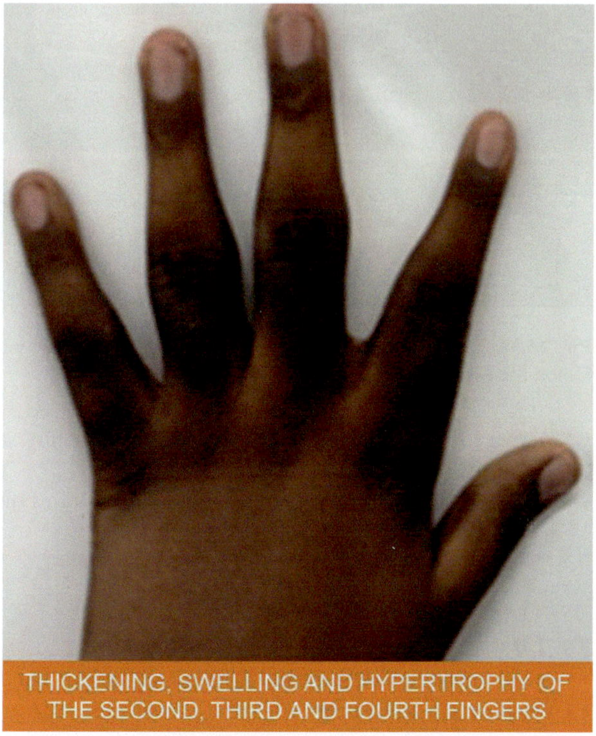

Fig. 13.72 Clinical photograph of patient with pachydermodactyly

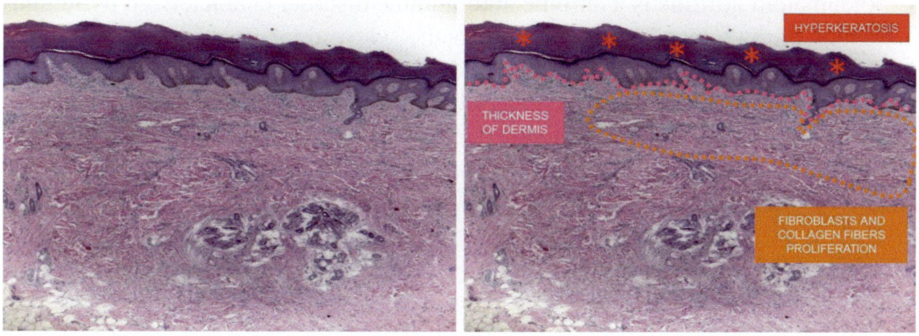

Fig. 13.73 Histological findings of pachydermodactyly (H&E x4)

13.3.8.6 MRI

- T2-weighted images typically show increased signal intensity in the affected skin and subcutaneous tissues due to edema and thickening.
- Hyperintense areas indicating increased thickness of the skin and subcutaneous tissues. The dermal layer may appear thickened.

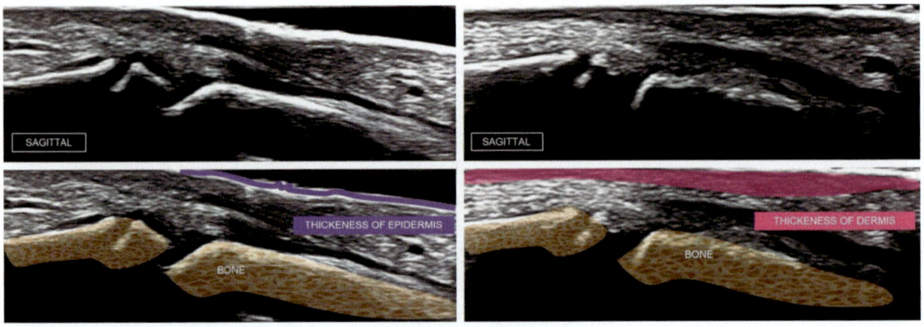

Fig. 13.74 Ultrasonographic findings of pachydermodactyly with a 24 MHz probe (Aplio i800, Canon Medical Systems)

- Increased signal on T1-weighted images may reflect fibrotic changes in the dermis.
- MRI may help identify any associated lesions or complications, such as secondary infections or structural abnormalities.

13.3.9 Rheumatoid Skin Lesions

13.3.9.1 Definition [79]

- Rheumatoid arthritis is a chronic autoimmune disorder characterized by inflammation of the joints. It primarily affects the synovial membrane, leading to joint pain, swelling, stiffness, and eventual destruction of joint cartilage and bone.
- Cutaneous involvement in rheumatoid arthritis includes a variety of skin manifestations, reflecting the systemic nature of the disease. The most common conditions that can be evaluated by imaging modalities is the rheumatoid nodule and the rheumatoid bursitis.

13.3.9.2 Epidemiology [80, 81]

- Rheumatoid Nodules.
  - Seven percent of patients with rheumatoid arthritis.
  - Rheumatoid nodules are found anytime during the disease course in 30 to 40 percent of patients.
- Rheumatoid Bursitis.
  - Approximately 5–10% of individuals with rheumatoid arthritis develop rheumatoid bursitis.
  - Affects bursae near joints commonly involved in RA, such as the shoulders, elbows, hips, and knees.

13.3.9.3 Clinical Presentation (Fig. 13.75) [80, 81]

- Rheumatoid Nodules.
  - Subcutaneous nodules vary from 2 to 5 mm, firm, nontender and most commonly found on pressure points or areas of repeated trauma (olecranon process and other extensor areas such as hands and fingers).
  - Can be painful or disfiguring, interfere with function, or cause compressive neuropathies. The nodules may also ulcerate and may be a site for local infection or other distant infectious complications by hematogenous spread of bacteria.
  - Mainly in patients with positive rheumatoid factor and more severe disease.
- Rheumatoid Bursitis.
  - The most common affected site is the olecraneal bursae.
  - Painful and tender to touch bursae, especially during movement or pressure.
  - Swelling over the affected bursa due to fluid accumulation, associated with erythema and warm temperature.

13.3.9.4 Dermoscopy [21]

- Dermoscopy is mainly used for rheumatoid nodules.
- White structureless areas, linear vessels with or without branches (of unspecific distribution), and brown lines (in reticular distribution).

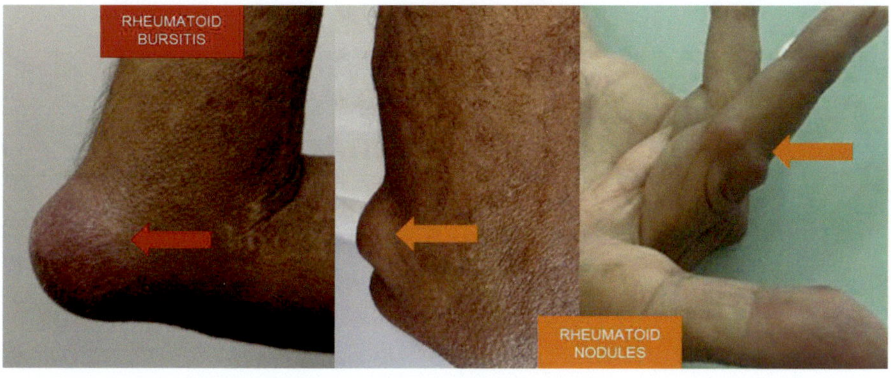

Fig. 13.75 Clinical photograph of patient with olecranon bursitis and rheumatoid nodules

13.3.9.5 Histopathology [80]

- Presence of large nodular areas when compared to granuloma annulare, consisting of palisade granuloma, with rare gigantocytes and presence of central fibrinoid necrosis, characteristically present in the deep dermis or hypodermis.
- They are rarely fully sampled in the punch and can be confused with deep granuloma annulare and rheumatoid pseudonodule, and the correlation with clinical aspects is important.
- Variable presence of neutrophils, secondary vascular changes including thrombosis, lymphocytic infiltrate, and fibrosis may occur.

13.3.9.6 Radiography and Computed Tomography (Fig. 13.76)

- Heterogeneous soft tissue high density adjacent to extensor areas or at the olecraneal bursae.
- Bone erosion has been reported in association with rheumatoid nodules and bursitis.

13.3.9.7 Ultrasonography (Fig. 13.77)

- Rhematoid Nodule.
  - Well-defined hypoechoic mass with hyperechogenic walls, presenting hypoechoic and anechoic areas, reflecting solid or cystic nature.
  - Without power Doppler vascularization.
  - Hypervascularization on power Doppler of the surrounding soft tissue indicating inflammatory process sometimes associated with "panniculitis pattern".

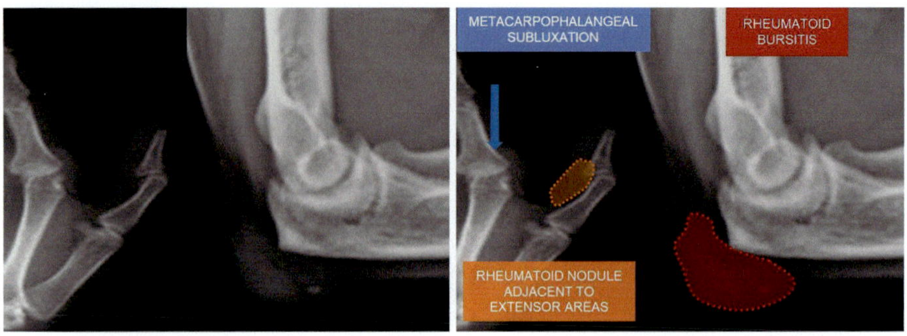

Fig. 13.76 Radiographic findings of olecranon bursitis and rheumatoid nodules (Philips Duo Diagnost R&F Room Digital RF and Tomo System)

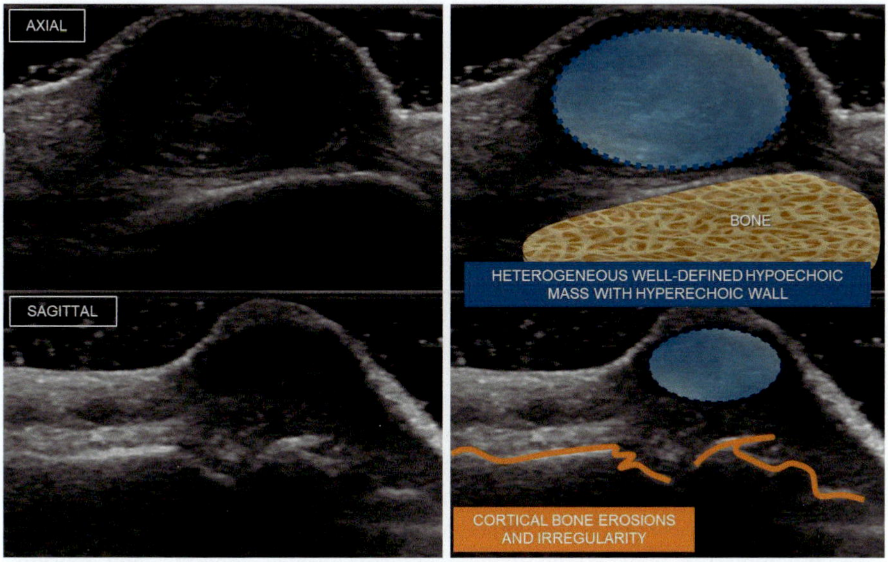

Fig. 13.77 Ultrasonographic findings of olecranon bursitis with a 24 MHz probe (Aplio i800, Canon Medical Systems)

- Rheumatoid Bursitis.
  - Presence of anechoic or hypoechoic fluid within the bursa, indicating fluid accumulation and inflammation.
  - Thickening of the bursal wall, often appearing as hypoechoic or echogenic areas, sometimes with "bodies rice pattern".
  - power Doppler ultrasonography may show increased blood flow in the thickened synovium, indicating active inflammation.
  - Presence of internal echoes or septations within the bursal fluid suggests chronic inflammation or secondary infection.
  - signs of inflammation extending into adjacent tissues, with a "panniculitis pattern".

13.3.9.8 MRI (Fig. 13.78)

- Rheumatoid Nodule.
  - Low to intermediate signal intensity masses on T1-Weighted images and high signal intensity on T2-Weighted images due to the presence of fluid or necrotic material within the nodule.
  - After administration of gadolinium contrast, rheumatoid nodules often enhance, indicating active inflammation or vascularity within the nodule.

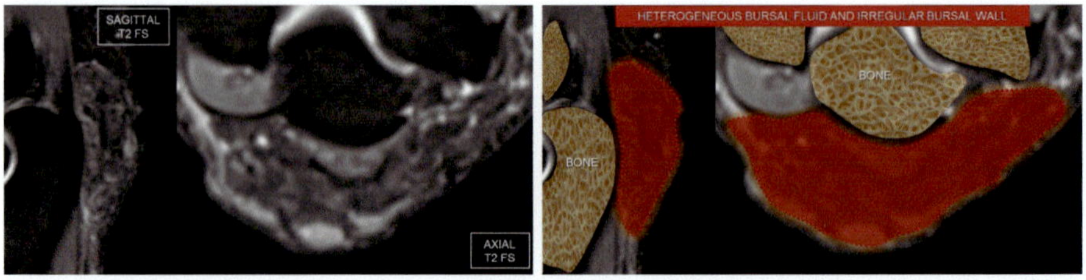

Fig. 13.78 MRI findings of olecranon bursitis on T2 FS-weighted sequence (Magnetom Avanto 1.5T MRI, Siemens)

- Rheumatoid Bursitis.
  - Bursal fluid appears as low signal intensity on T1-Weighted Images and high signal intensity on T2-Weighted Images.
  - Thickened synovium within the bursa appears as intermediate to high signal intensity on T2-weighted images and may enhance with gadolinium contrast.
  - Bursal wall may appear thickened and irregular due to chronic inflammation.
  - Inflammation may extend to adjacent soft tissues, tendons, and muscles, which can be seen as areas of increased signal intensity on T2-weighted images and enhancement post-contrast.

13.3.10 Lymphomatoid Papulosis

13.3.10.1 Definition [82]

- A self-healing recurrent papulonodular skin eruption.
- $CD30^+$ lymphoid proliferation of atypical T cells.

13.3.10.2 Epidemiology [82]

- 1.2 to 1.9 cases per million persons per year.
- No racial predilection.
- Bimodal distribution by sex and age with a male predominance among pediatric cases and female predominance among adult cases.

13.3.10.3 Clinical Presentation (Fig. 13.79) [82, 83]

- Recurrent eruption of nodules and papules, generally smaller than 2 cm, that have a chronic pattern and periods of spontaneous regression. May have pruritus associated with the eruption.

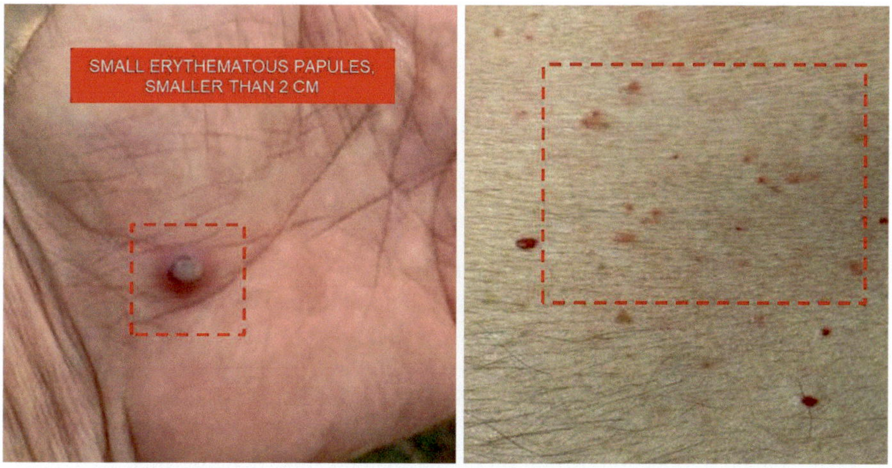

Fig. 13.79 Clinical photograph of patient with lymphomatoid papulosis

- The eruption coexists in different stages of evolution:
  - Early lesions appear as small erythematous or violaceous papules.
  - Evolutes to larger papules or nodules.
  - Develops central hemorrhage, necrosis, and crusting and subsequently disappear in 3–8 weeks.
- Lesions typically occur on the extremities.
- The presence of systemic symptoms, including fever, sweats, weight loss, raises the suspicion of an associated systemic lymphoma.

13.3.10.4 Dermoscopy [84]

- Dermoscopy varies with the different phases of the disease:
  - Initial inflammatory papular lesion: a vascular pattern of tortuous radially disposed irregular vessels surrounded by a white structureless area.
  - Hyperkeratotic papules: The whitish area progressively predominates on the vessels that become less evident.
  - Necrotic ulceration: Replaces the whitish structureless area, with vessels visible only at the extreme periphery of each lesion.

13.3.10.5 Histopathology [83]

- Skin often arose with paleness of the keratinocytes in relation to the surrounding epidermis, presenting wedge-shaped cellular infiltrate composed of atypical T lymphocytes and polymorphous background infiltrate.

- Occur six major patterns:
  - A (mixed infiltrate).
  - B (mycosis fungoides-like).
  - C (anaplastic large cell lymphoma-like).
  - D (cytotoxic T-cell variant).
  - E (angioinvasive variant).
  - F (folliculotropic variant).
- Immunohistochemical examination is typically positive for CD3, CD30 and CD4, negative for CD8, ALK, EMA and cytotoxic markers.

13.3.10.6 Ultrasonography (Fig. 13.80)

- Oval-shaped hypoechoic lesion on epidermis and superficial dermis.
- Hyperechogenic dots and irregularity on the surface of the lesion suggesting hyperkeratotic component.
- Some cases showed hypervascularity on power Doppler.
- Ultrasonography can also evaluate lymph nodes near areas affected by lymphomatoid papulosis, searching for lymph nodes presenting increased size, loss of the characteristic oval shape, echogenic centers, or increased blood flow as visualized by power Doppler, indicating hyperactivity.

13.3.11 Sarcoidosis

13.3.11.1 Definition [85–87]

- Multisystem disease of unknown etiology characterized by the infiltration of various organs by non-necrotizing granulomas.

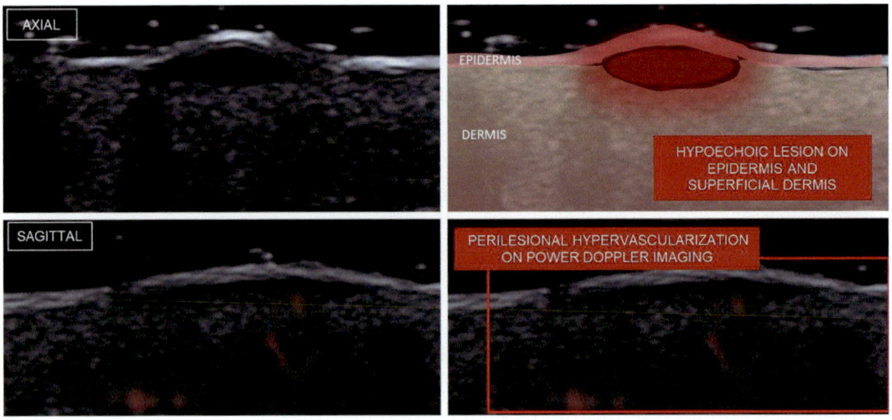

Fig. 13.80 Ultrasonographic findings of lymphomatoid papulosis with a 24 MHz probe (Aplio i800, Canon Medical Systems)

- Predominantly affects the lungs, but the skin is often cited as the second most frequently involved organ.
- The cutaneous manifestations of sarcoidosis are classified as specific and non-specific:
  - Specific skin lesions: Non-caseating granulomas.
  - Nonspecific lesion: Erythema nodosum, characterized histopathologically by panniculitis.

13.3.11.2 Epidemiology [85–87]

- Prevalence of about 2,17 to 160 per 100,000 individuals, and an incidence between 2,3 and 11 per 100,000 individuals per year. Sarcoidosis can occur regardless of ethnicity or age.
- More common in populations of African origin, women and ages between 45 and 65.
- Around 30% of patients with sarcoidosis present with the isolated cutaneous form.

13.3.11.3 Clinical Presentation (Fig. 13.81) [85, 86]

- The most commonly affected organs in sarcoidosis are the lungs and intrathoracic lymph nodes.
- General symptoms are frequent, like fatigue, fever and weight loss.
- The skin lesions may occur in scar tissue, at traumatized sites and around embedded foreign bodies, such as in tattoos.

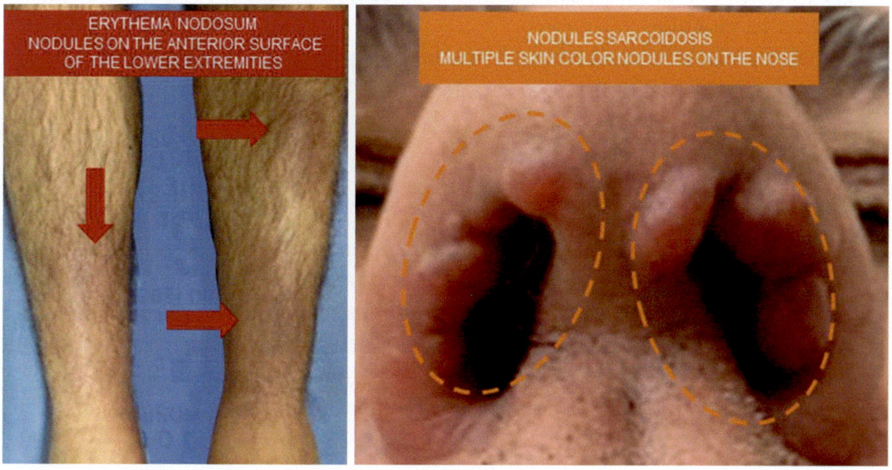

Fig. 13.81 Clinical photograph of patient with sarcoidosis (erythema nodosum and nasal nodules)

- Specific lesions most commonly appear as papules or nodules, but can be multiple erythematous macules, plaques or subcutaneous nodules.
  - Papular sarcoidosis: presents with numerous non scaly papules, can be skin colored, yellow-brown, red-brown, violaceous, or hypopigmented. Most frequently occurs on the face, nasolabial folds and eyelids.
  - Lupus pernio: presents as shiny erythematous or violaceous to blue papules or nodules on the nose, ears or cheeks.
  - Plaque sarcoidosis: often presents with oval or annular, indurated, discrete plaques that are skin colored, erythematous or brown. Most frequently occurs on the shoulders, back, and buttocks.
  - Subcutaneous nodules: is also known as Darier-Roussy sarcoidosis, are usually multiple and painless without overlying erythema. Most frequently occurs on the extremities and trunk.
  - Psoriasiform lesions: is a form of plaque sarcoidosis that presents with well-demarcated, erythematous, scaly plaques that may be clinically indistinguishable from psoriasis.
  - Verrucous sarcoidosis: consist of well demarcated, exophitic, hyperkeratotic plaques.
  - Hypopigmented sarcoidosis: Lesions manifest as hypopigmented, well-demarcated, round to oval macules, patches, or barely raised plaques.
- Erythema nodosum is the most frequent nonspecific cutaneous disorder associated with sarcoidosis. It typically presents as painful, erythematous nodules predominantly found on the anterior surface of the lower extremities.

13.3.11.4 Dermoscopy [88]

- Translucent, round or ovoid, yellowish or reddish-orange, focally or diffusely distributed globules.
- Linear vessels, branching vessels, or arborizing vessels.
- Less common vascular findings are glomerular or dotted structures.

13.3.11.5 Histopathology [28, 86, 89]

- The epidermis is usually normal and may present parakeratosis and acanthosis.
- Epithelioid cell granulomas with little or no lymphocytic crown, forming a histopathological pattern called naked granulomas, which may be restricted to the dermis at any level or extend to the hypoderma (uncommon in granuloma annulare).
- Sarcoid granulomas are well demarcated and have few gigantocytes and no central necrosis.

- Lesions in the late phase present exuberant fibrosis surrounding each granuloma.
- There may be asteroid bodies, a eosinophilic inclusion with an apparent halo around it, or, rarely, Schaumann bodies that are lamellar or concentric calcified inclusions within gigantocytes.

13.3.11.6 Ultrasonography (Fig. 13.82) [90]

- Well-defined lesions in the upper dermis with heterogeneous hypoechogenicity and surrounded by a hyperechoic surrounding edema compressing the adjacent dermis and subcutaneous tissue.
- Hypervascularity on power Doppler.
- "Cobblestone pattern" may be observed, signifying septal involvement and suggesting inflammatory process.

13.3.11.7 MRI (Fig. 13.83)

- Well-defined lesions in the upper dermis with heterogeneous signal intensity surrounded by edema.
- Enhancement after gadolinium administration.
- "Cobblestone pattern" due to septal involvement and suggesting inflammatory process.

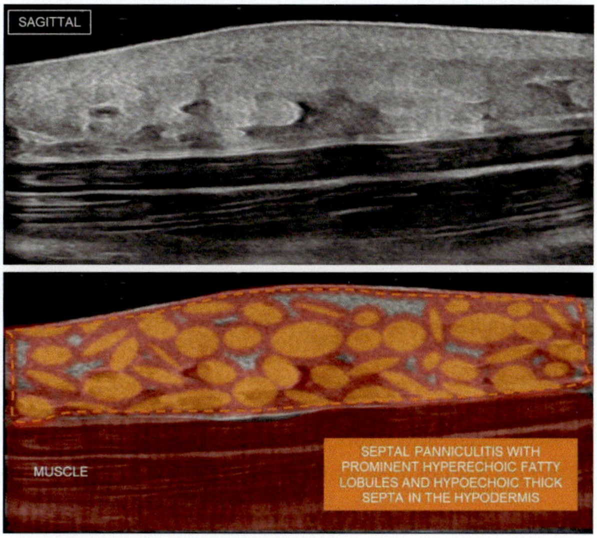

Fig. 13.82 Ultrasonographic findings of erythema nodosum due sarcoidosis with a 24 MHz probe (Aplio i800, Canon Medical Systems)

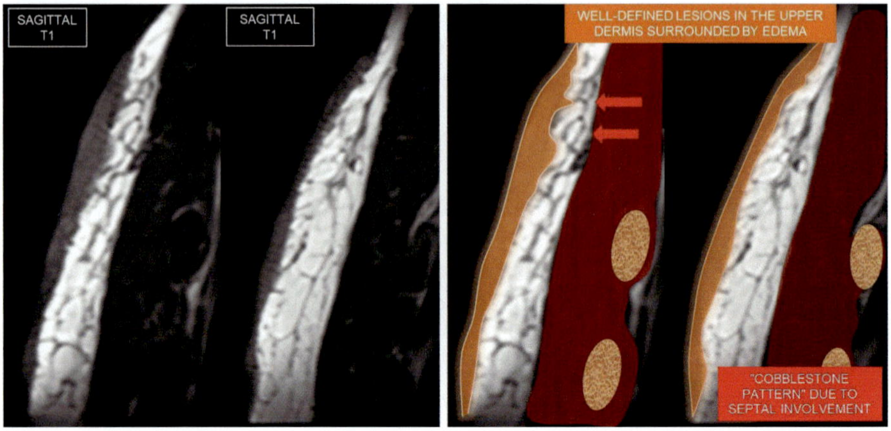

Fig. 13.83 MRI findings of erythema nodosum due sarcoidosis on T1-weighted sequence (Magnetom Avanto 1.5T MRI, Siemens)

13.3.12 Morell-Lavalee Lesion

13.3.12.1 Definition [91, 92]

- Closed degloving injuries associated with severe trauma when the skin and subcutaneous fatty tissue traumatically and abruptly separate from the underlying fascia.
- Hemolymphatic collections on deep to subcutaneous plane due to disruption of capillaries.

13.3.12.2 Epidemiology [92]

- Classically occur over the greater trochanter of the femur, in the thigh.
- Similar biomechanical forces to the lumbar region, scapula and knee can result in identical lesions and are often called Morel-Lavallée-like lesions.

13.3.12.3 Clinical Presentation (Fig. 13.84) [91, 92]

- Painful soft fluctuant area of contour deformity, which may have skin mobility.
- Decreased cutaneous sensation is often associated with the skin over the area of degloving because of shearing injury to the cutaneous nerves.

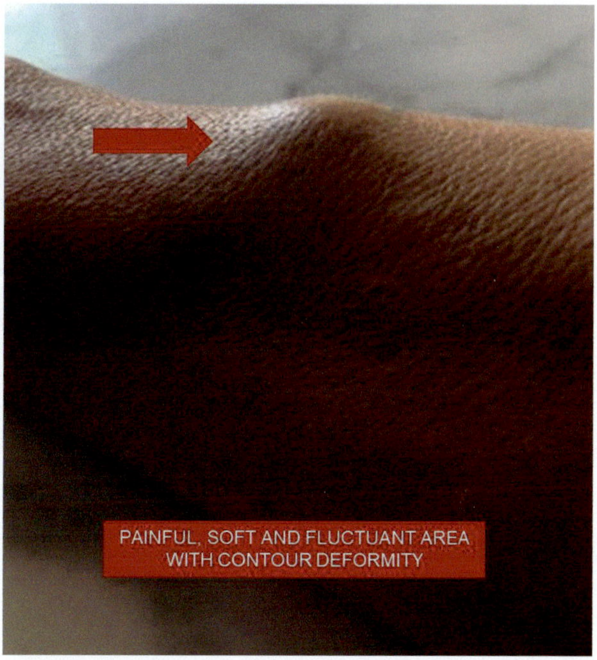

Fig. 13.84 Clinical photograph of patient with Morel–Lavalee lesion

13.3.12.4 Histopathology [92]

- These are liquid collections, seroma, that can induce surrounding fibrosis and are rarely biopsied.

13.3.12.5 Ultrasonography (Fig. 13.85)

- Fluid collections with heterogeneous echogenicity, compressible, without flow on power Doppler:
  - Acute and subacute (less than 1 month) lesions have a heterogeneous appearance with irregular margins and lobular shape, predominantly echogenic.
  - Chronic lesions (older than 18 months) are more often homogeneous with smooth margins and flat or fusiform shape, becoming more hypoechoic as blood products liquefy over time.

13.3.12.6 MRI (Fig. 13.86)

- Fluid collection is of variable signal intensity that even show a fluid-fluid level.
- The age of the blood within the Morel-Lavallée lesion is an essential factor for determining its MRI appearance:
  - Acute stages show T2 hyperintense appearance explained by the fluid and lymph collection that initially develops.

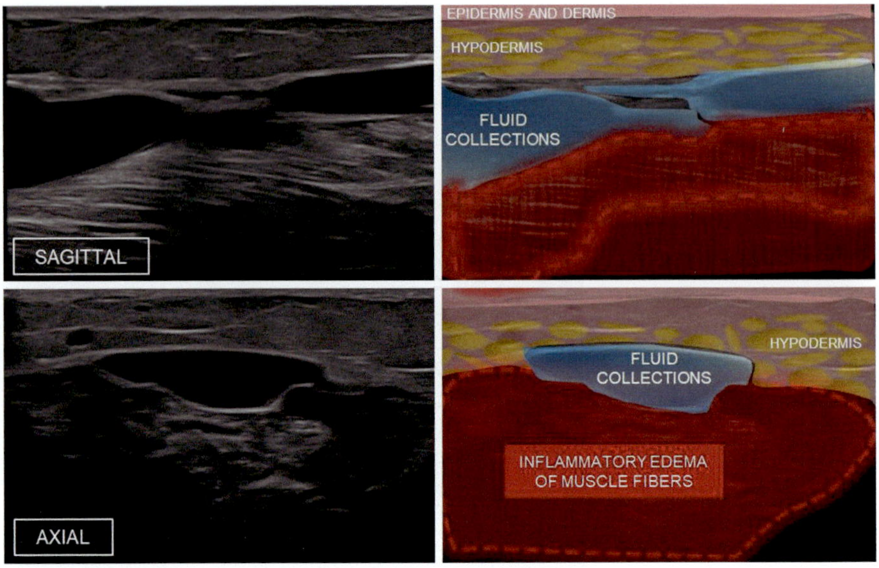

Fig. 13.85 Ultrasonographic findings of Morel–Lavalee lesion with a 24 MHz probe (Aplio i800, Canon Medical Systems)

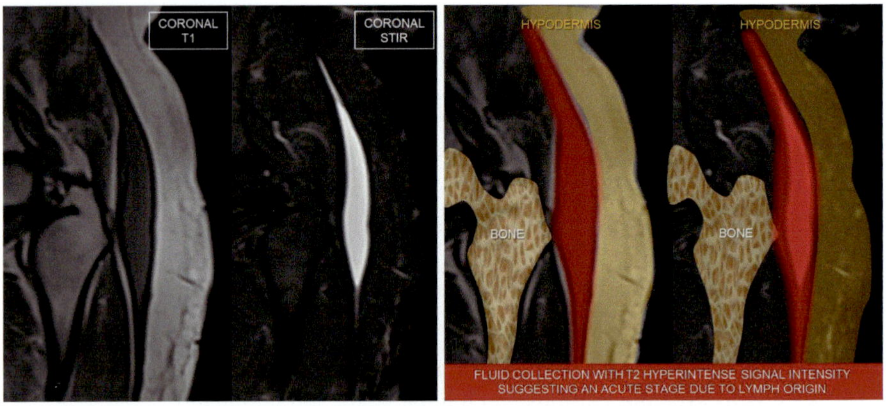

Fig. 13.86 MRI findings of Morel–Lavalee lesion on T1-weighted and STIR sequences (Magnetom Avanto 1.5T MRI, Siemens)

- Subacute stages demonstrate predominantly hypointense on T1-weighted images when comparing to the signal intensity of muscle.
- Chronic stages, hematoma organizes, and deoxyhemoglobin is converted into methemoglobin, which will demonstrate hyperintensity on T1-weighted images.

13.3.13 Livedoid Vasculopathy

13.3.13.1 Definition [93]

- Livedoid vasculopathy is a rare, chronic skin condition characterized by the inflammation and occlusion of small blood vessels, primarily affecting the skin.
- It leads to a distinctive pattern of skin lesions such as painful, violaceous or reddish-brown areas, ulcerations, necrotic areas, and Livedo reticularis.

13.3.13.2 Epidemiology [93]

- The exact prevalence of livedoid vasculopathy is not well established due to its rarity. It is considered an uncommon disorder, and precise epidemiological statistics are lacking.
- Livedoid vasculopathy can occur at any age, but it is most frequently diagnosed in adults. It is less common in children and the elderly.
- There is no strong evidence suggesting a significant gender preference, though some studies and case reports may show a slight female predominance.
- The condition does not appear to have strong geographical or ethnic predilections. However, variations in diagnosis rates and case reporting can influence perceived prevalence in different regions.
- Livedoid vasculopathy is often associated with other systemic conditions, including autoimmune disorders like systemic lupus erythematosus (SLE), antiphospholipid syndrome, and various coagulation disorders. The prevalence of livedoid vasculopathy in these contexts may vary based on the underlying condition.

13.3.13.3 Clinical Presentation (Fig. 13.87) [93]

- These are typically painful, violaceous (purplish) or reddish-brown skin lesions that can evolve into ulcerations or necrotic lesions. They often appear on the lower extremities, especially the legs and ankles.
- Many patients exhibit livedo reticularis, which is a mottled, net-like discoloration of the skin. This pattern is due to the irregular blood flow in the small vessels near the skin's surface.
- Lesions can lead to the development of ulcers. These ulcers are often very painful, persistent and difficult to heal.
- The lesions and ulcers associated with livedoid vasculopathy can be painful, and the pain may be a significant symptom for patients.
- The condition primarily affects the small blood vessels, leading to impaired blood flow and ischemia in the affected areas.
- Livedoid vasculopathy is a chronic condition with lesions that can persist for long periods. It often has a relapsing-remitting course, with new lesions appearing over time.

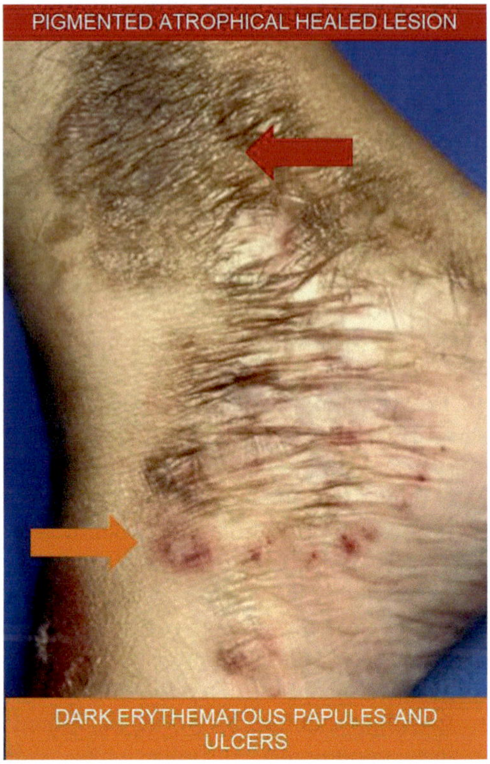

Fig. 13.87 Clinical photograph of patient with livedoid vasculopathy

13.3.13.4 Histopathology [93]

- The most significant finding is the occlusion of small dermal blood vessels. This can be observed as fibrin thrombi within the vessel lumens, leading to impaired blood flow and ischemia.
- There is often associated edema in the dermis surrounding the occluded vessels.
- Mild perivascular inflammatory infiltrate, usually consisting of lymphocytes and sometimes neutrophils, may be present. This inflammation is usually less pronounced compared to other types of vasculitis.
- Fibrinoid necrosis, where fibrin deposits accumulate in the walls of the small blood vessels, may be seen. This is indicative of damage to the vessel walls and is a common feature in various types of vasculitis.
- Changes in the epidermis can include atrophy or hyperkeratosis, often secondary to chronic ischemia and ulceration.
- Areas of hemorrhage and necrosis can be observed in more advanced or chronic lesions, reflecting tissue damage due to prolonged ischemia.

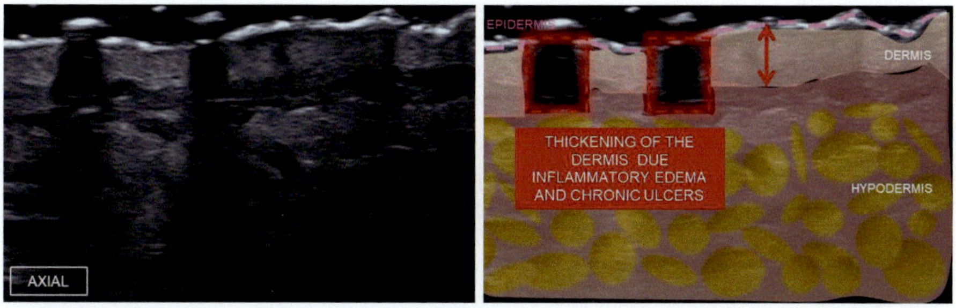

Fig. 13.88 Ultrasonographic findings of livedoid vasculopathy with a 24 MHz probe (Aplio i800, Canon Medical Systems)

13.3.13.5 Ultrasonography (Fig. 13.88)

- Ultrasonography may reveal thickening of the skin due to edema and inflammatory changes in the dermis.
- Power Doppler ultrasonography might show changes in the blood flow within the affected areas such as reduced or altered blood flow in the small vessels, which correlates with the histopathological findings of vessel occlusion.
- There might be evidence of subcutaneous edema or fluid accumulation in the area surrounding the affected lesions.
- If there are chronic ulcers present, ultrasonography can help assess the depth and extent of these ulcers. It may show disruption of the skin layers and involvement of the underlying tissues.

References

1. Niebel D, de Vos L, Fetter T, Brägelmann C, Wenzel J. Cutaneous lupus erythematosus: an update on pathogenesis and future therapeutic directions. Am J Clin Dermatol. 2023;24:521–40.
2. Fijalkowska A, Kadziela M, Zebrowska A. The spectrum of cutaneous manifestations in lupus erythematosus: a comprehensive review. J Clin Med. 2024;13:2419.
3. do Vale ECS, Garcia LC. Cutaneous lupus erythematosus: a review of etiopathogenic, clinical, diagnostic and therapeutic aspects. An Bras Dermatol. 2023;98:355–72.
4. Zychowska M, Reich A. Dermoscopic features of acute, subacute, chronic and intermittent subtypes of cutaneous lupus erythematosus in Caucasians. J Clin Med. 2022;11:4088.
5. Patel J, Borucki R, Werth VP. An update on the pathogenesis of cutaneous lupus erythematosus and its role in clinical practice. Curr Rheumatol Rep. 2020;22:69.
6. Wortsman X. Atlas of dermatologic ultrasound. Cham: Springer International; 2018. https://doi.org/10.1007/978-3-319-89614-4.
7. DeWane ME, Waldman R, Lu J. Dermatomyositis: clinical features and pathogenesis. J Am Acad Dermatol. 2020;82:267–81.
8. Volc-Platzer B. Dermatomyositis—update. Hautarzt. 2015;66:604–10.
9. Dalakas MC, Hohlfeld R. Polymyositis and dermatomyositis. Lancet. 2003;362:971–82.

10. Ashton C, Paramalingam S, Stevenson B, Brusch A, Needham M. Idiopathic inflammatory myopathies: a review. Intern Med J. 2021;51:845–52.
11. Namiki T, Hashimoto T, Hanafusa T, Miura K, Yokozeki H. Case of dermatomyositis with Gottron papules and mechanic's hand: dermoscopic features. J Dermatol. 2018;45:e19.
12. Molina E, Albayda J. Getting under the skin: ultrasound in dermatomyositis. Scand J Rheumatol. 2021;50:497–9.
13. Christen-Zaech S, Hakim MD, Afsar FS, Paller AS. Pediatric morphea (localized scleroderma): review of 136 patients. J Am Acad Dermatol. 2008;59:385–96.
14. De Luca DA, Papara C, Vorobyev A, Staiger H, Bieber K, Thaçi D, et al. Lichen sclerosus: the 2023 update. Front Med. 2023;10:1106318.
15. Hubail R, Karaidi N, Al AA. Idiopathic atrophoderma of Pasini and Pierini: a case report and literature review. Cureus. 2022;14:e26571.
16. Arif T, Fatima R, Sami M. Extragenital lichen sclerosus: a comprehensive review. Australas J Dermatol. 2022;63:452–62.
17. Borghi A, Corazza M, Minghetti S, Bianchini E, Virgili A. Dermoscopic features of vulvar lichen Sclerosus in the setting of a prospective cohort of patients: new observations. Dermatology. 2016;232:71–7.
18. Abbas L, Joseph A, Kunzler E, Jacobe HT. Morphea: progress to date and the road ahead. Ann Transl Med. 2021;9:437.
19. Ihn H. Eosinophilic fasciitis: from pathophysiology to treatment. Allergol Int. 2019;68:437–9.
20. Mertens JS, Seyger MMB, Thurlings RM, Radstake TRDJ, de Jong EMGJ. Morphea and eosinophilic fasciitis: an update. Am J Clin Dermatol. 2017;18:491–512.
21. Slawinska M, Zólkiewicz J, Behera B, Ding DD, Lallas A, Chauhan P, et al. Dermoscopy of inflammatory dermatoses (Inflammoscopy) in skin of color—a systematic review by the International Dermoscopy society "imaging in skin of color" task force. Dermatol Pract Concept. 2023;13:e2023297S.
22. Kaliyadan F, Errichetti E, Lallas A, Swaroop K, Alabdulsalam A. Dermoscopy of idiopathic atrophoderma of Pasini and Pierini. Australas J Dermatol. 2020;61:e120.
23. Pérez-López FR, Vieira-Baptista P. Lichen sclerosus in women: a review. Climacteric. 2017;20:339–47.
24. Chai K, Zhu R, Luo F, Shi Y, Liu M, Xiao Y, et al. Updated role of high-frequency ultrasound in assessing dermatological manifestations in autoimmune skin diseases. Acta Derm Venereol. 2022;102:adv00765. https://medicaljournalssweden.se/actadv/article/view/1969.
25. Castelino M, Eyre S, Barton A. Psoriasis and psoriatic arthritis. In: The microbiome in rheumatic diseases and infection; 2018. p. 239–50.
26. Boehncke W-H, Schön MP. Psoriasis. Lancet. 2015;386:983–94.
27. Griffiths CEM, Armstrong AW, Gudjonsson JE, Barker JNWN. Psoriasis. Lancet. 2021;397:1301–15.
28. Barnhill RL, Neil Crowson A, Magro CM, Piepkorn MW, Kutzner H, Desman GT. Barnhill's dermatopathology. 4th ed. New York: McGraw Hill/Medical; 2019. https://dermatology.mhmedical.com/content.aspx?bookid=2802&sectionid=238125236. Accessed 3 Aug 2024.
29. Yan B-X, Chen X-Y, Ye L-R, Chen J-Q, Zheng M, Man X-Y. Cutaneous and systemic psoriasis: classifications and classification for the distinction. Front Med. 2021;8:649408.
30. Greiling TM, Brown F, Syed HA. Pityriasis Rubra Pilaris. 2024.
31. Kumar S, Vinay K, Radotra B. Dermoscopy of erythrodermic pityriasis rubra pilaris. Indian Dermatol Online J. 2019;10:500.
32. Wang D, Chong VC-L, Chong W-S, Oon HH. A review on Pityriasis Rubra pilaris. Am J Clin Dermatol. 2018;19:377–90.
33. Rogner DF, Lammer J, Zink A, Hamm H. Darier and Hailey-Hailey disease: update 2021. J Dtsch Dermatol Ges. 2021;19:1478–501.
34. Patel TS, Herrera-Martinez M. Darier disease. Mayo Clin Proc. 2021;96:688–9.
35. Pani B, Singh BB. Darier's disease: a calcium-signaling perspective. Cell Mol Life Sci. 2008;65:205–11.

36. Takagi A, Kamijo M, Ikeda S. Darier disease. J Dermatol. 2016;43:275–9.
37. Messersmith L, Krauland K. Pemphigus vegetans [Internet]. Treasure Island, FL: StatPearls; 2024. http://www.ncbi.nlm.nih.gov/pubmed/30983604.
38. Radaschin DS, Laurentiu TA. Pemphigus vegetans. J Cutan Med Surg. 2021;25:443.
39. Lakhmiri M, Maouni S, Znati K, Meziane M, Ismaïli N, Benzekri L, et al. Pemphigus végétant. Ann Dermatol Venereol. 2020;147:78–9.
40. Almuhanna N, Wortsman X, Wohlmuth-Wieser I, Kinoshita-Ise M, Alhusayen R. Overview of ultrasound imaging applications in dermatology [formula: see text]. J Cutan Med Surg. 2021;25:521–9. https://pubmed.ncbi.nlm.nih.gov/33682489.
41. Engin B, Kutlubay Z, Çelik U, Serdaroglu S, Tüzün Y. Hailey-Hailey disease: a fold (intertriginous) dermatosis. Clin Dermatol. 2015;33:452–5.
42. Mandava A, Ravuri PR, Konathan R. High-resolution ultrasound imaging of cutaneous lesions. Indian J Radiol Imaging. 2013;23:269–77.
43. Sabat R, Jemec GBE, Matusiak L, Kimball AB, Prens E, Wolk K. Hidradenitis suppurativa. Nat Rev Dis Primers. 2020;6:18. https://www.nature.com/articles/s41572-020-0149-1.
44. Ballard K, Shuman VL. Hidradenitis Suppurativa. Treasure Island, FL: StatPearls; 2024. http://www.ncbi.nlm.nih.gov/pubmed/34057384.
45. Jemec GBE. Hidradenitis Suppurativa. N Engl J Med. 2012;366:158–64. https://doi.org/10.1056/NEJMcp1014163.
46. Goldburg SR, Strober BE, Payette MJ. Hidradenitis suppurativa. J Am Acad Dermatol. 2020;82:1045–58. https://linkinghub.elsevier.com/retrieve/pii/S0190962219328270.
47. Wortsman X. Imaging of Hidradenitis suppurativa. Dermatol Clin. 2016;34:59–68. https://linkinghub.elsevier.com/retrieve/pii/S0733863515000996.
48. Lopes AA, Moraes GN, Dias BMMDL, Souza GD, De Souza LQ. Preoperative imaging assessment of hidradenitis suppurativa. Rev Bras Cir Plást. 2019;34:264–7. https://doi.org/10.5935/2177-1235.2019RBCP0143.
49. Fernandez JM, Rizvi OH, Marr KD, Hendricks AJ, Maarouf M, Price KN, et al. Topography of lesion progression in hidradenitis suppurativa. Int J Dermatol. 2021;60:e323–5. http://www.ncbi.nlm.nih.gov/pubmed/33369730.
50. Der Sarkissian S, Frew JW. Ultrasound-guided de-roofing of epithelialised tunnels of hidradenitis suppurativa. Aust J Dermatol. 2021;62:360–3. https://doi.org/10.1111/ajd.13600.
51. Elkin K, Daveluy S, Avanaki K. Review of imaging technologies used in hidradenitis suppurativa. Skin Res Technol. 2020;26:3–10. https://doi.org/10.1111/srt.12772.
52. Hessam S, Scholl L, Sand M, Schmitz L, Reitenbach S, Bechara FG. A novel severity assessment scoring system for hidradenitis suppurativa. JAMA Dermatol. 2018;154:330–5.
53. Kelly AM, Cronin P. MRI features of hidradenitis suppurativa and review of the literature. AJR Am J Roentgenol. 2005;185:1201–4. http://www.ncbi.nlm.nih.gov/pubmed/16247134.
54. Nazzaro G, Calzari P, Vaienti S, Passoni E, Marzano AV. The role of imaging technologies in the diagnosis of hidradenitis suppurativa. Clin Dermatol. 2023;41:611–21. https://linkinghub.elsevier.com/retrieve/pii/S0738081X23001025.
55. Gil LA, Deans KJ, Minneci PC. Management of pilonidal disease. JAMA Surg. 2023;158:875.
56. Rosin D. Pilonidal disease: keep it simple! Isr Med Assoc J. 2022;24:120.
57. Nixon AT, Garza RF. Pilonidal cyst and sinus continuing education activity. In: StatPearls [Internet]. Treasure Island, FL: StatPearls; 2024. https://www.ncbi.nlm.nih.gov/books/NBK557770/?report=printable.
58. Gilchrist H, Patterson JW. Erythema nodosum and erythema induratum (nodular vasculitis): diagnosis and management. Dermatol Ther. 2010;23:320–7.
59. Pérez-Garza DM, Chavez-Alvarez S, Ocampo-Candiani J, Gomez-Flores M. Erythema Nodosum: a practical approach and diagnostic algorithm. Am J Clin Dermatol. 2021;22:367–78.
60. Miteva M, Romanelli P, Kirsner RS. Lipodermatosclerosis. Dermatol Ther. 2010;23:375–88.
61. Kirsner RS, Pardes JB, Eaglstein WH, Falanga V. The clinical spectrum of lipodermatosclerosis. J Am Acad Dermatol. 1993;28:623–7.

62. Demitsu T, Okada O, Yoneda K, Manabe M. Lipodermatosclerosis—report of three cases and review of the literature. Dermatology. 1999;199:271–3.
63. Hodak E, David M, Sandbank M. Semicircular lipoatrophy-a pressure-induced lipoatrophy? Clin Exp Dermatol. 1990;15:464–5.
64. Ángel-Ortega AO, Sierra-Santos L. Lipoatrofia semicircular: 3 casos clínicos. Semergen. 2017;43:154–5.
65. Ogino J, Saga K, Tamagawa M, Akutsu Y. Magnetic resonance imaging of semicircular lipoatrophy. Dermatology. 2004;209:340–1.
66. Nasr H, Scriven JM. Superficial thrombophlebitis (superficial venous thrombosis). BMJ. 2015;350:h2039.
67. Czysz A, Higbee SL. Superficial thrombophlebitis continuing education activity [Internet]. https://www.ncbi.nlm.nih.gov/books/NBK556017/?report=printable.
68. Comarmond C, Cacoub P. Granulomatosis with polyangiitis (Wegener): clinical aspects and treatment. Autoimmun Rev. 2014;13:1121–5.
69. Jennette JC, Falk RJ, Bacon PA, Basu N, Cid MC, Ferrario F, et al. 2012 Revised International Chapel Hill consensus conference nomenclature of vasculitides. Arthritis Rheum. 2013;65:1–11.
70. Ramos LO, Mattos PC, de Figueredo GLP, Maia AAA, Romero SAR. Pre-tibial myxedema: treatment with intralesional corticosteroid. An Bras Dermatol. 2015;90:143–6.
71. Cohen B, Cadesky A, Jaggi S. Dermatologic manifestations of thyroid disease: a literature review. Front Endocrinol. 2023;14:14.
72. Rodríguez-Garijo N, Tomás-Velázquez A, Estenaga A, Antoñanzas J, Segurado-Rodríguez MA, García-Tobar L, et al. Granuloma annulare subtypes: sonographic features and clinicopathological correlation. J Ultrasound. 2022;25:289–95.
73. Pellicano R, Caldarola G, Filabozzi P, Zalaudek I. Dermoscopy of necrobiosis Lipoidica and granuloma Annulare. Dermatology. 2013;226:319–23.
74. Errichetti E, Lallas A, Apalla Z, Di Stefani A, Stinco G. Dermoscopy of granuloma Annulare: a clinical and histological correlation study. Dermatology. 2017;233:74–9.
75. Joshi TP, Duvic M. Granuloma Annulare: an updated review of epidemiology, pathogenesis, and treatment options. Am J Clin Dermatol. 2022;23:37–50.
76. Elangovan S, Tan YK. The role of musculoskeletal ultrasound imaging in rheumatoid arthritis. Ultrasound Med Biol. 2020;46:1841–53.
77. do Vale LRG, Coeli FR, Michalany N, Hassun KM, Porro AM. Paquidermodactilia transgressiva: relato de um caso. An Bras Dermatol. 2009;84:190–3.
78. Chamberlain AJ, Venning VA, Wojnarowska F. Pachydermodactyly: a forme fruste of knuckle pads? Australas J Dermatol. 2003;44:140–3.
79. Sayah A, English JC. Rheumatoid arthritis: a review of the cutaneous manifestations. J Am Acad Dermatol. 2005;53:191–209.
80. Highton J, Hessian PA, Stamp L. The rheumatoid nodule: peripheral or central to rheumatoid arthritis? Rheumatology. 2007;46:1385–7.
81. Chua-Aguilera CJ, Möller B, Yawalkar N. Skin manifestations of rheumatoid arthritis, juvenile idiopathic arthritis, and Spondyloarthritides. Clin Rev Allergy Immunol. 2017;53:371–93.
82. Martinez-Cabriales SA, Walsh S, Sade S, Shear NH. Lymphomatoid papulosis: an update and review. J Eur Acad Dermatol Venereol. 2020;34:59–73.
83. Nowicka D, Mertowska P, Mertowski S, Hymos A, Forma A, Michalski A, et al. Etiopathogenesis, diagnosis, and treatment strategies for Lymphomatoid papulosis with particular emphasis on the role of the immune system. Cells. 2022;11:3697.
84. Piccolo V, Russo T, Agozzino M, Vitiello P, Caccavale S, Alfano R, et al. Dermoscopy of cutaneous lymphoproliferative disorders: where are we now? Dermatology. 2018;234:131–6.
85. Ezeh N, Caplan A, Rosenbach M, Imadojemu S. Cutaneous sarcoidosis. Dermatol Clin. 2023;41:455–70.
86. Mañá J, Marcoval J. Skin manifestations of sarcoidosis. Presse Med. 2012;41:e355–74.

87. Moore SL, Teirstein AE. Musculoskeletal sarcoidosis: spectrum of appearances at MR imaging. Radiographics. 2003;23:1389–99.
88. Errichetti E, Stinco G. Dermatoscopy of granulomatous disorders. Dermatol Clin. 2018;36:369–75.
89. Hubail A, Belkharoeva R, Tepluk N, Belerosova T. Lupus pernio (Besnier-Tenneson syndrome). A rare form of sarcoidosis. Dermatol Rep. 2018;10:7696.
90. Dybiec E, Pietrzak A, Bartosinska J, Kieszko R, Kanitakis J. Ultrasound findings in cutaneous sarcoidosis: report of a case. Adv Dermatol Allergol. 2015;1:51–5.
91. Bonilla-Yoon I, Masih S, Patel DB, White EA, Levine BD, Chow K, et al. The Morel-Lavallée lesion: pathophysiology, clinical presentation, imaging features, and treatment options. Emerg Radiol. 2014;21:35–43.
92. Molina BJ, Ghazoul EN, Janis JE. Practical review of the comprehensive management of Morel-Lavallée Lesions. Plast Reconstr Surg Glob Open. 2021;9:e3850.
93. Leeolou MC, Rieger KE, Yeh JE. Livedoid vasculopathy. Dermatol Online J. 2023;29.
94. Chan CC, Yang CY, Chu CY. Magnetic resonance imaging as a diagnostic tool for extensive lipodermatosclerosis. J Am Acad Dermatol. 2008 Mar;58(3):525–7. https://doi.org/10.1016/j.jaad.2006.08.068.
95. Wortsman X. Update on ultrasound diagnostic criteria and new ultrasound severity and activity scorings of hidradenitis suppurativa: modified SOS-HS and US-HSA. J Ultrasound Med. 2024;43(1):207–13. https://doi.org/10.1002/jum.16351).

Chapter 14
Clinical, Imaging, and Histological Findings in Infectious Lesions of Trunk and Limbs

Ana Luisa Sampaio, Camila Silveira Nobre, Ludmila do Valle Vieira Gusmão, André da Silva Cartell, Tatiana Venâncio Nakamura, Simone Guarçoni, Glauber Voltan, Manuela Boleira Sieiro Guimarães, Marcia Castilho Farme de Amoedo, Alejandra Galeano España, Ana Paula Stutz, Curt Mafra Treu, and Clarissa Canella Moraes do Carmo

14.1 Viral Warts

14.1.1 Definition [1–4]

- Cutaneous and mucosal epithelial proliferations are caused by various types of Human Papillomavirus (HPV).
- There are over 200 distinct HPV subtypes, some tend to infect specific body sites:
  - HPV type 1 commonly infects the soles of the feet and produces plantar wart.
  - HPV types 6 and 11 infect the anogenital area.

A. L. Sampaio
Department of Dermatology, Hospital Universitario Pedro Ernesto, Universidade Estadual do Rio de Janeiro—UERJ, Rio de Janeiro, Brazil

C. S. Nobre
State University of Rio de Janeiro—UERJ, Hospital Universitario Pedro Ernesto, Rio de Janeiro, RJ, Brazil

L. do Valle Vieira Gusmão
Marcilio Dias Naval Hospital, Dermatological Imaging Department of DASA - Rio de Janeiro, Rio de Janeiro, Brazil

A. da Silva Cartell
Adjunct Professor at Faculdade de Medicina da Universidade Federal do Rio Grande do Sul, Rio de Janeiro, Brazil

Dermatologist and Dermatopathologist in Private Practice, Rio de Janeiro, Brazil

T. V. Nakamura
Instituto Humanizare in Juína, Juína, Brazil

S. Guarçoni
Clinica ALTA—Botafogo, Rio de Janeiro, Brazil

© The Author(s), under exclusive license to Springer Nature Switzerland AG 2025

C. Canella Moraes do Carmo (ed.), *Atlas of Diagnostic Imaging in Dermatology*, https://doi.org/10.1007/978-3-031-77987-9_14

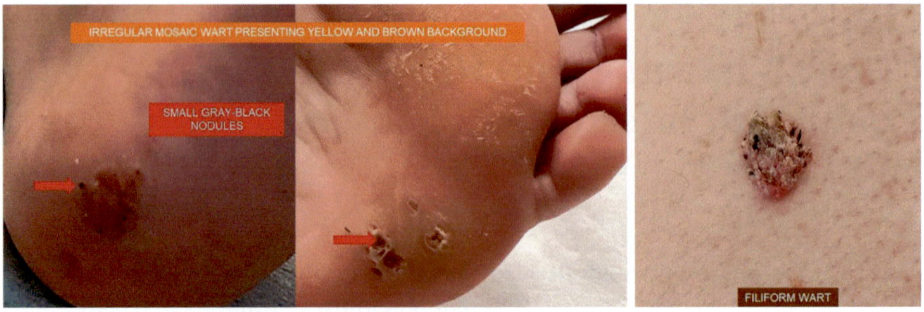

Fig. 14.1 Clinical photograph of patients with viral warts

14.1.2 Epidemiology [2, 4, 5]

- Cutaneous warts are most commonly observed in children and young adults.
- Certain occupations, such as handlers of meat, poultry, and fish, demonstrate a higher prevalence of cutaneous warts.

14.1.3 Clinical Presentation (Fig. 14.1) [2, 3, 5]

- Cutaneous warts may manifest as:
  - Common warts (verruca vulgaris)
  - Plantar warts (verruca plantaris)
  - Flat (plane) warts (verruca plana).

G. Voltan
Instituto Humanizare in Juína, NervUS Project, Juína, Brazil

M. B. S. Guimarães
The Dermatology Department at Policlinica Geral do Rio de Janeiro, Rio de Janeiro, Brazil

M. C. F. de Amoedo
Private Dermatology Practice, Rio de Janeiro, Brazil

A. G. España
Clinica Dermobarra, Rio de Janeiro, Brazil

A. P. Stutz
Department of Radiology, Universidade Federal Fluminense—UFF, Centro, Niterói, Brazil

C. M. Treu
Department of Dermatologic Surgery and Cutaneous Oncology, Policlinica Geral do Rio de Janeiro (PGRJ), Hospital Federal de Bonsucesso, Rio de Janeiro, Brazil

C. Canella Moraes do Carmo (✉)
Fluminense Federal University—UFF, Rio de Janeiro, Brazil

Federal University of Rio de Janeiro—UFRJ, Rio de Janeiro, Brazil

Diagnóstico das Américas—DASA—RJ, Rio de Janeiro, Brazil

Biodesign Laboratory, DASA-PUC, Rio de Janeiro, Brazil

- Cutaneous warts are also described based upon location and morphology (filiform or mosaic warts), usually presenting sharply demarcated, rough, round or irregular, firm, and light gray, yellow, brown, or gray-black nodules 2–10 mm in diameter.
- Warts may occur singly, in groups, or as coalescing warts forming plaques. Mosaic warts are coalescing plantar warts.

14.1.4 Dermoscopy (Fig. 14.2) [6]

- Dermoscopy of common warts exhibits the "frogspawn" pattern, which is the aspect of thrombosed vessels in the center of a papillomatous area.
- Flat warts (verruca plana) have dotted or globular vessels with regular distribution on a yellowish-brown background.
- Plantar warts demonstrated blackish dots with irregular distribution on the surface, which means dilated and thrombosed capillaries.

14.1.5 Histopathology (Fig. 14.3) [7]

- Epithelial hyperplasia with acanthosis and papillomatosis.
- Parakeratosis columns on the upward projections of the rete ridges.
- Vacuolated epidermal cells in the granular layer and upper spinous layer are called koilocytes.
- Larger, irregular, and hyperchromatic atypical nuclei may be binucleation.
- Presence of eosinophilic granulations (viral inclusion bodies) in the early lesions.
- Hypergranulosis with keratohyaline granules larger and larger, resembling a charcoal stone.

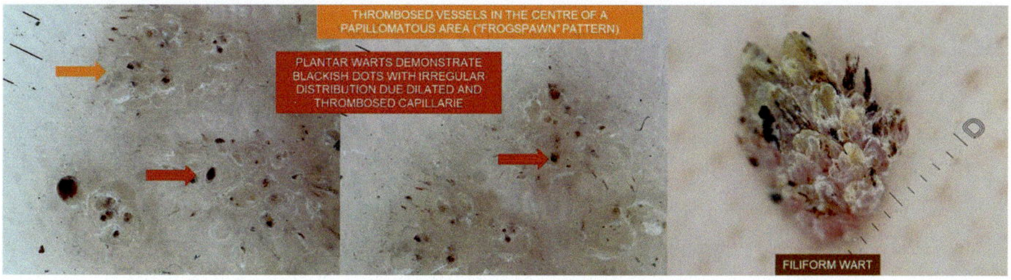

Fig. 14.2 Dermoscopic findings in patients with viral warts (x10 and x20)

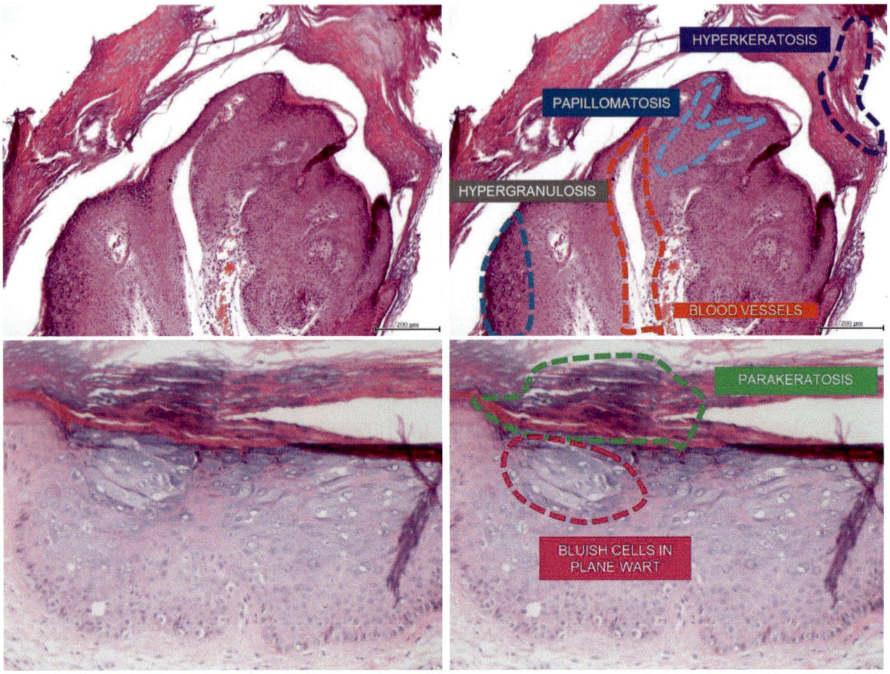

Fig. 14.3 Histological findings of viral warts (H&E x10 and x20)

- Interpapillary cones converging toward the center of the lesion are called collarette.
- Dilated or ectatic and tortuous capillaries in the papillary derma. There may be thrombosis of the superficial vessels and intracorneal hemorrhage, clinically appearing as black dots and chronic.
- Superficial perivascular and nonspecific inflammatory infiltrate.

14.1.6 Ultrasonography (Figs. 14.4 and 14.5) [8]

- Well-defined and hypoechoic lesion with a fusiform and exophytic morphology in epiderms and dermis.
- May present spots of posterior acoustic shadowing due to hyperkeratosis areas
- Prominent SLEB can also be identified due to inflammatory process.
- Often demonstrate hypovascularity, but painful and active warts tend to exhibit prominent blood flow.

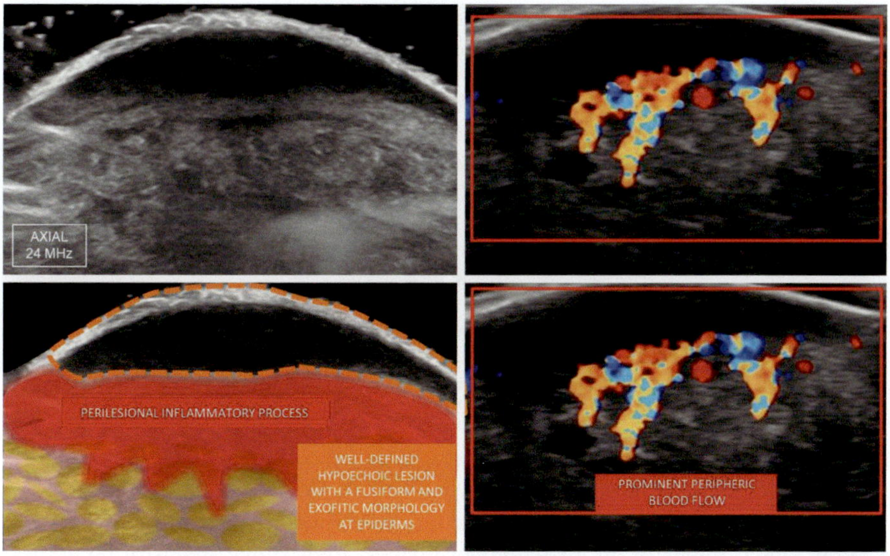

Fig. 14.4 Ultrasonographic images of viral warts with 24 MHz probe (Aplio i800, Canon Medical Systems)

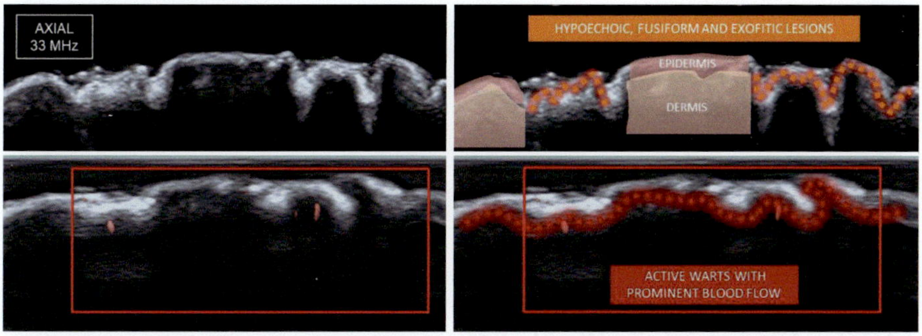

Fig. 14.5 Ultrasonographic findings of viral warts with 33 MHz probe (Aplio 1800, canon Medical Systems)

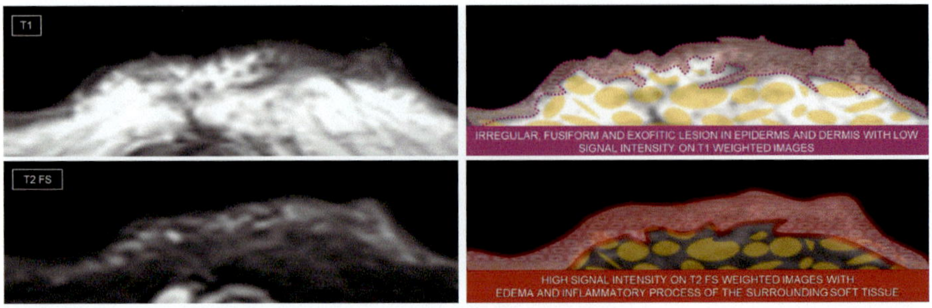

Fig. 14.6 MRI findings of viral warts on axial T2 FS and T1-weighted sequences (Magnetom Prisma 3T MRI, Siemens)

14.1.7 MRI (Fig. 14.6)

- Well-defined, fusiform, and exophytic lesion in epiderms and dermis.
- Low signal intensity on T1-weighted images, high signal intensity on T2-FS-weighted images, and variable contrast enhancement.
- Edema and inflammatory process of the surrounding soft tissue.

14.2 Cutaneous Histoplasmosis

14.2.1 Definition [4, 9, 10]

- Histoplasmosis is a systemic mycosis caused by the dimorphic fungus Histoplasma capsulatum.

14.2.2 Epidemiology [9, 11, 12]

- The infection predominantly affects men between the fourth and fifth decades of life [1, 2].
- Most patients who develop the disease have a history of immunosuppression, of which more than 90% are associated with HIV infection [1, 2].
- Histoplasmosis has a worldwide distribution, with high endemicity in the Ohio and Mississippi river valleys (USA) and most parts of Latin America [1, 2].

14.2.3 Clinical Presentation (Fig. 14.7) [9–12]

- There are three possible clinical forms of histoplasmosis: acute pulmonary, chronic cavitary, and disseminated disease. Cutaneous manifestations occur in the disseminated form, which is the most severe [1].
- Skin lesions predominantly result from secondary skin invasion by hematogenic dissemination, but they may also occur due to traumatic inoculation of the fungus into the skin [1, 3].
- Skin lesions are highly polymorphic, and may manifest with umbilicated papules, plaques, nodules, erosions, ulcers, and acneiform eruptions. Ulcerated mucosal lesions can occur in up to 1/3 of cases [1, 3, 4].

14.2.4 Histopathology [11, 13]

- Agent: Histoplasma capsulatum.
- Presentation in two forms, anergic as histiocytic infiltrate and classic granulomatous reactive form in immunocompetent patient
- Tendency to ulcerate the epiderma, often arranged around hair follicles, mimicking necrotizing acne.
- Diffuse mixed dermal inflammatory infiltrate without gigantocytes in immunocompromised patients with a predominance of foamy histiocytes and few leukocytoclastic neutrophils around.
- Numerous intracellular spores with 2–4 (2–4 μm) and discrete mucopolysaccharide capsule form a clear halo around the spores; the spores may be protruded on phase microscopy (lower the entire condenser of the microscope).

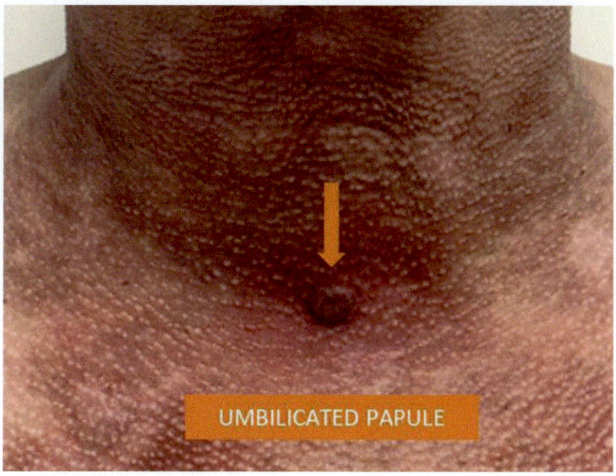

Fig. 14.7 Clinical photograph of patients with histoplasmosis showing a raised, round lesion with a central depression

14.2.5 Radiography and Computed Tomography [4]

- Findings are unspecific.
- Soft tissue thickening.
- Obliteration of fat planes surrounding the joints.

14.2.6 Ultrasonography (Fig. 14.8) [4]

- Although the findings are not specific, they help assess changes in affected skin layers, identify foreign bodies and abscesses, and exclude musculoskeletal involvement.
- The affected areas may exhibit heterogeneous increased echogenicity, with hypoechoic regions intermingled with adipose tissue, indicating peripheral reactional panniculitis.
- Fluid collections in the surrounding tissue may also be observed, as well as complications such as arthritis and bone destruction.

14.2.7 MRI (Fig. 14.9) [4]

- MRI is essential for detecting the extension of the infection into deep soft tissues and identifying complications such as arthritis, osteomyelitis, embolic endovascular involvement, and myositis.

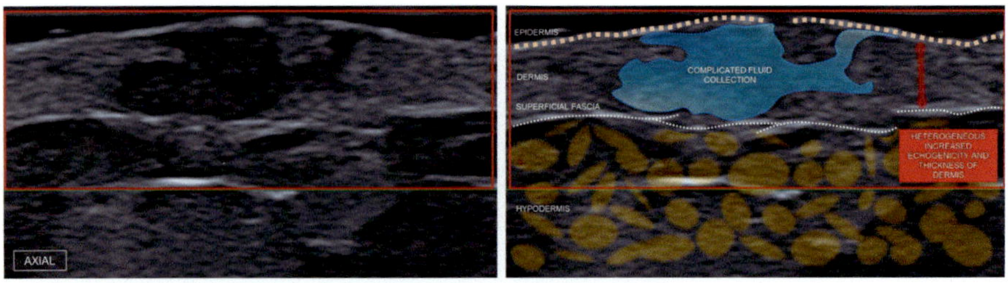

Fig. 14.8 Ultrasonographic findings of histoplasmosis with 24 MHz probe (Aplio i800, Canon Medical Systems)

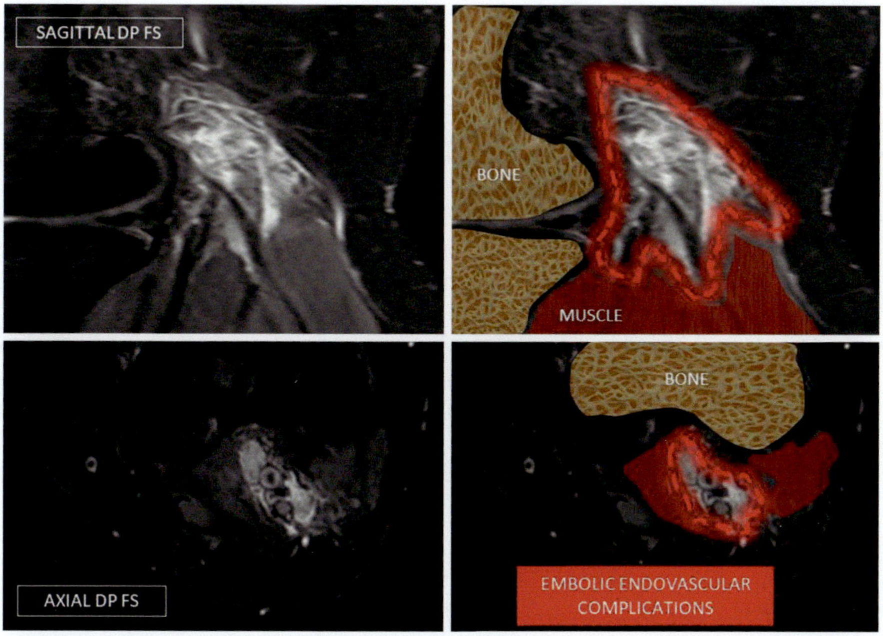

Fig. 14.9 MRI findings of an embolic complication of histoplasmosis on sagittal and axial DP FS weighted sequence (Magnetom Avanto 1.5T MRI, Siemens)

- The affected cutaneous areas may show nonspecific heterogeneous thickening of the dermis and hypodermis with high signal intensity on T2 FS sequences, indicating an inflammatory origin, and may be associated with collections, abscesses, and fistula tracts.

14.3 Sporotrichosis

14.3.1 Definition [14, 15]

- Sporotrichosis is a subacute or chronic infection, caused by a thermodimorphic fungi of the genus Sporothrix.
- The traditional route of infection is traumatic inoculation via plant thorns and decaying wood. Zoonotic transmission, especially from infected cats, and fungal conidial inhalation from the environment are other routes of infection.
- Infection usually involves cutaneous and subcutaneous tissues but can occasionally occur in other sites.

14.3.2 Epidemiology [14–17]

- It is the most common subcutaneous mycosis across the globe, and it is caused by dimorphic fungi belonging to the genus Sporothrix.
- The epidemiological profile is mainly characterized by children, elderly, and women.
- In Brazil, there are two important disease transmission routes for humans, a sapronotic route involving direct contact with the soil and decomposing organic matter; and a zoonotic route, in which felines participate actively in the disease transmission.
- In Asia, especially China, *S. globosa* is estimated to be the etiological agent in 99.3% of the human sporotrichosis cases. In other endemic areas, such as Australia and South Africa (94%), also in North America and part of South America (89%), *S. schenckii* is the predominant species. In the South and Southeast Brazilian regions, *S. brasiliensis* (88%) is the main etiological agent of human and animal sporotrichosis.

14.3.3 Clinical Presentation (Fig. 14.10) [14, 16, 18, 19]

- Sporotrichosis was classified in the following forms:
  - Lymphocutaneous form: Initially, the lesion has a papulonodular appearance where the fungus was introduced into the skin, appearing between two to four

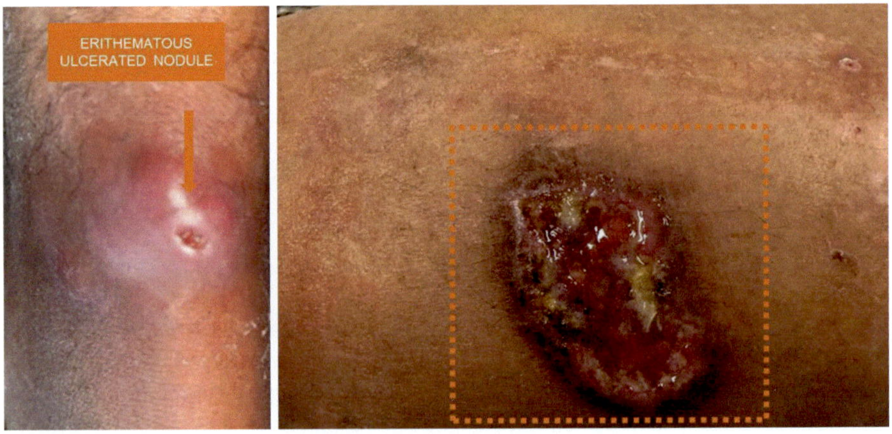

Fig. 14.10 Clinical photograph of patients with sporotrichosis

weeks after the trauma. Afterward, the lesion may ulcerate, and fistulize draining a purulent discharge. This is so-called the inoculation chancre. The lesions, usually nodules, progress along the regional lymphangitic channels, upwards or downwards depending on the anatomical site. Later, these nodules may ulcerate, fistulize, and heal, characterizing a gumma.

- Fixed cutaneous form: Consists of a single lesion, usually similar to the inoculation chancre, with no regional lymphatic spreading. Some patients exhibit multiple skin lesions, disseminated on the tegument, with no systemic invasion.
- Mucous membrane: Any mucous membrane may be affected by sporotrichosis, the ocular mucosa is more commonly involved, causing conjunctivitis, episcleritis, uveitis, choroiditis, and retrobulbar lesions, among others.
- Multifocal disease is most likely to occur in immunosuppressed patients, including patients living with the human immunodeficiency virus (PLHIV), transplant recipients, patients receiving corticosteroids or tumor necrosis factor antagonists, alcoholism, or diabetes.

14.3.4 Dermoscopy (Fig. 14.11) [20, 21]

- Orange-yellow background with erythema corresponding to the dermal granuloma with inflammation, hemorrhages, yellowish crusts, white structureless areas showing dermal scarring, superficial ulcerations, scaling, and polymorphic vessels.

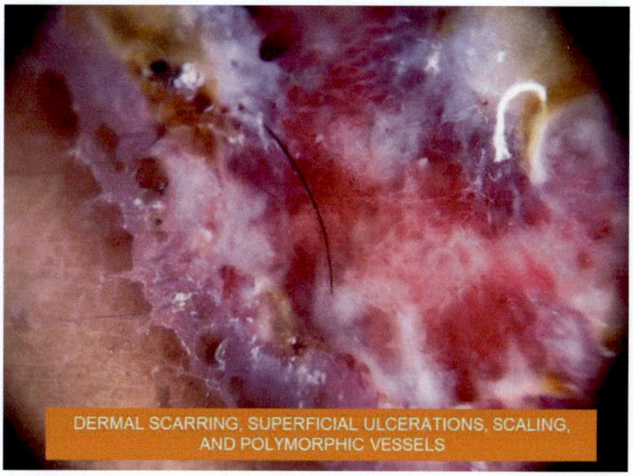

Fig. 14.11 Dermoscopic findings in patients with sporotrichosis (x20)

- Yellow tears have been described specifically for the facial lesions and correspond to follicular plugs due to compression of follicular openings from the lesional growth.
- Scattered yellowish-orange areas corresponding to the dermal granulomas.
- Yellowish-orange areas are not specific for cutaneous sporotrichosis and are a finding described generously in various granulomatous dermatoses.

14.3.5 Histopathology (Fig. 14.12) [13]

- Agent: Sporothrix sp., a dematiaceous fungus, i.e., expressing melanic pigmentation (see table).
- It often presents with pseudoepithelial hyperplasia.
- May present with intraepidermal neutrophilic microabscesses.
- There may be ulceration and gum formation clinically forming a rosario pattern.
- Presence of a very variable dermal inflammatory infiltrate, which may exhibit neutrophils, lymphocytes, histiocytes, plasma cells, and Langhans gigantocytes in variable amounts; Suppurative granulomas are generally rare, unlike other deep granulomatous mycoses, and are located in the upper or middle dermis.
- Fungal spore-rich forms occur more in acute infections, commonly seen in veterinarians.
- Spores that are very scarce or even absent in the sections, best visualized in the HE, oval or cigar-shaped and brownish in color, called fumagoid bodies, measuring between 1 and 2 μm in diameter.

14.3.6 Radiography and Computed Tomography

- Soft tissue thickening.
- Obliteration of fat planes surrounding the joints.

14.3.7 Ultrasonography (Fig. 14.13) [4]

- Ultrasonography is the initial imaging modality of choice for evaluating sporotrichosis.

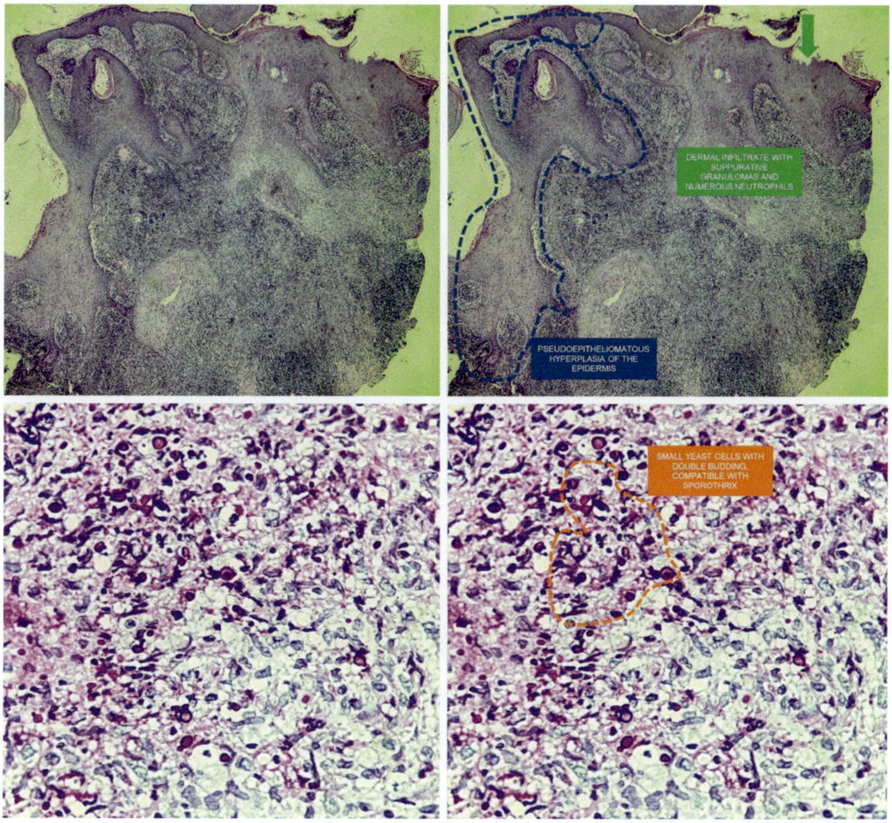

Fig. 14.12 Histological findings of sporotrichosis (H&E x4 and x40)

- Although the findings are not specific to sporotrichosis, but help assess changes in affected skin layers, identify foreign bodies and abscesses, and exclude musculoskeletal involvement.
- The affected areas may exhibit heterogeneous increased echogenicity, with hypoechoic regions intermingled with adipose tissue, indicative of peripheral reactional panniculitis. This pattern may correspond to the dilation of lymphatic vessels seen in lymphocutaneous involvement of sporotrichosis

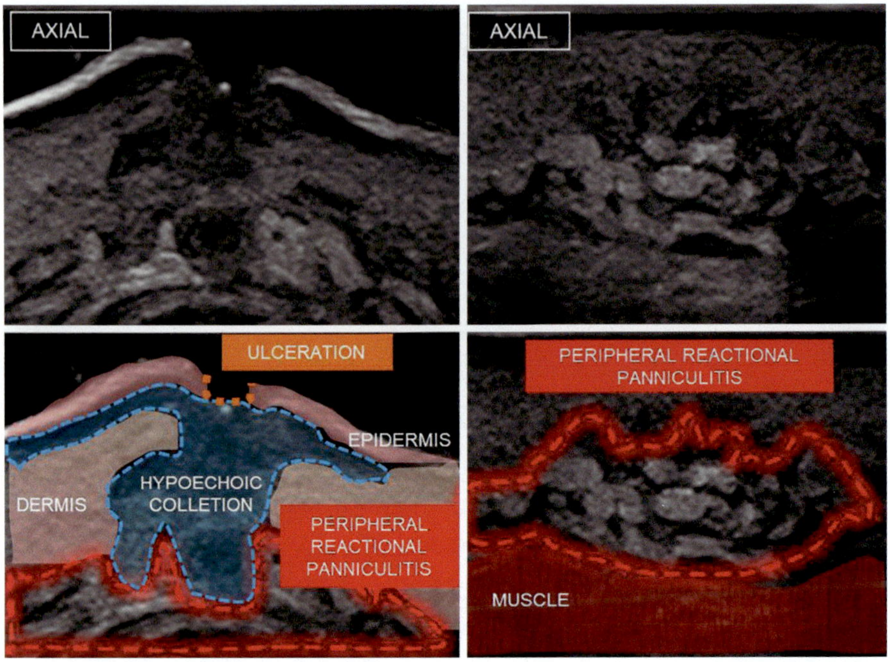

Fig. 14.13 Ultrasonographic findings of sporotrichosis with 24 MHz probe (Aplio i800, Canon Medical Systems)

14.3.8 MRI (Fig. 14.14)

- MRI plays a vital role in identifying the extension of infection into deep soft tissues and diagnosing complications like arthritis, osteomyelitis, embolic endovascular involvement, and myositis.
- Areas of affected skin may show nonspecific thickening of the dermis and hypodermis with high signal intensity on T2 FS sequences, suggesting an inflammatory origin, often accompanied by collections, abscesses, and fistula tracts.

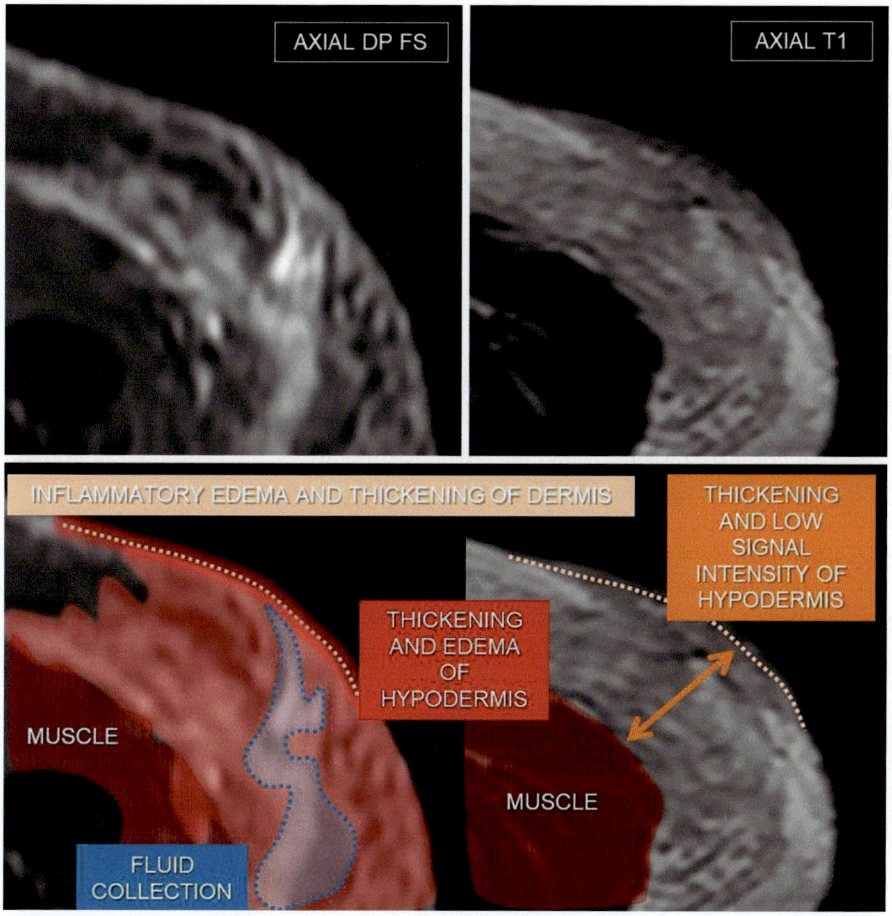

Fig. 14.14 MRI findings of sporotrichosis on axial DP FS and T1-weighted sequences (Magnetom Avanto 1.5T MRI, Siemens)

14.4 Cutaneous Leishmaniasis

14.4.1 Definition [22–24]

- Leishmania is a vector-borne, obligate intracellular, protozoan parasite, family Trypanosomatidae, causing cutaneous, mucocutaneous, and visceral disease in the Old and New World.

14.4.2 Epidemiology [22, 23]

- While likely underreported, current estimates of cutaneous leishmaniasis incidence range from 700,000 to 1.2 million cases per year with approximately 95% of cases occurring in the Americas, the Mediterranean basin, the Middle East, and Central Asia.

14.4.3 Clinical Presentation (Fig. 14.15) [22–24]

- Mucocutaneous leishmaniasis: Leishmania causes a spectrum of cutaneous diseases.
  - Mucosal leishmaniasis and leishmaniasis recidivans are caused by oligoparasitic disease associated with a marked cellular immune response.
  - Diffuse cutaneous leishmaniasis is caused by polyparasitic disease with a predominance of parasitized macrophages and no granulomatous inflammation.
  - The center of the spectrum consists of localized cutaneous leishmaniasis, which is the most common clinical presentation. It consists of cutaneous lesions on exposed areas of the skin. It begins as a pink-colored papule that enlarges and develops into a nodule or plaque-like lesion leading to a painless ulceration with an indurated border.
- Visceral leishmaniasis (VL): The infection can be asymptomatic or symptomatic infection.
  - Asymptomatic infection—Many leishmanial infections are asymptomatic, reflecting the ability of the host immune system to control the parasite. Despite this, one can develop reactivation disease if immunosuppression occurs.

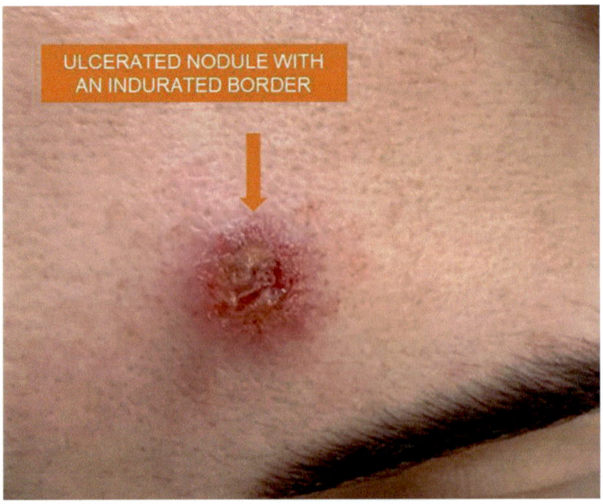

Fig. 14.15 Clinical photograph of patients with leishmaniasis showing an ulcerated nodule with an indurated border

– Symptomatic infection—The most important clinical manifestation of VL is the syndrome known as kala-azar (Hindi for "black fever"). Onset of symptoms is usually insidious or subacute, with slow progression of malaise, fever, weight loss, and splenomegaly (with or without hepatomegaly) over a period of months. Less frequently, acute febrile illness can occur with rapidly progressive symptoms. Post-kala azar dermal leishmaniasis: Skin lesions (always starts on face) 6 months following VL.

14.4.4 Dermoscopy (Fig. 14.16) [24, 25]

- Most frequently in cutaneous leishmaniasis: Generalized erythema and vascular structures (irregular linear, hairpin, coma, and arborizing vessels) almost constantly, followed by a white starburst-like pattern (between 58.3–87%), yellow tears (41.7–75%) and central hyperkeratosis (33.3–35.3%).
- Other findings: Presence of yellowish hue, central ulcerations, and millium pseudocysts that appear as small yellowish-white circular structures.

14.4.5 Histopathology [13]

- Normal, atrophic, or hyperplastic epidermis is irregularly shaped and may even present pseudoepitheliomatous hyperplasia, or ulcerated.
- They occur most often in the deep derma.
- Mixed dermal inflammatory infiltrate consisting mainly of histiocytes with variable amounts of lymphocytes, plasma cells, neutrophils, and eventually multinucleated giant cells. It has clear histiocytes surrounded by small mature lymphocytes, a histopathological pattern called a clearing of Montenegro or a macrophage clearing.

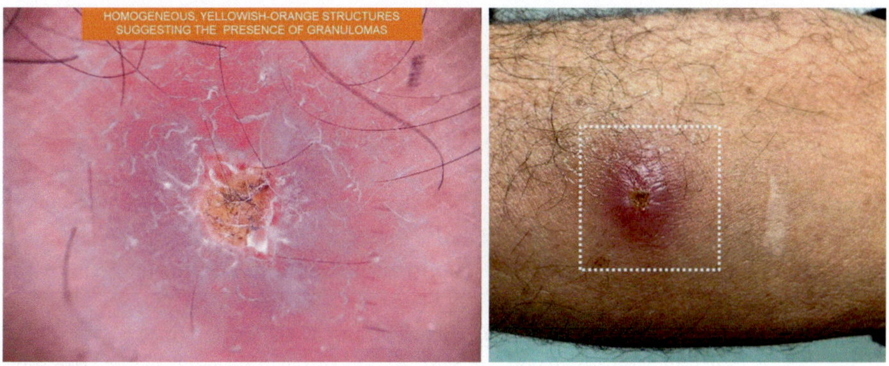

Fig. 14.16 Dermoscopic findings in patients with leishmaniasis (x10)

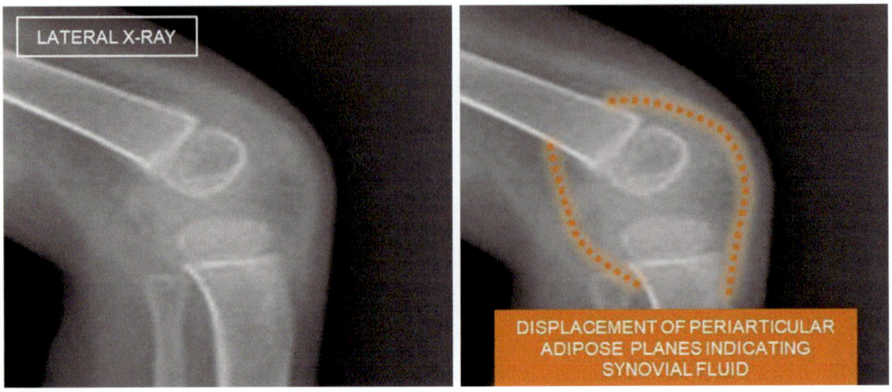

Fig. 14.17 Radiographic findings of articular leishmaniasis (Philips Duo Diagnost R&F Room Digital RF and Tomo System)

- It usually does not present central necrosis in the inflammatory process.
- Swollen stroma with vascular proliferation and/or ectasia and fibrosis in later lesions.
- Intracytoplasmic organisms (amastigotes) in histiocytes, measuring between 1 and 2 μm, to be seen under immersion at 1000-fold magnification, with a nucleus and a paranucleus, also called quinethoplast; are best visualized by Giemsa's coloring.

14.4.6 Radiography and Computed Tomography (Fig. 14.17)

- Soft tissue thickening.
- Obliteration of fat planes surrounding the joints.

14.4.7 Ultrasonography (Fig. 14.18) [8, 26, 27]

- Although the findings are not specific, they assist in evaluating changes in affected skin layers, identifying foreign bodies and abscesses, and ruling out musculoskeletal involvement.
- The affected areas might show heterogeneous increased echogenicity, with hypoechoic thickening, peripheral reactional panniculitis, ruptured areas of the hypodermis, and fistulae.
- Fluid collections in the surrounding tissue, along with perilesional hypervascularization, may also be observed, as well as complications such as arthritis and bone destruction.

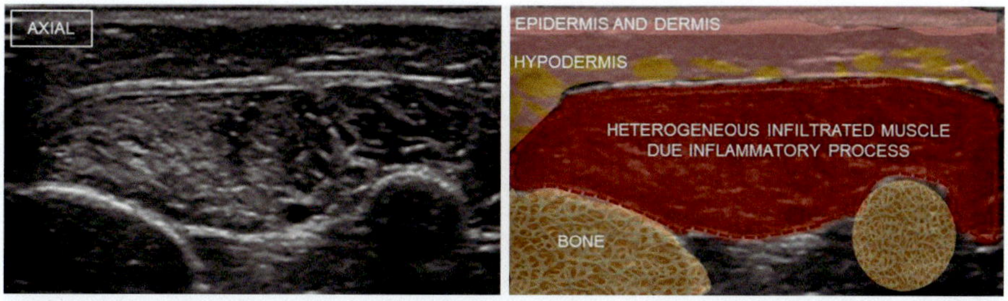

Fig. 14.18 Ultrasonographic findings of cutaneous leishmaniasis with 24 MHz probe (Aplio i800, Canon Medical Systems)

14.4.8 MRI (Fig. 14.19)

- MRI is crucial for identifying the spread of infection into deep soft tissues and diagnosing complications such as arthritis, osteomyelitis, embolic endovascular involvement, and myositis.
- Affected skin areas may display nonspecific thickening of the dermis and hypodermis with high signal intensity on T2 FS sequences, indicating an inflammatory origin, often associated with collections, abscesses, and fistula tracts.

14.5 Tuberculosis

14.5.1 Definition [28–30]

- Indolent infection caused by *Mycobacterium tuberculosis*.
- The cutaneous tuberculosis (CTB) can be categorized into multibacillary and paucibacillary forms.

14.5.2 Epidemiology [29]

- Approximately one-third of cutaneous tuberculosis is associated with systemic involvement.
- In total, 1.5–3% of all extrapulmonary cases are CTB.
- HIV is a predisposing factor to the disease (and also the coinfection TB and HIV addresses to more severe disease, higher mortality, and drug resistance).

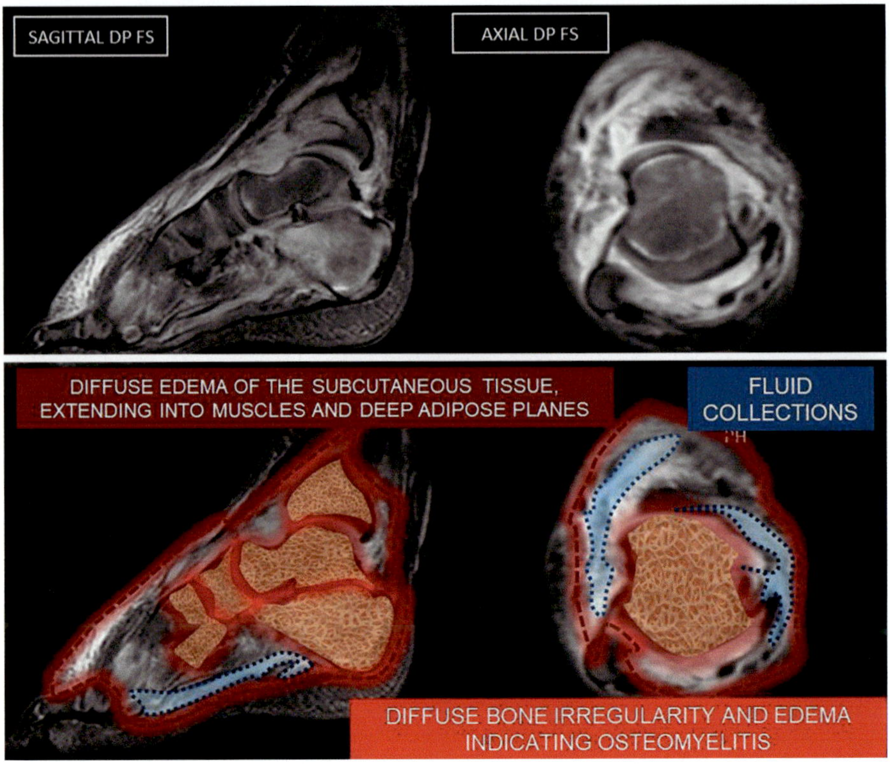

Fig. 14.19 MRI findings of articular leishmaniasis on sagittal and axial DP FS sequences (Magnetom Avanto 1.5T MRI, Siemens)

14.5.3 Clinical Presentation (Fig. 14.20) [28–30]

- CTB can vary depending on the route of infection and the host immunity.
- Primary cutaneous inoculation on the host with no prior exposure leads to tuberculous chancre; and if the host has good immunity, he can develop TB verrucosa cutis.
- If the source of inoculation is hematogenous, the patient can have lupus vulgaris or TB gumma.
- The contiguous infection leads to scrofuloderma and contiguous or autoinoculation to orificial TB.
- Lesions caused by hypersensitivity reaction (lichen scrofulosorum, erythema induratum of Bazin, and papulonecrotic tuberculid) will not be discussed in this chapter.

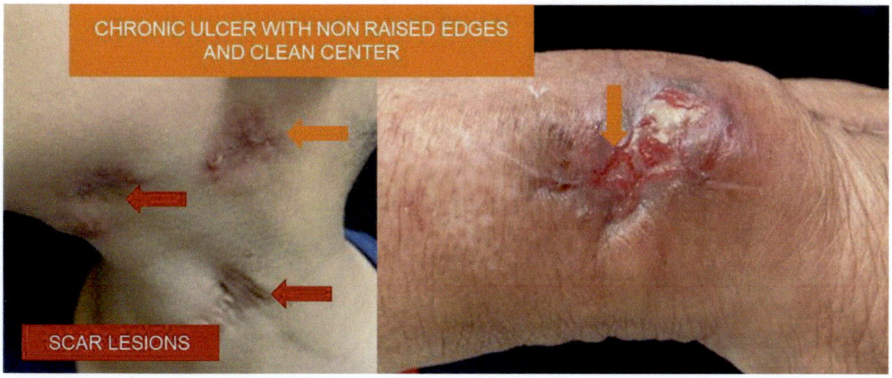

Fig. 14.20 Clinical photograph of patients with tuberculosis lesions at cervical and arm regions (Images courtesy from Prof, Luna Azulay)

14.5.4 Dermoscopy [31]

- Lupus vulgaris has yellow-orange structureless areas that represent the epithelioid granulomas seen in histopathology. Linear vessels and focal white scales are also present.
- Scrofuloderma: Linear vessels with and without branches, white structureless areas, and yellow-orange structureless areas.
- Tuberculosis verrucosa cutis: Dirty white thick scales with a papillated surface that resembles common warts.

14.5.5 Histopathology [13]

- It has a generally hyperplastic and ulcerated epidermis.
- Presence of a granulomatous component with caseification and the characteristic tuberculoid pattern in immunocompetent patients, showing a thick lymphocytic crown.
- The atypical and anergic forms present many leukocytoclastic neutrophils, extensive necrosis of the fibrinoid pattern, dystrophic calcification (quite common in Boruli ulcer) and are markedly rich in bacilli in AFB research. Tuberculosis in immunocompromised patients tends to present with a lot of necrosis, foamy histiocytic infiltrate, or little inflammatory infiltrate.
- The reactional forms show classical tuberculoid granulomas in the derma and hypodermis, different from granulomatous deep mycoses.
- The intensity of mycobacteria is inversely related to the ability to develop granulomas, which is valid for all infectious granulomatous lesions.
- Presence of fibrosis in late lesions.

14.5.6 Radiography and Computed Tomography [4, 8]

- Soft tissue thickening.
- Obliteration of fat planes surrounding the joints.
- In case of dactilitis:
  - Lytic lesion of the phalanx associated with bone expansion.
  - Trabecular destruction.
  - Cortical thinning.
  - Similar to an inflated balloon = "spina ventosa."

14.5.7 Ultrasonography (Fig. 14.21) [4]

- High-frequency ultrasonography can show a hypoechoic, hypodermic structure, containing prominent echogenic foci and posterior enhancement.
- Furthermore, HFUS can reveal dermics sinus tracts with or without hyperechoic content, due to the caseous material.
- Additionally, there is perilesional hypervascularization upon evaluation with power Doppler.

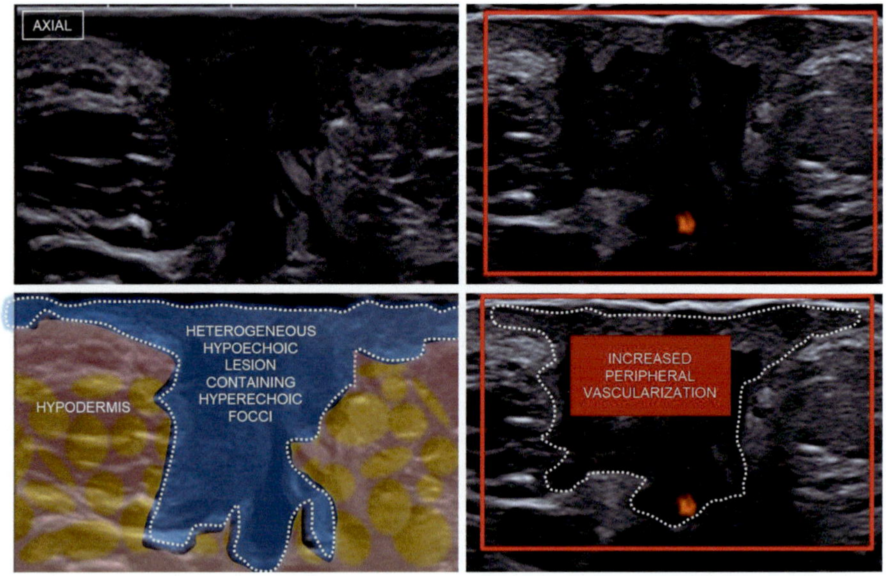

Fig. 14.21 Ultrasonographic findings of tuberculosis with 24 MHz probe (Aplio i800, Canon Medical Systems)

14.5.8 MRI

- MRI plays a critical role in identifying the extension of infection into deep soft tissues and diagnosing complications such as arthritis, osteomyelitis, embolic endovascular involvement, and myositis.
- Affected skin areas may exhibit nonspecific thickening of the dermis and hypodermis with high signal intensity on T2 FS sequences, suggesting an inflammatory origin and frequently accompanied by collections, abscesses, and fistula tracts.

14.6 Leprosy

14.6.1 Definition [32, 33]

- Chronic infectious disease caused by the bacterium *Mycobacterium leprae*.
- Primarily affects the skin, peripheral nerves, upper respiratory tracts, and eyes.

14.6.2 Epidemiology [34]

- According to the World Health Organization (WHO), as of 2019, there were 176,176 new cases reported globally.
- Brazil, India, and Indonesia are the countries with the highest number of cases.
- The disease is most prevalent in tropical and subtropical regions, particularly in areas with inadequate healthcare and subpar living conditions. It is more common in rural areas than urban areas.
- Transmission is thought to occur through respiratory droplets from close and prolonged contact with untreated individuals who have the disease.

14.6.3 Clinical Presentation (Figs. 14.22, 14.23, and 14.24) [33]

- Tuberculoid hanseniasis (TT)
  - Paucibacillary, predominant Th-1 immune response, BAAR: negative, Mitsuda: positive.
  - Features: well-circumscribed skin lesions (reddish, erythematous plaques) with numbness. The initial loss is thermal and posterior tactil and pain. The last symptom is deep pressure hypoesthesia. The lesions present with elevated edges, and there may be a loss of pigmentation or hair in the affected areas. Nerve involvement is usually limited.

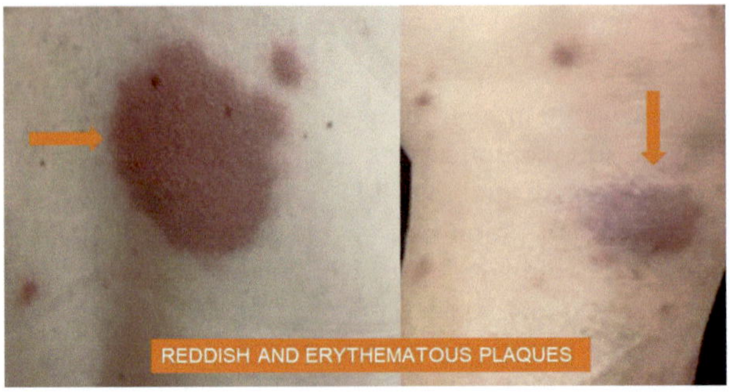

Fig. 14.22 Clinical photograph of patients with erythematous plaques from leprosy

Fig. 14.23 Clinical photograph of patients with ear infiltration from leprosy

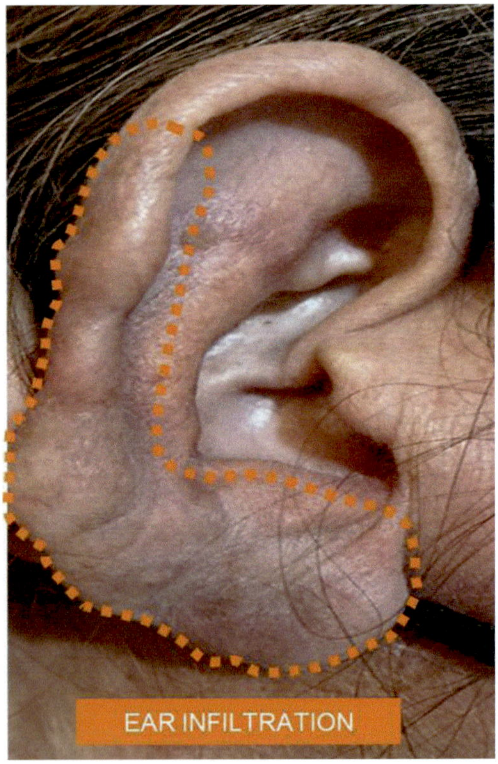

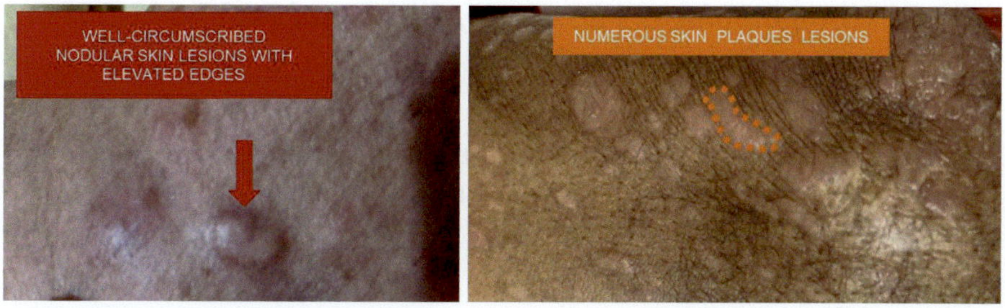

Fig. 14.24 Clinical photograph of patients with cutaneous nodular and plaque lesions

- Borderline tuberculoid (BT):
  - Intermediate immune response.
  - This form lies between TT and the mid-spectrum forms.
  - Skin lesions are larger plaques and more numerous when compared to TT.
  - Nerve involvement is more frequent.
- Borderline borderline (BB):
  - Intermediate form. The immune response is less intense when compared to TT and BT forms.
  - Skin lesions are more widespread.
  - Nerve involvement is significant, leading to sensory and motor impairments, muscle weakness, and deformities.
- Borderline lepromatous (BL):
  - Skin lesions become more widespread and prominent.
  - Poorly defined, irregularly shaped, and may be occasionally nodular.
- Lepromatous leprosy:
  - The more severe and widespread form.
  - Predominant Th-2 immune response.
  - Multibacillary form. BAAR: positive; Mitsuda: negative
  - Skin involvement is marked by numerous skin lesions, nerve damage, and potential disfigurement.
  - The skin lesions are usually marked by nodules, plaques, and infiltration, which can lead to classic late findings like the leonine facies and madarosis.
  - Lepromatous leprosy can affect various organs, including the eyes, nose, and respiratory tract.

14.6.4 Histopathology (Figs. 14.25, 14.26, and 14.27) [13, 35]

- Indeterminate:
  - Granulomas are undeveloped or consist of few cells with preserved epidermis.
  - Discrete and nonspecific chronic inflammatory infiltrate, sometimes periadnexal and perineural.
  - Perineural and perieccrine lymphocytic infiltrate.
- Tuberculoid:
  - Presence of non-caseifying granulomas (necrosis is uncommon in leprosy), with a sarcoid pattern with a tendency to stay along the cutaneous nerves and the erector pili muscle, eccrine glands, or vessels, as if forming cords, giving a rosary-like appearance by confluence.
  - Injury to the erector pili muscle, when present, favors the diagnosis of tuberculoid leprosy.

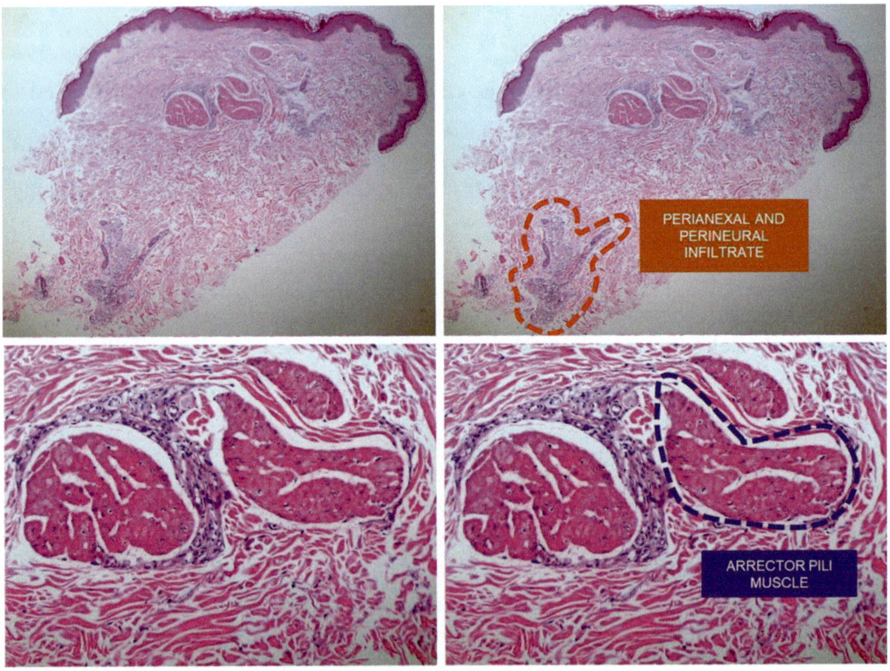

Fig. 14.25 Histological findings of indeterminate leprosy (H&E x4 and x20)

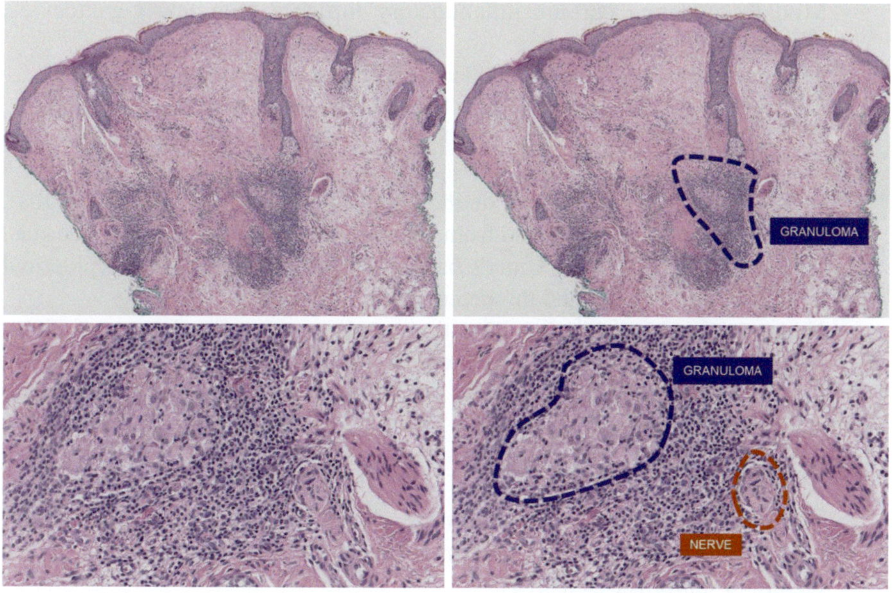

Fig. 14.26 Histological findings of tuberculoid leprosy (H&E x4 and x20)

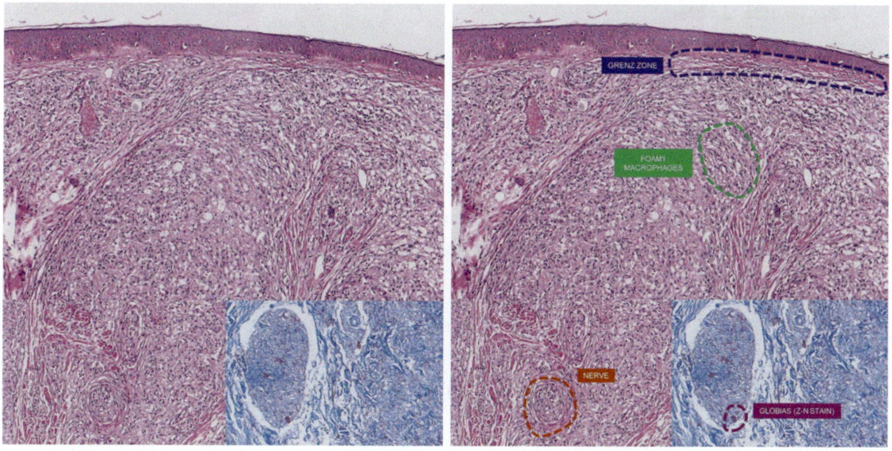

Fig. 14.27 Histological findings of lepromatous leprosy (H&E x10 and Ziehl Neelsen x100)

- Mild to moderate chronic inflammatory infiltrate with few gigantocytes, absence of the Grenz zone.
- May be fibrous and lamellar thickening of the nerve sheaths.
- Bacilli research usually shows few fragmented-looking bacilli.

- Lepromatous diffuse infiltrate
  - Predominating foamy cells (xanthomatous histiocytes or Virchow cells), without granulomas, separated from the epiderma by a spared band of dermis, also called grenz zone or Unna's band, appearing as a narrow subepidermal hyaline band, rectified and thinned epiderma.
  - Numerous acid-resistant bacilli with strongly positive Fite-Faraco or Ziehl-Neelsen staining, sometimes grouped into globias.
  - Can present prominent fibrosis in the histoid form which is an uncommon subpattern of MHV.
- Dimorphic:
  - The microscopic aspects vary according to the predominant pole and may have a mixture types, but the infiltrate is more localized, without the diffuse pattern of lepromatous leprosy,
  - The search for bacilli is usually positive of weak to moderate intensity
  - May appear like the tuberculoid form at small magnification, but more diffuse and mixed with foam cells.
- Reactional states
  - Erythema nodosum leprosum with panniculitis pattern is a late manifestation.
  - In the early phase, it presents leukocytoclastic vasculitis with eosinophils, which involves small vessels of the deep dermis and subcutaneous adipose tissue with endothelial edema and fibrinoid material around the vascular wall.
  - In the late phase, it progresses to mixed panniculitis, superimposed on histopathological findings of lepromatous leprosy, with strongly positive bacilli testing.

14.6.5 Ultrasonography (Figs. 14.28, 14.29, 14.30, and 14.31) [36]

- Skin lesions in leprosy present unspecific patterns on imaging methods
- Ultrasonography is especially important to assess neuropathy, studying structural changes in nerves

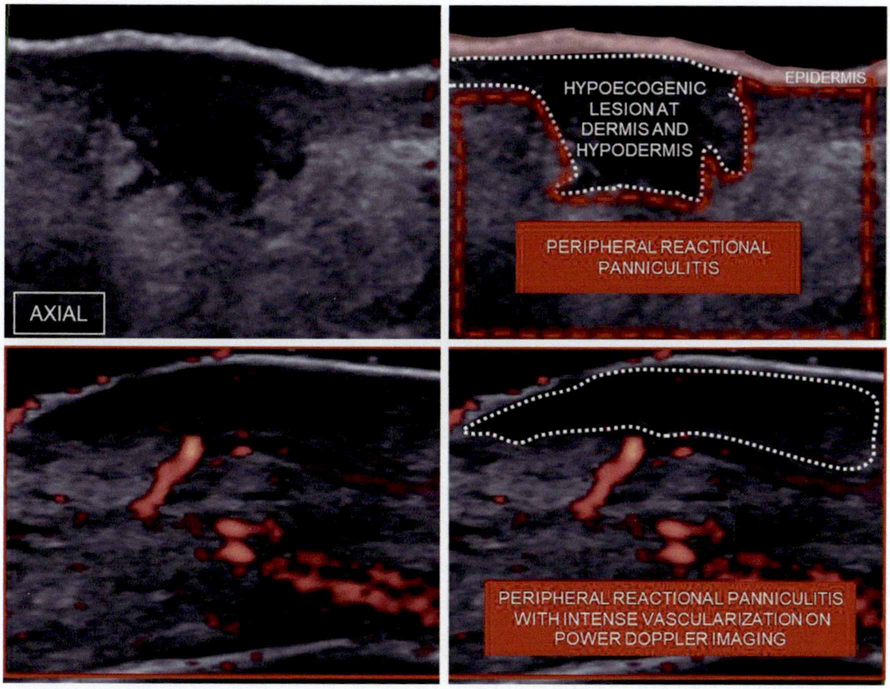

Fig. 14.28 Ultrasonographic findings of cutaneous leprosy with 24 MHz probe (Aplio i800, Canon Medical Systems)

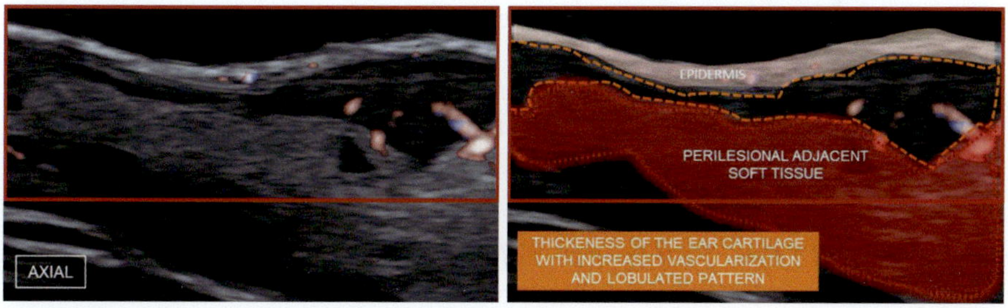

Fig. 14.29 Ultrasonographic findings of ear infiltration from leprosy with 24 MHz probe (Aplio i800, Canon Medical Systems)

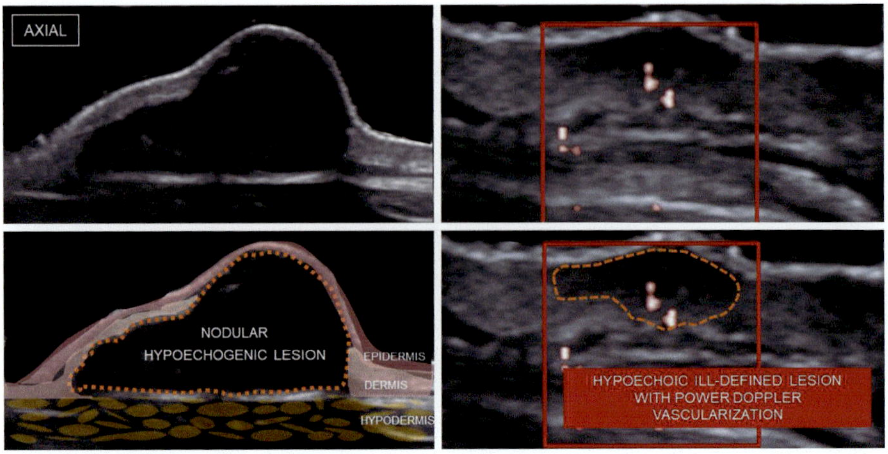

Fig. 14.30 Ultrasonographic findings of lip lesion from leprosy with 24 MHz probe (Aplio i800, Canon Medical Systems)

- Normal peripheral nerves reveal a characteristic pattern on ultrasonography:
  - Tubular structure with multiple hypoechoic but discontinuous linear areas separated by hyper-echoic bands
  - Multiple rounded hypo-echoic areas in a homogenous background in transverse plane (fascicular or honeycomb pattern)
- Nerve ultrasonography in leprosy can demonstrate five changes:
  - Nerve enlargement
  - Increased hypoechogenicity or hyperechogenicity
  - Enlarged fascicles
  - Increased thickness of the epineurium
  - Increased endo- or epineural blood flow

14.6.6 MRI (Fig. 14.32) [36, 37]

- MR neurography is a well-established and more objective diagnostic modality for peripheral neuropathy, especially leprosy.
- Thickened of the nerve caliber.
- High signal intensity on T2W image of the nerve.
- Focal abscess formation surrounding the nerve.
- Secondary denervation and fatty infiltration of corresponding muscles.

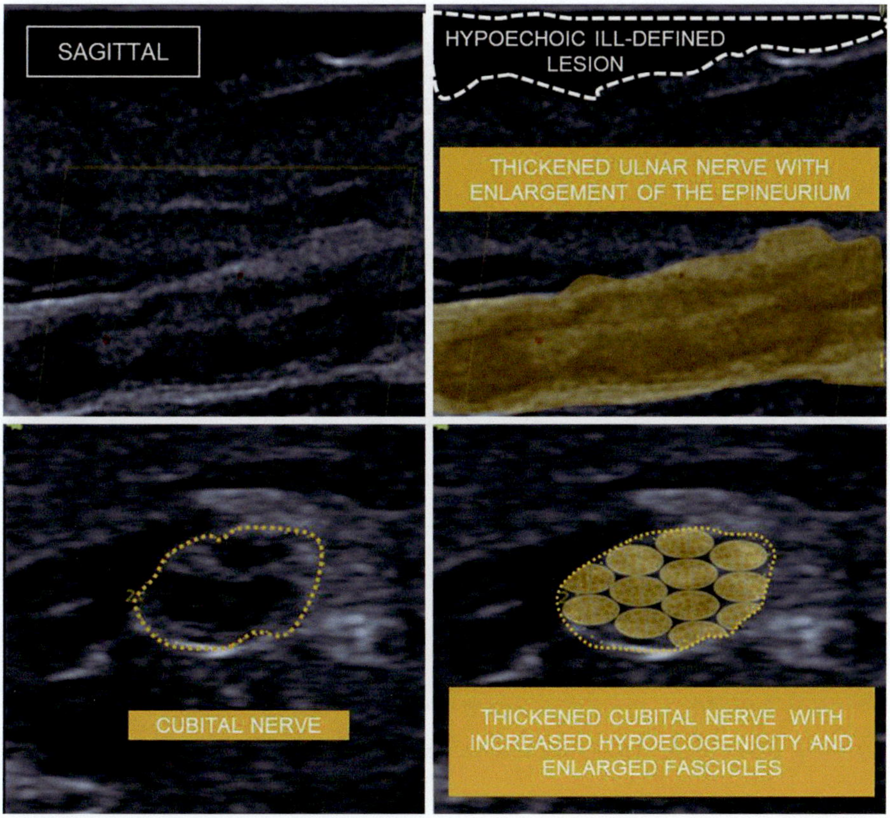

Fig. 14.31 Ultrasonographic findings of neural thickening from leprosy with 24 MHz probe (Aplio i800, Canon Medical Systems)

14.7 Actinomycosis

14.7.1 Definition [38–42]

- Actinomycosis is a bacterial infection caused mostly by Actinomyces israelii, a Gram-positive, filamentous bacterium that is part of the normal flora of the mouth and intestines.
- These bacteria can cause opportunistic infections and are found in soil, where they can be acquired exogenously.
- There are six species of Actinomyces known to infect humans, with *Actinomyces israelii* being the most common.

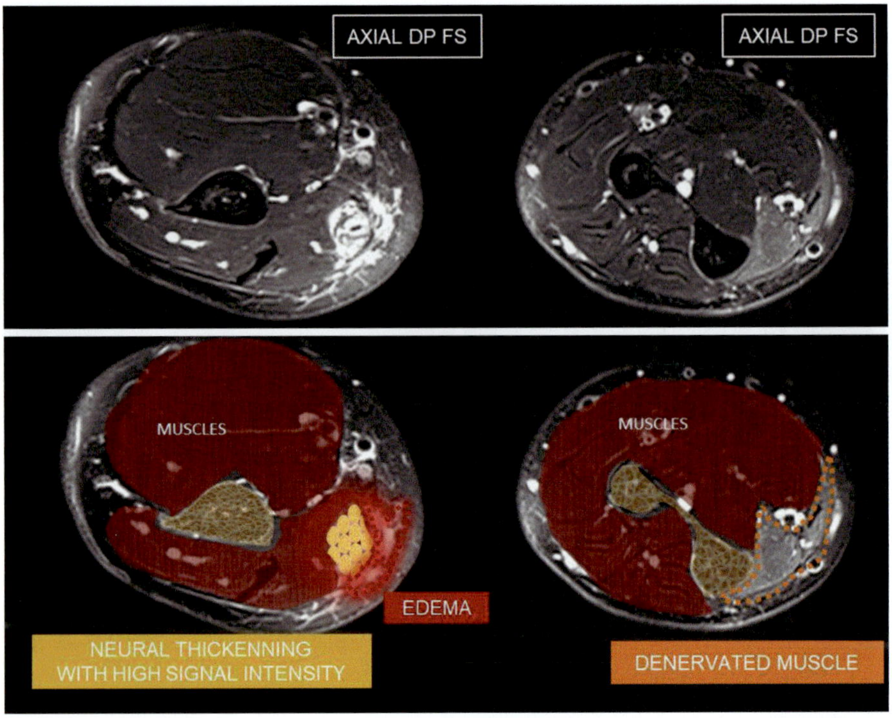

Fig. 14.32 MRI findings of neural thickening from leprosy on axial DP FS sequences (Magnetom Avanto 1.5T MRI, Siemens)

14.7.2 Epidemiology [38–41]

- Actinomycosis is a challenging infection to diagnose, often being mistaken for tuberculosis, fungal infections, botryomycosis, and malignancies.
- It can occur due to trauma, penetrating wounds, and compound fractures.
- The infection is more common in populations with poor oral hygiene, in individuals using intrauterine devices (IUDs), and in immunocompromised patients.

14.7.3 Clinical Presentation (Fig. 14.33) [38–41]

- Cervicofacial actinomycosis, while rare, is the most common form of actinomycosis, accounting for approximately 50–70% of cases.

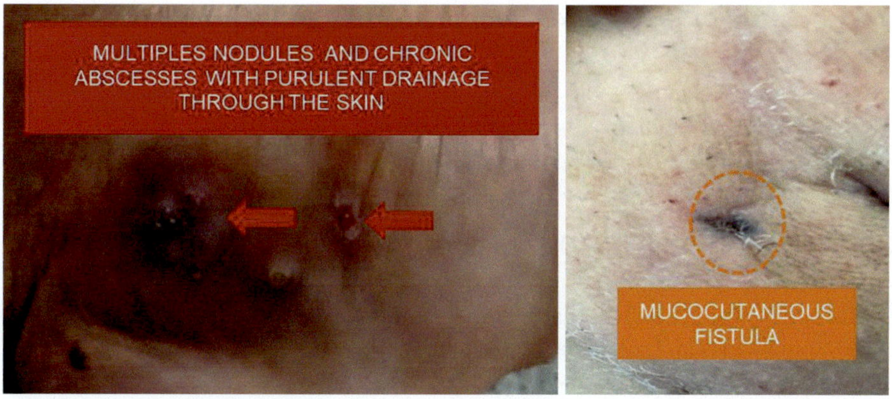

Fig. 14.33 Clinical photograph of patients with actinomycosis of the foot and the neck

- It is frequently associated with poor dental conditions, oral trauma, or dental procedures. This form of the disease is characterized by chronic abscesses with purulent drainage through the skin, often involving the jaw. Infections are typically polymicrobial, involving other bacteria such as Aggregatibacter actinomycetemcomitans, Fusobacterium nucleatum, and Streptococcus species.

14.7.4 Histopathology [13, 43]

- It usually occurs in the deep dermis and subcutaneous adipose tissue in a zone of granulation tissue with a fibrous capsule in the late phase when it is usually biopsied.
- The inflammatory infiltrate has a chronic mixed pattern, including plasma cells, macrophages, and fibroblasts surrounding a central abscessed area, containing neutrophils and fibrinous exudate.
- Inside the abscess are the basophilic lobulated bodies, called sulfur granules, measuring an average of 300 μm, surrounded by an eosinophilic cuticle called the Splendore–Hoeppli phenomenon and which involves small peripheral projections (clubs). The Splendore–Hoeppli phenomenon, an immune response of the body, is not exclusive to actinomycosis but also occurs in botriomycosis and eumycetomas.
- Filamentous organisms are best observed by staining for fungi (PAS and silver) or Gram but are not acid-fast.

14.7.5 Radiography and Computed Tomography

- Soft tissue thickening.
- Obliteration of fat planes surrounding the joints.

14.7.6 Ultrasonography (Fig. 14.34) [4]

- In eumycetoma (lesions caused by yeasts such as Madurella mycetomatis, Madurella grisea, Exophiala jeanselmei, and others), the grains produce numerous sharp, hyper-reflective echoes, resembling black grains and a grain-cement substance. There are single or multiple thick-walled cavities without acoustic enhancement.
- In actinomycetoma (caused by Gram-positive bacteria such as Actinomadura madurae, Streptomyces pelletieri, Streptomyces somaliensis, and Nocardia species), the findings are similar, but the hyper-reflective echoes are fine, closely aggregated, and often settle at the bottom of the cavities. The less distinct hyper-reflective echo of actinomycetoma grains may be attributed to their consistency, typically smaller size, individual embedding of the grains, and the absence of a cement substance in certain types of actinomycetoma.
- While the findings may not be specific, they are useful for detecting changes in affected skin layers as well as complications like arthritis and bone destruction.

14.7.7 MRI (Fig. 14.35) [4, 44]

- "Dot-in-circle" sign is specific.

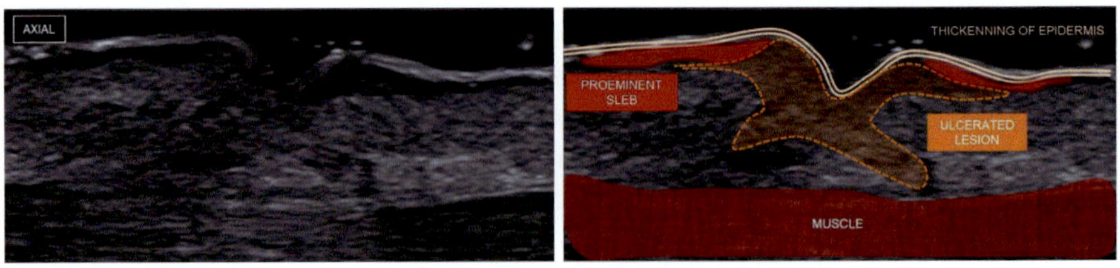

Fig. 14.34 Ultrasonographic findings of actinomycosis with 24 MHz probe (Aplio i800, Canon Medical Systems)

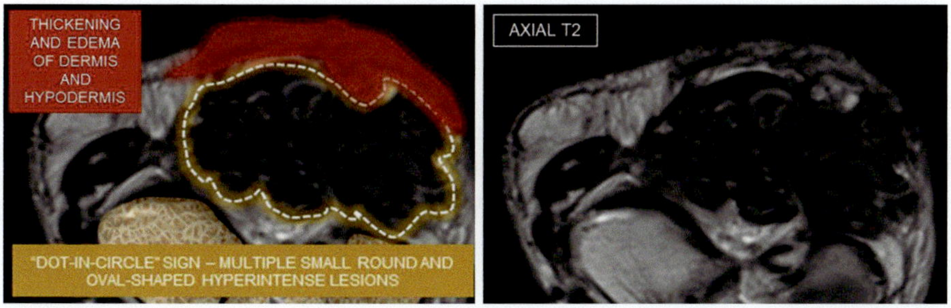

Fig. 14.35 MRI findings of actinomyces on axial T2-weighted sequences (Magnetom Avanto 1.5T MRI, Siemens)

- Conglomerate masses forming of multiple small round and oval-shaped hyperintense lesions, measuring a few millimeters across each (dot) involving the subcutaneous tissue, muscles, and intermuscular fascial planes.
- The lesions were separated by a hypointense rim (circle). Additionally, a central hypointense dot was observed within many of these lesions.
- MRI is crucial for detecting the spread of infection into deep soft tissues and diagnosing complications such as bone and joint involvement.

14.8 Myiasis

14.8.1 Definition [45]

- Myiasis refers to a parasitic infestation caused by the larvae of flies.
- It is generally categorized into two forms: furuncular and cavitary.
- Furuncular myiasis is most frequently linked with the Dermatobia hominis fly and typically affects the skin.

14.8.2 Epidemiology [45]

- Furuncular myiasis is prevalent in tropical regions, particularly in rural areas of tropical America.
- The condition occurs when fly eggs are transferred to the skin by phoretic insects like mosquitoes.
- These eggs penetrate the skin through hair follicles or bite wounds, developing into larvae within the subcutaneous tissue.

14.8.3 Clinical Presentation (Fig. 14.36)

- Clinically, furuncular myiasis appears as a painful or itchy, erythematous nodule with a central opening that secretes serous fluid.
- This condition is often misdiagnosed as an abscessed lesion.
- Secondary bacterial infections may complicate the primary infestation, requiring prompt diagnosis and treatment.

14.8.4 Dermoscopy [45]

- The anterior part of the larva, where the respiratory spiracles are located, can be observed through the cavity orifice. The larva makes recurrent movements toward the surface to breathe.
- A yellowish central structure with surrounding spikes may be visible, depending on the size of the larva.
- Dermoscopy also aids in diagnosing the sucess of furuncular myiasis treatment. Occlusion of the orifice (e.g., with adhesive tape) prevents the larva from breathing, leading to its death. The absence of respiratory movements, confirmed via dermoscopy, indicates successful treatment.

14.8.5 Histopathology (Fig. 14.37) [46]

- The larva can be identified during macroscopic examination.
- The larva's exoskeleton consists of a wavy chitinous cuticle with pigmented spines.

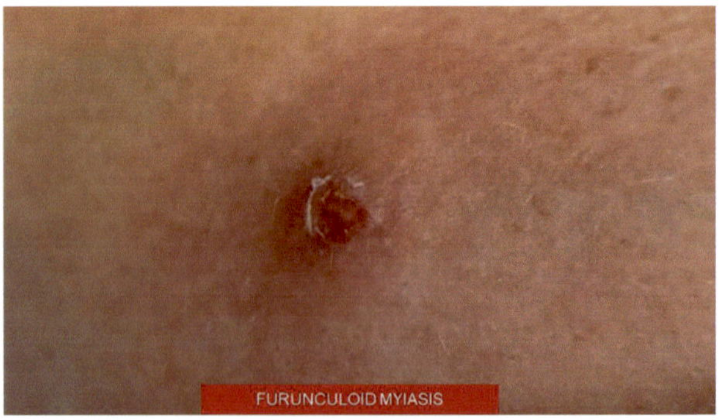

Fig. 14.36 Clinical photograph of patients with furunculoid myiasis

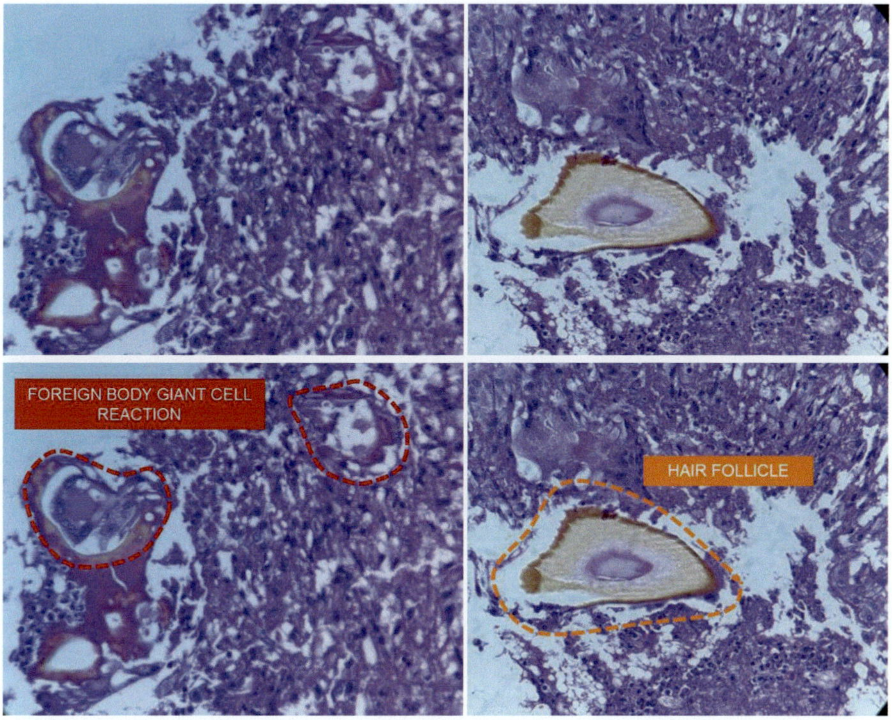

Fig. 14.37 Histological findings of giant cell reaction from myiasis (H&E x20)

- The exoskeleton contains intestinal epithelium, striated muscle, and blood-filled luminal spaces.
- There is a variable density of infiltration by neutrophils, lymphocytes, histiocytes, and eosinophils in the surrounding tissue.

14.8.6 Ultrasonography (Fig. 14.38) [45, 47–49]

- Hyperechoic area suggests the presence of a larva with hypoechoic inflammatory rim surrounding the hyperechoic area.
- A distinct tract through the dermis to the skin surface, representing the larval communication pore with the external environment.
- Hypoechoic area in superficial layers: Visualizes the communication pore.
- Vascularization on power Doppler indicates an inflammatory reaction due to the foreign body response.

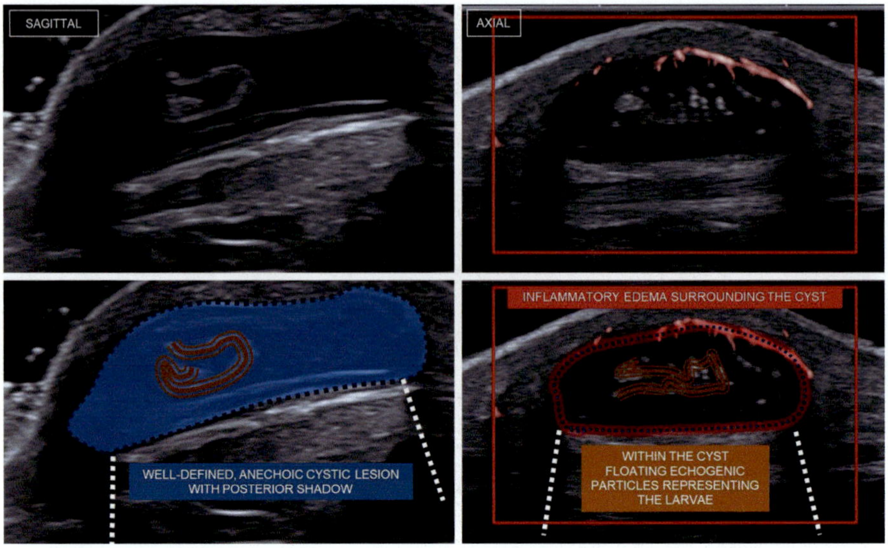

Fig. 14.38 Ultrasonographic findings of retained myiasis with 24 MHz probe (Aplio i800, Canon Medical Systems)

- Bubbling Sign: occurs when the central pore of the furuncular lesion is occluded with ultrasonography gel.
- The circulation of larva and fluid within the central core causes a bubbling or fizzing appearance on the ultrasonography screen, indicating the presence of a live larva within the lesion.

14.8.7 MRI (Fig. 14.39)

- Lesion characteristics:
  - Hypointense on T1-weighted images.
  - Hyperintense on T2-weighted images, indicating fluid or edema.
- Cystic or cavitary lesion:
  - A well-defined cavity may be present, with the larva appearing as a low-signal area.
- Edema and Iinflammation:
  - Surrounding tissues show hyperintense signals on T2, indicating inflammation.
- Sinus tract:

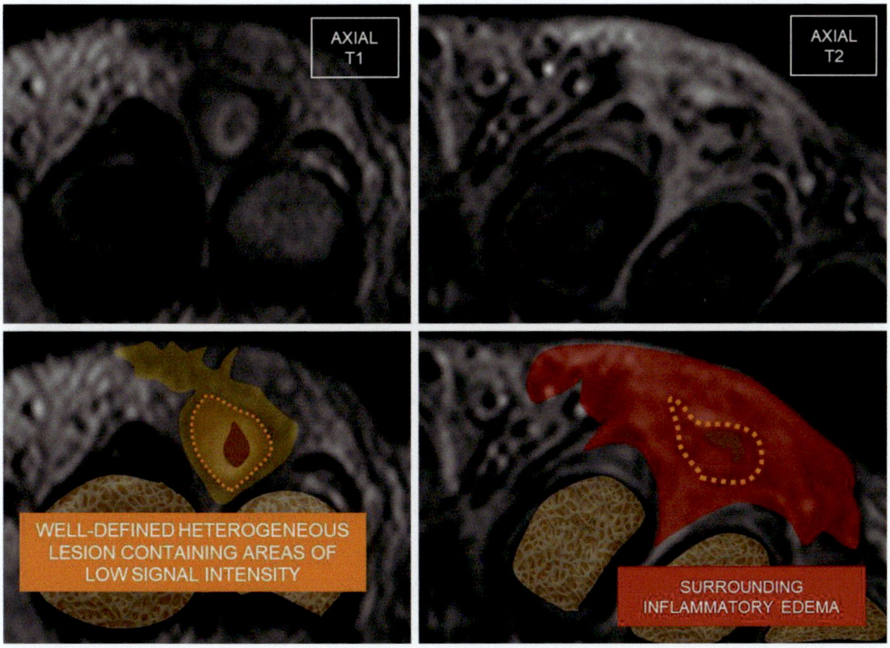

Fig. 14.39 MRI findings of myiasis on axial T2 and T1-weighted sequences (Magnetom Avanto 1.5T MRI, Siemens)

  - A possible sinus tract may be visible, connecting the surface to the deeper lesion.
- Contrast enhancement:
  - Peripheral enhancement may occur, indicating active inflammation.
- Soft tissue involvement:
  - Potential involvement of surrounding soft tissues, including muscle.

14.9 Lesions Caused by Venomous Animals

14.9.1 Definition [50, 51]

- Skin manifestations resulting from the injection of venom through bites or stings. These lesions can vary in appearance and severity, depending on the type of venomous animal, the amount of venom injected, and the individual's immune response.
- The most common venomous animals are the spiders and snakes.
  - Spiders

    - Brown recluse spider (Loxosceles reclusa): Causes necrotic lesions, which may develop into deep ulcers.
    - Black Widow Spider (Latrodectus spp.): Bites can cause pain, redness, and systemic symptoms, though significant skin damage is less common.

  - Snakes

    - Vipers (Rattlesnakes, Bothrops species): Venom can cause severe local tissue damage, including swelling, blistering, and necrosis.
    - Cobras and other elapids: Bites can lead to local necrosis and systemic effects, including neurotoxicity.

- Most common effects:

  - The venom can cause local inflammation, leading to redness, swelling, and pain at the site of the bite or sting.
  - In some cases, the venom may cause tissue damage, resulting in necrosis (death of skin cells), which can lead to ulceration.
  - Allergic reactions: Some individuals may develop allergic reactions to the venom, ranging from mild irritation to severe anaphylaxis.
  - Although primarily affecting the skin, some venomous bites or stings can have systemic effects, including fever, muscle pain, or more severe reactions like shock.

14.9.2 Epidemiology [50, 51]

- Tropical and subtropical regions: Higher incidence of venomous bites and stings, particularly from spiders (Loxosceles species), snakes (Bothrops species), and scorpions (Centruroides species).
- Temperate regions: Lower incidence, with venomous bites from animals like brown recluse spiders and certain snakes (rattlesnakes in North America) being more common.
- Coastal areas: Higher incidence of jellyfish stings, particularly from species like the box jellyfish and Portuguese man o'war.

14.9.3 Clinical Presentation (Fig. 14.40) [50, 51]

- Bites from Snakes

  - Local findings:

    - Usually two puncture wounds; sometimes only one or multiple small marks.

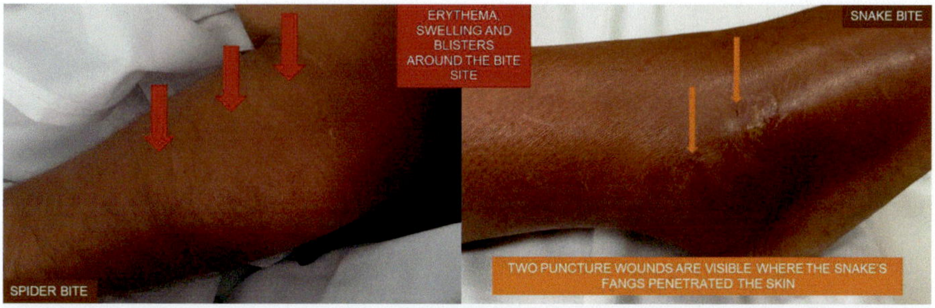

Fig. 14.40 Clinical photograph of patients with lesions caused by venomous animals

- Immediate pain, intense, and localized, possibly radiating.
- Rapid swelling around the bite, possibly spreading to the entire limb.
- Erythema and ecchymosis: Redness and bruising that may expand.
- Blisters or bullae may form quickly due to venom damage.
- Tissue death can occur in severe cases, leading to ulcers.

– Systemic findings:

- Severe envenomation may cause shock with low blood pressure and rapid heart rate.
- Some venoms cause blood clotting issues, leading to bleeding and prolonged clotting times.
- Neurotoxic venoms may cause muscle weakness, respiratory paralysis, and potentially respiratory failure.
- Some venoms can cause kidney injury, directly or via muscle breakdown.
- Muscle breakdown leads to pain, weakness, and dark urine due rhaddomyolysis.

– Bites from Spiders

- Usually two small puncture marks, though often only a red bump or irritation is visible.
- Mild to moderate pain, often with itching, that may radiate from the bite site. Onset can be immediate or delayed.
- The bite site may become red, swollen, and warm; swelling is typically localized.
- Blisters, which may be clear or blood-filled, can develop at the bite site.
- Some spider bites, like those from the brown recluse, can cause tissue necrosis, leading to ulceration and potentially slow-healing sores.
- Fever, nausea, vomiting, and general malaise may occur as part of the body's response to venom.

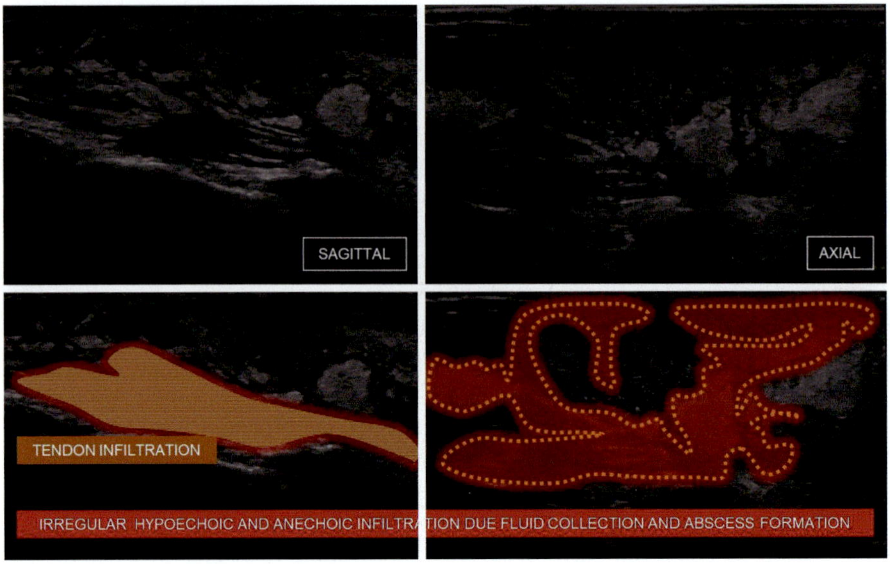

Fig. 14.41 Ultrasonographic findings of cutaneous lesion after a snake bite (Logic E9, GE Healthcare)

14.9.4 Ultrasonography (Figs. 14.41 and 14.42)

- Hypoechoic areas in the subcutaneous tissue, indicating inflammation and swelling.
- Increased power Doppler signals, indicating hyperemia and ongoing inflammation.
- A well-defined, dark area suggesting fluid collection or abscess, often due to secondary infection or tissue necrosis.
- Irregular hypoechoic areas with poorly defined margins, possibly with gas bubbles, indicating tissue necrosis, common in bites like those from the brown recluse spider.
- Thickened dermal layers with a bright appearance, reflecting an inflammatory response in the skin.
- A linear, bright structure with posterior shadowing, indicating a possible retained fang or other material.
- Enlarged lymph nodes with a hypoechoic center and hyperechoic cortex, indicating systemic involvement or significant local inflammation.

14.9.5 MRI (Fig. 14.43)

- Hyperintense on T2-weighted images, indicating inflammation and swelling, which helps assess the bite's severity.

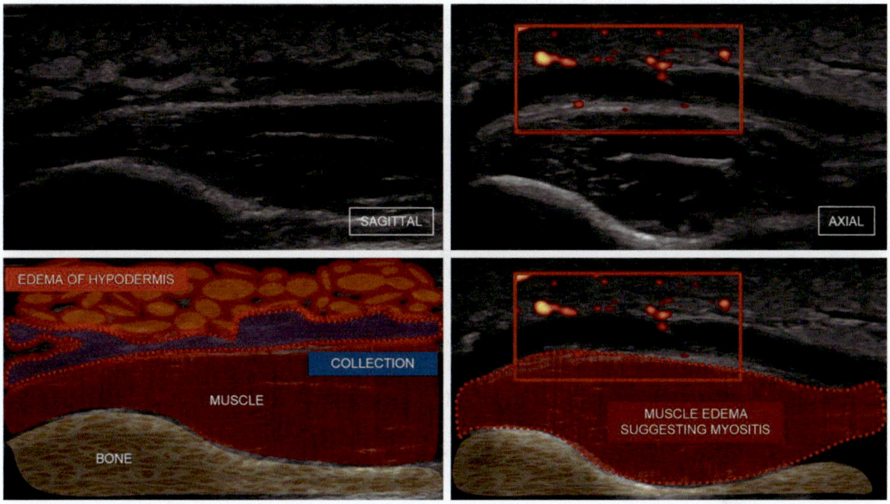

Fig. 14.42 Ultrasonographic findings of cutaneous lesion after a spider bite (Aplio i800, Canon Medical Systems)

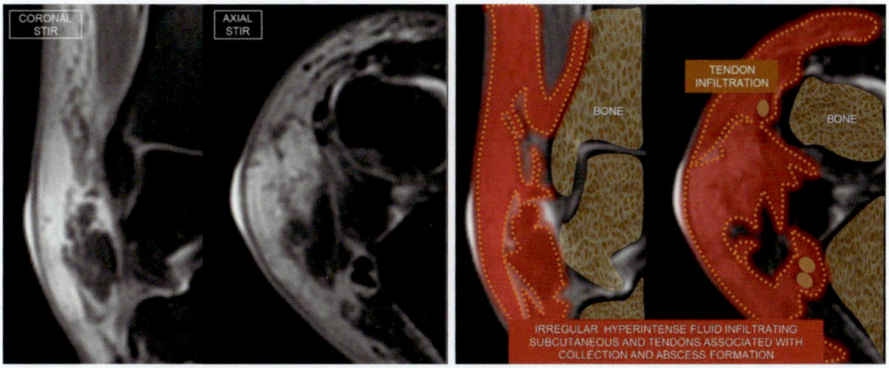

Fig. 14.43 MRI findings of cutaneous soft tissue lesions after snake bite on STIR sequences (Magnetom Avanto 1.5T MRI, Siemens)

- Increased signal on T2-weighted and decreased signal on T1-weighted images of muscles suggest inflammation (myositis) or muscle damage, significant for bites with cytotoxic venom.
- Hyperintense signal in fascial planes on T2-weighted images inside bones, indicating inflammation or involvement, contributing to pain and restricted movement.
- Increased signal in muscle compartments with possible loss of normal architecture, showing interstitial fluid accumulation and indicating a surgical emergency.

- Nonenhancing regions on post-contrast T1-weighted images and heterogeneous hyperintensity on T2-weighted images, indicating tissue death, crucial for surgical planning.
- Mixed signal intensity areas, with acute hemorrhage appearing hypointense on T2*-weighted images, reflecting venom-induced coagulopathy.
- Well-defined fluid collections with rim enhancement on contrast-enhanced T1-weighted images and hyperintense signals on T2-weighted images, indicating secondary infection.
- Increased signal on T2-weighted images inside bones, suggesting marrow edema or osteomyelitis, rare but possible in deeper tissue involvement.
- MRI angiography may show thrombosis, reduced blood flow, or vascular compression, which can lead to ischemia and increase the risk of necrosis.

14.10 Infectious Bursitis

14.10.1 Definition [52]

- It is the inflammation and infection of a bursa, which is a synovial membrane-lined space present overlying a number of joints.
- Superficial bursitis, such as olecranal, prepatellar, infrapatellar and retrocalcaneal bursitis can lead to dermatological manifestations.
- Superficial infectious bursitis most often occurs in the olecranon and prepatellar bursae.

14.10.2 Epidemiology [52]

- The clinical features of infectious bursitis are sometimes indistinguishable from noninfectious bursitis.
- Identifying infectious bursitis is crucial as bursal aspiration should be performed and fluid examined using Gram stain, crystal analysis, glucose measurement, blood cell count, and culture.
- More commonly in males with the mean age at onset approximately 50 years.
- The etiology is the inoculating of the bursa with infectious bacteria. This happens most often:
  - Micro-trauma.
  - Direct puncture of the overlying skin.
  - Contiguous spread of overlying cellulitis of the skin.

- In 80–90% of cases, *Staphylococcus aureus* is the most common organism in acute infectious bursitis.

14.10.3 Clinical Presentation (Fig. 14.44) [52]

- Tender and fluid-filled olecranon bursa.
- Inflammatory skin changes such as erythema and edema.
- May happen systemic symptoms such as fever in worst prognostic cases.

14.10.4 Histopathology [52]

- Infectious bursitis has no characteristic pattern unless a special agent causes it. It usually exhibits the classic forms of acute and chronic inflammation with late-stage fibrosis.

14.10.5 Radiography and Computed Tomography (Fig. 14.45) [52]

- Radiography shows soft tissue edema with effacement of the normal adjacent fat planes and is helpful to discard foreign bodies.
- CT reveals bursal distension with fluid and peri-bursal fat stranding.
- The contrast enhancement of the thickened wall might be irregular, compared to the wall of a cyst.
- Bursitis may be acute or chronic, in the latter, calcifications at the bursal sites may be apparent on plain radiographs.

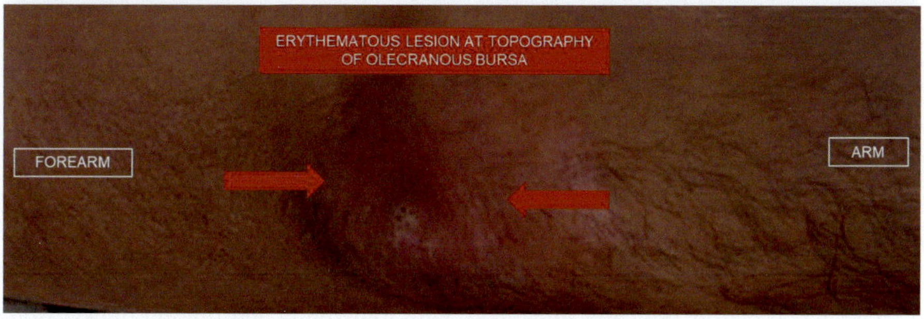

Fig. 14.44 Clinical photograph of patient with infectious bursitis

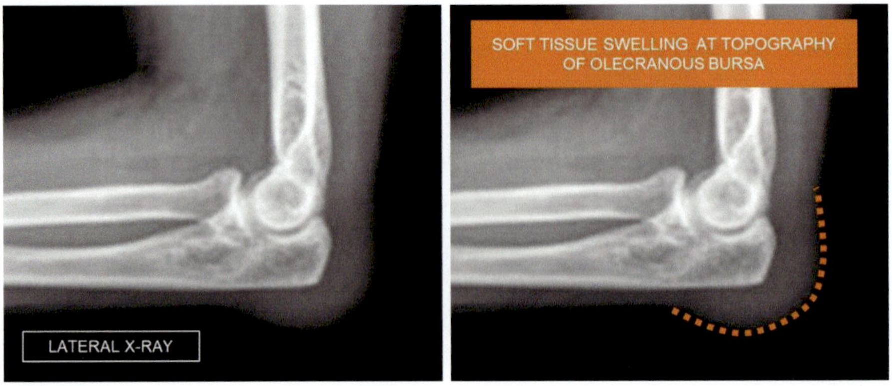

Fig. 14.45 Radiographic findings of infectious bursitis on lateral X-ray (Philips Duo Diagnost R&F Room Digital RF and Tomo System)

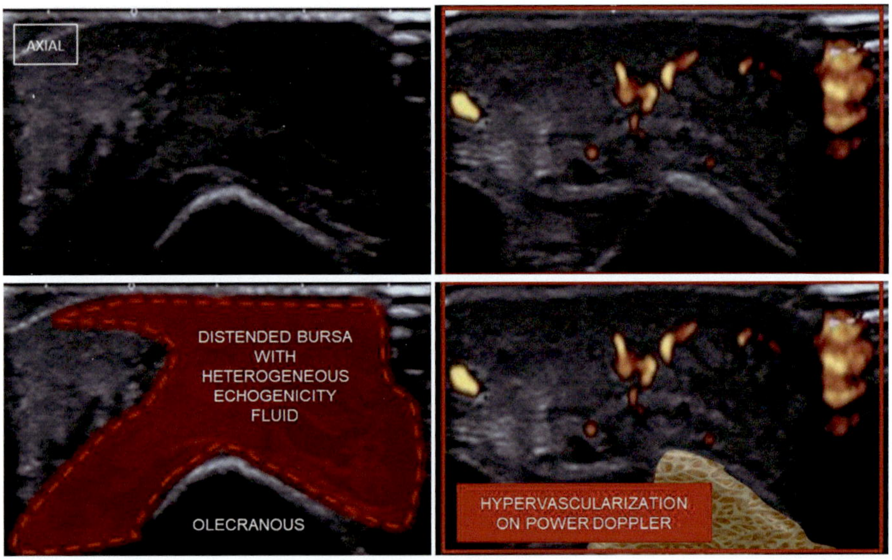

Fig. 14.46 Ultrasonographic findings of infectious bursitis with 24 MHz probe (Aplio i800, Canon Medical Systems)

14.10.6 Ultrasonography (Fig. 14.46) [53]

- An infected bursa is surrounded by peribursal edema and is distended, with mixed echogenicity fluid with possible internal debris and septations.
- The bursal wall is typically thickened, with hyperemia and present hypervascularization on power Doppler evaluation.

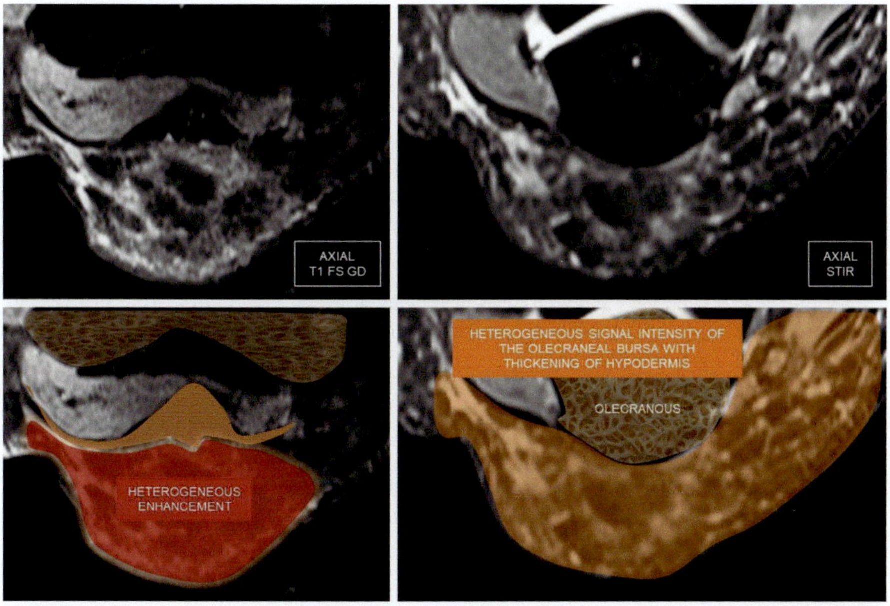

Fig. 14.47 MRI findings of infectious bursitis on STIR and T1 FS weighted sequences after gadolinium administration (Magnetom Avanto 1.5T MRI, Siemens)

14.10.7 MRI (Fig. 14.47) [54]

- Bursa is distended with either fluid, which may be simple or complex, and usually enhances synovitis.
- Simple fluid is hypointense in signal on T1-weighted images and hyperintense signal on T2 FS-weighted images and demonstrates smooth, thin peripheral synovial enhancement following intravenous contrast administration. If the fluid is complex, due to the presence of blood or debris, it will have a more heterogeneous appearance.
- Thick enhancement of bursal wall and peribursal soft tissues on post-contrast sequences.

References

1. Viac J, Thivolet J, Chardonnet Y. Specific immunity in patients suffering from recurring warts before and after repetitive intradermal tests with human papilloma virus. Br J Dermatol. 1977;97:365–70.
2. Sterling JC, Gibbs S, Haque Hussain SS, Mohd Mustapa MF, Handfield-Jones SE, Hughes JR, et al. British Association of Dermatologists' guidelines for the management of cutaneous warts 2014. Br J Dermatol. 2014;171:696–712.

3. Lynch MD, Cliffe J, Morris-Jones R. Management of cutaneous viral warts. BMJ. 2014;348:g3339.
4. de Almeida CÁ, Nakamura R, Leverone A, Costa F, Estrada BD, Haui P, et al. Imaging features for the evaluation of skin and nail infections. Skeletal Radiol. 2024;53(10):2051–65. https://link.springer.com/10.1007/s00256-023-04557-4.
5. Herschthal J, McLeod MP, Zaiac M. Management of ungual warts. Dermatol Ther. 2012;25:545–50. https://doi.org/10.1111/j.1529-8019.2012.01509.x.
6. Bakos RM, Leite LL, Reinehr C, Escobar GF. Dermoscopy of skin infestations and infections (entomodermoscopy) – part II: viral, fungal and other infections. An Bras Dermatol. 2021;96:746–58.
7. Ball SLR, Winder DM, Vaughan K, Hanna N, Levy J, Sterling JC, et al. Analyses of human papillomavirus genotypes and viral loads in anogenital warts. J Med Virol. 2011;83:1345–50.
8. Wortsman X. Atlas of dermatologic ultrasonography. Cham: Springer; 2018. https://doi.org/10.1007/978-3-319-89614-4.
9. de Almeida MA, Almeida-Silva F, Guimarães AJ, Almeida-Paes R, Zancopé-Oliveira RM. The occurrence of histoplasmosis in Brazil: a systematic review. Int J Infect Dis. 2019;86:147–56.
10. Saheki MN, de Schubach AO, de Salgueiro MM, Conceição-Silva F, Wanke B, Lazera M. Histoplasmose cutânea primária: relato de caso em paciente imunocompetente e revisão de literatura. Rev Soc Bras Med Trop. 2008;41:680–2.
11. Ahuja A, Bhardwaj M, Agarwal P. Cutaneous histoplasmosis in HIV seronegative patients: a clinicopathological analysis. Dermatology. 2021;237:934–9.
12. Kumari M, Udayakumar M, Kaushal M, Madaan GB. Unusual presentation of disseminated histoplasmosis in an immunocompetent patient. Diagn Cytopathol. 2017;45:848–50.
13. Barnhill RL, Neil Crowson A, Magro CM, Piepkorn MW, Kutzner H, Desman GT. Barnhill's dermatopathology. 4th ed. New York: McGraw Hill; 2019. https://dermatology.mhmedical.com/content.aspx?bookid=2802&sectionid=238125236.
14. Yu L, Zhang T-D. Skin lesions caused by sporotrichosis. Can Med Assoc J. 2021;193:E1139. https://doi.org/10.1503/cmaj.202688.
15. Orofino-Costa R, de Macedo PM, Rodrigues AM, Bernardes-Engemann AR. Sporotrichosis: an update on epidemiology, etiopathogenesis, laboratory and clinical therapeutics. An Bras Dermatol. 2017;92:606–20.
16. Zhu H, Xia X, Zhi H, Shen H, Lv W, Sang B, et al. Retrospective analysis of 71 patients with cutaneous sporotrichosis. Mycoses. 2023;66:621–31.
17. Morgado DS, Castro R, Ribeiro-Alves M, Corrêa-Moreira D, Castro-Alves J, Pereira SA, et al. Global distribution of animal sporotrichosis: a systematic review of Sporothrix sp. identified using molecular tools. Curr Res Microb Sci. 2022;3:100140.
18. Schwalb A, Carcamo PM, Seas C. Lymphocutaneous sporotrichosis. Am J Trop Med Hyg. 2022;106:758–9.
19. Pinto-Almazán R, Sandoval-Navarro KA, Damián-Magaña EJ, Arenas R, Fuentes-Venado CE, Zárate-Segura PB, et al. Relationship of sporotrichosis and infected patients with HIV-AIDS: an actual systematic review. J Fungi. 2023;9:396.
20. Kothari R, Varghese J, Bhatnagar A, Kishore K, Kumar R. Dermoscopy of fixed cutaneous sporotrichosis with a follow-up till cure: a case report. Cureus. 2024;16(3):e55960.
21. Vinay K, Bhattacharjee R, Bishnoi A, Chatterjee D, Rudramurthy S, Dogra S. Dermatoscopic features of cutaneous sporotrichosis. J Eur Acad Dermatol Venereol. 2020;34:16539. https://doi.org/10.1111/jdv.16539.
22. Singh OP, Hasker E, Sacks D, Boelaert M, Sundar S. Asymptomatic leishmania infection: a new challenge for leishmania control. Clin Infect Dis. 2014;58:1424–9.
23. Gurel MS, Tekin B, Uzun S. Cutaneous leishmaniasis: a great imitator. Clin Dermatol. 2020;38:140–51.
24. Mann S, Frasca K, Scherrer S, Henao-Martínez AF, Newman S, Ramanan P, et al. A review of leishmaniasis: current knowledge and future directions. Curr Trop Med Rep. 2021;8:121–32.

25. García-Gil MF, Monte Serrano J, Matovelle C, Ara-Martín M. Dermatoscopia e impronta en la leishmaniasis cutánea. An Pediatr. 2021;94:118–9.
26. Vergara-de-la-Campa L, Cembrero-Saralegui H, Luna-Bastante L, Martínez-Lorenzo ER, Alfageme-Roldán F. Usefulness of ultrasonography for treatment and follow-up of cutaneous leishmaniasis. J Ultrasonography. 2021;24:573–6.
27. Sechi A, Neri I, Patrizi A, Di Altobrando A, Clinca R, Caro RDC, et al. Ultrasonography patterns of localized cutaneous leishmaniasis and clinical correlations. J Ultrasonography. 2022;25:343–8.
28. Da Silva Sousa AC, Sousa M, Tente D, Menezes N, Baptista A, Guedes R. Ungual tuberculosis: a unique clinical case. Skin Appendage Disord. 2019;5:386–9.
29. Kaul S, Kaur I, Mehta S, Singal A. Cutaneous tuberculosis. Part I: pathogenesis, classification, and clinical features. J Am Acad Dermatol. 2023;89:1091–103.
30. Nguyen KH, Alcantara CA, Glassman I, May N, Mundra A, Mukundan A, et al. Cutaneous manifestations of Mycobacterium tuberculosis: a literature review. Pathogens. 2023;12:920.
31. Jindal R, Chauhan P, Sethi S. Dermoscopy of the diverse spectrum of cutaneous tuberculosis in the skin of color. Dermatol Pract Concept. 2022;12:e2022203.
32. da Reis AS, de Souza EA, Ferreira AF, da Silva GV, de Macedo SF, de Araújo OD, et al. Sobreposição de casos novos de hanseníase em redes de convívio domiciliar em dois municípios do Norte e Nordeste do Brasil, 2001-2014. Cad Saude Publica. 2019;35:10.
33. Maymone MBC, Laughter M, Venkatesh S, Dacso MM, Rao PN, Stryjewska BM, et al. Leprosy: clinical aspects and diagnostic techniques. J Am Acad Dermatol. 2020;83:1–14.
34. Yang J, Li X, Sun Y, Zhang L, Jin G, Li G, et al. Global epidemiology of leprosy from 2010 to 2020: a systematic review and meta-analysis of the proportion of sex, type, grade 2 deformity and age. Pathog Glob Health. 2022;116:467–76.
35. Massone C, Belachew WA, Schettini A. Histopathology of the lepromatous skin biopsy. Clin Dermatol. 2015;33:38–45.
36. Jain S, Visser LH, Suneetha S. Imaging techniques in leprosy clinics. Clin Dermatol. 2016;34:70–8.
37. Aggarwal A, Das CJ, Khanna N, Sharma R, Srivastava DN, Goyal V, et al. Role of diffusion tensor imaging in the evaluation of ulnar nerve involvement in leprosy. Br J Radiol. 2022;95:20210290.
38. Kamath RR, Kura MM, Basumatary R. Primary cutaneous actinomycosis mimicking cutaneous leishmaniasis. Indian Dermatol Online J. 2024;15:496–9.
39. Könönen E, Wade WG. Actinomyces and related organisms in human infections. Clin Microbiol Rev. 2015;28:419–42.
40. Khan S, Khan B, Batool W, Khan M, Khan AH. Primary cutaneous actinomycosis: a diagnostic enigma. Cureus. 2023;15:e37261.
41. Fronek L, Brazen B, Ross R, Miller R. Cervicofacial actinomycosis: a unique diagnostic challenge. Dermatol Online J. 2021;27:7.
42. Vasilovici A, Ungureanu L, Grigore L, Cojocaru E, Senila S. Actinic Cheilitis—from risk factors to therapy. Front Med. 2022;9:805425.
43. Guerrant RL, Walker DH, Weller PF. Tropical infectious diseases: principles, pathogens and practice. Amsterdam: Elsevier; 2011.
44. Laohawiriyakamol T, Tanutit P, Kanjanapradit K, Hongsakul K, Ehara S. The "dot-in-circle" sign in musculoskeletal mycetoma on magnetic resonance imaging and ultrasonography. Springerplus. 2014;3:671. https://doi.org/10.1186/2193-1801-3-671.
45. Papineni V, Dieu S, Rennie WJ. The human botfly "bubbling sign": ultrasonography features of cutaneous Furuncular myiasis. Indian J Radiol Imaging. 2023;33:121–3. https://doi.org/10.1055/s-0042-1758203.
46. Hausdörfer-Scheiff S, Bourlond A, Pirard C. Histopathological aspects of myiasis. Dermatology. 1993;186:298–300.

47. Bouer M, Rodriguez-Bandera AI, Albizuri-Prado F, Lobos A, Gubeling W, Wortsman X. Real-time high-frequency colour Doppler ultrasonography detection of cutaneous *Dermatobia hominis* myiasis. J Eur Acad Dermatol Venereol. 2016;30:e180–1. https://doi.org/10.1111/jdv.13492.
48. Nazzaro G, Germiniasi F, Passoni E, Veraldi S. The role of high-frequency ultrasonography in diagnosing myiasis: report of a case and review of the literature. Skin Res Technol. 2019;25:238–9. https://doi.org/10.1111/srt.12620.
49. Jones CH, Leon M, Auerbach J, Portillo-Romero J. Ultrasonography detection of human botfly myiasis of the scalp: a case report. Cureus. 2020;12(12):e11905. https://www.cureus.com/articles/44847-ultrasonography-detection-of-human-botfly-myiasis-of-the-scalp-a-case-report.
50. Yuenyongviwat V, Laohawiriyakamol T, Suwanno P, Kanjanapradit K, Tanutit P. Calcific myonecrosis following snake bite: a case report and review of the literature. J Med Case Rep. 2014;8:193.
51. Zamare Y, Mendhe D. An unusual representation of spider bite with erythema and facial puffiness: a rare clinical image. Pan Afr Med J. 2024;47:106.
52. Chin TY, Peh WC. Imaging update on musculoskeletal infections. J Clin Orthop Trauma. 2021;22:101600.
53. Weaver JS, Omar I, Epstein K, Brown A, Chadwick N, Taljanovic MS. High-resolution ultrasonography in the evaluation of musculoskeletal infections. J Ultrason. 2023;23:270–82.
54. Weaver JS, Omar IM, Mar WA, Klauser AS, Winegar BA, Mlady G, et al. Magnetic resonance imaging of musculoskeletal infections. Pol J Radiol. 2022;87:141–62.

Chapter 15
Clinical, Imaging, and Histological Findings in Tumoral Lesions of Trunk and Limbs

Ana Luisa Sampaio, Viviane Maria Maiolini, Maria de Oliveira Buffara, Camila Silveira Nobre, Haizza Cristina de Almeida Cabral Monteiro, Elisa de Oliveira Barcaui, Manuela Boleira Sieiro Guimarães, Curt Mafra Treu, Romer Braga da Silva, André da Silva Cartell, Alessandro Aita, Flávio Barbosa Luz, Tadeu de Rezende Vergueiro, Silvana Machado Mendonça, Flavia Martins Costa, Marcelo Bragança dos Reis Oliveira Seba, Fernanda Philadelfo Arantes Pereira, Livia Guidoni, Leila Riedel, Caroline Brandão, Ana Maria Doffémond Costa, Carolina Andrea Fernández Quiroga, Thais Emanuelle Freire Barbosa, Ellyete de Oliveira Canella, and Clarissa Canella Moraes do Carmo

Tumoral lesions of the trunk and limbs encompass a wide range of pathologies, from benign growths to aggressive malignancies. Imaging plays a crucial role in the diagnosis, characterization, and management of these lesions, offering insights that guide clinical decision-making. In this chapter, we delve into the imaging analysis of tumoral lesions affecting the trunk and limbs, exploring the various modalities and techniques used to assess these abnormalities. From the identification of key

Supplementary Information The online version contains supplementary material available at https://doi.org/10.1007/978-3-031-77987-9_15.

A. L. Sampaio
Department of Dermatology, Hospital Universitario Pedro Ernesto, Universidade Estadual do Rio de Janeiro—UERJ, Rio de Janeiro, Brazil

M. de Oliveira Buffara · C. S. Nobre
State University of Rio de Janeiro—UERJ, Pedro Ernesto Hospital—HUPE, Rio de Janeiro, RJ, Brazil

V. M. Maiolini
Cancer Institute of the State of São Paulo—ICESP and Faculty of Medicine, University of São Paulo—FMUSP, São Paulo, RJ, Brazil

H. C. de Almeida Cabral Monteiro
State University of Rio de Janeiro—UERJ, Pedro Ernesto Hospital—HUPE, Rio de Janeiro, RJ, Brazil

Department of Dermatology, Hospital Rio-Barra and Rede D'Or São Luiz, Rio de Janeiro, Brazil

© The Author(s), under exclusive license to Springer Nature Switzerland AG 2025

C. Canella Moraes do Carmo (ed.), *Atlas of Diagnostic Imaging in Dermatology*, https://doi.org/10.1007/978-3-031-77987-9_15

E. de Oliveira Barcaui
Ultrasonography, Clinica Dermatologica de Ipanema—CDI—Rio de Janeiro, Ipanema, Rio de Janeiro, Brazil

M. B. S. Guimarães
Dermatology Department at Policlinica Geral do Rio de Janeiro Centro, Castelo, Brazil

C. M. Treu
Department of Dermatologic Surgery and Cutaneous Oncology, Policlinica Geral do Rio de Janeiro—PGRJ, Hospital Federal de Bonsucesso Centro, Rio de Janeiro, Brazil

R. B. da Silva
Rede Amil, DASA and Prevent—Rio de Janeiro Centro, Rio de Janeiro, Brazil

A. da Silva Cartell
Adjunct Professor at Faculdade de Medicina da Universidade Federal do Rio Grande do Sul, Rio de Janeiro, Brazil

Dermatologist and Dermatopathologist in Private Practice, Rio de Janeiro, Brazil

A. Aita
Musculoskeletal and Dermatological Imaging, Universidade Federal do Piaui—UFPI Ininga, Teresina, Brazil

F. B. Luz
Department of Dermatology, Universidade Federal Fluminense—UFF, Dermatologic Surgery and Mohs Micrographic Surgery—UFF, Niterói, Brazil

Centro de Cirurgia da Pele, Rio de Janeiro, Brazil

T. de Rezende Vergueiro
Centro de Cirurgia da Pele, Rio de Janeiro, Brazil

S. M. Mendonça
Clinica Cavallieri, Rio de Janeiro, Brazil

Diagnóstico das Américas—DASA—RJ, Rio de Janeiro, Brazil

F. M. Costa
Universidade Federal do Rio de Janeiro—UFRJ, Cidade Universitária, Rio de Janeiro, Brazil

Diagnóstico das Américas—DASA—RJ, Rio de Janeiro, Brazil

M. B. dos Reis Oliveira Seba
Universidade Federal do Rio de Janeiro—UFRJ, Rio de Janeiro, Brazil

Trauma-Orthopaedics Service, Orthopaedic Oncology, Federal University of Rio de Janeiro—UFRJ, Rio de Janeiro, Brazil

F. P. A. Pereira
Alta Excelência Diagnóstica and Clínica de Diagnóstico por Imagem, DASA Barra da Tijuca, Rio de Janeiro, Brazil

L. Guidoni
DERMUS Specialized Ultrasound, Hospital Universitario Cassiano Antonio Moraes—UFES Santos Dumont, Vitória, Brazil

L. Riedel
Doppler Imaging Diagnostic Clinic—Niterói, Postgraduate Program in Dermatological Ultrasound at Lapidare—São Paulo, General Ultrasound at Unissom—Rio de Janeiro, Niterói, Brazil

C. Brandão
Oncological Dermatology Gávea, Rio de Janeiro, Brazil

A. M. D. Costa
Clinica Ana Doffemond, Belo Horizonte, Brazil

radiological features to the evaluation of lesion extent and involvement of surrounding structures, this chapter provides a comprehensive overview that is essential for accurate diagnosis and effective treatment planning.

15.1 Epidermal Cyst

15.1.1 Definition [1, 2]

- Common cutaneous lesions are characterized by the proliferation of squamous epithelium within a confined space in the dermis or subdermis.

15.1.2 Epidemiology [1, 2]

- Epidermal cysts are the most common cutaneous cysts, typically appearing in the third and fourth decades of life.
- They are more commonly found in males than females, with a ratio of 2:1.
- In neonates, epidermal cysts are referred to as milia.

15.1.3 Clinical Presentation (Fig. 15.1) [1, 3]

- Epidermal cysts are typically discovered incidentally or present as firm, painless nodules.

  When they rupture, the release of necrotic debris can trigger a localized inflammatory reaction that resembles an infection.

  They are most commonly found on the scalp, face, neck, trunk, and back.
- Etiology:
  - Traumatic or surgical implantation of epidermal cells.

C. A. F. Quiroga
Internal Medicine Radiology and Dermatological Imaging, Cutaneous Ultrasound Unit, Dermatology Department, Hospital Moisès Broggi, Barcelona, Spain

T. E. F. Barbosa
Marcilio Dias Naval Hospital and National Cancer Institute—INCA, Rio de Janeiro, Brazil

E. de Oliveira Canella
Breast Radiology Center, Hospital Quinta d'Or, Rio de Janeiro, Brazil

C. Canella Moraes do Carmo (✉)
Fluminense Federal University—UFF, Rio de Janeiro, Brazil

Federal University of Rio de Janeiro—UFRJ, Rio de Janeiro, Brazil

Diagnóstico das Américas—DASA—RJ, Rio de Janeiro, Brazil

Biodesign Laboratory, DASA-PUC, Rio de Janeiro, Brazil

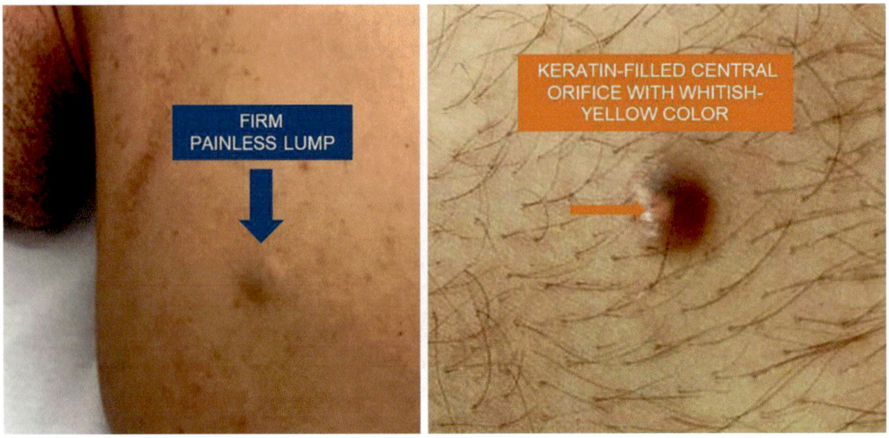

Fig. 15.1 Clinical photograph of patients with epidermic cyst

- Obstruction of the pilosebaceous unit.
- Congenital inclusion of epidermal remnants.

15.1.4 Dermoscopy [2]

- Presence of a central pore:
  - Typically appears as a keratin-filled orifice.
  - Colors can vary: whitish, yellow, brown, or black.
  - Clinically visible in most cases but better distinguished with dermoscopy.
- Wobble sign:
  - Movement of the cyst with respect to surrounding tissues when the dermoscope is moved horizontally.
  - Indicates the site of anchorage of the cyst to the overlying epidermis.
- Visibility variations:
  - Pore visibility is less in facial lesions due to their smaller size and earlier development phase.
  - Dermoscopy increases the detection rate of pores in epidermal cysts compared to clinical examination alone.

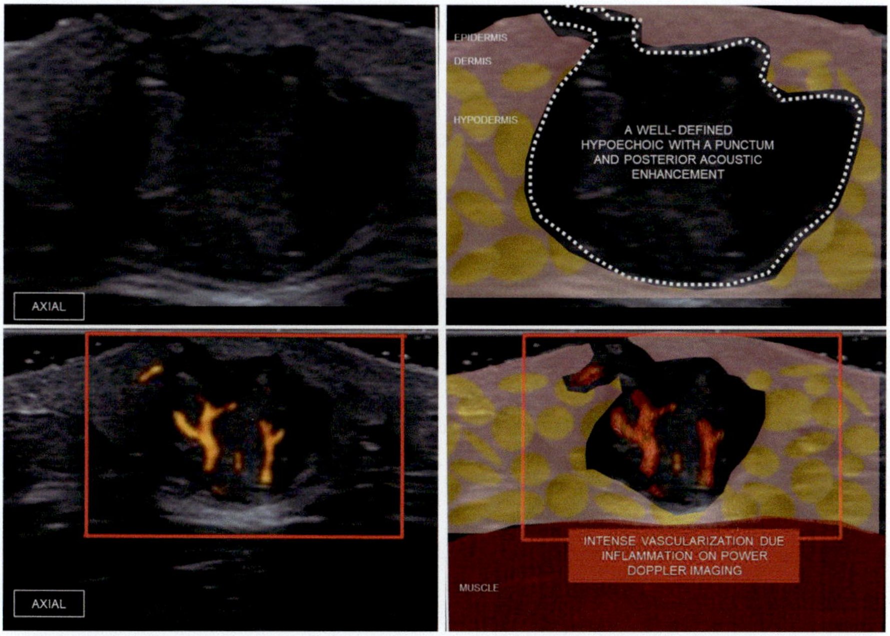

Fig. 15.2 Ultrasonographic findings of epidermic cyst with a 24 MHz probe (Aplio i800, Canon Medical Systems)

15.1.5 Histopathology [3]

- Cystic epithelial proliferation is located entirely in the dermis or subcutaneous adipose tissue.
- The lining epithelium is similar to the interadnexal epidermis with a preserved granular layer and a loose lamellar corneal material content, resembling seagulls flocking on the beach.
- As the lesion enlarges, the lining epithelium becomes flattened, making it difficult to see the layers.
- Absence of adnexal structures around the wall, differentiating it from dermoid cyst.
- When the cyst ruptures, the lesions are surrounded by acute suppurative or there may be chronic inflammation, dystrophic calcification or foreign body granuloma (corneal lamellae).
- Surrounding fibrosis or total replacement of the cyst by a fibrosis nodule marks the late phase of the lesion.

15.1.6 Ultrasonography (Fig. 15.2) [4]

- Appearance:
  - Well-defined, predominantly hypoechoic mass.
  - Common shapes: ovoid to spherical (70%), lobulated (20%), tubular (8%).
  - Anechoic or hypoechoic in dermis and subcutaneous tissue.
  - Internal echoes or debris.
  - Well-circumscribed with posterior acoustic enhancement.
  - May contain calcium or compact hair shafts with central linear hyperechogenicity.
- Characteristic feature:
  - Anechoic or hypoechoic tract extending to the subepidermal layer (punctum).

15.1.7 MRI (Fig. 15.3) [5]

- T1-weighted images displaying low to intermediate signal intensity.
- T2-weighted images showing high signal intensity.
- DWI (diffusion-weighted imaging) indicating true restricted diffusion on ADC (Apparent Diffusion Coefficient).
- T1 with contrast (Gadolinium) typically presents no central enhancement, however a possible thin peripheral enhancement can be observed.
- Ruptured cysts:
  - May exhibit septations and thick, irregular rim enhancement.
  - Potential for diffuse enhancement in the surrounding subcutaneous tissues.

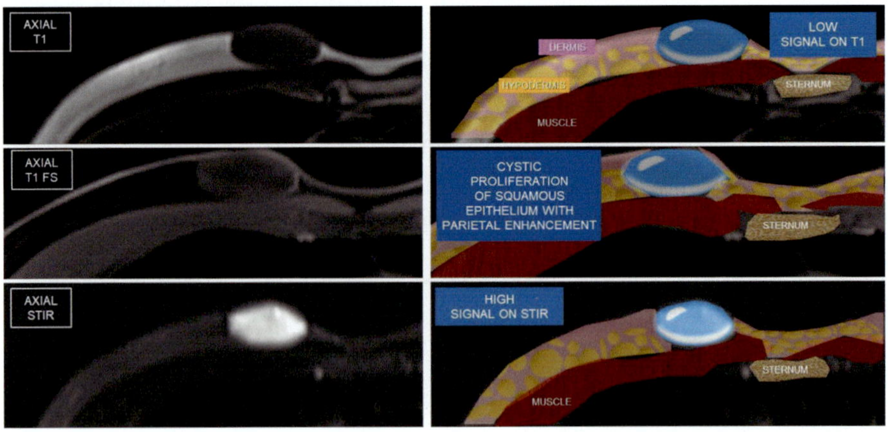

Fig. 15.3 MRI with surface coil findings of epidermic cyst on T1, T1 FS, and STIR sequences (Magnetom Prisma 3T MRI, Siemens)

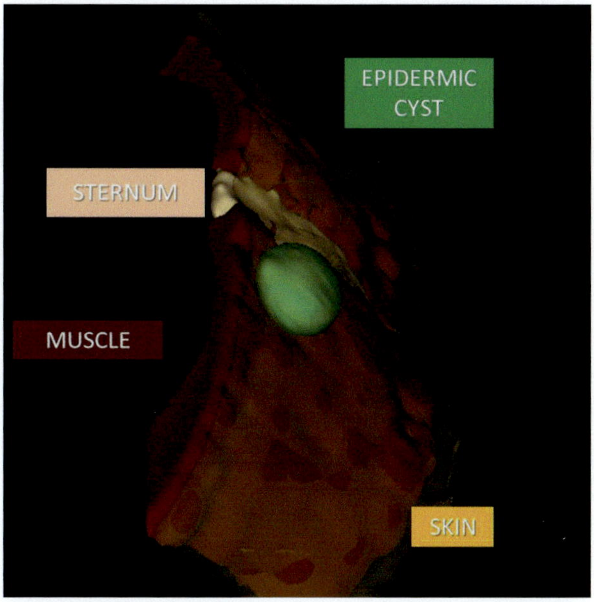

Fig. 15.4 3D images of epidermic cyst after segmentation of MRI isotropic images for surgical planning

15.1.8 3D Images (Fig. 15.4, Video 15.1)

- Highly effective for small lesions or recurrent, challenging cases.
- Provides clear visualization of the lesion's extent, helping to evaluate its severity and its relationship with nearby structures, particularly any surrounding vascular structures.

15.2 Lipoma

15.2.1 Definition [6, 7]

- Lipoma is a benign tumor composed of mature adipocytes.

15.2.2 Epidemiology [7, 8]

- Lipomas are relatively common, affecting approximately 2% of the population.
- Typically found in adults aged 40–60 years and are slightly more common in women.

15.2.3 Clinical Presentation (Fig. 15.5) [8]

- Lipomas are usually asymptomatic and present as soft, mobile, and painless subcutaneous masses.
- They can occur anywhere in the body but are most commonly found on the trunk, shoulders, and neck.

15.2.4 Histopathology [8]

- Lipomas consist of mature adipocytes that are identical to normal fat cells.
- They are usually encapsulated and have a yellowish appearance on gross examination.

15.2.5 Radiography [9]

- On radiographs, large lipomas may be appreciated as a region of low density exerting a mass effect.
- Calcification may be present in up to 11% of cases, although it is more commonly associated with well-differentiated liposarcoma.

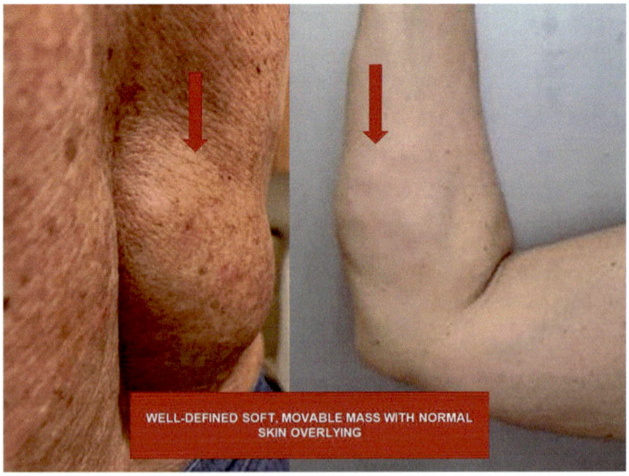

Fig. 15.5 Clinical photograph of patients with lipoma

15.2.6 Computed Tomography (Fig. 15.6) [9]

- CT scans show lipomas as well-defined, homogenous masses with fat attenuation values (attenuation values between -65 and - 120 Hounsfield units).
- They do not enhance with contrast.

15.2.7 Ultrasonography (Fig. 15.7) [6]

- Ultrasonography images show lipomas as variably echogenic masses. Superficial lipomas most commonly appear isoechogenic and homogeneous.
- Features may include no acoustic shadowing, minimal power Doppler flow, and no or minimal encapsulation visibility.
- Heterogeneous echotexture, more than minimal power Doppler flow, or large size is suspicious for liposarcoma.

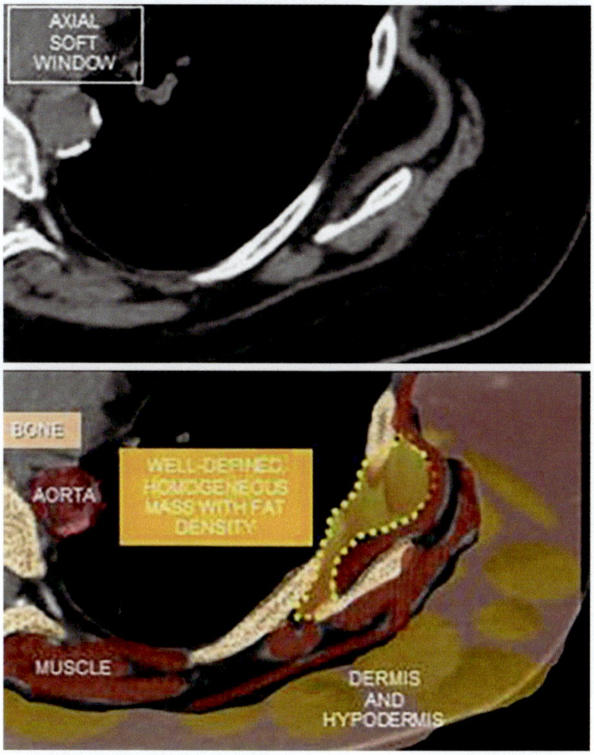

Fig. 15.6 Computed tomography findings of lipoma (Philips Brilliance CT 64-slice)

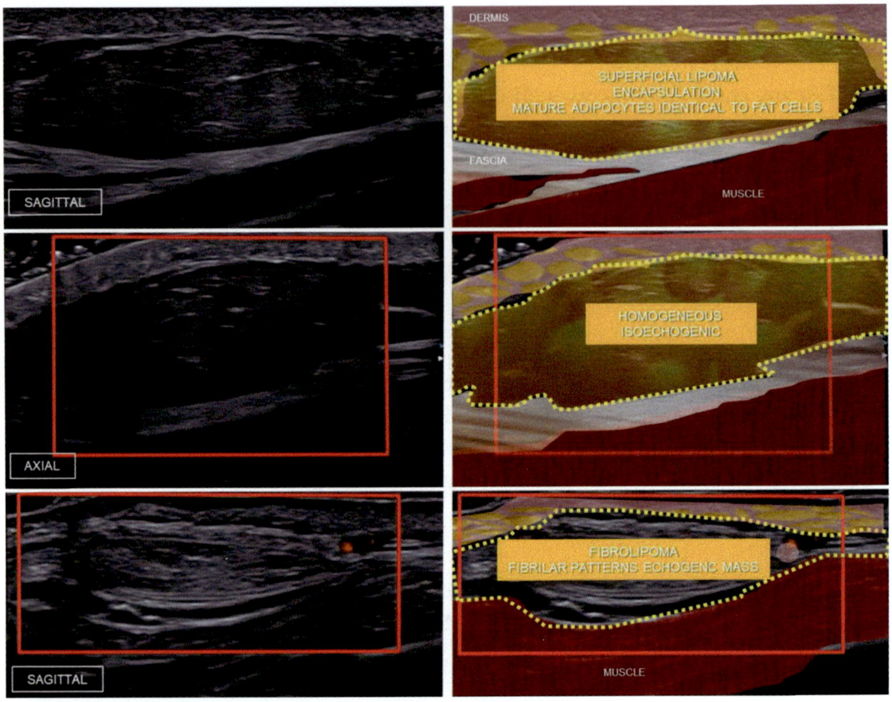

Fig. 15.7 Ultrasonographic findings of lipoma with a 24 MHz probe (Aplio i800, Canon Medical Systems)

15.2.8 MRI (Figs. 15.8 and 15.9) [6]

- MRI is the imaging modality of choice for lipomas, confirming the diagnosis suggested by ultrasonography and CT and assessing for atypical features suggesting liposarcoma. Lipomas follow subcutaneous fat signal on all sequences:
- High signal on T1-weighted sequences, saturates on fat-saturated sequences, no or minimal enhancement.
- High signal on FSE T2-weighted sequences, saturates on fat-saturated sequences; persistent areas of high T2 signal are worrisome.

15.3 Dermatofibroma

15.3.1 Definition [10]

- Also recognized as benign fibrous histiocytoma.
- Prevalent soft tissue lesions are characterized by the proliferation of benign spindle cells within the dermis.

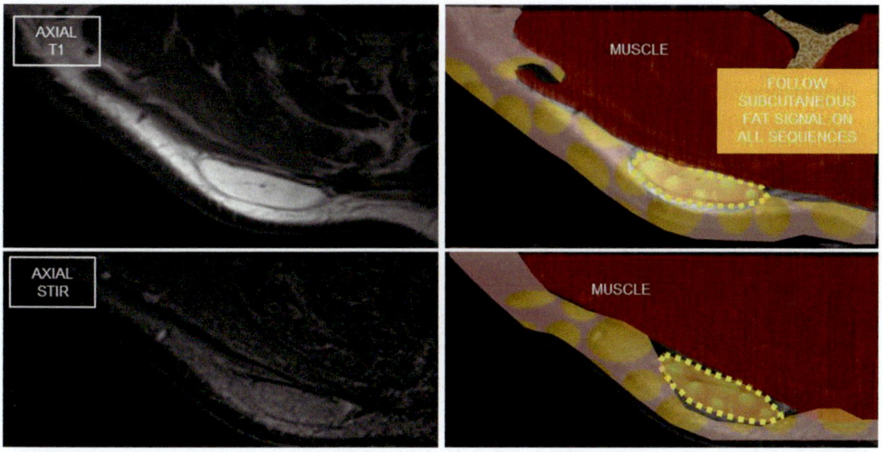

Fig. 15.8 MRI with surface coil findings of lipoma on T1-weighted and STIR sequences (Magnetom Prisma 3T MRI, Siemens)

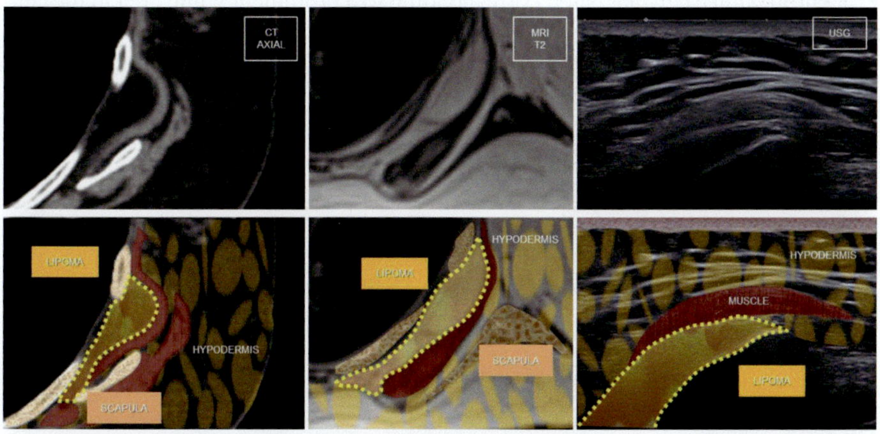

Fig. 15.9 Computed tomography, ultrasonography, and MRI findings of subscapular lipoma on T2-weighted sequence

15.3.2 Epidemiology [11]

- Dermatofibromas rank among the most frequently encountered cutaneous lesions.
- Aged 20–40 years, with a notable predominance in females.

15.3.3 Clinical Presentation (Fig. 15.10) [10, 11]

- Most dermatofibromas are thought to be a reactive process secondary to local trauma including, but not limited to, insect bites, puncture wounds due to splinters, and ingrown hairs.
- Present as slow-growing, dermal papules with colors ranging from pink or tan/brown to black, exhibiting firmness.
- Usually, these lesions measure <2 cm in diameter and are commonly located on the limbs.
- Dermatofibromas characteristically display the “dimple sign,” wherein applying lateral pressure results in central dimpling of the lesions.

15.3.4 Dermoscopy (Fig. 15.11) [10–12]

- A delicate network of pigmentation around the periphery of the lesion.
- Central white scar-like patch corresponding to a prominent white area in the center, resembling a scar.

15.3.5 Histopathology [11]

- Overlying epidermis usually presents with lentiginous hyperplasia (about 80%).
- The lesion corresponding to a poorly circumscribed dermal proliferation composed of spindle cells, with variable cellularity, rarely extending to the hypodermis.

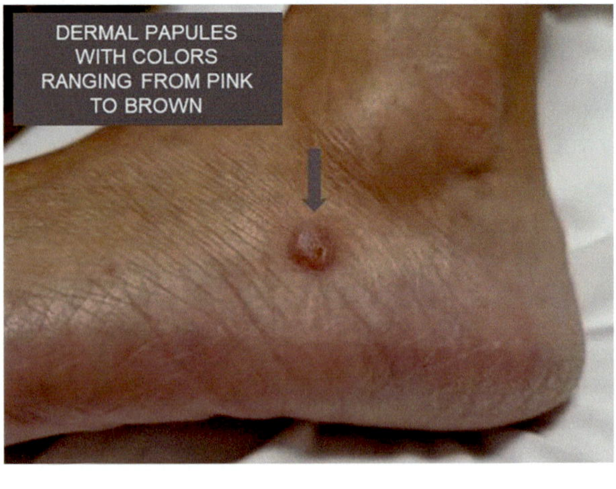

Fig. 15.10 Clinical photograph of patient with dermatofibroma

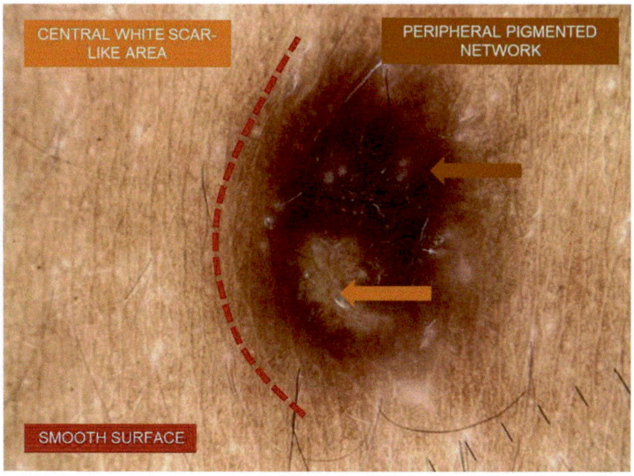

Fig. 15.11 Dermoscopic findings of patient with dermatofibroma (x10)

- Collagen may be enveloped by proliferating cells, with an entrapped appearance; rarely it may exhibit giant cells, foamy cells, or Touton cells.

15.3.6 Radiography and Computed Tomography

- Nonspecific soft tissue mass with avid enhancement.

15.3.7 Ultrasonography (Fig. 15.12) [13]

- A dermal structure that is hypoechoic with poorly defined contours can protrude into the hypodermis. In these cases, the tumor does not exhibit lobulations or prominent convexity at the deep hypodermal margins.
- On power Doppler, vascularization can range from mild to marked.
- Nodular subtypes typically present with a more intense pseudo nodular hypoechoic center and distortion of regional hair follicles.
- Aneurysmal variants may display anechoic cystic spaces due to hemorrhage.
- Atrophic variants may appear as solid hypoechoic lesions with dermal atrophy.

15.3.8 MRI

- The mass exhibits avid contrast enhancement and increased vascularity.
- It is mostly homogeneous but contains areas of internal necrosis and hemorrhage, with central vascularity.

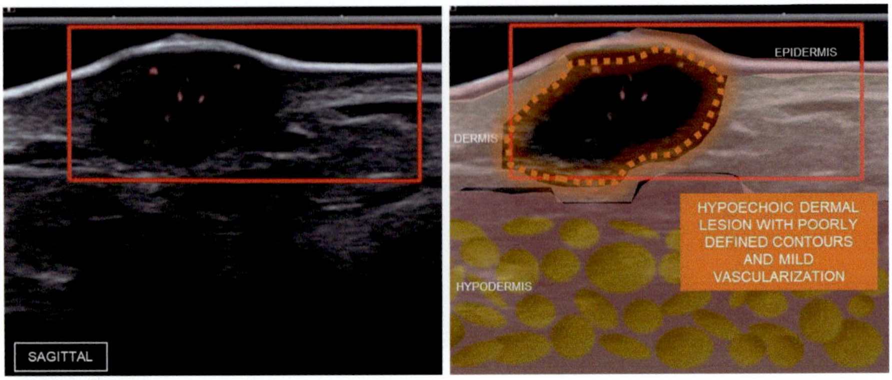

Fig. 15.12 Ultrasonographic findings of dermatofibroma with a 24 MHz probe (Aplio i800, Canon Medical Systems)

- There is no definite hypointense pseudocapsule or T2-hyperintense peritumoral edema on MRI.
- T1-weighted images show signal intensity similar to muscle.
- T2-weighted images show heterogeneity and intermediate to high signal intensity.
- Cystic lesions exhibit hypointense central areas on T1-weighted images post-contrast.
- Solid areas demonstrate intermediate signal intensity.

15.3.9 3D Images

- Particularly useful for detecting small lesions or addressing recurrent and complex cases.
- Offers precise visualization of the lesion's boundaries, aiding in the assessment of its severity and its proximity to adjacent structures, especially surrounding blood vessels.

15.4 Poroma

15.4.1 Definition [14]

- A rare benign adnexal tumor, derived from the eccrine gland.
- Poroma is referred to be the great imitator because its clinical and dermoscopical findings can share features of benign and malignant tumors.

15.4.2 Epidemiology [14]

- Middle-aged to elderly patients.
- No sex predilection.
- 10% of the eccrine and apocrine sweat glands (which are 1% of all primary cutaneous lesions).

15.4.3 Clinical Presentation (Fig. 15.13) [14–16]

- The tumor is usually a normochromic or erythematous papule.
- The most common locations are the volar skin (palms and soles), but we can find it also on head and neck, and lower extremities. Less common locations have been described, such as the eyelids and the vulva.
- EP on non-volar sites is challenging and can mimic other malignant tumors, such as melanoma, basal cell carcinoma (BCC), or squamous cell carcinoma (SCC).

15.4.4 Dermoscopy (Fig. 15.14) [17]

- Poromas can exhibit dermoscopic features similar to those of pyogenic granulomas, seborrheic keratosis, nevi, malignant melanoma, basal cell carcinoma (BCC), and squamous cell carcinoma (SCC).
- In nonpigmented poromas, the vascular pattern is a key dermoscopic feature that aids in diagnosis.
- Specific findings:
  - White interlacing areas around vessels.

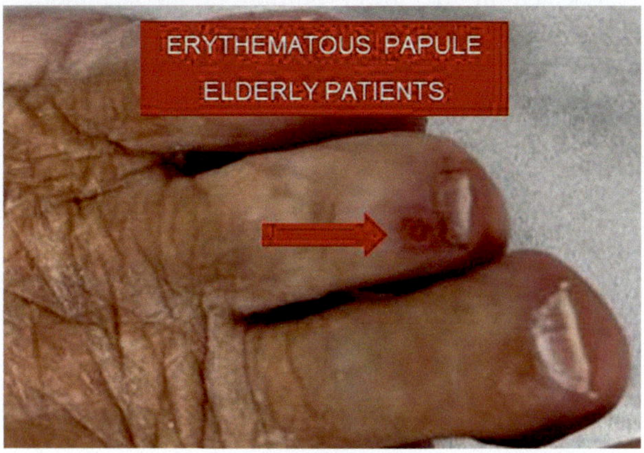

Fig. 15.13 Clinical photograph of patient with poroma

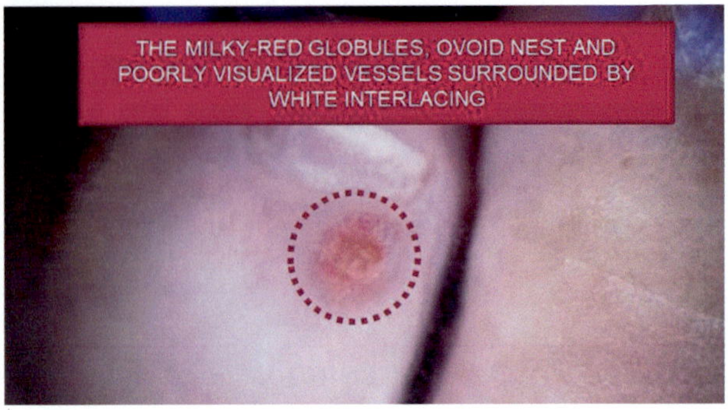

Fig. 15.14 Dermoscopic findings of patient with poroma (x10)

- Yellow structureless areas.
- Milky-red globules.
- Poorly visualized vessels.
- Branched vessels with rounded endings.

- The presence of any of these five features indicates poroma with a sensitivity of 62.8% and specificity of 82.0%.

15.4.5 Histopathology (Fig. 15.15) [17]

- Poroma can be categorized into four types based on the localization of poroid cells:
  - Hidracanthoma simplex.
  - Eccrine poroma (EP).
  - Dermal duct tumor.
  - Poroid hidradenoma.
- Tumor of basaloid or cuboidal cells, called poroid cells, with pale eosinophilic cytoplasm and which are clearly distinguished at the junction with the epidermis.
- Located in the lower portion of an acanthotic epiderma, forming anastomotic cords.
- May have eccrine ducts within the tumor mass, detached by the PAS.
- May present areas of coagulation necrosis (necrosis en masse) and atypia, which do not characterize malignancy.
- Porocarcinoma shows marked pleomorphism and a high mitotic index.
- Vascularized fibrous stroma; there may be mild chronic inflammation.
- Simple hydroacanthoma, nodular hydroadenoma, and dermal duct tumor are considered poroma variants.

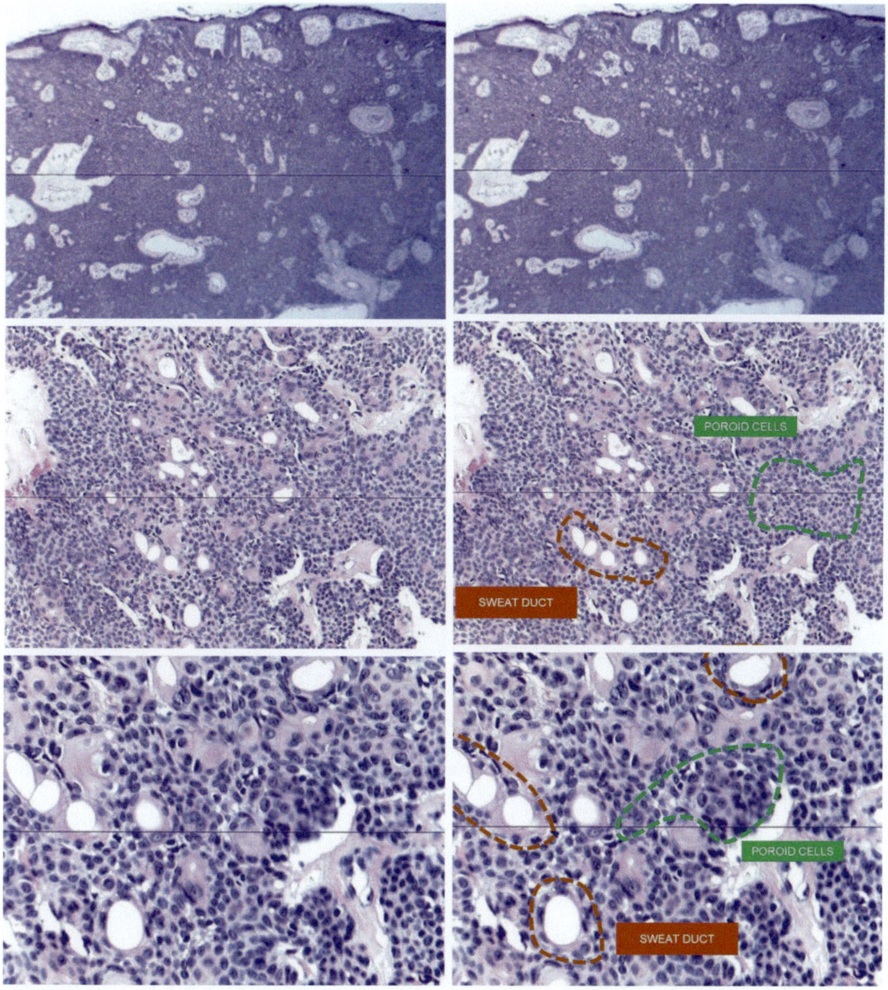

Fig. 15.15 Histological findings of poroma. Image kindly provided by Dr. Olga Harris—Brazil (H&E x20)

15.4.6 Ultrasonography (Fig. 15.16) [16]

- Well-defined, oval-shaped dermal lesion.
- Heterogeneous internal echo.
- Presence of hyperechoic spots.

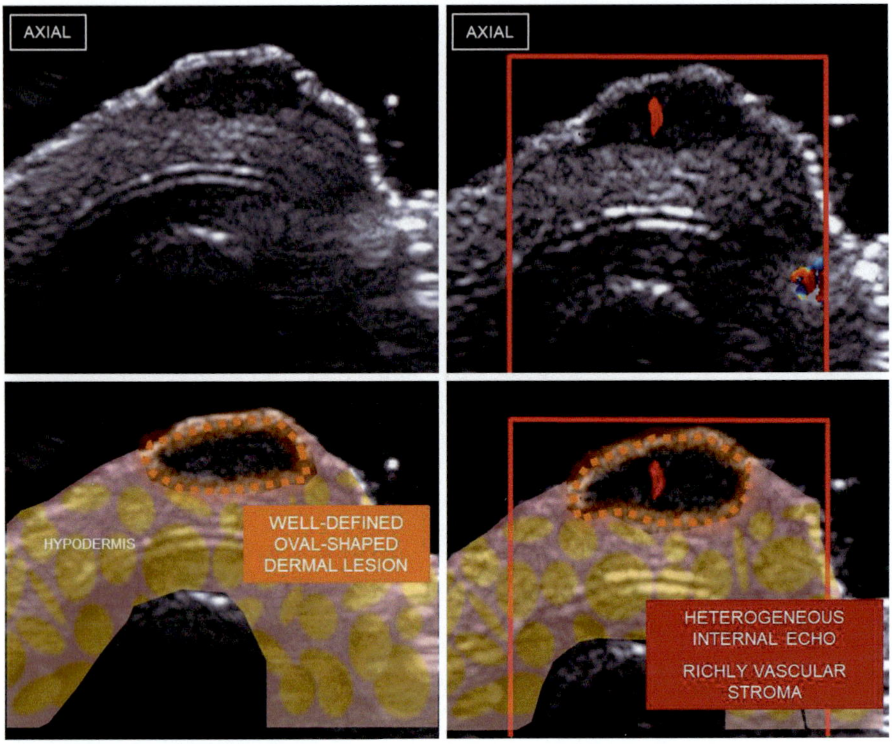

Fig. 15.16 Ultrasonographic findings of poroma with a 24 MHz probe (Aplio i800, Canon Medical Systems)

15.4.7 MRI (Fig. 15.17) [16]

- Common features:
  - Both poromas and porocarcinomas exhibit intratumoral T1 hyperintensity due to richly vascular stroma with dilated vessels.
- Porocarcinoma features:
  - Pedunculated solid lesions measuring =30 mm in diameter.
  - Protrusion into subcutaneous fat.

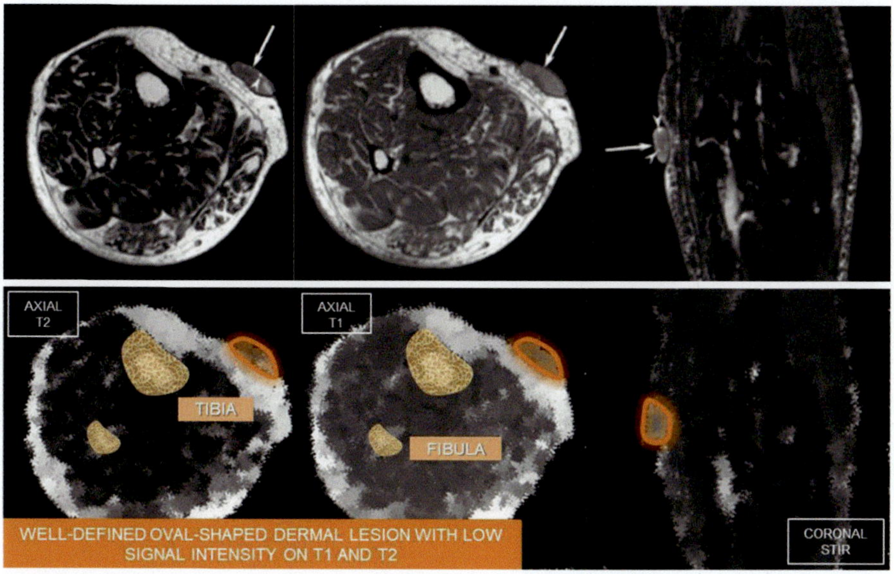

Fig. 15.17 MRI with surface coil findings of poroma on T1, T2-weighted, and STIR sequences. (*From* Kawaguchi et al. [113]; *with permission*)

15.5 Elastoma

15.5.1 Definition [18]

- Elastoma, also known as elastic nevus, is a dermatological condition characterized by the formation of yellow or normochromic papules and plaques.
- It belongs to the connective tissue nevus group (CTNs) and typically manifests in childhood, either congenitally or acquired later in life.
- The condition arises from embryological dysgenesis affecting dermal mesenchyme, leading to abnormal development of elastic fibers.

15.5.2 Epidemiology [18]

- Elastoma is rare, predominantly diagnosed in childhood, though sporadic cases may occur in adulthood.
- It may present as an isolated condition or be associated with Buschke–Ollendorff syndrome (BOS), characterized by the presence of osteopoikilosis and other CTNs.
- The incidence varies, with familial cases linked to autosomal dominant inheritance patterns.

15.5.3 Clinical Presentation (Fig. 15.18) [18]

- Clinically, elastoma appears as normochromic or yellow papules and plaques of varying sizes, commonly found on the lower back, thighs, legs, and abdomen.
- Lesions are asymptomatic and may proliferate over time, often appearing asymmetrical in distribution.

15.5.4 Histopathology [18]

- Histopathological examination reveals increased interstitial spaces between collagen fibers in the dermis.
- Staining for elastic fibers, such as Verhoeff's stain, demonstrates fragmented and irregularly shaped fibers (elastolysis and elastorrhexis), particularly in the reticular dermis.

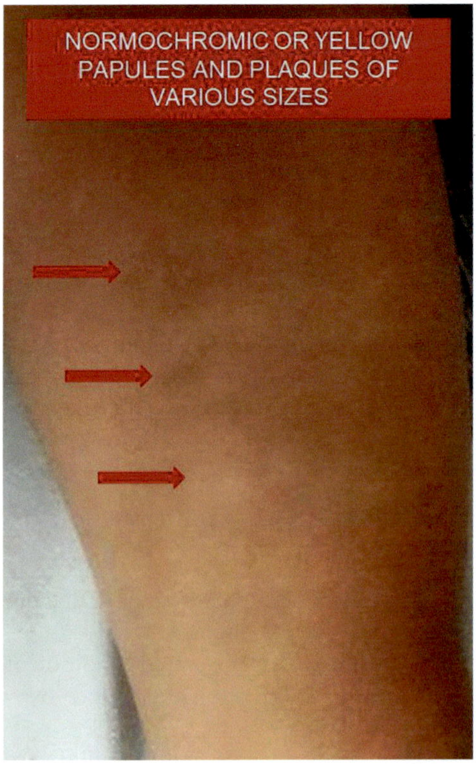

Fig. 15.18 Clinical photograph of patient with elastoma

15.5.5 Ultrasonography (Fig. 15.19)

- Elastomas typically appear as well-defined hypoechoic areas within the dermis. This reduced echogenicity reflects the increased elastin content and the dense connective tissue structure.
- The lesion often presents with well-defined, sharp margins that distinguish it from the surrounding normal tissue. This clear boundary can be seen between the elastoma and the adjacent dermis.
- The lesion is confined to the dermis, with no extension into the subcutaneous fat or deeper structures. This localization is important in distinguishing elastomas from other skin lesions that may involve multiple layers of the skin.
- Using power Doppler ultrasonography, elastomas usually show minimal to no internal vascularity. This absence of significant blood flow helps differentiate them from other types of nevi or skin tumors, which might have increased vascularity.
- The internal texture of the elastoma on ultrasonography tends to be relatively homogeneous, without the heterogeneous patterns often seen in malignant lesions or other types of connective tissue disorders.
- Unlike some other skin lesions, elastomas generally do not contain calcifications, which would appear as bright, echogenic spots on the ultrasonography.

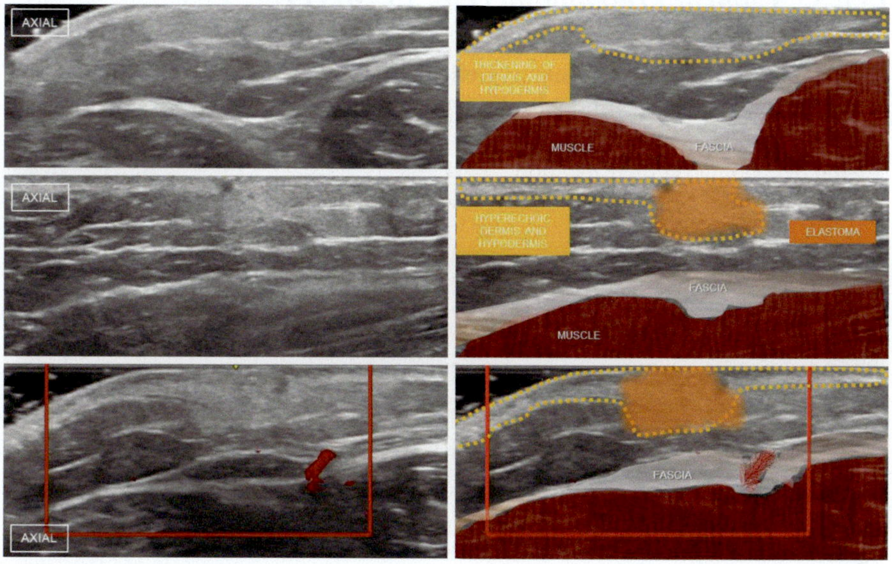

Fig. 15.19 Ultrasonographic findings of elastoma with a 24 MHz probe (Aplio i800, Canon Medical Systems)

15.6 Hibernoma

15.6.1 Definition [19]

- Hibernomas are uncommon benign soft tissue tumors composed of brown adipocytes, resembling the brown fat typically found in hibernating animals.
- Originally referred to as pseudolipomas due to their histological resemblance to lipomas, they were later formally named hibernomas by Gery in 1914.

15.6.2 Epidemiology [19]

- Hibernomas account for approximately 2% of benign tumors containing fat.
- They typically manifest between the ages of 20 and 40, with a slightly higher prevalence in males.
- These tumors often arise in residual deposits of brown fat, which persist in various anatomical sites including the thigh, retroperitoneum, and periscapular regions.

15.6.3 Clinical Presentation (Fig. 15.20) [19]

- Clinically, hibernomas present as well-defined, soft, lobulated masses that grow within fascial planes without infiltrating adjacent tissues.
- While usually asymptomatic, they can cause symptoms related to local compression depending on their location.

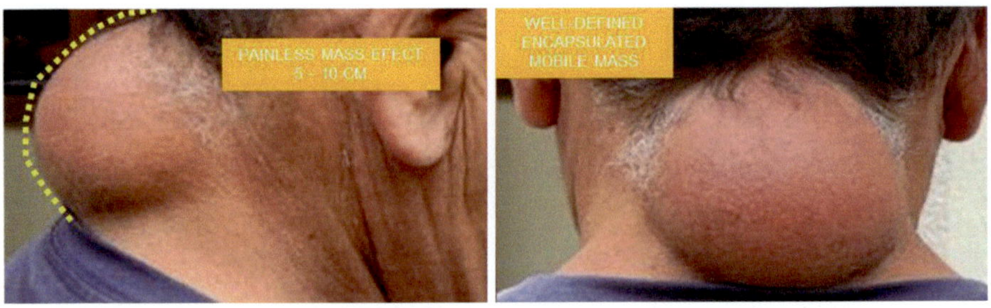

Fig. 15.20 Clinical photograph of patient with hibernoma

15.6.4 Histopathology [19]

- Hibernomas are characterized by multivacuolated adipocytes with centrally located nuclei and eosinophilic cytoplasm.
- They typically stain positive for S100 and CD31, and negative for CD34 and p53.
- Hibernomas exhibit several variants, including typical (classic), myxoid, lipoma-like, and spindle-cell types.

15.6.5 Radiography [19]

- Conventional radiography commonly reveals hibernomas as radiolucent masses without internal calcifications or osseous abnormalities, indicating their soft tissue origin.

15.6.6 Computed Tomography [19]

- On CT scans, hibernomas appear as well-defined masses with internal septations and attenuation values that vary between fat and muscle.
- Enhancement with intravenous contrast can highlight internal septa to varying degrees.

15.6.7 Ultrasonography (Fig. 15.21) [19]

- Ultrasonography imaging typically depicts hibernomas as well-circumscribed, solid masses with hyperechoic features and increased internal vascular flow, although these characteristics are not exclusive to hibernomas.

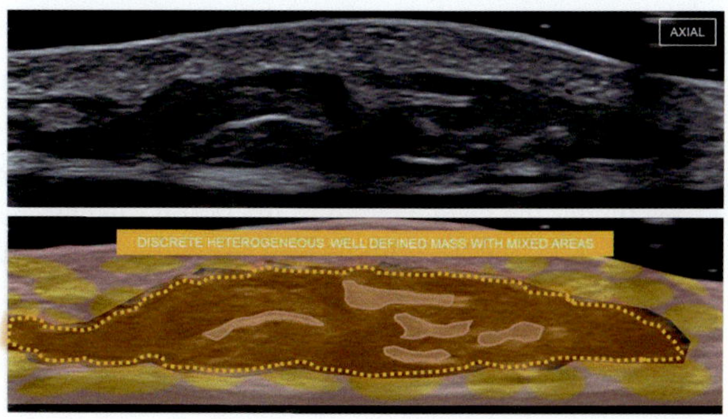

Fig. 15.21 Ultrasonographic findings of hibernoma with a 24 MHz probe (Aplio i800, Canon Medical Systems)

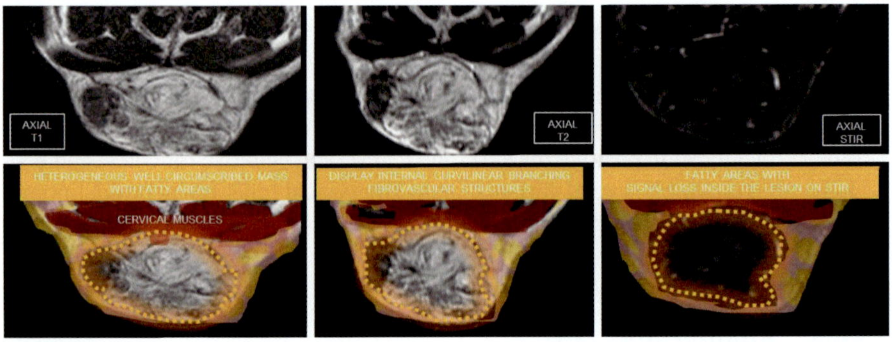

Fig. 15.22 MRI with surface coil findings of hibernoma on T1, T2-weighted and STIR sequences (Magnetom Prisma 3T MRI, Siemens)

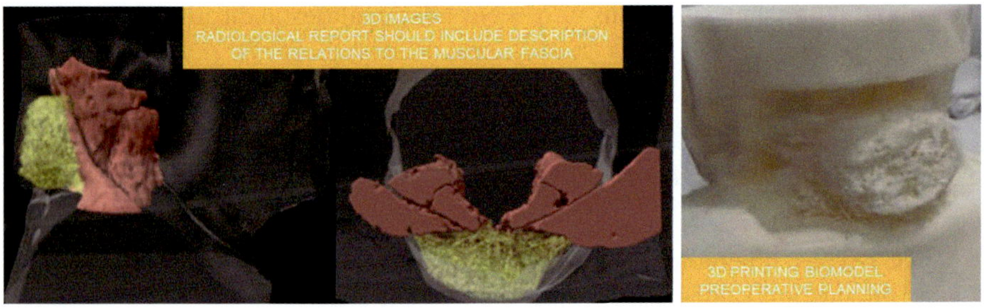

Fig. 15.23 3D images of hibernoma after segmentation of MRI isotropic images for surgical planning

15.6.8 MRI (Fig. 15.22) [19]

- On MRI, hibernomas typically appear hyperintense relative to skeletal muscle on T1-weighted images and slightly hypointense relative to subcutaneous fat due to differences in gyromagnetic ratios.
- T2-weighted and STIR images often show high signal intensity, particularly in myxoid variants.

15.6.9 3D Imaging (Fig. 15.23, Video 15.2)

- Particularly beneficial for managing challenging and recurrent cases.
- Facilitates the visualization of the lesion's extent, helping to evaluate its severity and its relationship with nearby structures, especially any surrounding vascular dilatation and fascial tissue.
- Enhances the precision of surgical procedures.

- Biomodels can be employed to create physical replicas of the affected area, providing valuable representations that assist in surgical planning and patient education.

15.7 Xanthomas

15.7.1 Definition [20, 21]

- Sebum-containing cysts measuring from less than 3 mm in diameter to 3 cm or more.
- Steatocystoma multiplex is a rare condition that is characterized by cutaneous cysts and may be inherited in an autosomal dominant manner or may occur sporadically.

15.7.2 Epidemiology [21]

- Lesions typically manifest during adolescence or early adulthood.
- Lesions can appear anywhere on the body, including the scalp, intertriginous areas, and genitalia, with a notable predilection for the chest.
- While predominantly a sporadic disorder, autosomal dominant inheritance is observed in some cases.

15.7.3 Clinical Presentation (Fig. 15.24) [20, 21]

- The clinical variants of cutaneous xanthomas include eruptive xanthomas, tuberous xanthomas, tendinous xanthomas, plane xanthomas (including xanthelasma), and verruciform xanthomas.
- Most xanthomas present as erythematous to yellow papules, plaques, or nodules, indicative of lipid deposition in the skin.
- Koebnerization (the appearance of eruptive xanthomas at sites of skin trauma) can occur.

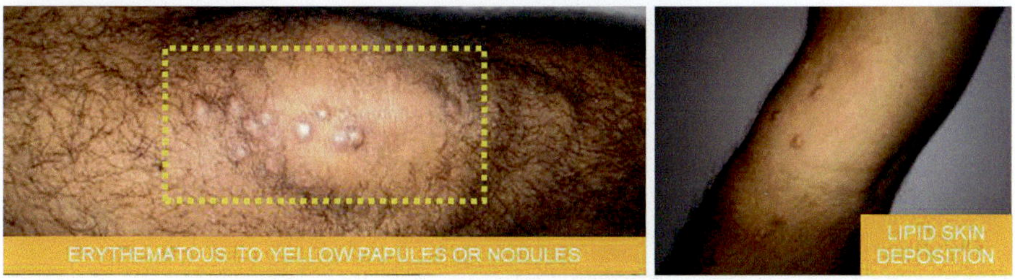

Fig. 15.24 Clinical photograph of patient with xanthoma

15.7.4 Dermoscopy (Fig. 15.25) [20]

- Nonpolarized dermoscopy findings:
  - Displays a circumscribed, yellowish, structureless area.
  - Margins appear diffuse.
  - Vellus hairs surround the area.
- Polarized dermoscopy findings:
  - Shows a distinctive central yellowish glow.
  - Lesions have a darker rim surrounding the yellow center.
  - Background exhibits a pseudoreticular pigmentary pattern.
  - The yellow structureless area correlates with the sebum contained in the cyst cavity.
  - Entrapped vellus hairs within the cystic cavity impart a greenish tinge to the yellow area.

15.7.5 Histopathology [21]

- Infiltrate composed only of foamy macrophages arranged close to venular spaces, from few cells to confluent nodular clusters.
- Rarely, there is a relevant associated chronic inflammatory process.

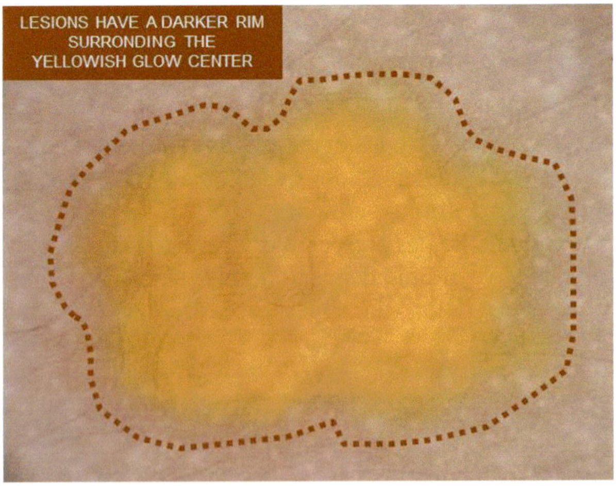

Fig. 15.25 Dermoscopic findings of patient with xanthoma (x20)

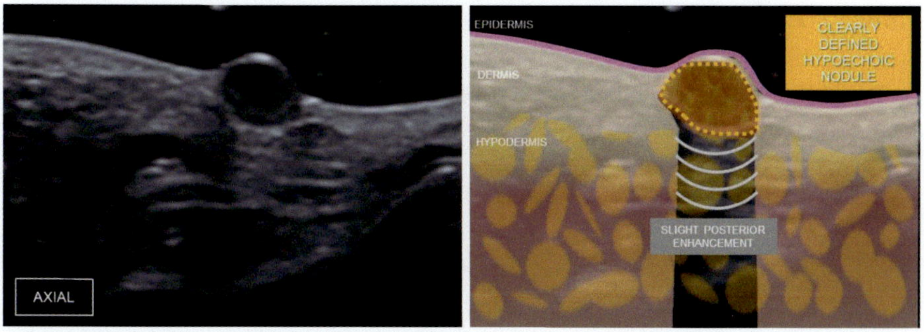

Fig. 15.26 Ultrasonographic findings of xanthoma with a 24 MHz probe (Aplio i800, Canon Medical Systems)

15.7.6 Ultrasonography (Fig. 15.26)

- Clearly defined hypoechoic nodules with slight posterior enhancement are located in the dermal and subcutaneous layers.
- More than half of the cases exhibit hypervascularity around the edges of the nodules.

15.7.7 MRI

- Well-defined heterogeneous nodules display intermediate signal intensity on T1-weighted sequences and hyperintense signal intensity on T2-weighted images, located in the dermal and subcutaneous layers.
- Fibrous tissue and calcifications can be observed.
- Peripheral homogeneous enhancement is seen after gadolinium administration.

15.8 Hidradenoma

15.8.1 Definition [22]

- Clear cell hidradenoma is a rare tumor originating from sweat gland tissues, traditionally identified with eccrine differentiation but also displaying apocrine features.

15.8.2 Epidemiology [22]

- Typically seen in individuals aged between the fourth and eighth decades of life.
- It affects women more frequently, with a female-to-male ratio of approximately 2:1.
- Usually solitary and slow-growing, with sizes ranging from 5 to 30 mm.

15.8.3 Clinical Presentation (Fig. 15.27) [22]

- Commonly presents as small, superficial, painless, palpable masses.
- Predominantly found on the trunk, lower limbs, and head.
- Often diagnosed incidentally or due to aesthetic concerns, rarely necessitating radiological evaluation.

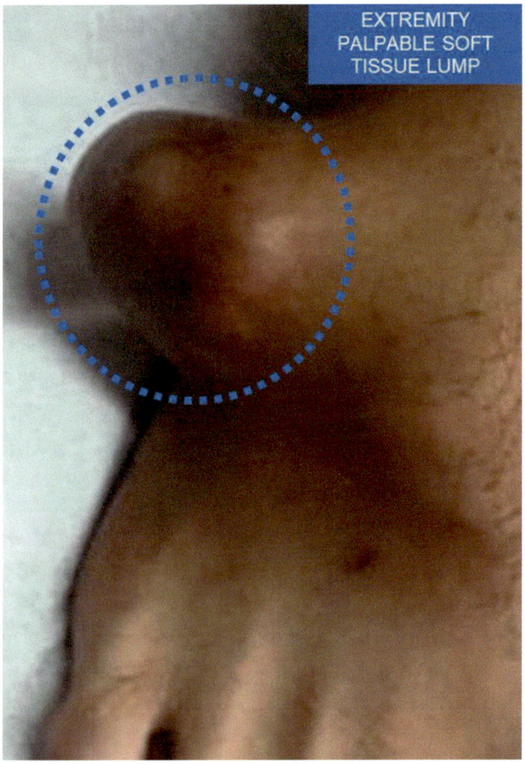

Fig. 15.27 Clinical photograph of patient with hidradenoma

15.8.4 Histopathology [22]

- Microscopic examination reveals cystic structures interspersed with solid components.
- Solid areas comprise polygonal to short spindle cells with clear cytoplasm.
- Typically encapsulated, lobulated masses with well-defined margins on histopathological analysis.

15.8.5 Computed Tomography [22]

- Presents with low attenuation of the mass.
- Displays heterogeneous enhancement of the peripheral wall and internal nodule post-contrast.
- No evidence of calcification is typically noted.

15.8.6 Ultrasonography (Fig. 15.28) [22]

- Shows heterogeneous echo texture with anechoic and echogenic areas.
- Exhibits posterior acoustic enhancement.
- Demonstrates vascularity with both central and peripheral flow observed on Doppler imaging.

15.8.7 MRI (Fig. 15.29) [22]

- Indicates low signal intensity on T1-weighted images.
- Shows high signal intensity on T2-weighted images.
- Demonstrates heterogeneous enhancement of the peripheral wall, septa, and central nodule following contrast administration.

15.8.8 3D Imaging

- Especially useful for complex, exuberant, and recurrent cases.
- Enables detailed visualization of the lesion's extent, allowing for accurate assessment of its severity and its connection to surrounding structures, particularly in areas with exuberant vascular supply.
- Improves the accuracy of surgical interventions.

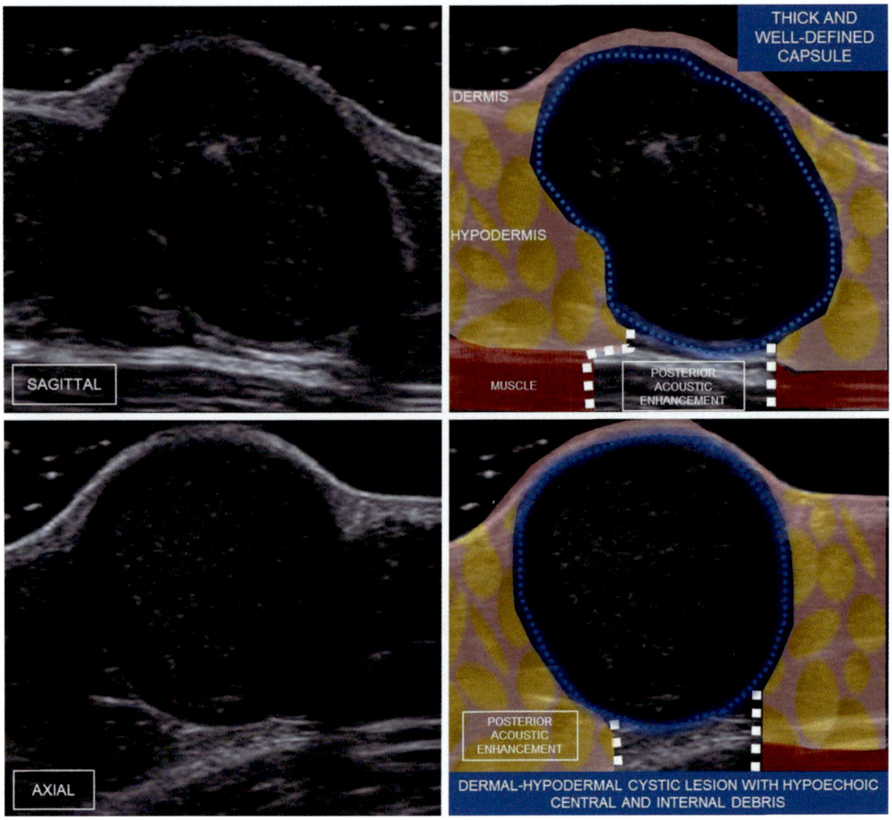

Fig. 15.28 Ultrasonographic findings of hidradenoma with a 24 MHz probe (Aplio i800, Canon Medical Systems)

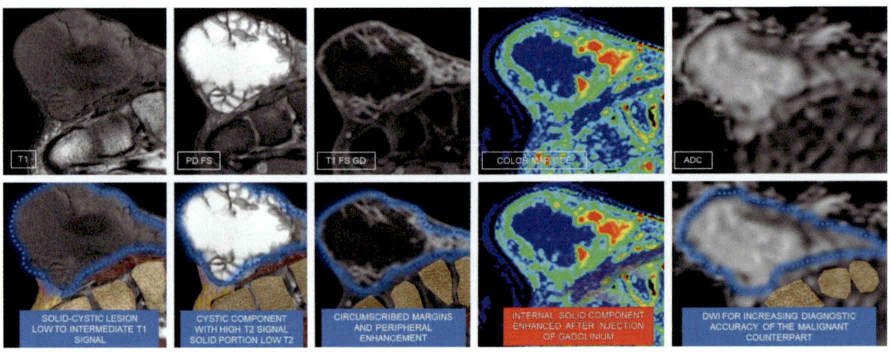

Fig. 15.29 MRI findings of hidradenoma on T1, DP FS, DWI, and T1 FS-weighted sequences after administration of gadolinium (Magnetom Prisma 3T MRI, Siemens)

- Biomodels can be utilized to produce physical replicas of the affected region, offering helpful representations for both surgical planning and patient education.

15.9 Acrochordon

15.9.1 Definition [23]

- Acrochordons, also known as fibroepithelial polyps, skin tags, or papillomas, are common benign skin neoplasms frequently associated with obesity.
- These small, pedunculated polyps can be bothersome to patients, typically developing in areas like the neck, axillae, and groin.
- They may cause discomfort due to symptoms such as itching, rubbing against clothing, or simply due to their appearance.
- There is a well-established association between acrochordons and insulin resistance, obesity, as well as a familial predisposition to developing these lesions.

15.9.2 Epidemiology [23]

- Acrochordons are extremely common, particularly among adults.
- They are most prevalent in middle-aged and elderly individuals, affecting both genders equally.
- Risk factors include obesity, diabetes mellitus, and metabolic syndrome. The prevalence increases with age, and there is a higher occurrence in areas prone to friction, such as the neck, armpits, and groin.

15.9.3 Clinical Presentation (Fig. 15.30) [23]

- Acrochordons present as small, soft, usually pedunculated lesions most commonly located on the neck, axillae, and inguinal folds (typically in intertriginous areas), though they can appear on almost any part of the skin.
- They may range in color from skin-toned to hyperpigmented and generally measure between 2 and 5 mm, although larger lesions can occur.
- They are usually asymptomatic but can become pruritic, painful, or inflamed due to catching on clothing or jewelry.

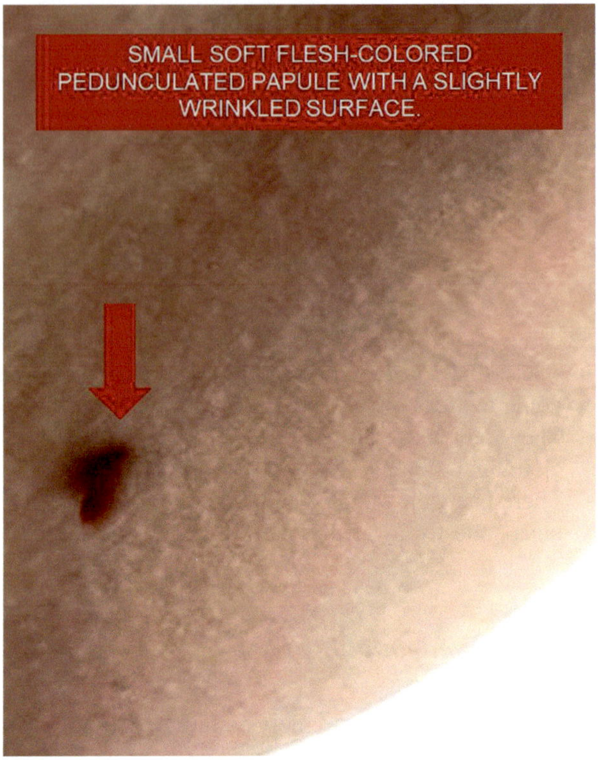

Fig. 15.30 Clinical photograph of patient with acrochordon

15.9.4 Histopathology [23]

- Acrochordons are composed of loose collagen fibers, a variable number of dilated capillaries, and adipose tissue within the dermis.
- The overlying epidermis is usually unremarkable but can show slight hyperkeratosis or acanthosis.
- The presence of a fibrovascular core within the stalk is characteristic.

15.9.5 Ultrasonography (Fig. 15.31)

- Acrochordons typically appear as well-defined, hypoechoic, or isoechoic lesions with a thin stalk connecting them to the skin.
- Power Doppler imaging may reveal minimal vascularity, consistent with the fibrovascular structure seen histologically.
- Although ultrasonography is generally not required for diagnosis due to the small size and superficial location of acrochordons, it can be useful in atypical cases.

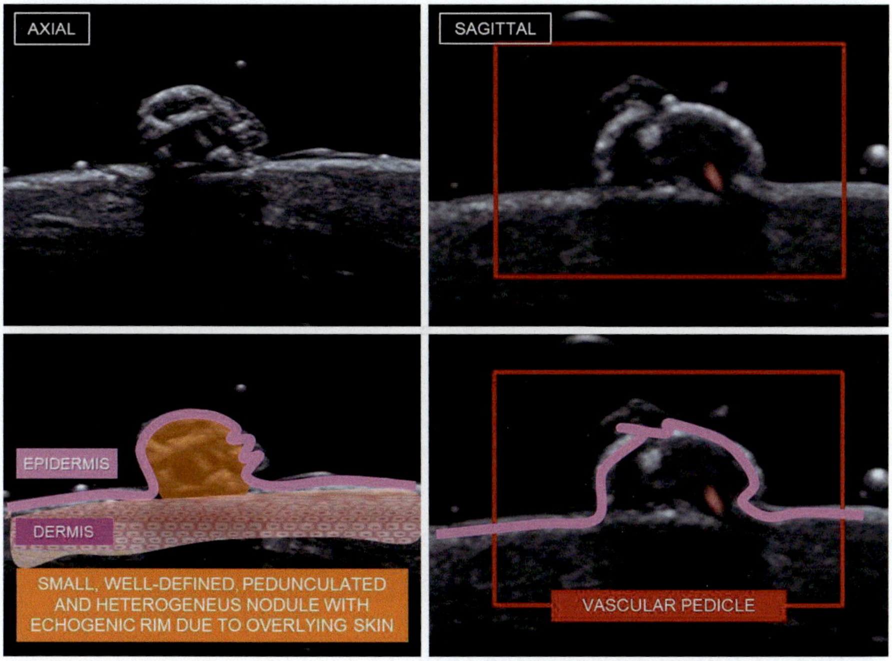

Fig. 15.31 Ultrasonographic findings of acrochordon with a 24 MHz probe (Aplio i800, Canon Medical Systems)

15.10 Desmoid Tumor

15.10.1 Definition [24]

- Desmoid tumors, also known as aggressive fibromatoses, are uncommon soft-tissue tumors characterized by proliferative fibroblastic and myofibroblastic cells and invasive growth, often recurring locally. The term originates from the Greek "desmos," highlighting their tendon-like or band-like consistency.

15.10.2 Epidemiology [24]

- Desmoid tumors primarily affect young adults, typically between 25 and 35 years old.
- They are categorized into extraabdominal, abdominal, and intraabdominal types, with specific associations such as Gardner syndrome in the intraabdominal cases.

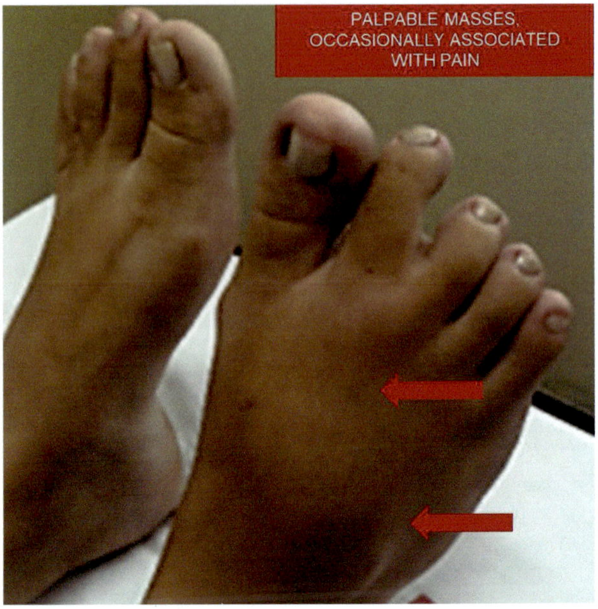

Fig. 15.32 Clinical photograph of patient with desmoid tumor

15.10.3 Clinical Presentation (Fig. 15.32) [24]

- Patients commonly present with palpable masses, occasionally associated with pain.
- Unusual presentations include rapid enlargement during pregnancy or suspicion of breast malignancies.

15.10.4 Histopathology [24]

- Histologically, desmoid tumors consist of spindle-shaped cells surrounded by collagen.
- Macroscopically, they appear as whitish bands indicative of collagen-rich areas.

15.10.5 Computed Tomography [24, 25]

- CT imaging provides detailed anatomical information and is integral to the diagnostic evaluation of desmoid tumors.

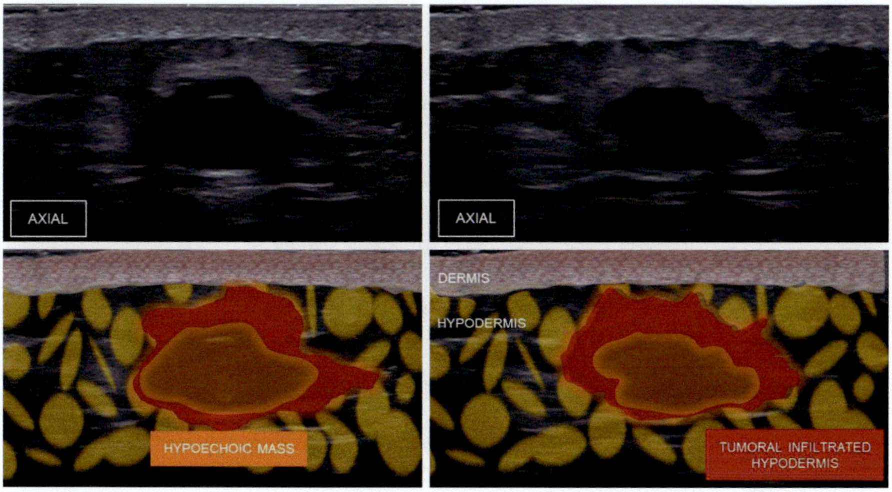

Fig. 15.33 Ultrasonographic findings of desmoid tumor with a 24 MHz probe (Aplio i800, Canon Medical Systems)

15.10.6 Ultrasonography (Fig. 15.33) [24, 25]

- High-Resolution ultrasoonography has emerged as a valuable tool due to its cost-effectiveness, high resolution, and ability to assess tumor vascularity and extension.
- Shows fibrillar hyperechogenic areas within tumors, reflecting collagen-rich regions observed on MRI.
- Useful for assessing tumor extensions and vascularization, guiding biopsies.

15.10.7 MRI (Fig. 15.34) [24, 25]

- MRI offers superior soft tissue contrast and is essential for evaluating desmoid tumors, particularly in assessing their relationships with adjacent structures such as vessels and nerves.
- Desmoids exhibit irregular stellar-like appearance with "fascial tail" extensions along fascial planes and subcutaneous fat.
- They appear isointense to muscle on T1-weighted and hyperintense on water-sensitive images.
- Bands of low signal intensity correlate with collagenized areas.

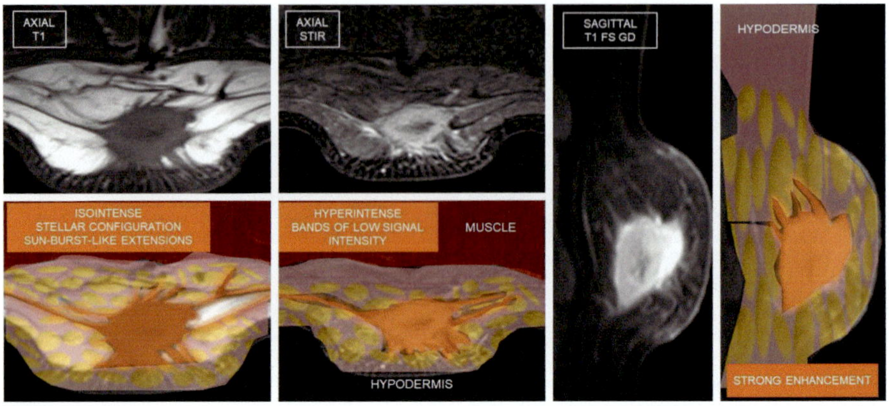

Fig. 15.34 MRI with surface coil findings of desmoid tumor on T1, STIR, and T1 FS-weighted sequences after administration of gadolinium (Magnetom Prisma 3T MRI, Siemens)

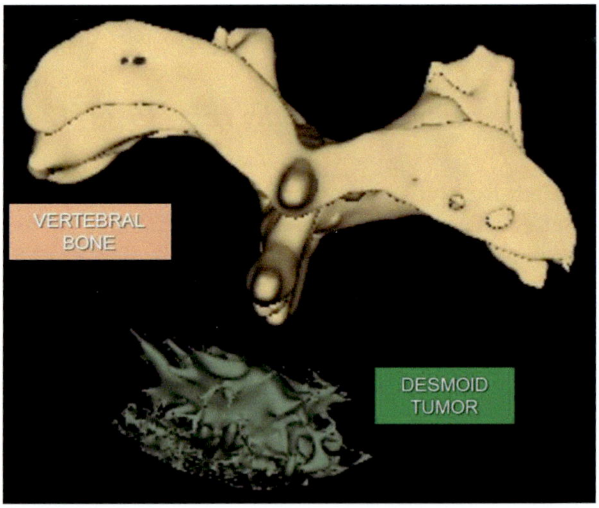

Fig. 15.35 3D images of desmoid tumor after segmentation of MRI isotropic images for surgical planning

15.10.8 3D Imaging (Fig. 15.35, Video 15.3)

- Especially useful for handling complex and persistent cases.
- Aids in visualizing the full extent of the lesion, assisting in assessing its severity and how it interacts with adjacent structures, including any nearby blood vessel expansions and connective tissues.
- Improves the accuracy of surgical interventions, especially in delicate areas.
- Biomodels can be used to generate physical replicas of the affected area, offering valuable insights for surgical planning and patient education.

15.10.9 Nodular Fasciitis

15.10.9.1 Definition [26]

- Nodular fasciitis (NF), also known as nodular fasciitides when multiple lesions are present, is a rapidly spreading, nonneoplastic soft tissue lesion commonly found deep within the subcutaneous layer or fascia.
- Initially termed subcutaneous pseudosarcomatous fibromatosis, it was formally designated as nodular fasciitis in 1966.

15.10.10 Epidemiology [26]

- NF is the most prevalent benign fibroblastic proliferative lesion affecting soft tissue, typically occurring in individuals aged between the third and fourth decades of life.
- It commonly manifests as a single, rapidly growing tumor predominantly located in the upper limbs, trunk, and lower limbs.

15.10.11 Clinical Presentation (Fig. 15.36) [26]

- NF presents as a swiftly enlarging solitary tumor, often reaching sizes up to 2–3 cm within a span of 2–6 weeks.

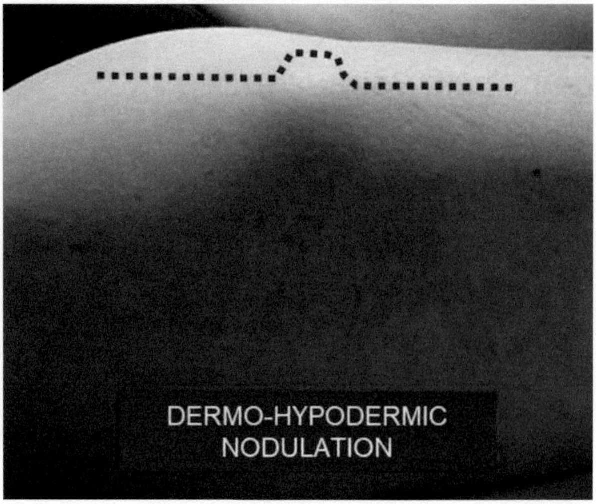

Fig. 15.36 Clinical photograph of patient with nodular fascitis

- Symptoms may include pain or occasional bleeding. It can appear in unusual sites such as the head and neck, and rarely in locations like the lower female genital tract or bladder.

15.10.12 Histopathology [27]

- Nodular fasciitis appears as a dermohypodermic nodulation characterized by a proliferation of myofibroblasts in a storiform pattern, typically within the hypodermis.
- Histological patterns include myxoid, cellular, or fibrous variants, often presenting with typical mitotic activity and occasional osteoclast-like giant cells.
- These lesions may exhibit sparse lymphocytic infiltrates and foci of hemorrhage, often seen as hemosiderin deposits.

15.10.13 Ultrasonography (Fig. 15.37) [26]

- NF lesions typically display well-defined isoechoic to hypoechoic nodules with mild vascular flow enhancement in deep subcutaneous fat or within fascial planes.
- They are predominantly hypoechoic with mixed echogenicity and poorly defined margins on ultrasonography.

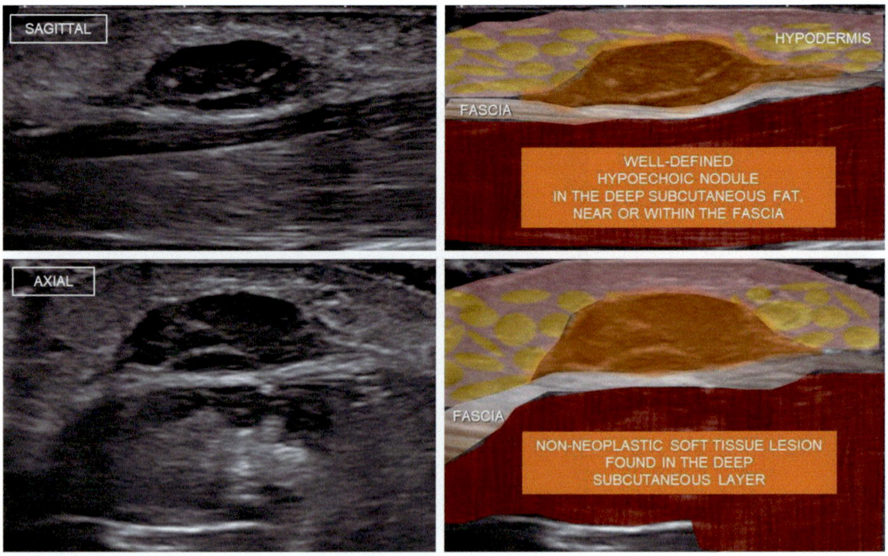

Fig. 15.37 Ultrasonographic findings of nodular fascitis with a 24 MHz probe (Aplio i800, Canon Medical Systems)

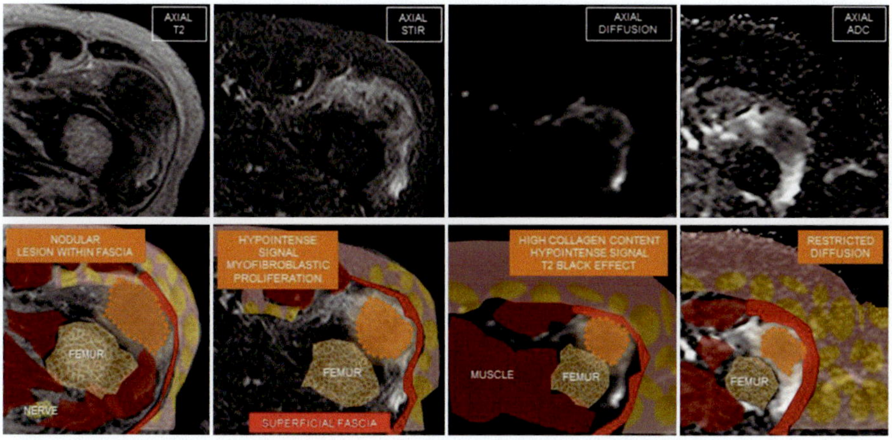

Fig. 15.38 MRI findings of nodular fascitis on T1-weighted, STIR, and DWI sequences (Magnetom Avanto 1.5T MRI, Siemens)

15.10.14 MRI (Fig. 15.38) [28]

- NF can exhibit various characteristics depending on its type (myxoid, cellular, fibrous).
- Hypercellular lesions typically appear isointense to skeletal muscle on T1-weighted images and hyperintense compared to adipose tissue on T2-weighted images
- Lesions rich in collagen content show hypointense signals across all sequences, with contrast enhancement usually diffuse, occasionally peripheral.
- NF lesions are typically surrounded by adipose tissue with poorly defined borders on MRI.

15.10.15 3D Images

- Particularly effective for managing intricate and ongoing cases.
- Helps in visualizing the lesion's full extent, crucial for evaluating its severity and its relationship with surrounding structures, such as nearby vascular expansions and connective tissues.
- Enhances the precision of surgical procedures, especially in sensitive areas.
- Biomodels can create tangible replicas of the affected region, providing essential insights for surgical planning and educating patients.

15.11 Hematoma

15.11.1 *Definition [29]*

- A hematoma is a localized collection of blood outside the blood vessels, typically caused by an injury to the wall of a blood vessel, allowing blood to leak into surrounding tissues.
- Hematomas can occur in any tissue or organ and vary in size, ranging from small, superficial bruises to large, life-threatening accumulations of blood.

15.11.2 *Epidemiology [29]*

- Hematomas are common and can occur in individuals of all ages.
- The incidence of hematomas is often associated with trauma, anticoagulant therapy, or conditions that predispose individuals to bleeding, such as hemophilia or other clotting disorders.
- Elderly individuals and those with a history of falls or high-impact injuries are particularly at risk.

15.11.3 *Clinical Presentation (Fig. 15.39) [29]*

- Hematomas present as a swollen, painful area, often with discoloration of the overlying skin ranging from red to purple or blue.
- The size, location, and severity of the hematoma determine the specific symptoms.
- For instance, a subcutaneous hematoma might present as a simple bruise.
- Hematomas can be associated with tenderness, restricted movement if near joints, and in severe cases, symptoms related to compression of nearby structures.

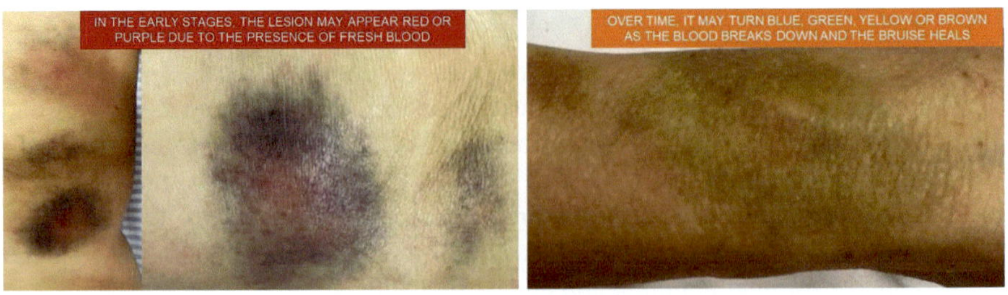

Fig. 15.39 Clinical photograph of patients with hematoma

15.11.4 Histopathology [29]

- Hematoma is characterized by the presence of clotted blood within tissues.
- Over time, the blood undergoes various stages of organization and resorption.
- Early stages show fresh blood cells, while older hematomas may demonstrate the breakdown of red blood cells, with hemosiderin-laden macrophages and fibrosis as the body attempts to repair the area.

15.11.5 Radiography and Computed Tomography (Fig. 15.40)

- Appears as a well-defined, often hyperdense mass within the soft tissues.
- The density can vary depending on the age of the hematoma—acute hematomas are typically hyperdense, while older ones may become hypodense.
- Hematomas generally do not enhance with contrast, helping differentiate them from other soft tissue masses.
- May be associated with surrounding soft tissue swelling or edema.
- In some cases, there may be fluid–fluid levels due to layering of blood components.

15.11.6 Ultrasonography (Fig. 15.41) [29]

- Ematomas appear as heterogeneous, hypoechoic to hyperechoic masses depending on the age of the hematoma and the degree of clot organization.
- Acute hematomas may appear more hypoechoic, while chronic hematomas, as they become more organized, tend to show mixed echogenicity with potential calcifications.
- Power Doppler ultrasonography may be used to assess for any ongoing bleeding or to differentiate a hematoma from other types of masses.

15.11.7 MRI (Fig. 15.42) [30]

Acute Skin Hematoma (within 0–3 days):

- The hematoma may appear isointense or slightly hypointense relative to muscle tissue on T1-weighted images, as the blood is in its early stage with intact red blood cells and deoxyhemoglobin.
- Typically hypointense on T2-weighted images, though it may also appear slightly hyperintense depending on the surrounding tissue.

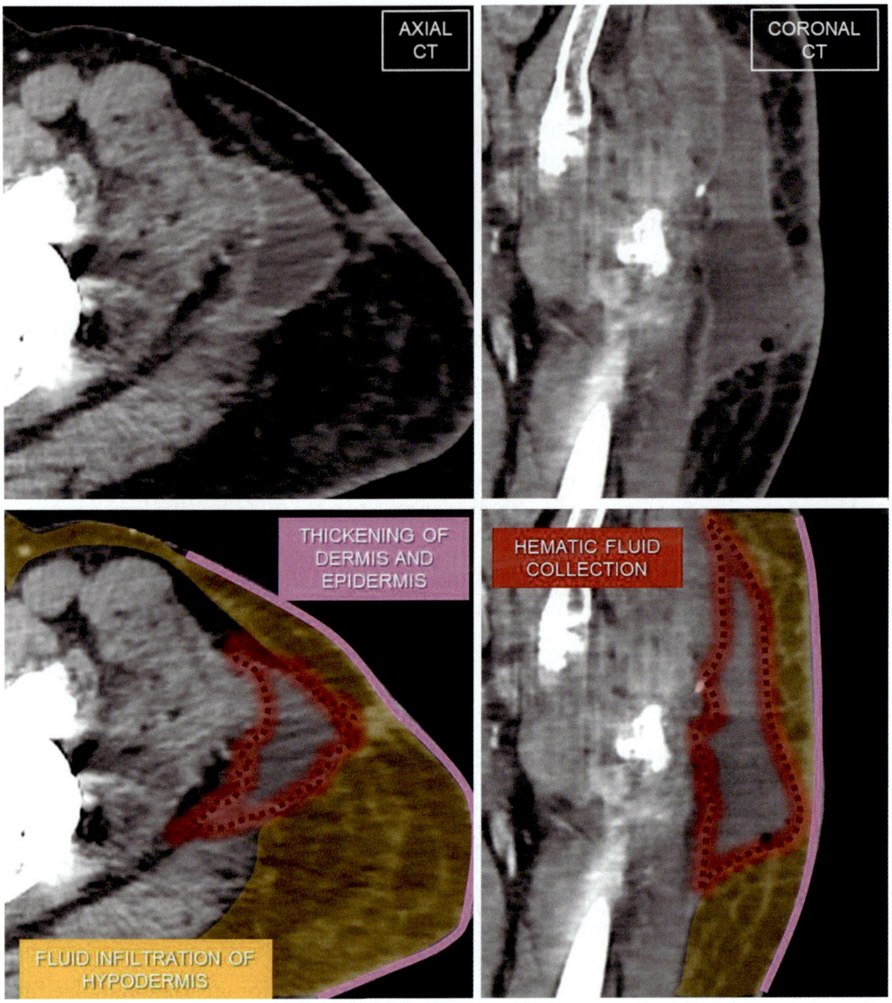

Fig. 15.40 Computed tomography findings of hematoma after axial and coronal reconstructions (Philips Brilliance CT 64-slice)

Subacute Skin Hematoma (3 days to 2 weeks):

- Early Subacute (3–7 days):
  - The hematoma becomes hyperintense on T1-weighted images due to the presence of intracellular methemoglobin.
  - It may appear hypointense to isointense on T2-weighted images as methemoglobin is still within cells.
- Late Subacute (1–2 weeks):
  - Remains hyperintense on T1-weighted images as methemoglobin continues to dominate.

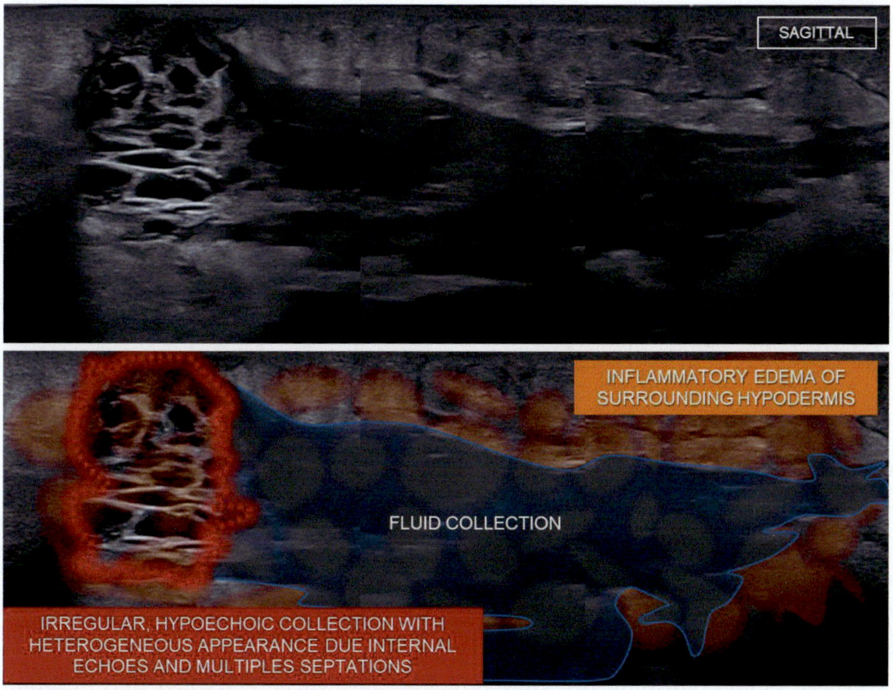

Fig. 15.41 Ultrasonographic findings of hematoma with a 24 MHz probe (Aplio i800, Canon Medical Systems)

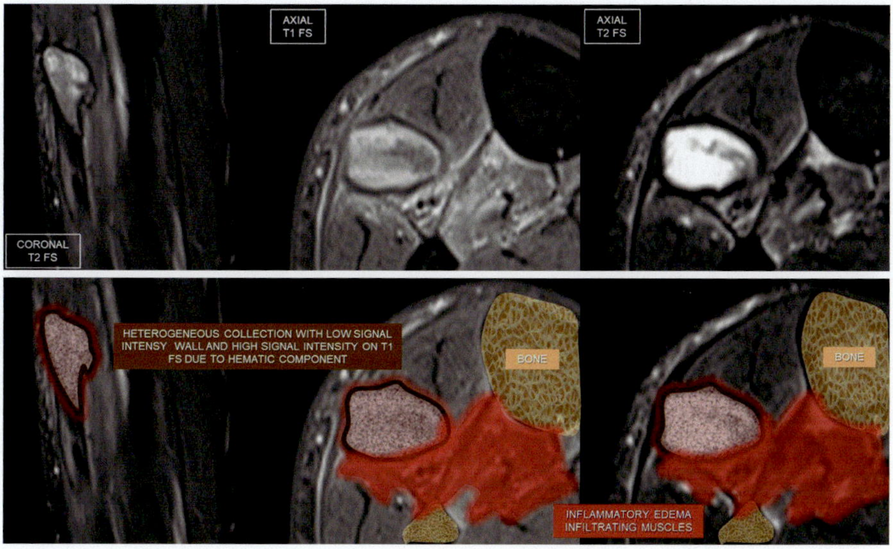

Fig. 15.42 MRI findings of hematoma on T1 FS and T2 FS-weighted images (Magnetom Avanto 1.5T MRI, Siemens)

  - Becomes hyperintense on T2-weighted images as methemoglobin transitions to the extracellular space.

Chronic Skin Hematoma (over 2 weeks):

- May return to being isointense or slightly hypointense on T1-weighted images as the hematoma resolves and hemosiderin begins to deposit.
- Often shows a hypointense rim due to hemosiderin deposition on T2-weighted images, with a possible surrounding hyperintense area indicating fibrosis or fluid content. The "blooming effect" on gradient echo sequences may be more prominent due to hemosiderin.

15.12 Neurofibroma

15.12.1 Definition [31]

- A neurofibroma is a benign peripheral nerve sheath tumor primarily composed of Schwann cells, fibroblasts, and perineural cells.
- Neurofibromas can occur sporadically or as part of a genetic condition known as Neurofibromatosis type 1 (NF1).
- These tumors are typically slow-growing and can be classified into different types, including cutaneous, subcutaneous, and plexiform neurofibromas.

15.12.2 Epidemiology [31, 32]

- Neurofibromas are relatively common, with a higher incidence in individuals with NF1, an autosomal dominant genetic disorder that affects approximately 1 in 3000 individuals worldwide.
- Sporadic neurofibromas, occurring in individuals without NF1, are less common.
- The tumors can develop at any age but are most frequently diagnosed in young adults and individuals with NF1.

15.12.3 Clinical Presentation (Fig. 15.43) [31, 32]

- Neurofibromas usually present as soft, fleshy nodules that may be skin-colored or slightly hyperpigmented.
- They are typically painless but can cause discomfort if they compress adjacent nerves or tissues.

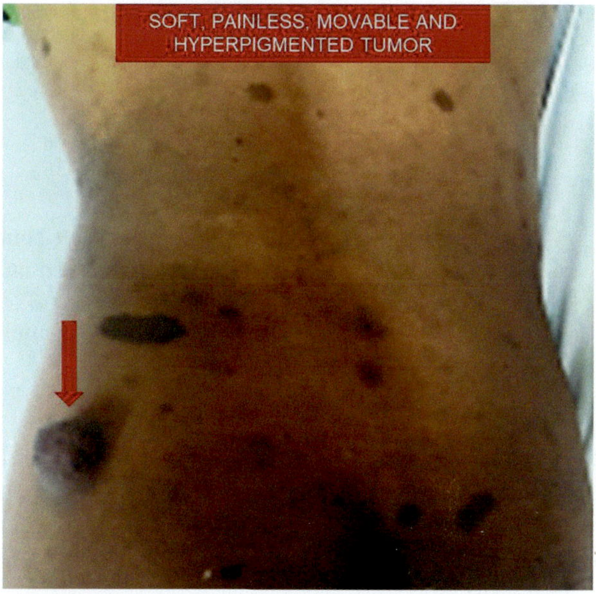

Fig. 15.43 Clinical photograph of patient with neurofibroma

- Cutaneous neurofibromas are often solitary in sporadic cases, while individuals with NF1 may have multiple lesions.
- Plexiform neurofibromas, which involve multiple nerve fascicles and can grow large, are associated with NF1 and may cause significant disfigurement or functional impairment.
- Neurofibromas are usually asymptomatic but can become symptomatic if they affect nerve function, leading to pain, numbness, or weakness.

15.12.4 Histopathology [33]

- Neurofibromas are characterized by a mixture of spindle-shaped Schwann cells, fibroblasts, and perineural cells within a myxoid stroma.
- The tumor is often well-demarcated but not encapsulated.
- The cells are arranged in a wavy or serpentine pattern, and the stroma may contain collagen bundles and mast cells.
- Plexiform neurofibromas, associated with NF1, have a more complex architecture with multiple nerve fascicles involved, and they can show diffuse growth, often making complete surgical resection challenging.

15.12.5 Radiography and Computed Tomography (Fig. 15.44) [32]

- Computed tomography:
  - Appears as a well-defined, homogeneous, low- to intermediate-density soft tissue mass.
  - The mass may show mild enhancement after contrast administration.
  - Typically, no bone erosion or invasion is seen unless associated with a larger plexiform neurofibroma.
  - In cases of neurofibromatosis type 1 (NF1), multiple neurofibromas may be present.
- Radiography:
  - May appear as a nonspecific soft tissue shadow.
  - Generally, no calcification or bony involvement is seen on plain radiographs.
  - In NF1, radiographs might show scoliosis or other skeletal deformities related to the disease.

15.12.6 Ultrasonography (Fig. 15.45) [34]

- Neurofibromas typically appear as well-defined, hypoechoic masses with a homogenous texture.
- They may show the "target sign," which consists of a hypoechoic peripheral rim with a central hyperechoic area, indicative of their nerve origin.
- This sign is more commonly seen in deeper or larger lesions.

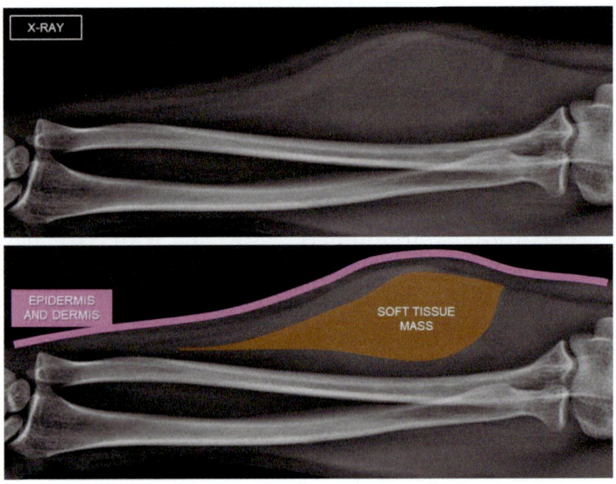

Fig. 15.44 Radiographic findings of neurofibroma (Philips Duo Diagnost R&F Room Digital RF and Tomo System)

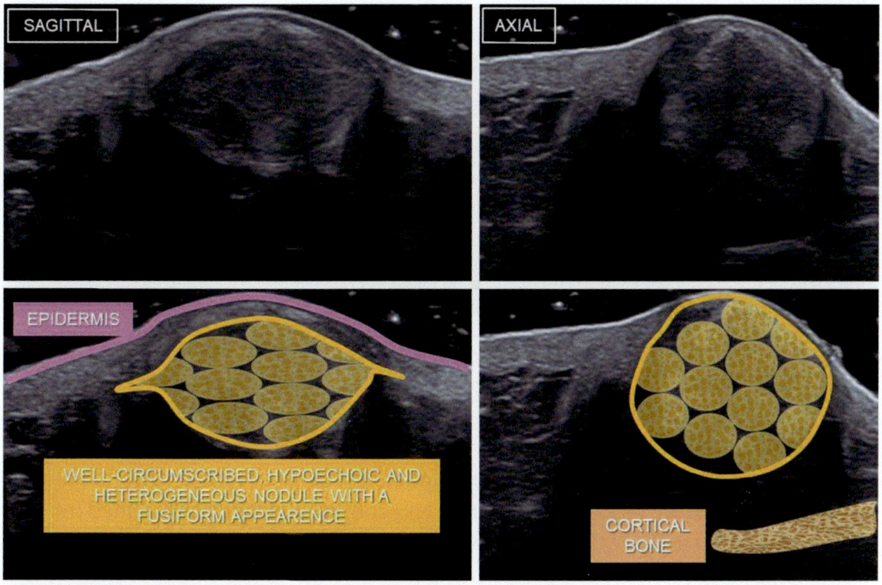

Fig. 15.45 Ultrasonographic findings of neurofibroma with a 24 MHz probe (Aplio i800, Canon Medical Systems)

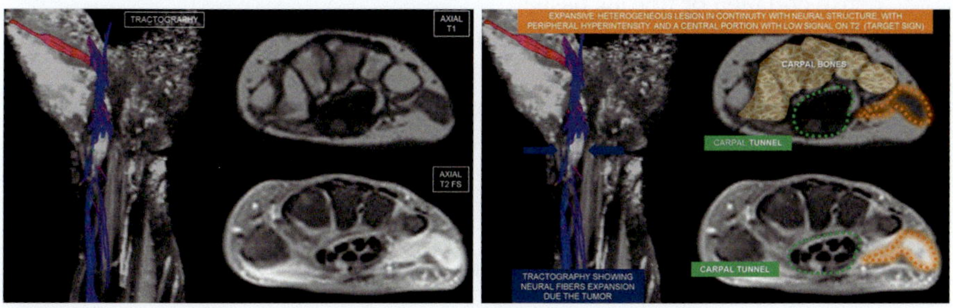

Fig. 15.46 MRI neurography findings of neurofibroma on T1, tractography, and T2 FS-weighted sequences (Magnetom Prisma 3T MRI, Siemens)

- Power Doppler imaging may reveal some vascularity, though neurofibromas are generally poorly vascularized.
- Plexiform neurofibromas may appear as larger, more heterogeneous masses, often with a characteristic "bag of worms" appearance due to their complex, intertwining structure.

15.12.7 MRI (Figs. 15.46 and 15.47) [31]

- Cutaneous and subcutaneous neurofibromas:

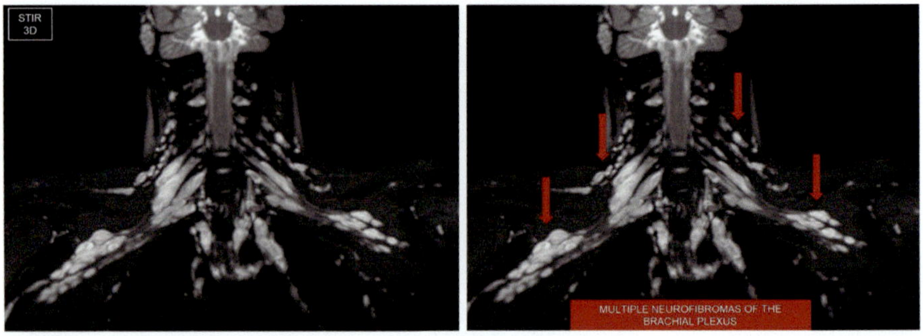

Fig. 15.47 MRI neurography findings of neurofibromatosis on STIR 3D sequence (Magnetom Prisma 3T MRI, Siemens)

- Neurofibromas generally appear as isointense or slightly hypointense relative to muscle on T1-weighted images. Cutaneous neurofibromas often blend with the surrounding tissue, making them less conspicuous on T1-weighted images.
- They are usually hyperintense on T2-weighted images, with a characteristic "target sign," where the peripheral portion of the tumor is hyperintense, and the central portion is hypointense. This pattern reflects the heterogeneous composition of the tumor, with the central hypointense area corresponding to dense collagen or fibrous tissue.
- Neurofibromas typically show uniform, but mild to moderate enhancement after gadolinium administration. The enhancement pattern can help distinguish neurofibromas from malignant peripheral nerve sheath tumors (MPNSTs), which tend to enhance more irregularly.

15.13 Post-Trauma Neuroma (Fig. 15.48)

15.13.1 Definition [35]

- A post-trauma neuroma, also known as a traumatic neuroma, is a benign nerve lesion that forms after a nerve injury or surgical procedure.
- It occurs due to abnormal regeneration of nerve fibers following trauma, where the regenerating axons encounter a physical barrier or a disruption in the nerve sheath, leading to disorganized nerve tissue growth.
- This condition can cause pain and sensory disturbances.

15.13.2 Epidemiology [35]

- Post-trauma neuromas are relatively common, particularly after surgical procedures involving nerves or accidental injuries.
- They can occur at any age but are more frequently reported in adults, especially in areas where nerves are more likely to be injured, such as the limbs or head and neck regions.
- The prevalence varies depending on the type and location of trauma or surgery.

15.13.3 Clinical Presentation [35]

- Patients with post-trauma neuromas typically present with localized pain at the site of the injury or surgery.
- The pain may be sharp, burning, or tingling and is often exacerbated by touch or pressure.
- In addition to pain, patients may experience numbness, hypersensitivity, or a sensation of a foreign body at the site of the neuroma.
- The symptoms can be persistent and significantly impact the patient's quality of life, especially if the neuroma forms in a weight-bearing area or a region frequently subjected to pressure.

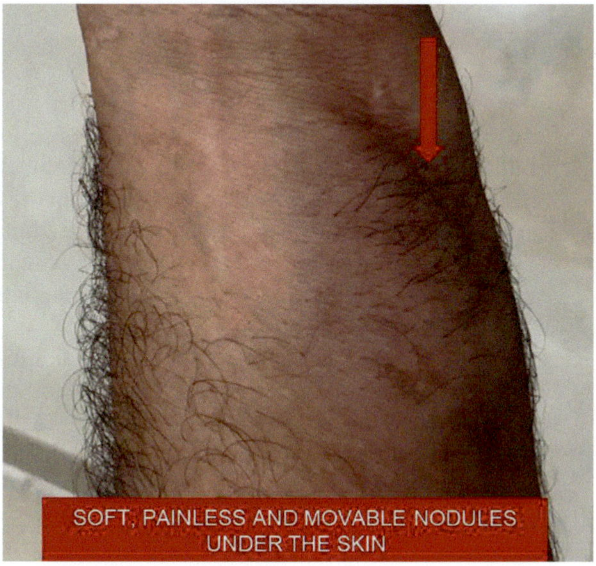

Fig. 15.48 Clinical photograph of patient with post-traumatic neuroma

15.13.4 Histopathology [35]

- Post-trauma neuroma is characterized by a disorganized proliferation of nerve fibers, Schwann cells, fibroblasts, and connective tissue.
- The lesion consists of tangled nerve fascicles surrounded by a fibrous stroma, with irregular axonal growth.
- Inflammatory cells may be present, reflecting the body's response to injury.
- The absence of an organized nerve sheath is a hallmark of post-trauma neuromas.
- The histopathological appearance is nonneoplastic, differentiating it from other nerve-related tumors.

15.13.5 Ultrasonography [36, 37]

- Post-trauma neuroma typically appears as a well-defined, hypoechoic mass at the site of the nerve injury.
- The mass may be ovoid or fusiform, often located at the end of a severed nerve.
- Power Doppler imaging may show increased vascularity around the neuroma due to associated inflammation.
- Ultrasonography is particularly useful in identifying the relationship between the neuroma and the surrounding structures, and it can help in guiding needle interventions or planning surgical excision.

15.13.6 MRI (Fig. 15.49) [31]

- Post-trauma neuromas usually appear isointense to slightly hypointense compared to surrounding muscle tissue on T1-weightetd images. The lesion may be well-circumscribed, with clear delineation from the adjacent tissues.
- The neuroma generally exhibits hyperintense signals on T2-weighted images due to the presence of myxoid and fibrous tissue within the lesion. The hyperintensity on T2-weighted images helps in differentiating the neuroma from other soft tissue masses.
- Neuromas typically show mild to moderate, uniform enhancement after gadolinium administration, reflecting the lesion's vascularity. The enhancement pattern can help in distinguishing neuromas from malignant tumors, which tend to show more heterogeneous and intense enhancement.

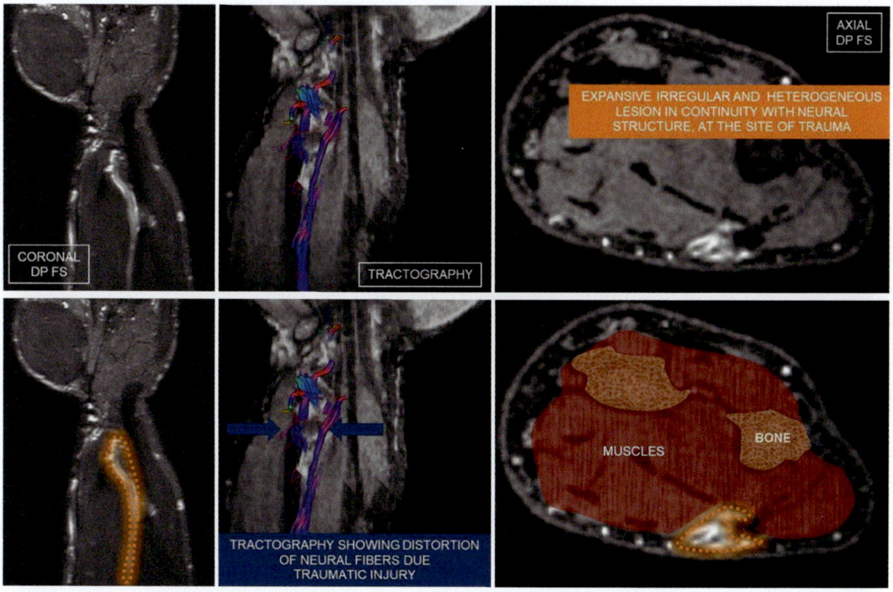

Fig. 15.49 MRI findings of post-traumatic neuroma on T1, tractography, and DP FS-weighted sequences (Magnetom Prisma 3T MRI, Siemens)

15.14 Schwannoma

15.14.1 Definition [38]

- A schwannoma, also known as a neurilemmoma, is a benign tumor that originates from Schwann cells, which are the cells that form the myelin sheath around peripheral nerves.
- Schwannomas are typically encapsulated and slow-growing, and they can occur along any peripheral nerve, though they most commonly arise from cranial nerves (especially the vestibular nerve) and spinal nerve roots.

15.14.2 Epidemiology [38]

- Schwannomas are the most common benign peripheral nerve sheath tumors, with an incidence of about 1 in 100,000 people per year.
- They can occur at any age but are most commonly diagnosed in adults between the ages of 20 and 50.
- Schwannomas are usually solitary and sporadic, but they can be associated with genetic conditions such as Neurofibromatosis type 2 (NF2), where multiple schwannomas may develop, particularly involving the vestibular nerves.

15.14.3 Clinical Presentation (Fig. 15.50) [38, 39]

- The clinical presentation of schwannomas depends on their size, location, and the nerves they affect.
- Common symptoms include:
  - Peripheral nerve schwannomas: Localized pain, palpable mass, and nerve compression symptoms such as numbness, tingling, or weakness in the distribution of the affected nerve. Schwannomas are often painless unless they become large enough to compress adjacent structures.

15.14.4 Histopathology (Fig. 15.51) [38, 39]

- Histologically, schwannomas are characterized by two distinct patterns:
  - Antoni A areas: These regions are composed of densely packed, elongated Schwann cells arranged in a palisading pattern around central acellular areas known as Verocay bodies.
  - Antoni B areas: These regions are less cellular, with a looser, myxoid stroma and scattered Schwann cells.
- Schwannomas are typically encapsulated, which distinguishes them from neurofibromas. They also lack significant mitotic activity, confirming their benign nature.

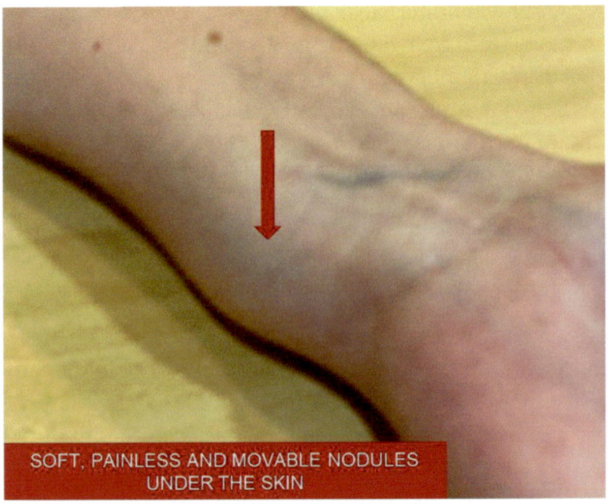

Fig. 15.50 Clinical photograph of patients with schwannoma

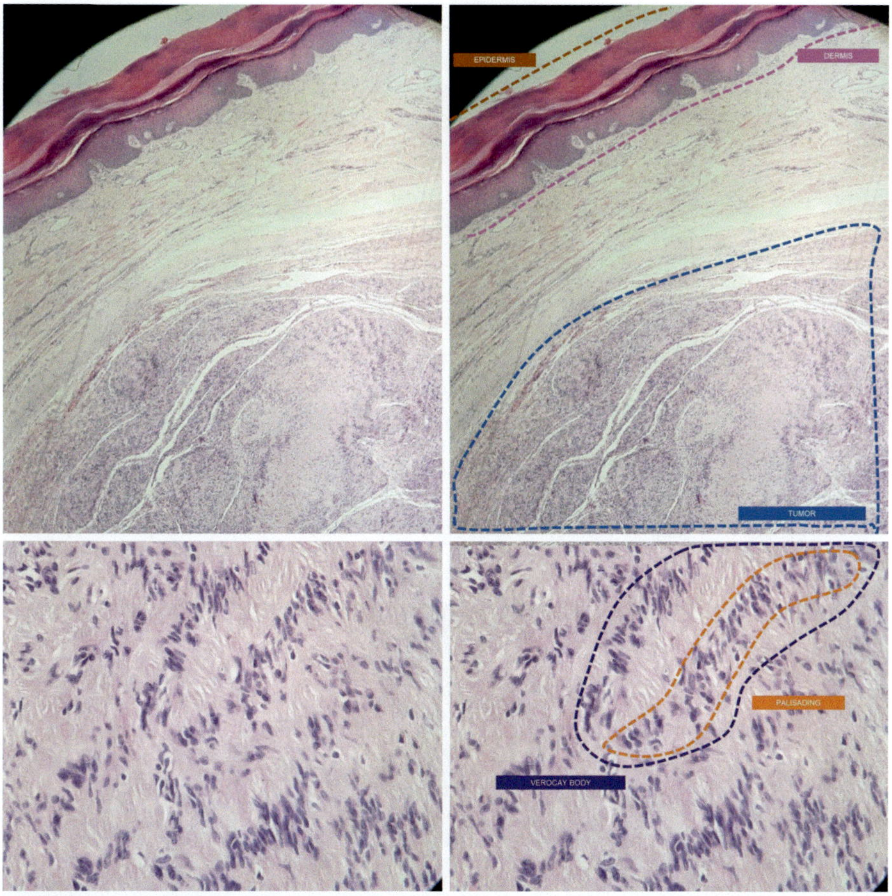

Fig. 15.51 Histological findings of schwannoma (H&E x10 and x20)

15.14.5 Ultrasonography (Fig. 15.52) [40]

- Schwannomas usually appear as well-defined, hypoechoic, homogenous masses.
- They are often ovoid and may show posterior acoustic enhancement due to their solid, soft-tissue nature.
- Larger schwannomas might display cystic degeneration, giving them a heterogeneous appearance.
- Power Doppler imaging may reveal some internal vascularity, especially at the periphery.
- The tumor's relationship with the adjacent nerve is often evident, and the nerve can sometimes be seen entering and exiting the mass.

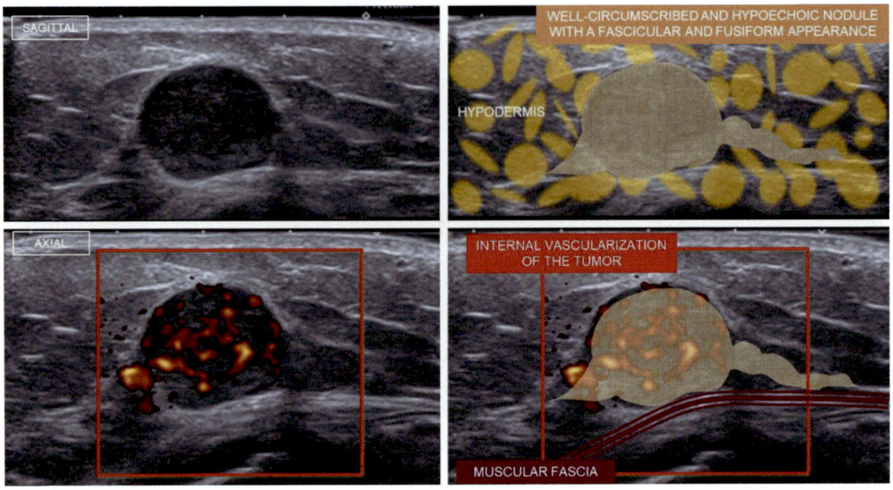

Fig. 15.52 Ultrasonographic findings of schwannoma with a 24 MHz probe (Aplio i800, Canon Medical Systems)

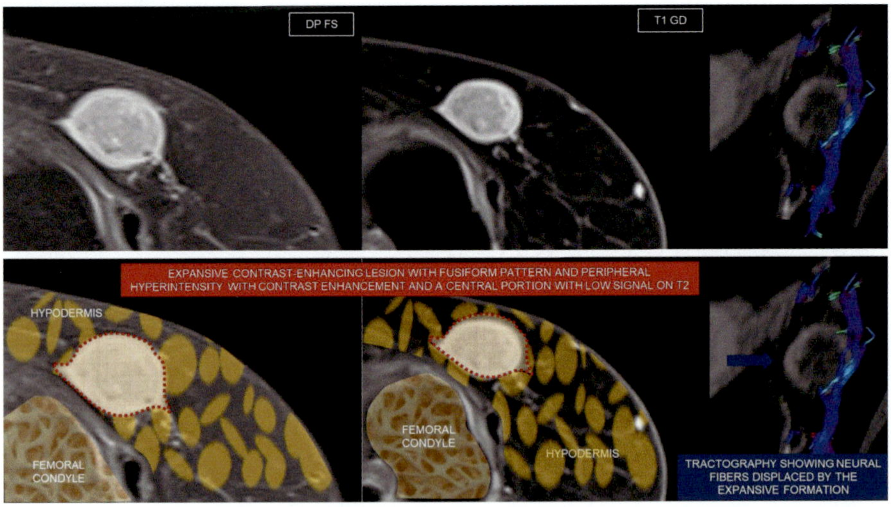

Fig. 15.53 MRI with surface coil findings of schwannoma on T2 FS, T1 FS-weighted images after gadolinium administration and tractography sequences (Magnetom Prisma 3T MRI, Siemens)

15.14.6 MRI (Fig. 15.53) [41]

- Schwannomas typically appear isointense or slightly hypointense relative to muscle on T1-weighted images. They are usually well-circumscribed, and in some cases, the "split-fat sign" (a rim of fat surrounding the tumor) can be seen, which is characteristic of peripheral nerve sheath tumors.

- Schwannomas often appear hyperintense with a heterogeneous signal on T2-weighted images due to areas of cystic degeneration or myxoid change within the tumor. The "target sign" may be observed, where a central low-signal area (corresponding to dense collagen) is surrounded by a high-signal rim (due to the more myxoid peripheral tissue).
- Schwannomas typically show strong, homogeneous enhancement after gadolinium administration due to their vascularity. In larger tumors, areas of cystic degeneration may not enhance, leading to a heterogeneous enhancement pattern.

15.15 Porokeratosis

15.15.1 Definition [42, 43]

- Porokeratosis is an uncommon disorder of keratinization that can be either inherited or acquired.
- It is characterized by the presence of one or more atrophic patches or macules surrounded by a hyperkeratotic, ridge-like border known as a "cornoid lamella."
- The disorder exhibits multiple clinical variants.
- Although rare, some cases may undergo malignant transformation.

15.15.2 Epidemiology [42, 43]

- The exact incidence and prevalence are not well-documented.
- Porokeratosis typically affects adults and older adults, with a higher prevalence in males.

15.15.3 Clinical Presentation (Fig. 15.54) [42, 43]

- The hallmark of porokeratosis is the presence of a cornoid lamella, which appears as a keratotic rim around a slightly atrophic skin lesion.
- Characterized by erythematous, hyperpigmented, or skin-colored well-defined macules, typically less than 1 cm in diameter. These lesions commonly appear on the extensor surfaces of the legs, shoulders, arms, or back, sparing the palms and soles. The cornoid lamella in these cases is often subtle.
- Porokeratosis of Mibelli: Begins as a small, asymptomatic, or mildly pruritic papule that expands slowly over years. Developed lesions are usually a few centimeters in diameter but can occasionally grow to 10–20 cm. The cornoid lamella is often prominent, and lesions typically occur on the extremities.

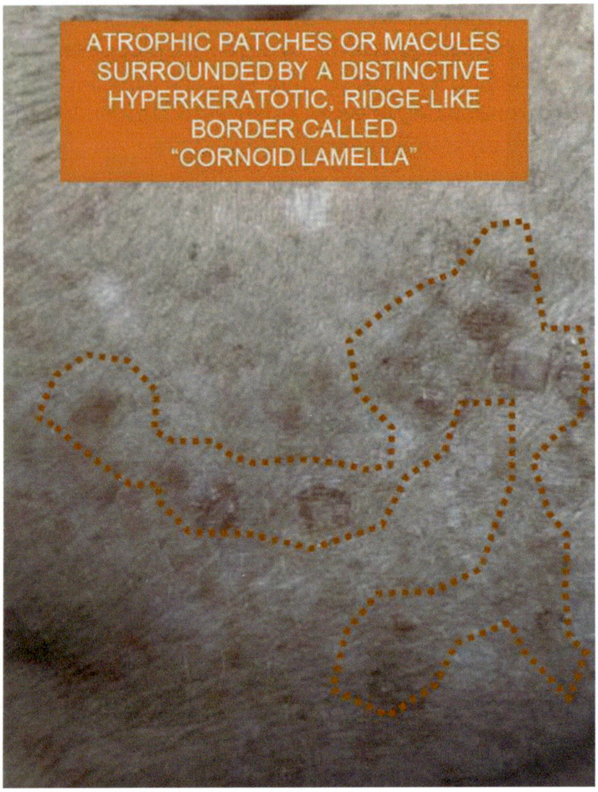

Fig. 15.54 Clinical photograph of patients with porokeratosis

- Linear porokeratosis: This rare form typically presents during infancy, but can also develop in adults. It can be subdivided based on lesion distribution into localized, zosteriform, systematized, or generalized variants.
- Other variants: Includes plantaris palmaris et disseminata, punctate, ptychotropica, genitogluteal, follicular, eruptive, giant, and filiform porokeratosis.

15.15.4 Dermoscopy (Fig. 15.55) [44]

- Dermoscopy reveals a characteristic pattern of a white or brown peripheral keratotic tract with a double free edge, often accompanied by pigmentary structures such as brown dots or areas.

Fig. 15.55 Dermoscopic findings of patient with porokeratosis (x20)

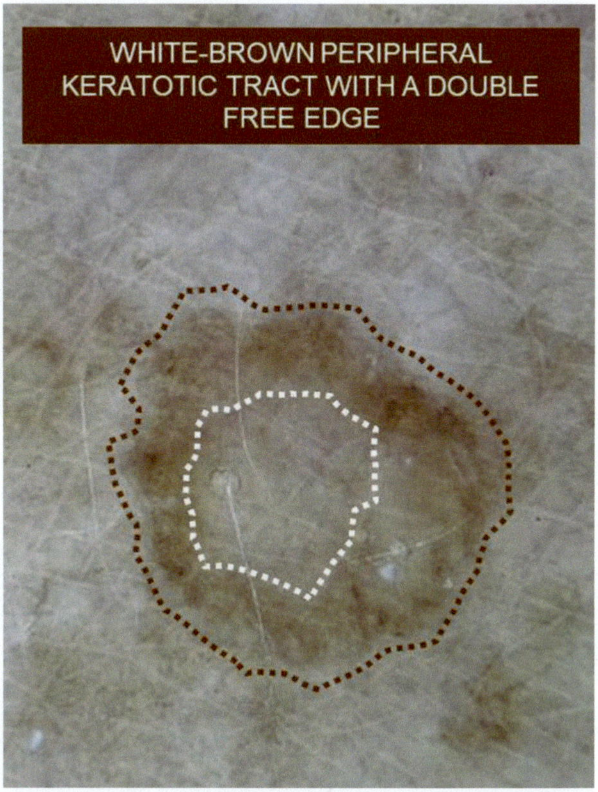

15.15.5 Histopathology (Fig. 15.56) [33]

- Histopathologic examination shows a superficial proliferation of small ectatic venules, which contain few or no red blood cells and are irregularly surrounded by hyperplastic epidermis. This appearance gives a false impression of the vessels being within the epidermis. Thrombosis may occasionally be present.

15.15.6 Ultrasonography (Fig. 15.57)

- Well-circumscribed, hypoechoic lesions on ultrasonography, however, it's necessary a high-resolution probe.
- The internal echotexture of a poroma is generally homogeneous, indicating uniformity within the lesion.

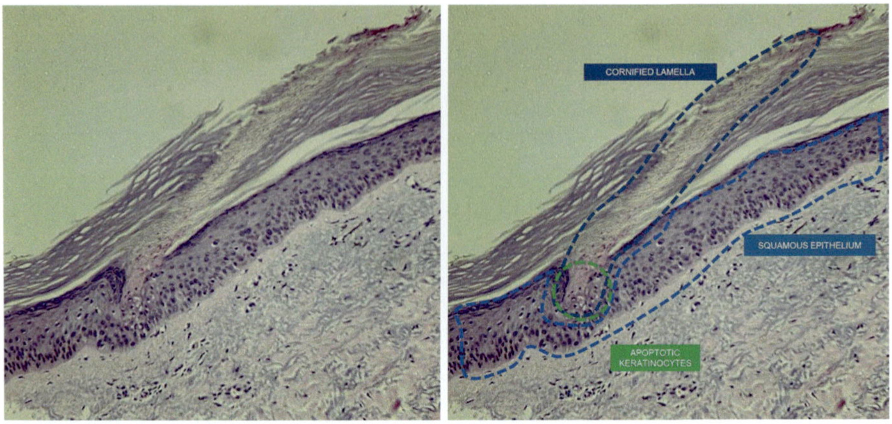

Fig. 15.56 Histological findings of porokeratosis (H&E x10)

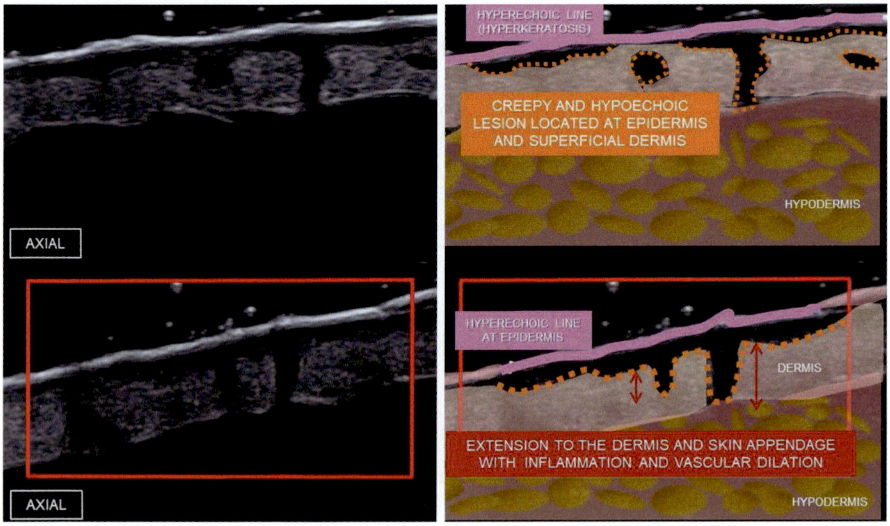

Fig. 15.57 Ultrasonographic findings of porokeratosis with a 24 MHz probe (Aplio i800, Canon Medical Systems)

- Poromas can vary in size and shape but are often round or oval.
- Calcifications are typically not present in poromas, distinguishing them from other types of skin lesions.
- On power Doppler ultrasonography, poromas usually show minimal to no significant blood flow within the lesion.

15.16 Steatocystoma

15.16.1 Definition [45]

- Sebum-containing cysts measuring from less than 3 mm in diameter to 3 cm or more.
- Steatocystoma multiplex is a rare condition that is characterized by cutaneous cysts and may be inherited in an autosomal dominant manner or may occur sporadically.

15.16.2 Epidemiology [45]

- Adolescence or early adulthood: Lesions typically manifest during adolescence or early adulthood.
- Lesions can appear anywhere on the body, including the scalp, intertriginous areas, and genitalia, with a notable predilection for the chest.
- Steatocystoma multiplex is associated with mutations in the KRT17 gene, also linked to a subtype of pachyonychia congenita.
- While predominantly a sporadic disorder, autosomal dominant inheritance is observed in some cases.

15.16.3 Clinical Presentation (Fig. 15.58) [45]

- The lesions are asymptomatic, with no malignant potentiaL.
- Despite the absence of symptoms, patients often seek treatment due to the psychological distress caused by cosmetically undesirable lesions.

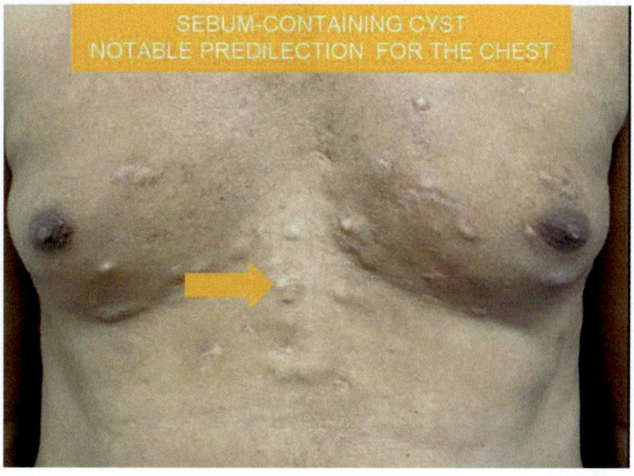

Fig. 15.58 Clinical photograph of patients with steatocystoma. Image kindly provided by Dr. Andre Luíz Vairo Donda, Rio de Janeiro—Brazil

15.16.4 Dermoscopy (Fig. 15.59) [45]

- Nonpolarized dermoscopy findings:
  - Displays a circumscribed, yellowish, structureless area.
  - Margins appear diffuse.
  - Vellus hairs surround the area.
- Polarized dermoscopy findings:
  - Shows a distinctive central yellowish glow.
  - Lesions have a darker rim surrounding the yellow center.
  - Background exhibits a pseudoreticular pigmentary pattern.
  - The yellow structureless area correlates with the sebum contained in the cyst cavity.
  - Entrapped vellus hairs within the cystic cavity impart a greenish tinge to the yellow area.

15.16.5 Histopathology [45]

- Superficial proliferation of small ectatic venules, containing few or no red blood cells.
- Surrounded by the hyperplastic epidermis, giving an appearance of being falsely inside the epidermis; may present thrombosis occasionally.

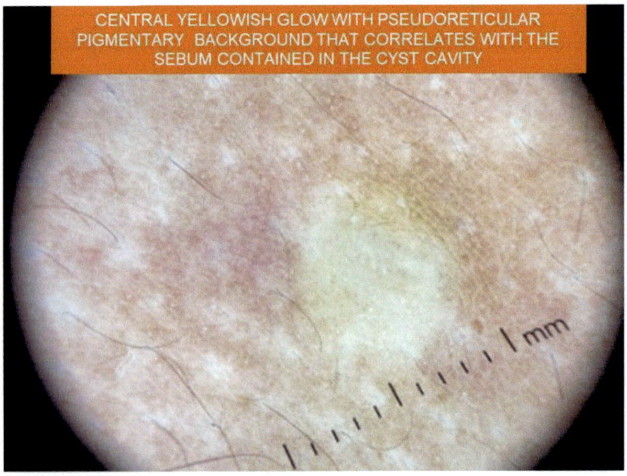

Fig. 15.59 Dermoscopic findings of patient with steatocystoma. Image kindly provided by Dr. Andre Luíz Vairo Donda, Rio de Janeiro—Brazil (x10)

15.16.6 Radiography

- Round nodules with a circumscribed margin, central fat density, and a peripheral high-density rim located in subcutaneous tissue.
- The maximum diameter was usually up to 1.5–2.0 cm.

15.16.7 Computed Tomography [46]

- Fat density cysts, well-defined, round to ovoid, in the subcutaneous layer, with no contrast enhancement.

15.16.8 Ultrasonography (Fig. 15.60) [47]

- Homogeneous echotexture and absent or mild posterior acoustic enhancement.
- It is frequently located in the subcutaneous or involves both dermal and subcutaneous layers and occurs principally on the anterior chest, epigastrium, axillae, groin, neck area, and on the proximal part of the extremities.
- Around 50% of the cases showed signs of hypervascularity in the edge of the nodules.
- In some cases the lesions were associated with another dermatologic condition, most frequent being hidradenitis suppurativa, followed by vellus hair cysts.

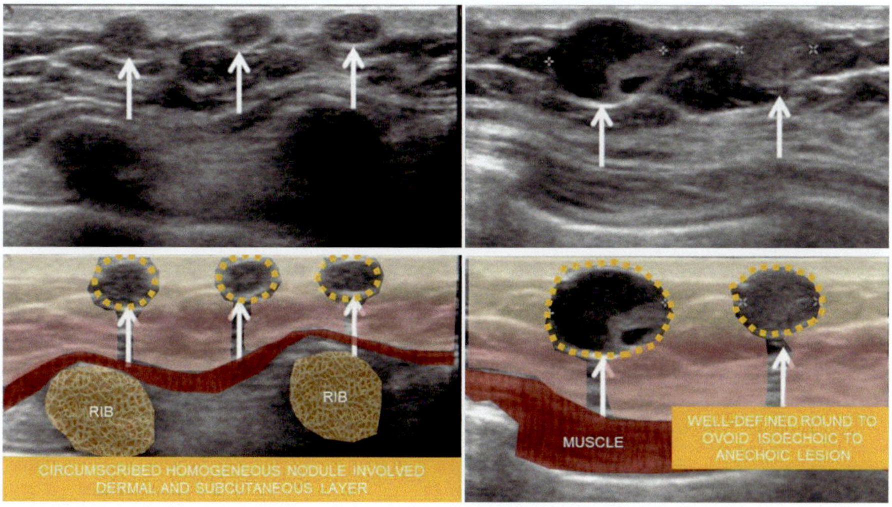

Fig. 15.60 Ultrasonographic findings of steatocystoma with a 24 MHz probe. (*From* Chotai and Lim [114]; *with permission*)

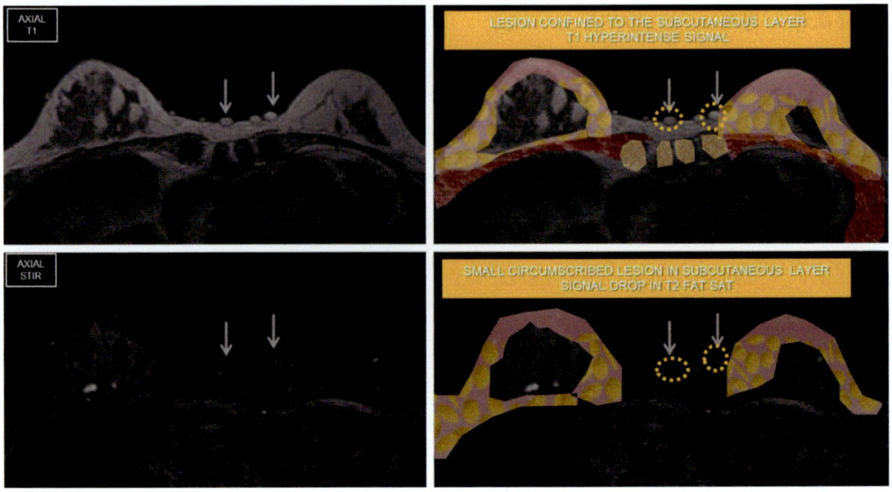

Fig. 15.61 MRI findings of steatocystoma on T2 FS, T1 FS-weighted images after gadolinium administration. (*From* Chotai and Lim [114]; *with permission*)

15.16.9 MRI (Fig. 15.61)

- T1-weighted hyperintense signal, and heterogeneous T2-weighted lesion with hypo and isointense signal.
- A significant signal drop in the T2-weighted fat saturation is frequently present.
- The lesion is usually confined to the subcutaneous layer, with no evidence of other tissue infiltration.

15.17 Eccrine Spiradenoma

15.17.1 Definition [48]

- Rare adnexal neoplasms are characterized by dual lineage cell proliferation within the dermis.
- Likely derived from apocrine cells in the hair follicle bulge, exhibiting a round, cylindrical morphology.
- Generally benign with slow growth, although malignant transformation and metastasis can occur, especially in Brooke–Spiegler syndrome.

15.17.2 Epidemiology [48]

- Rare, predominantly affecting females (9:1 ratio compared to males) and more common in Caucasian populations.
- Sporadic forms present as solitary lesions in older patients, while familial forms, associated with syndromes like Brooke–Spiegler syndrome, appear around puberty.
- Associated with other tumors such as spiradenomas, trichoepitheliomas, and parotid tumors.

15.17.3 Clinical Presentation (Fig. 15.62) [48]

- **Solitary lesions**: Slow-growing, painless, round nodules usually less than 1 cm in diameter, primarily on the scalp and face, with pinkish or tan coloration and small superficial blood vessels.
- **Multiple lesions**: Linked to familial syndromes, these can grow larger, exceed 20 cm, become painful, and ulcerate, predominantly found in the head and neck region with sparing of palms and soles.

15.17.4 Dermoscopy (Fig. 15.63) [48]

- Reveals round, well-defined nodules with a smooth surface, often showing small superficial blood vessels.
- Characteristic cylindrical shape supports diagnosis, especially on the scalp; multiple lesions may merge in syndromic cases.

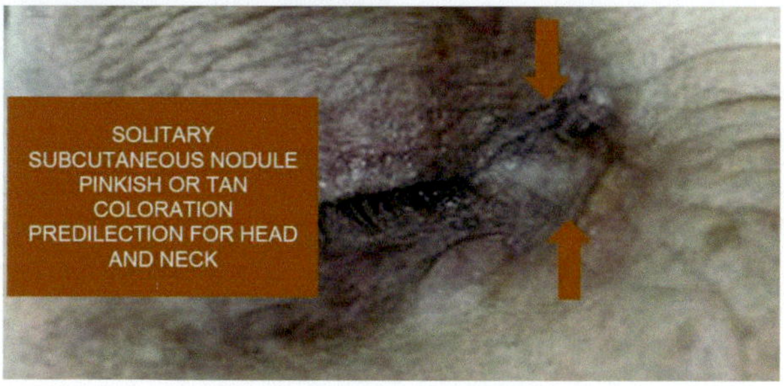

Fig. 15.62 Clinical photograph of patients with eccrine spiradenoma

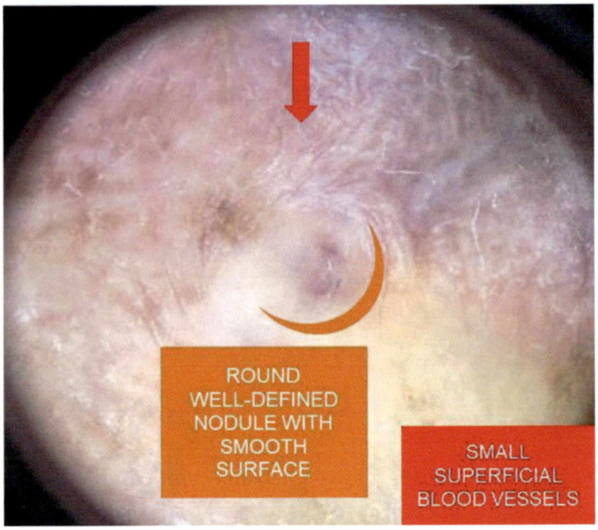

Fig. 15.63 Dermoscopic findings of patient with eccrine spiradenoma (x10)

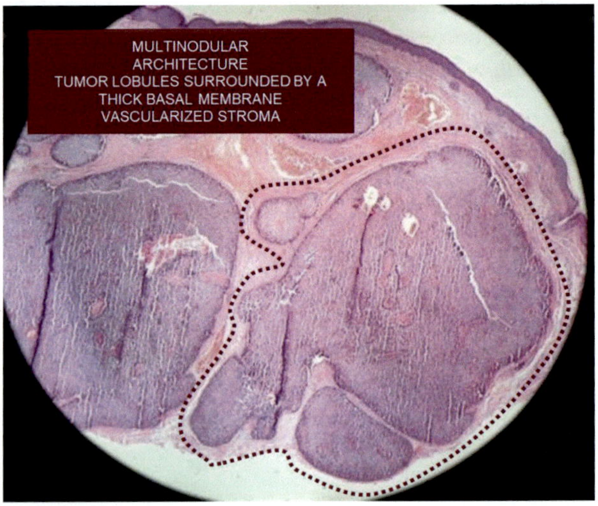

Fig. 15.64 Histological findings of eccrine spiradenoma (H&E x10)

15.17.5 Histopathology (Fig. 15.64) [48]

- Solid basophilic tumors in the dermis, well-circumscribed, forming cords and lobules with eventual ductal lumens.
- Two-phase pattern with small peripheral cells and larger central cells.
- Presence of ductal lumens and vascularized stroma with occasional hemorrhage; rare mitotic activity observed.

15.17.6 Ultrasonography (Fig. 15.65) [48]

- Tract-like appearance with a lobulated outline, well-defined, heterogeneous mass in the hypodermis, predominantly hypoechoic with posterior acoustic enhancement.
- Hypervascularity noted peripherally and centrally on power Doppler imaging; typically lacks invasion of adjacent structures.

15.17.7 MRI

- Tract-like appearance with a lobulated outline, low signal intensity on T1-weighted images, and intermediate to high signal intensity on T2-weighted images.

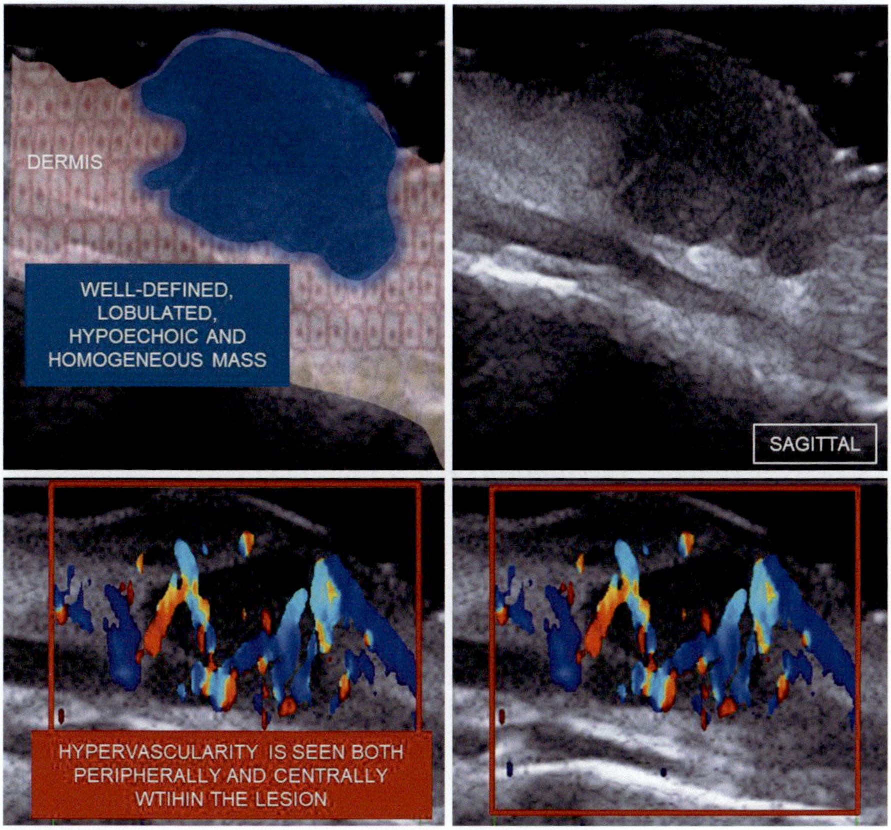

Fig. 15.65 Ultrasonographic findings of eccrine spiradenoma with a 24 MHz probe (Aplio i800, Canon Medical Systems)

- Homogeneous enhancement on contrast imaging; giant lesions may exhibit high vascularity and hemorrhagic features.

15.18 Infantile Mastocytoma

15.18.1 Definition [49]

- Mastocytoma is a tumor originating from mast cells, derived from myeloid stem cells predominantly located in connective tissues, including the skin and mucosal linings.
- It falls under the spectrum of mastocytosis, a clonal hematopoietic disorder characterized by neoplastic mast cell proliferation, which can be confined to the skin (cutaneous mastocytosis) or involve systemic tissues (systemic mastocytosis).

15.18.2 Epidemiology [49]

- The skin is the most commonly affected organ, followed by involvement of the bone marrow and gastrointestinal tract.
- Primary cutaneous mastocytosis typically manifests in childhood, with the majority of cases appearing within the first 2 years of life, often within the first 3 months or congenitally.
- Mastocytomas are usually solitary, but fewer than four lesions are categorized under mastocytoma.
- There is no significant gender or racial predilection, although adult-onset cutaneous mastocytoma is exceptionally rare.

15.18.3 Clinical Presentation (Fig. 15.66) [49]

- Ranges from solitary mastocytoma to diffuse erythrodermic mastocytosis, often appearing as maculopapular lesions (urticaria pigmentosa).
- Typically presents as 1–5 cm indurated, erythematous, yellow-brown, or reddish-brown macules, papules, plaques, or nodules. Often exhibits a peau d'orange appearance with leathery or rubbery consistency and variable margins.
- Lesions may be asymptomatic or moderately itchy, with potential for spontaneous urtication or aggravation with friction (Darier sign), particularly in large lesions.

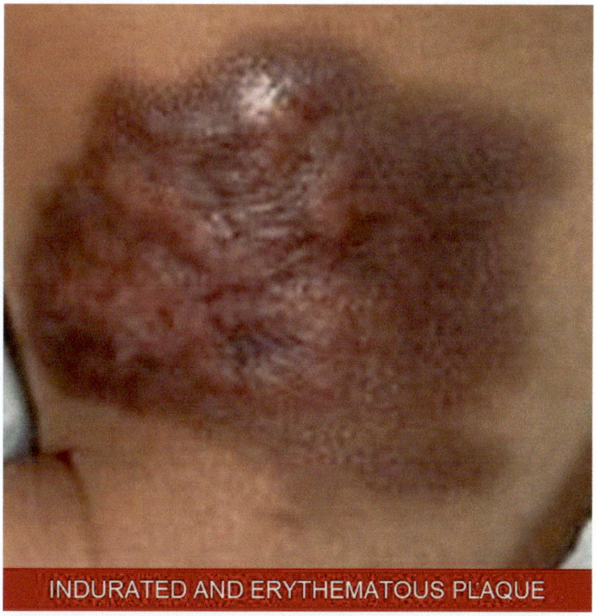

Fig. 15.66 Clinical photograph of patients with infantile mastocytoma

- Lesions generally grow proportionally with the child and may regress over time.
- Commonly found on the trunk, extremities, and flexural areas, sparing the palms and soles.
- While less common than in systemic mastocytosis, systemic symptoms such as flushing, dyspnea, nausea, and abdominal pain can occur.
- Primarily clinical based on lesion appearance, Darier sign, and absence of systemic involvement. Histological and molecular tests are necessary for definitive diagnosis, differentiating from reactive conditions or mast cell hyperplasia.
- Mastocytoma is differentiated from urticaria pigmentosa based on lesion count, with three or fewer nodules categorized as mastocytoma.

15.18.4 Dermoscopy [49]

- Dermoscopy typically reveals a light-brown blot and pigment network corresponding to melanin accumulation in basal keratinocytes.

15.18.5 Histopathology (Fig. 15.67) [49]

- Mastocytoma shows dermal clustering of mast cells without epidermotropism, usually dense and focal, with metachromasia evident on Giemsa staining and positive markers like CD117 and tryptase on immunohistochemistry.

15.18.6 Ultrasonography (Fig. 15.68)

- Ultrasonography reveals a heterogeneous hypoechoic area, suggesting mild subcutaneous edema indicative of localized inflammation.
- Additionally, punctate echogenicity with posterior acoustic shadowing can be observed, possibly indicating a small calcification or air focus.

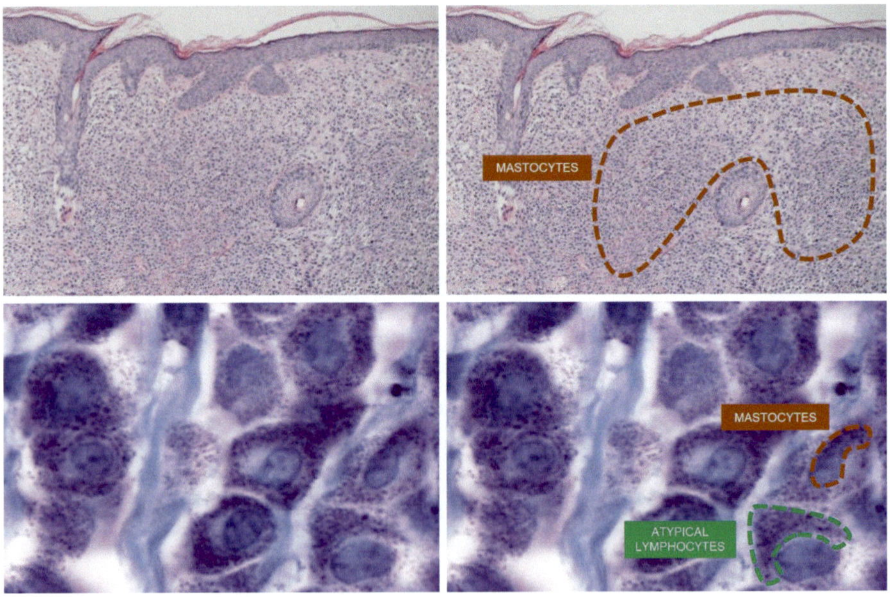

Fig. 15.67 Histological findings of infantile mastocytoma (H&E x4 and x40)

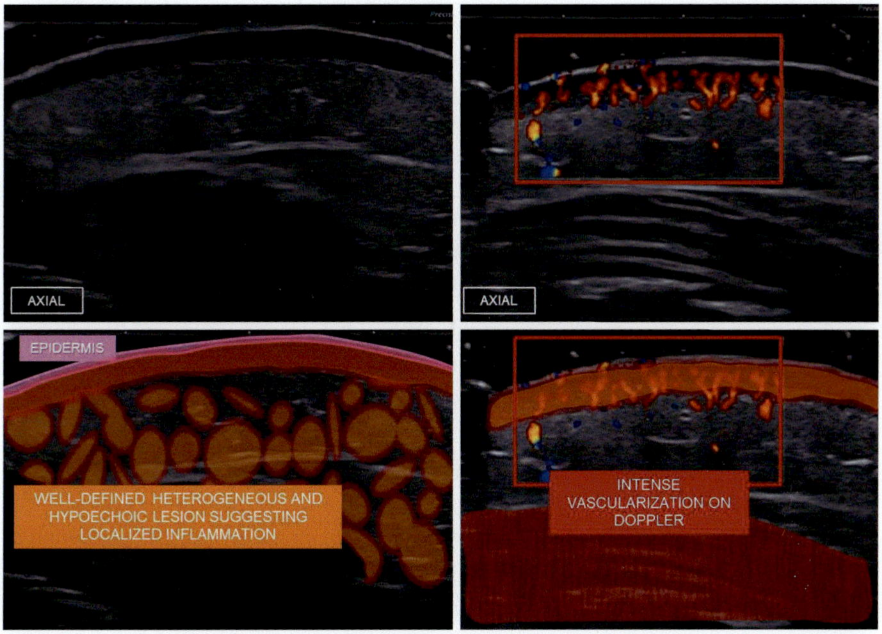

Fig. 15.68 Ultrasonographic findings of infantile mastocytoma with a 24 MHz probe (Aplio i800, Canon Medical Systems)

15.19 Surfers Knots

15.19.1 Definition [50]

- Uncommon acquired connective tissue nodules found on tibial tuberosities, dorsum of the feet, and occasionally on surfers' chests.
- Result from repeated low-grade trauma during long- and short-board surfing.

15.19.2 Epidemiology [50]

- First reported in the 1960s in warmer regions where surfers predominantly used larger, heavier surfboards while sitting on their knees.
- Surfers' knots are uncommon and have decreased in incidence since the introduction of shorter surfboards, which led to changes in surfing techniques.
- They primarily affect surfers who engage in both long- and short-board surfing activities.
- Typically, they develop over areas prone to repeated friction with surfboards, such as tibial tuberosities, dorsum of the feet, and occasionally on the chest.
- Most cases are benign and resolved with cessation or modification of surfing activities.

15.19.3 Clinical Presentation (Fig. 15.69) [50]

- Patients often present with palpable nodules or lumps on the lower extremities (e.g., feet) and sometimes on the chest.
- The nodules are usually slow-growing and painless, occasionally causing mild discomfort or tightness in shoes.
- They are smooth, non-tender, and do not exhibit signs of infection or inflammation.
- History typically includes a long-standing history of surfing, with nodules developing over years due to repeated microtrauma during surfing maneuvers.

15.19.4 Dermoscopy [50]

- Dermoscopic features of surfers' knots are not extensively described in the literature provided.
- Further examination with dermoscopy may reveal characteristic findings such as changes in skin texture, vascular patterns, or structural alterations indicative of fibrotic changes.

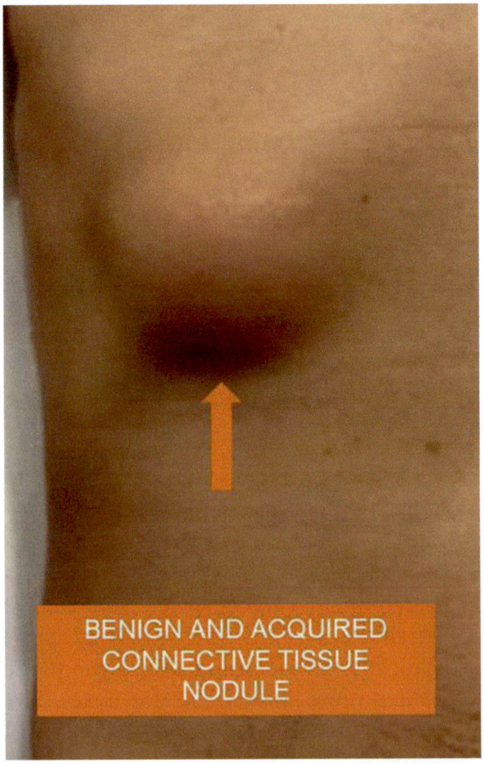

Fig. 15.69 Clinical photograph of patients with surfer's knots

15.19.5 Histopathology [51]

- Microscopic findings are nonspecific; lesions are rarely biopsied.
- Minimal chronic inflammation and characteristic fibrosis.

15.19.6 Radiography and Computed Tomography

- Non-contrast and contrast-enhanced CT scans revealed a soft tissue density mass with unclear margins in the subcutaneous area of the affected region.

15.19.7 Ultrasonography (Fig. 15.70) [50]

- High-frequency ultrasonography reveals ill-defined hypoechoic masses.
- The masses are surrounded by dermal and subcutaneous thickening.

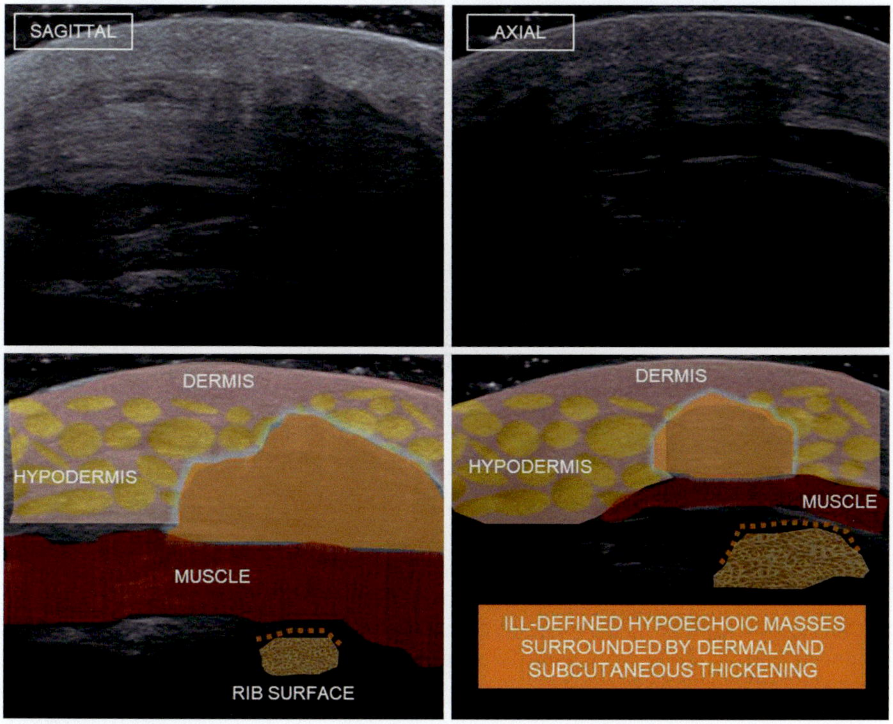

Fig. 15.70 Ultrasonographic findings of surfer's knots with a 24 MHz probe (Aplio i800, Canon Medical Systems)

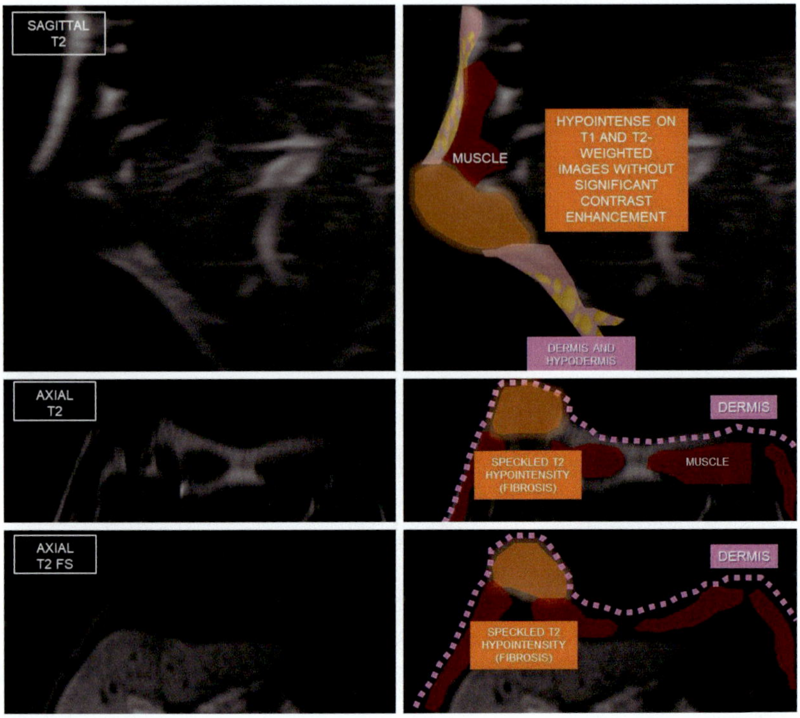

Fig. 15.71 MRI findings of surfer's knots on T2 and T2 FS-weighted sequences (Magnetom Prisma 3T MRI, Siemens)

15.19.8 MRI (Fig. 15.71) [51]

- T1-weighted images show hypointensity.
- T2-weighted images show speckled hypointensity.
- No significant contrast enhancement is observed.
- There are no joint erosions, infiltration into adjacent joints, or malignant features.

15.20 Foreign Bogy (Implants)

15.20.1 Definition [52]

- Soft tissue injuries frequently involve foreign bodies, which are objects introduced into the body from external sources, potentially leading to complications if not managed appropriately.

15.20.2 Epidemiology [52]

- According to recent data, soft tissue wounds constituted a primary reason for 6.8 million emergency department visits in the United States in 2016, with a notable incidence of associated foreign bodies.

15.20.3 Clinical Presentation (Fig. 15.72) [52]

- Patients often do not initially recognize the presence of foreign bodies, particularly following high-velocity injuries.
- Visual examination and careful palpation are essential for identification.

15.20.4 Dermoscopy [52]

- Dermoscopic examination plays a crucial role in identifying and managing superficial foreign bodies, aiding in minimizing tissue damage and patient discomfort.

15.20.5 Histopathology [33]

- Presence of macrophage aggregates, epithelioid cells, and/or giant foreign body cells surrounding the central foreign body.

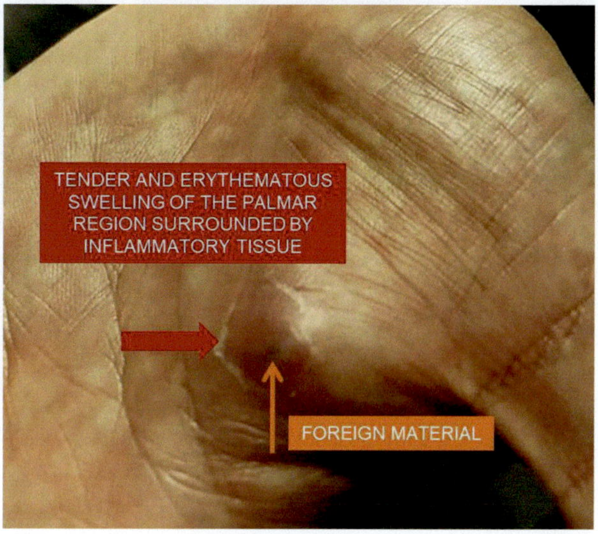

Fig. 15.72 Clinical photograph of patients with a foreign body

- Possible association with neutrophils and abscess formation depending on material and biopsy phase.
- Granulomatous process may obscure foreign body, especially in ruptured epidermal cysts.
- Chronic phase may feature fibrosis and dystrophic calcification.

15.20.6 Radiography [52]

- Effective for detecting radiopaque materials such as metal and glass.
- Low cost and reduced radiation exposure.
- Limitations in detecting radiolucent objects like wood or plastic.

15.20.7 Computed Tomography [52]

- Provides three-dimensional localization but with higher costs and radiation doses.
- Useful for visualizing objects obscured by bone or evaluating complications from retained foreign bodies.

15.20.8 Ultrasonography (Fig. 15.73) [53]

- Detects both radiopaque and radiolucent objects.

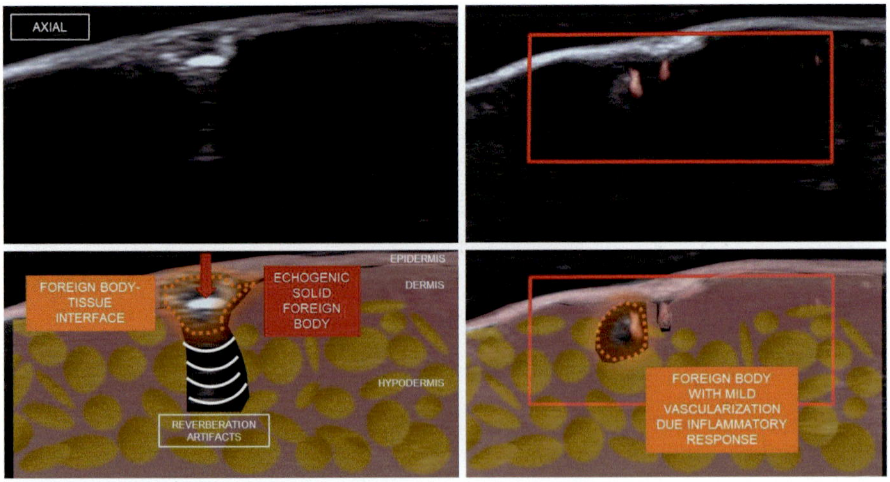

Fig. 15.73 Ultrasonographic findings of a foreign body with a 24 MHz probe (Aplio i800, Canon Medical Systems)

- Requires specialized training and may have limitations in deep tissues.
- Acoustic characteristics aid in distinguishing foreign body materials.
- A dark, circular region around the foreign object representing hypoechoic halo, indicates inflammation or a granulomatous reaction.
- Increased vascularity on power Doppler imaging around the object due to inflammation.
- Bright spots that can represent calcifications or fibrotic tissue around the foreign body observed as echogenic foci.
- Areas of fluid collections near the foreign object, suggesting an ongoing inflammatory response.

15.20.9 MRI (Fig. 15.74) [52]

- Magnetic resonance imaging, although less frequently utilized due to cost and availability constraints, can offer insights into small foreign bodies through soft tissue contrast and characterization of complex cases.
- Highly sensitive to organic materials but may exhibit magnetic susceptibility artifacts, making precise localization of metallic objects challenging.
- Sensitive for detecting metals through magnetic susceptibility artifacts.

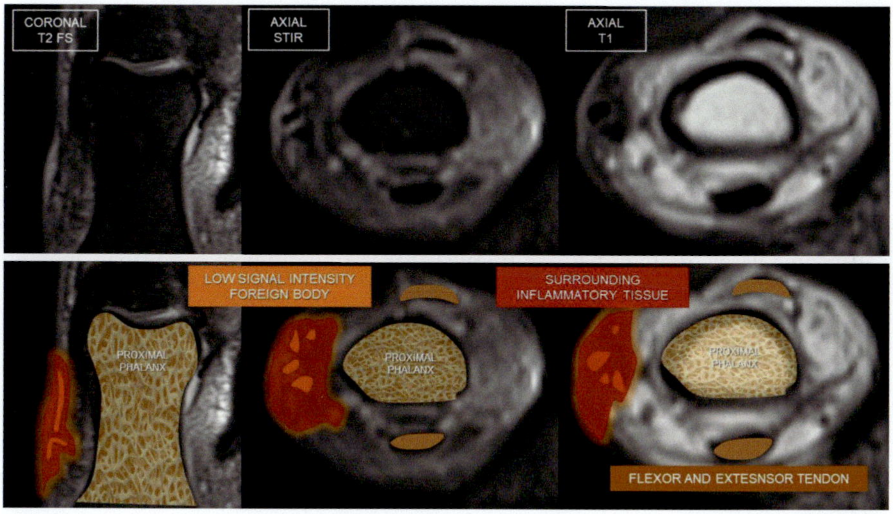

Fig. 15.74 MRI with surface coil findings of a foreign body on T1, T2, and T2 FS-weighted sequences (Magnetom Prisma 3T MRI, Siemens)

15.21 Foreign Body Reaction

15.21.1 Definition [54]

- Foreign body granulomas arise as a result of the body's immune system responding to materials it perceives as foreign and nondegradable.
- When objects such as implants, splinters, or other nonbiodegradable substances enter the body—whether through medical procedures or accidental means—the immune system initiates a complex inflammatory response.
- This reaction leads to the development of granulomas, which are aggregations of macrophages and other immune cells that form in an effort to encapsulate and manage the foreign material.

15.21.2 Epidemiology [54]

- Foreign body granulomas can arise from a variety of sources, including medical implants, tattoos, and accidental introduction of foreign materials during injuries.
- They can affect individuals of any age or gender, with specific types more common based on exposure risks.

15.21.3 Clinical Presentation (Fig. 15.75) [54]

- Patients with foreign body granulomas may present with nodules or masses at the site of foreign material introduction.
- These lesions can be painless or tender and may show signs of inflammation such as redness and swelling.
- In some cases, granulomas can mimic other dermatological conditions, making diagnosis challenging.

15.21.4 Dermoscopy [54]

- Foreign body granulomas may exhibit specific patterns depending on the type of foreign material.
- Common features include pigmented structures and vascular patterns indicative of inflammation.

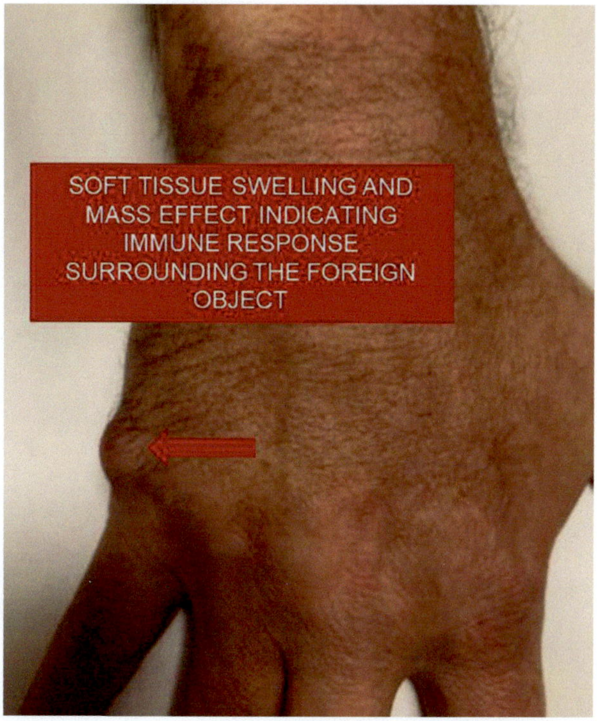

Fig. 15.75 Clinical photograph of patient with a foreign body reaction due to surgical implants

15.21.5 Histopathology [33]

- Presence of aggregates of macrophages, epithelioid cells or giant foreign body cells that tend to aggregate and shape around the central foreign body.
- Depending on the nature of the material and the biopsied phase, it may be associated with neutrophils and abscess formation.
- The process can be diffusely granulomatous with almost total destruction of the foreign body, making it difficult to recognize; this occurs in ruptured epidermal cysts, where it is important to perform polarization to highlight the corneal lamellae that are retractable, as well as surgical thread and hair fragments.
- In the chronic phase, it can be totally replaced by fibrosis and dystrophic calcification eventually.

15.21.6 Radiography (Fig. 15.76) [54]

- Radiographic imaging can identify foreign bodies and the extent of tissue reaction.

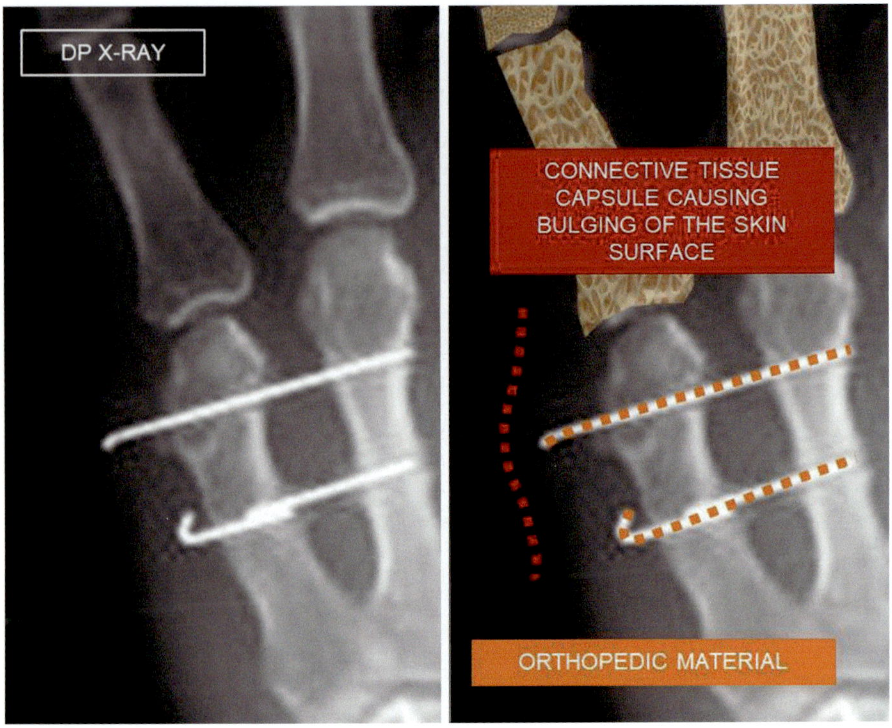

Fig. 15.76 Radiographic findings of a foreign body reaction due to surgical implants (Philips Duo Diagnost R&F Room Digital RF and Tomo System)

- Radiopaque materials such as metals are easily visible, while radiolucent materials may require advanced imaging techniques for detection.

15.21.7 Computed Tomography [54]

- CT scans provide detailed cross-sectional images and are particularly useful for locating foreign bodies within deeper tissues.
- They can reveal both the foreign material and the extent of the granulomatous response.

15.21.8 Ultrasonography (Fig. 15.77) [54]

- Ultrasonography imaging is effective in detecting foreign bodies and assessing the surrounding soft tissue reaction.

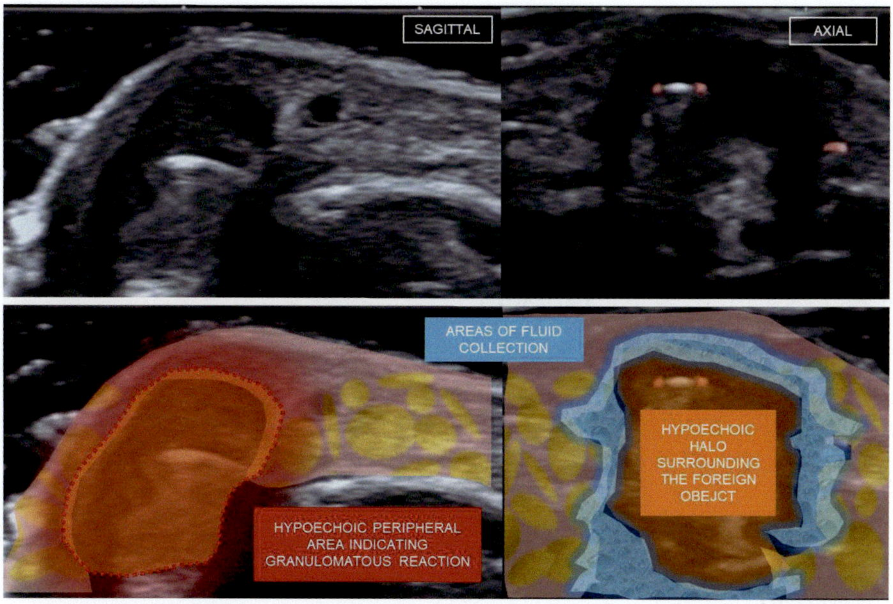

Fig. 15.77 Ultrasonographic findings of a foreign body reaction due to surgical implants with a 24 MHz probe (Aplio i800, Canon Medical Systems)

- Key features include hypoechoic halos indicating inflammation, increased vascularity on power Doppler imaging, echogenic foci representing calcifications, and fluid collections suggesting ongoing inflammation.

15.21.9 MRI [54]

- MRI is highly sensitive for detecting foreign bodies and the associated granulomatous response.
- It provides excellent soft tissue contrast, making it ideal for identifying inflammation, fibrosis, and other tissue changes resulting from the presence of foreign material.

15.21.10 3D Images (Fig. 15.78; Video 15.4)

- Highly advantageous for addressing minimal foreign body.
- Facilitates a comprehensive view of the lesion, aiding in the assessment of its severity and its interaction with nearby structures, including vascular expansions and connective tissues.
- Boosts the accuracy of surgical interventions, particularly in delicate regions.

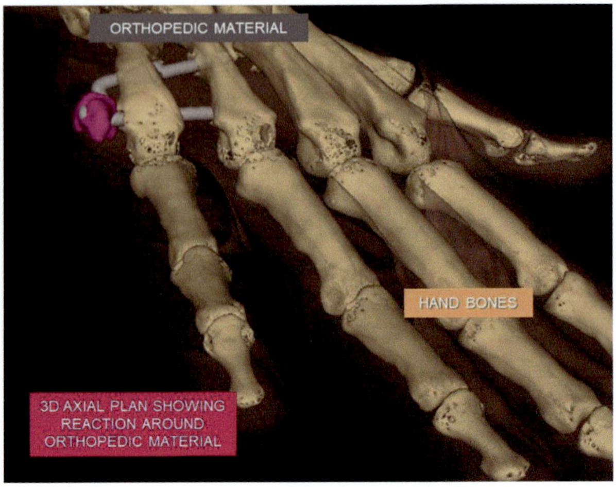

Fig. 15.78 3D images of a foreign body reaction due to surgical implants after segmentation of MRI isotropic images for surgical planning

15.22 Piezogenic Papules

15.22.1 Definition [55]

- Small, soft, yellowish, or skin-colored protrusions that appear on the heels when standing due to increased pressure.

15.22.2 Epidemiology [55]

- Common in adults, with higher prevalence in individuals who stand for prolonged periods.
- Can affect any age group and gender, though more frequently seen in adults due to occupational stress.

15.22.3 Clinical Presentation (Fig. 15.79) [55]

- Typically asymptomatic but can become painful.
- Firm papules that appear on the lateral, posterior, or medial aspects of the heel, becoming more pronounced under weight-bearing conditions.

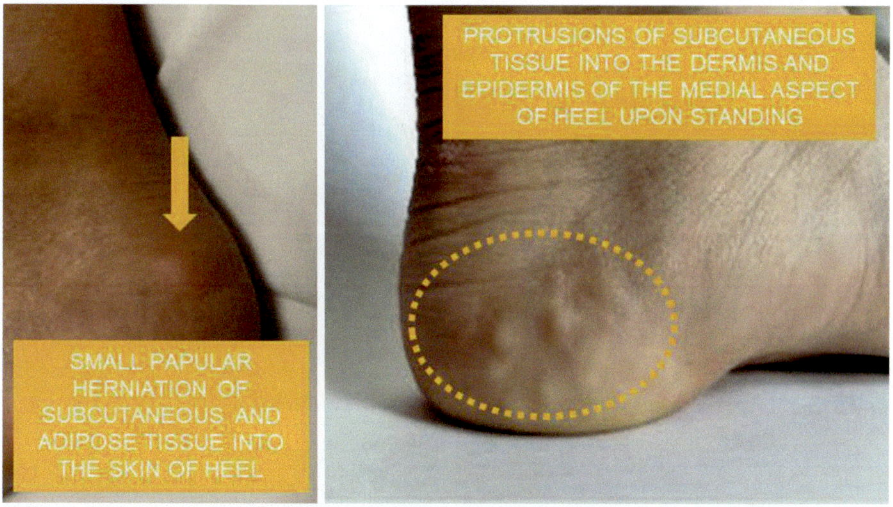

Fig. 15.79 Clinical photograph of patients with piezogenic papules

15.22.4 Dermoscopy [55]

- Not commonly used for diagnosis, as clinical history and physical examination are usually sufficient.

15.22.5 Histopathology [33, 55]

- Shelley and Rawnsley first described piezogenic pedal papules (PPP) in 1968. At that time, they were described as small papular herniations of subcutaneous tissue into the skin of the medial aspect of each heel that occurred only upon standing or upon application of pressure to the sole.
- As they are easily recognized in clinical examination and do not generate diagnostic.

15.22.6 Ultrasonography (Figs. 15.80 and 15.81)

- High-frequency ultrasonography can confirm clinical findings, showing isoechoic lesions that corresponds to the fat tissue herniating into dermis. Typically no fascial defect is observed.
- Differentiating intrafascial fat herniation from piezogenic papules can be subtle. Unlike piezogenic papules, intrafascial fat herniation occurs within the muscle fascia, protrudes with muscle contraction, can be painful (especially under pressure) and is usually not limited to the heel.

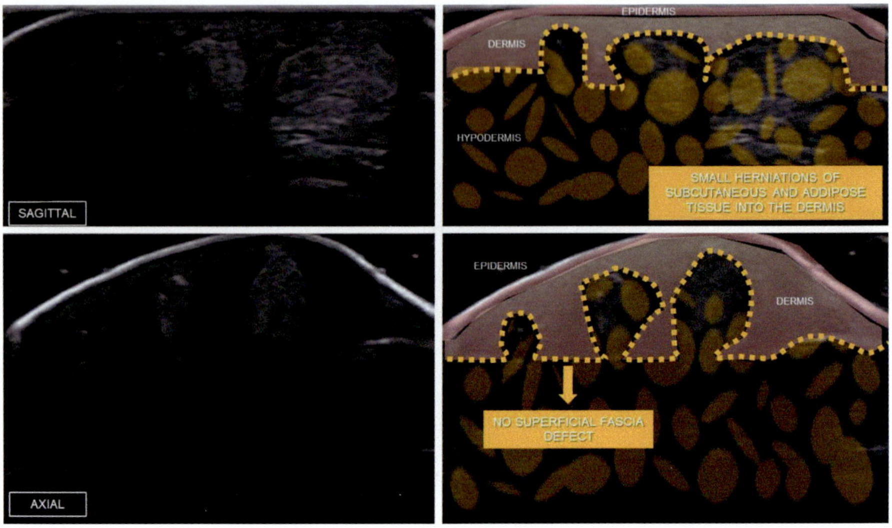

Fig. 15.80 Ultrasonographic findings of a piezogenic papule with a 24 MHz probe (Aplio i800, Canon Medical Systems)

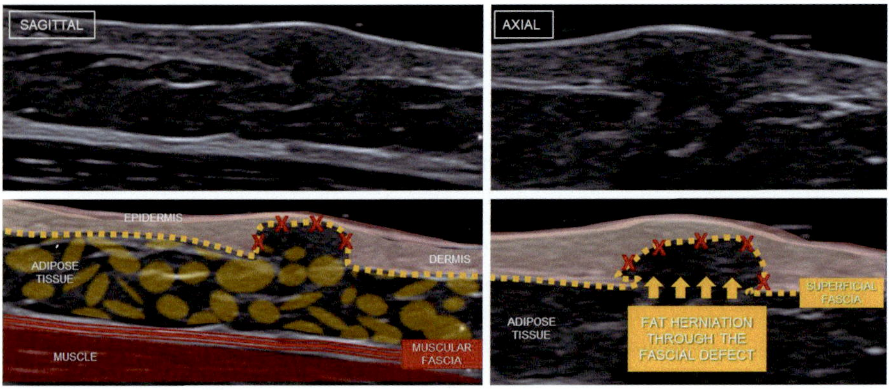

Fig. 15.81 Ultrasonographic findings of a intrafascial fat herniation that simulates a piezogenic papule with a 24 MHz probe (Aplio i800, Canon Medical Systems)

15.22.7 MRI

- MRI is not a primary diagnostic tool for piezogenic pedal papules but may be utilized in atypical cases.
- Imaging characteristics:
  - Lesions appear well-circumscribed with high signal intensity on T1-weighted sequences, attributed to their fat content.

- Signal intensity can vary on T2-weighted sequences, but the high-fat content generally results in a high signal.
- Typically, these lesions do not enhance after contrast administration, reflecting their benign nature and adipose tissue composition.
- MRI excels in differentiating these lesions from surrounding tissues due to its superior soft tissue contrast, clearly highlighting fat herniations.

15.23 Intrafascial Muscle Herniation

15.23.1 Definition [56]

- Intra-fascial muscle herniation involves the protrusion of muscle tissue through a defect in the overlying fascia, often resulting in a visible or palpable subcutaneous lump. This condition can arise from congenital weak points in the fascia or as a result of trauma, overuse, or increased intra-compartmental pressure.

15.23.2 Epidemiology [56]

- Although the precise prevalence of intra-fascial muscle herniation is not well-documented, it is generally more common in the lower extremities, especially among athletes or individuals with a history of lower limb trauma.
- Reports indicate a higher occurrence in males, but cases in females and adolescents have been documented.

15.23.3 Clinical Presentation (Fig. 15.82) [56]

- Patients with intra-fascial muscle herniation typically present with subcutaneous nodules that become more prominent with muscle contraction or standing.
- These nodules are usually asymptomatic but can be associated with pain, cramping, or a sensation of pressure during physical activity.

15.23.4 Radiography [56]

- Standard X-rays are generally not useful for diagnosing intra-fascial muscle herniation as they do not clearly depict soft tissue structures.

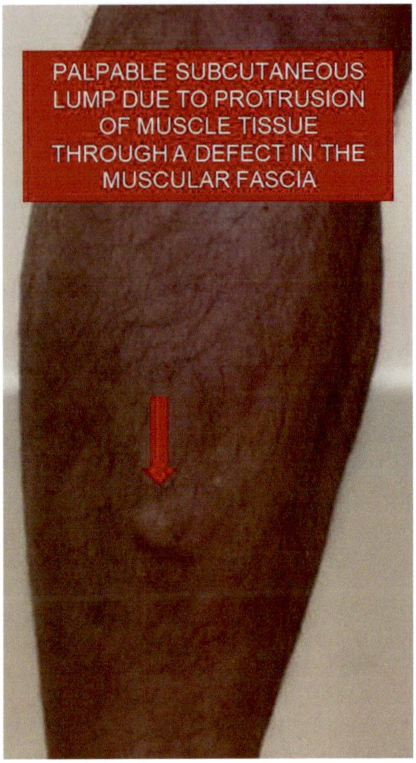

Fig. 15.82 Clinical photograph of patients with intrafascial muscle herniation

15.23.5 Computed Tomography [56]

- CT scans can provide detailed images of soft tissues and are sometimes employed to visualize the extent of fascial defects and herniated muscle. However, they are less commonly used due to the higher radiation exposure compared to other imaging modalities.

15.23.6 Ultrasonography (Fig. 15.83) [56]

- Ultrasonography is ideal for diagnosing intra-fascial muscle herniation, offering real-time, dynamic visualization:
- Identifies muscle bulging through a fascial defect as a hypoechoic mass during contraction.
- Highlights the continuity and breaks in the fascia, with defects appearing as interruptions in the hyperechoic fascia line.
- Observes herniation in real-time during muscle movements or positional changes, aiding diagnosis and muscle functionality assessment.

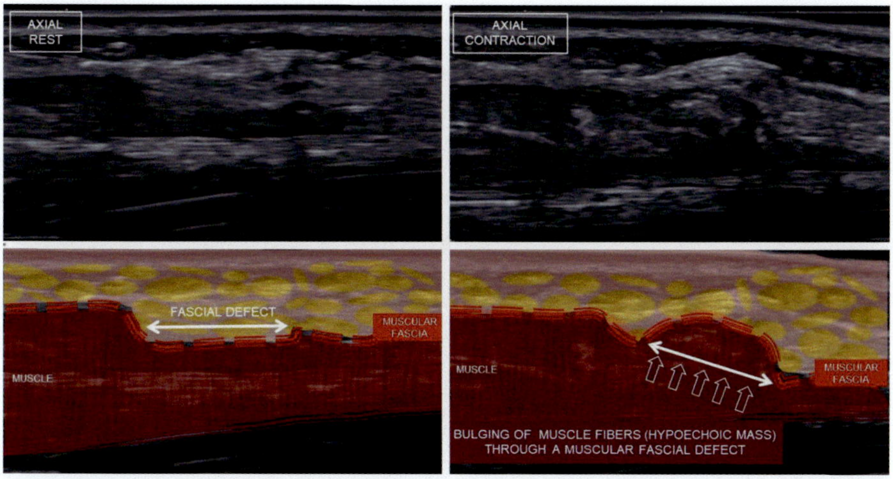

Fig. 15.83 Ultrasonographic findings of intrafascial muscle herniation with a 24 MHz probe (Aplio i800, Canon Medical Systems)

- Power Doppler ultrasonography assesses increased blood flow around the herniation, distinguishing between active inflammation and chronic changes.
- Evaluates adjacent tissues for secondary effects like compression or edema.
- Assesses the unaffected side for comparison to highlight abnormalities.

15.23.7 MRI (Fig. 15.84) [56]

- MRI excels in evaluating atypical muscle herniation cases, providing superior soft tissue contrast.
- Clearly shows muscle tissue extending through the fascial defect, disrupting the normal muscle fascia.
- Visualizes the fascial tear as a discontinuity in the low signal intensity line surrounding the muscle, detailing the extent and size of the defect.
- Herniated muscle retains similar signal intensity to surrounding muscle on T1 and T2-weighted images, with increased T2 signal potentially indicating edema or inflammation.
- Although typically not dynamic, MRI can include protocols showing herniation in both relaxed and contracted states.
- Post-contrast images may reveal enhancement at the herniation site, indicating inflammation or vascular changes, differentiating acute from chronic herniations.
- Offers a comprehensive view of herniated muscle relationships with surrounding structures, aiding surgical planning and assessing complications.

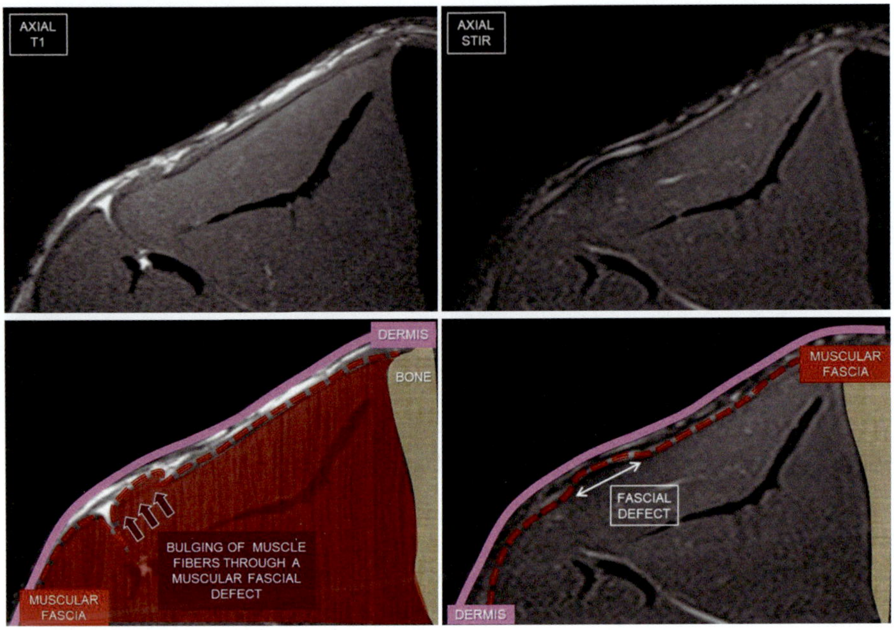

Fig. 15.84 MRI with surface coil findings of intrafascial muscle herniation on T1-weighted and STIR sequences (Magnetom Prisma 3T MRI, Siemens)

15.24 Endometriosis Implant

15.24.1 Definition [57, 58]

- Skin endometriosis is a rare condition characterized by the presence of endometrial stroma outside the uterus, often influenced by hormonal stimuli.
- While most cases of endometriosis occur in pelvic sites like ovaries and peritoneum, skin involvement is uncommon but typically linked to obstetric and gynecologic surgery.

15.24.2 Epidemiology [57, 58]

- Prevalence of endometriosis in the general female population ranges from 2–10%, increasing up to 50% in cases of pain, infertility, or abdomino-pelvic surgery.
- Cesarean section (C-section) is a common risk factor, with skin endometriosis occurring in about 1% of cases post-surgery.

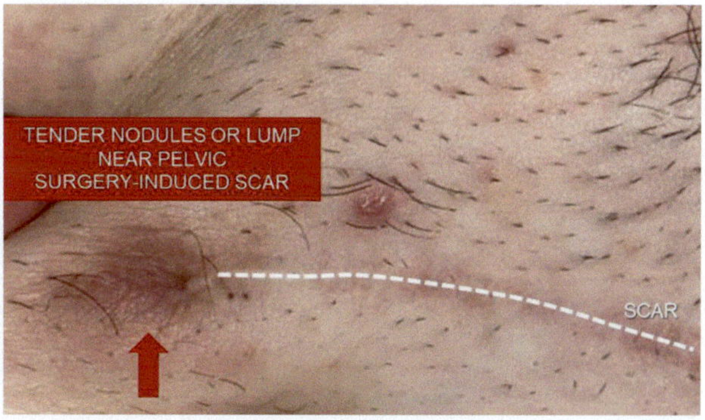

Fig. 15.85 Clinical photograph of patients with endometriosis implant at pelvis

15.24.3 Clinical Presentation (Fig. 15.85) [57, 58]

- Typically affects women of reproductive age, presenting as painful, tender nodules or lumps near pelvic surgery-induced scars.
- Symptoms may include cyclic or intermittent pain, with diagnosis often delayed due to nonspecific clinical appearance and lack of awareness among clinicians.

15.24.4 Dermoscopy [58]

- Endometriosis lesions often exhibit a varied vascular pattern under dermatoscopy.
- Milky red or pink structureless area is a characteristic feature observed in dermatoscopy, indicating the presence of endometrial tissue.
- White lines is also another common dermoscopic finding, although nonspecific, often seen in endometriosis lesions.
- Bluish blotch or clod is unique to cutaneous endometriosis, this feature correlates with haemosiderin deposition, aiding in diagnosis.

15.24.5 Histopathology [59]

- Endometriosis represents the presence of nonneoplastic endometrial tissue outside the uterus; however, the cutaneous form is less common, largely because it is less biopsied.
- Characteristically presents endometrial glands in the middle of the dermis or in fibrous tissue when deeper, often exhibiting recent hemorrhage or hemosiderin deposits.

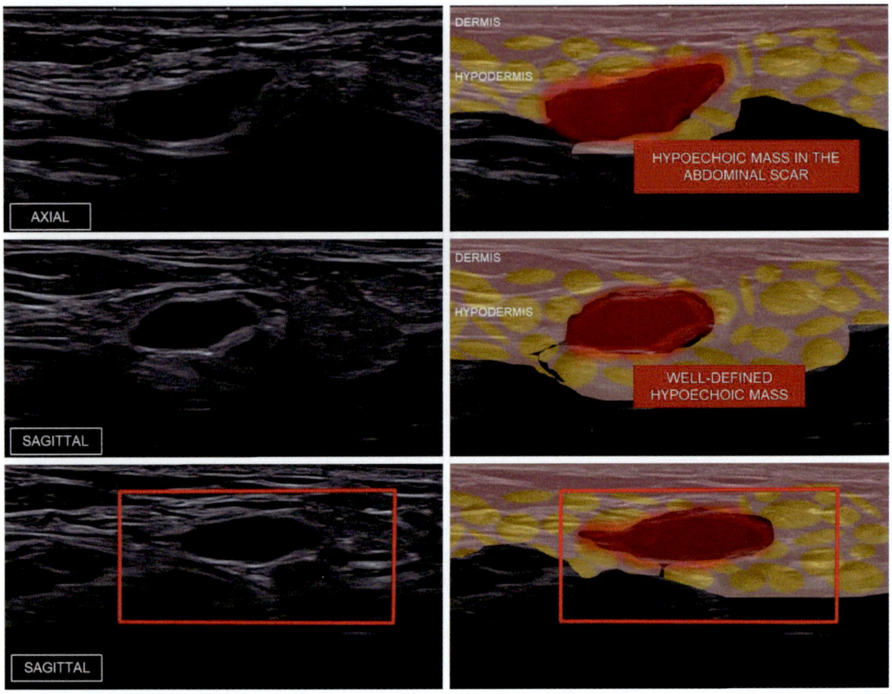

Fig. 15.86 Ultrasonographic findings of endometriosis implant at pelvis with a 24 MHz probe (Aplio i800, Canon Medical Systems)

15.24.6 Ultrasonography (Fig. 15.86) [58]

- Cutaneous endometriosis:
  - Well-defined hypoechoic mass in the abdominal scar.
  - Presence of intralesional vascular spots detected on power Doppler.
- Umbilical endometriosis:
  - Palpable nodule at the umbilicus.
  - Well-defined hypoechoic mass in the abdominal scar or umbilicus.
  - Presence of intralesional vascular spots on power Doppler.
  - Possibility of associated umbilical hernia.
- Subcutaneous endometriosis:
  - Heterogeneous hypoechoic mass with indistinct edges in the right or left inguinal region and subcutaneous tissue.
  - Presence of intralesional vascular spots on power Doppler.
  - Pattern of increased stiffness on elastography compared to surrounding tissues.
- Intramuscular Endometriosis:

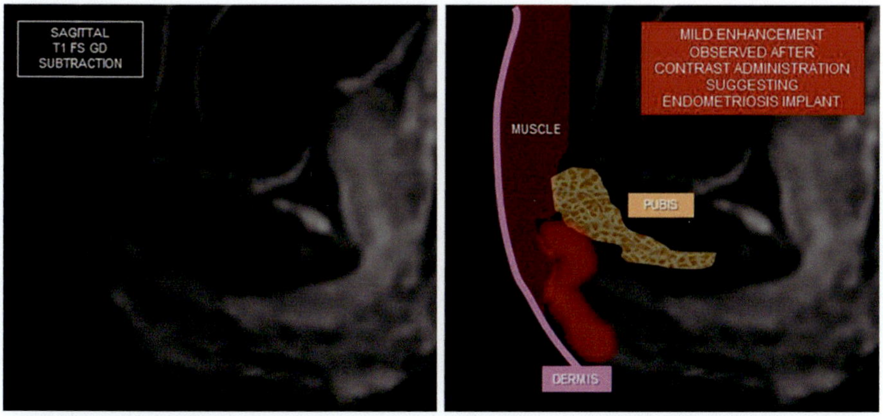

Fig. 15.87 MRI findings of endometriosis implant at abdominal wall on T1 FS-weighted sequences after gadolinium administration (Magnetom Prisma 3T MRI, Siemens)

- Hypoechoic mass located within the rectus abdominis muscle.
- Indistinct borders.
- Possible intralesional fluid collections.
- Presence of intralesional vascular spots on power Doppler.
- Pattern of increased stiffness on elastography compared to surrounding tissues.

15.24.7 MRI (Fig. 15.87) [60]

- Low signal intensity of the lesion on T2-weighted sequences.
- Presence of small hyperintense foci on T2-weighted sequences.
- Intermediate signal intensity of the lesion on T1-weighted sequences.
- Lesion appears isointense with skeletal muscle on T1-weighted sequences.
- Moderate enhancement was observed after administration of contrast.

15.25 Lipodystrophy

15.25.1 Definition [60]

- Lipodystrophy is a group of disorders characterized by abnormal or degenerative conditions of the body's adipose tissue, leading to the loss of fat from specific regions or, in some cases, an abnormal accumulation of fat in others.
- Lipodystrophy can be congenital or acquired and may involve partial or generalized loss of fat.

- The condition is often associated with metabolic complications, including insulin resistance, hyperlipidemia, and fatty liver disease.

15.25.2 *Epidemiology*

- The prevalence of lipodystrophy varies depending on the specific type.
- Congenital forms, such as congenital generalized lipodystrophy (CGL), are rare, with an estimated prevalence of 1 in ten million people.
- Acquired forms, such as acquired partial lipodystrophy (Barraquer–Simons syndrome) and acquired generalized lipodystrophy (AGL), are also rare but slightly more common than congenital types.
- The HIV-associated lipodystrophy, often seen in patients on antiretroviral therapy, has a more significant prevalence, affecting up to 30–50% of treated individuals.

15.25.3 *Clinical Presentation (Fig. 15.88) [60]*

- The clinical presentation of lipodystrophy varies widely depending on the type and extent of fat loss or accumulation:

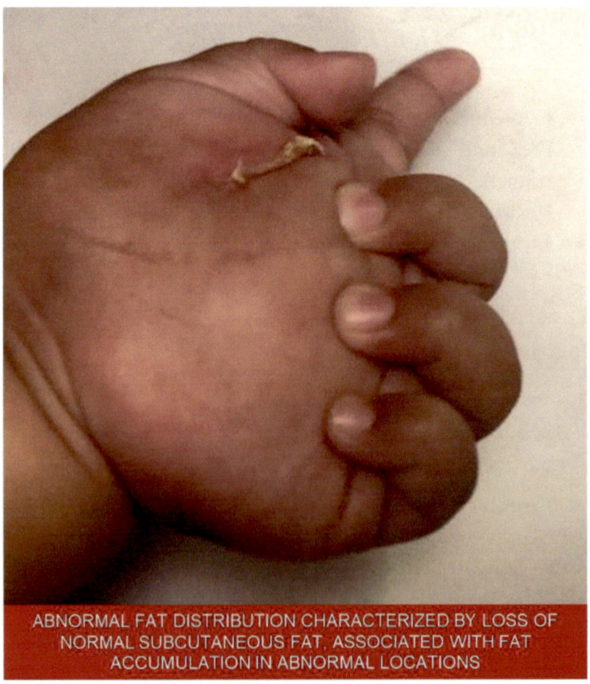

Fig. 15.88 Clinical photograph of patient with lipodystrophy

- Congenital generalized lipodystrophy (CGL): Patients present with a near-total absence of adipose tissue from birth or early infancy, leading to prominent muscles, acromegaloid features, and hepatomegaly. They often develop severe metabolic complications, including insulin resistance, diabetes, and hypertriglyceridemia.
- Acquired generalized lipodystrophy (AGL): Typically presents with a progressive loss of subcutaneous fat during childhood or adolescence, often after an infection or autoimmune event. Patients develop similar metabolic issues as seen in CGL.
- Acquired partial lipodystrophy (Barraquer–Simons syndrome): Characterized by fat loss from the upper body (face, arms, and trunk) with preservation or accumulation of fat in the lower body. This type often presents with complement system abnormalities and can be associated with autoimmune diseases.
- HIV-associated lipodystrophy: Patients may exhibit a combination of lipoatrophy (loss of fat from the face, limbs, and buttocks) and lipohypertrophy (fat accumulation in the abdomen, dorsocervical region, and breasts).

15.25.4 Histopathology [60]

- Histopathological findings in lipodystrophy depend on the specific type but generally include:
  - Lipoatrophy: Reduced or absent adipocytes in the affected areas, with possible fibrosis and a reduction in the overall volume of subcutaneous tissue. There may be an increase in connective tissue components, such as collagen, and a loss of adipose tissue architecture.
  - Lipohypertrophy: Enlarged adipocytes with an increased number of fat cells, particularly in areas of fat accumulation. In some cases, inflammatory cells may be present, particularly in HIV-associated lipodystrophy.
- Other findings: In autoimmune-associated forms of lipodystrophy, perivascular lymphocytic infiltrates can be observed in the affected tissues.

15.25.5 Ultrasonography (Fig. 15.89) [60]

- Ultrasonography can be useful in assessing lipodystrophy, particularly for evaluating the distribution and volume of subcutaneous fat:
  - Lipoatrophy: Ultrasonography may show a marked reduction or absence of the subcutaneous fat layer, with a corresponding increase in the visibility of underlying structures, such as muscles and blood vessels. The remaining fat tissue may appear hyperechoic compared to normal fat due to fibrotic changes.

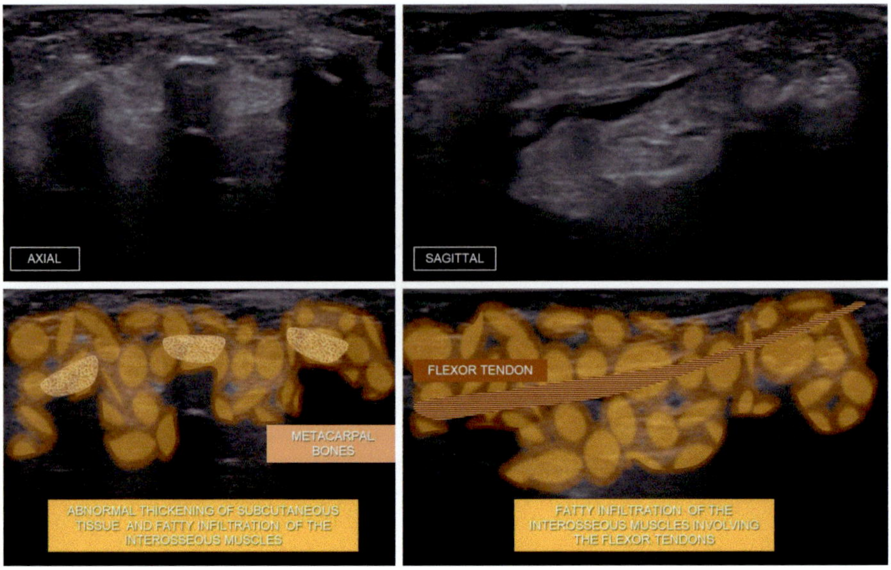

Fig. 15.89 Ultrasonographic findings of lipodystrophy with a 24 MHz probe (Aplio i800, Canon Medical Systems)

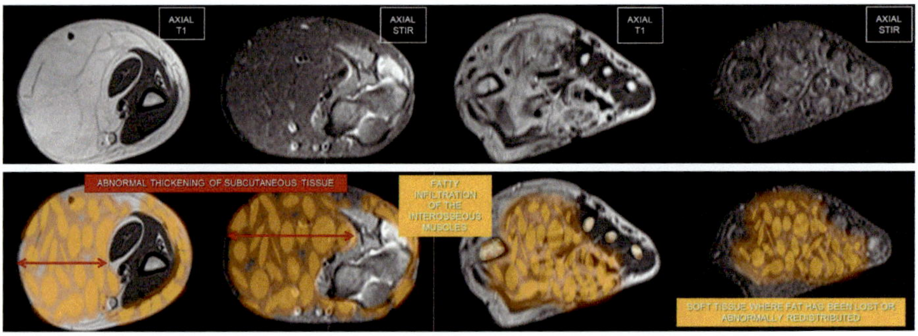

Fig. 15.90 MRI findings of lipodystrophy on T1-weighted and STIR sequences (Magnetom Avanto 1.5T MRI, Siemens)

- Lipohypertrophy: In areas of fat accumulation, ultrasonography may reveal increased thickness of the subcutaneous fat layer, which is typically hypoechoic and homogeneous. Power Doppler studies may show increased vascularity in some cases.

15.25.6 MRI (Fig. 15.90)

- MRI is a highly effective modality for evaluating the extent and distribution of fat in lipodystrophy:

- Lipoatrophy: MRI typically shows a loss of subcutaneous fat, which is normally hyperintense on T1-weighted images. The absence of this fat layer allows for better visualization of the underlying muscles and bone structures. In severe cases, muscle tissue may also show increased signal intensity due to fatty infiltration.
- Lipohypertrophy: MRI reveals increased volumes of adipose tissue, particularly in the abdomen and other affected areas. The fat appears hyperintense on T1-weighted images and may show varying degrees of intensity on T2-weighted images, depending on the presence of inflammation or fibrosis. MRI can also help assess fat infiltration in other organs, such as the liver (hepatic steatosis), which is common in generalized lipodystrophy.

15.26 Knuckle Pads

15.26.1 Definition [61]

- Knuckle pads are well-defined, firm, and often painless thickened areas of skin located over the dorsal aspect of the interphalangeal joints, particularly the proximal interphalangeal joints.
- They are a type of fibromatosis, characterized by the formation of nodules or plaques in the skin and subcutaneous tissue, and are considered a benign condition.

15.26.2 Epidemiology [61]

- Knuckle pads are relatively uncommon and can occur at any age, though they are most frequently seen in adults.
- There is no clear gender predilection.
- The exact prevalence is not well established due to the benign nature of the condition, which often leads to underreporting.
- Knuckle pads may be associated with repetitive trauma or pressure, certain occupations, or specific behaviors such as repetitive hand movements.
- There may also be an association with other forms of fibromatosis, including Dupuytren's contracture.

15.26.3 Clinical Presentation (Fig. 15.91) [33, 61]

- Knuckle pads present as localized, firm, and smooth or slightly raised plaques or nodules over the dorsal aspects of the PIP joints. They can vary in size from a few millimeters to several centimeters.

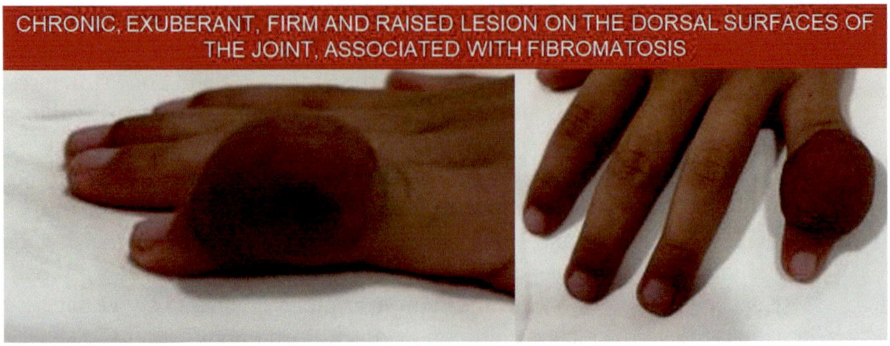

Fig. 15.91 Clinical photograph of patient with a giant knuckle pads

- Most knuckle pads are asymptomatic, though some patients may experience mild discomfort, particularly if the nodules are large or subjected to repeated trauma. The condition is typically bilateral and symmetrical.
- Knuckle pads may develop gradually over time, often in response to chronic friction or trauma. In some cases, they may stabilize and remain unchanged for years, while in others, they may slowly increase in size.

15.26.4 Histopathology [33]

Histopathological examination of knuckle pads reveals:

- Hyperkeratosis characterozed by thickening of the stratum corneum.
- Acanthosis observed as thickening of the epidermis.
- Increased collagen deposition in the dermis, due fibrosis often extending into the subcutaneous tissue.
- Unlike other fibromatoses, knuckle pads typically lack significant inflammatory infiltrate.
- These findings are consistent with other forms of fibromatosis and help to differentiate knuckle pads from other skin lesions.

15.26.5 Ultrasonography (Fig. 15.92)

- The nodules appear as hypoechoic areas, indicating the presence of dense fibrous tissue.
- The lesions are usually well-circumscribed and do not infiltrate surrounding structures.
- Power Doppler ultrasonography typically shows no increased blood flow within the nodules, which helps to differentiate them from inflammatory conditions.

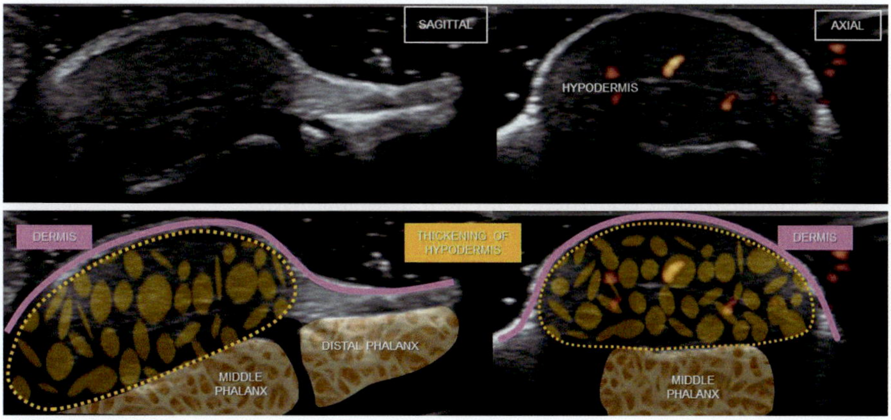

Fig. 15.92 Ultrasonographic findings of a giant knuckle pads with a 24 MHz probe (Aplio i800, Canon Medical Systems)

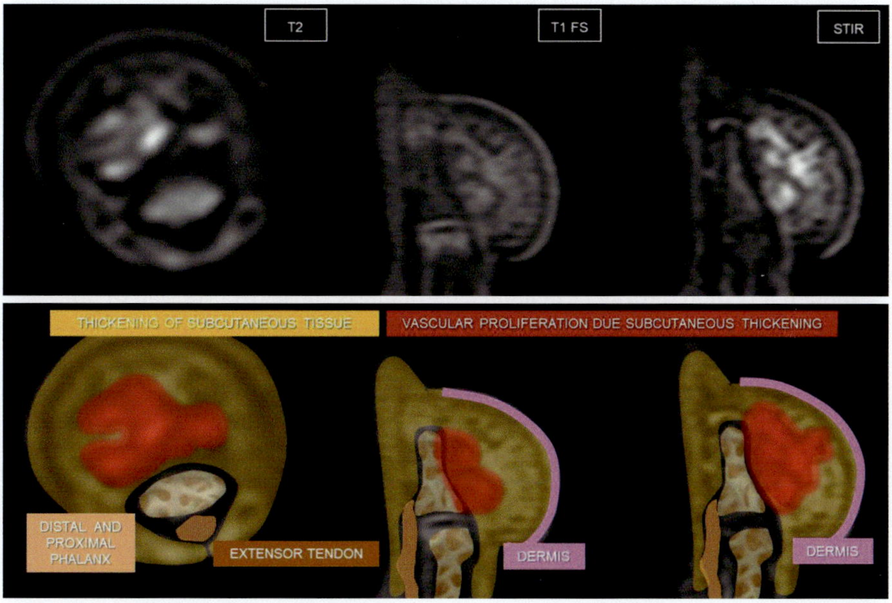

Fig. 15.93 MRI findings of a giant knuckle pads on T1, T2, and T1 FS-weighted sequences (Magnetom Avanto 1.5T MRI, Siemens)

15.26.6 MRI (Fig. 15.93)

- MRI can provide detailed imaging of knuckle pads, particularly in cases where a deeper fibrous component is suspected:

- Knuckle pads typically appear as isointense or slightly hypointense lesions on T1-weighted images compared to surrounding muscle tissue, reflecting their fibrous content.
- May appear as low to intermediate signal intensity areas on T2-weighted sequences due to the dense fibrous tissue, which contains little water.
- Knuckle pads generally show minimal or no enhancement after gadolinium contrast administration, consistent with their avascular nature.

15.27 Vascular Ectasia

15.27.1 Definition [62]

- Vascular ectasia refers to a localized dilation of blood vessels, usually capillaries or venules, within the skin.
- This condition results in visible red or purple discoloration, often appearing as macules, patches, or telangiectasias (spider veins).
- Vascular ectasia can occur as a primary condition or secondary to other underlying disorders.

15.27.2 Epidemiology [62]

- Vascular ectasia is a common condition that can affect individuals of all ages, though it is more prevalent in adults, particularly those over the age of 50.
- The condition is often associated with chronic sun exposure, aging, and certain genetic predispositions.
- It may also be seen in association with systemic conditions such as liver disease (e.g., spider angiomas in cirrhosis) or connective tissue disorders.
- There is no significant gender predilection.

15.27.3 Clinical Presentation (Fig. 15.94) [62]

- Vascular ectasia manifests as small, dilated blood vessels visible through the skin. These can appear as fine red or purple lines, often forming a branching pattern, particularly on the face, neck, chest, and extremities.
- The lesions are typically asymptomatic and are primarily a cosmetic concern. In some cases, they may be associated with mild discomfort or a burning sensation, especially if the underlying cause is related to systemic conditions.

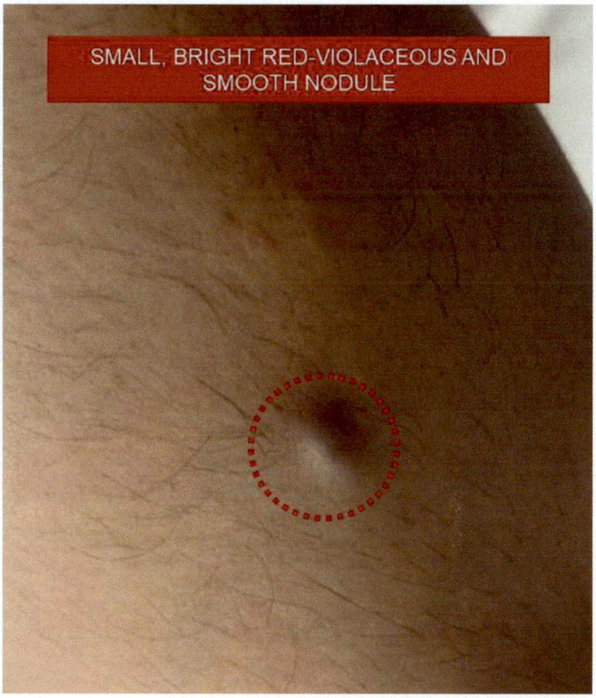

Fig. 15.94 Clinical photograph of patient with vascular ectasia

- The condition often affects sun-exposed areas and can be widespread or localized depending on the underlying cause. In systemic diseases, the distribution may follow a more characteristic pattern, such as spider angiomas on the upper body in patients with liver disease.

15.27.4 Histopathology [33]

- Histopathological examination of vascular ectasia reveals:
  - The primary feature is the dilation of capillaries or venules within the dermis. These vessels may have thin walls and are filled with red blood cells.
  - There is usually little to no inflammatory infiltrate surrounding the dilated vessels.
  - The overlying epidermis is typically normal, though in some cases, there may be mild hyperkeratosis or atrophy, especially in long-standing lesions.

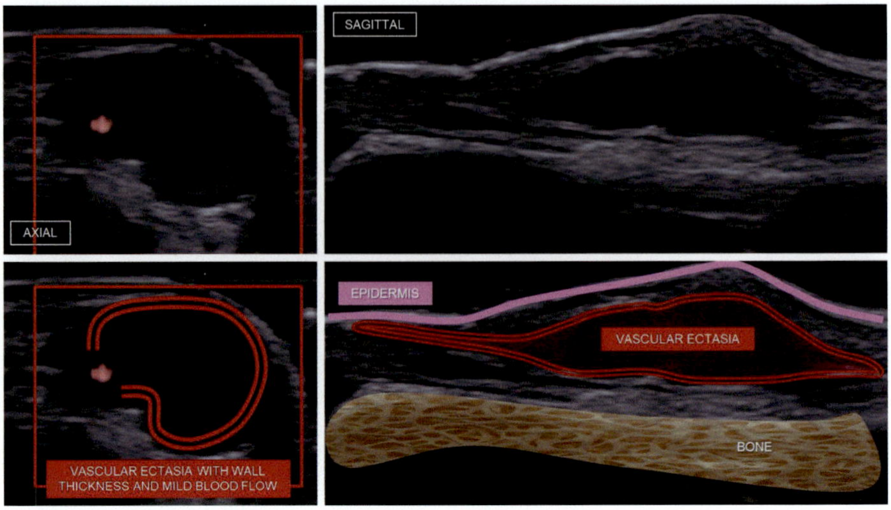

Fig. 15.95 Ultrasonographic findings of vascular ectasia with a 24 MHz probe (Aplio i800, Canon Medical Systems)

15.27.5 Ultrasonography (Fig. 15.95)

- Ultrasonography of vascular ectasia can provide detailed imaging of the dilated vessels:
  - The dilated blood vessels appear as hypoechoic or anechoic tubular structures within the dermis.
  - Power Doppler ultrasonography may reveal slow or stagnant blood flow within the ectatic vessels, and in some cases, the vessels may not demonstrate any significant flow.
  - The surrounding skin and subcutaneous tissue are usually unremarkable, helping to differentiate vascular ectasia from more infiltrative vascular lesions.

15.27.6 MRI

- MRI imaging of vascular ectasia, while not typically required, can provide additional information in complex cases:
  - The ectatic vessels may appear as low-signal intensity areas on T1-weighted images due to the presence of slow-moving blood or stagnant flow.
  - These lesions may appear hyperintense on T2-weighted images, reflecting the presence of blood within the dilated vessels.
  - Post-gadolinium enhancement is usually minimal or absent, as these vessels are not associated with neovascularization or significant inflammation.

15.28 Pseudoaneurysm

15.28.1 Definition [63]

- A pseudoaneurysm (also known as a false aneurysm) of the skin refers to a localized collection of blood that forms between the layers of an artery wall, typically after trauma or an invasive procedure.
- Unlike a true aneurysm, which involves all three layers of the arterial wall, a pseudoaneurysm occurs when blood leaks out of the vessel but is contained by the surrounding tissue, creating a pulsatile mass.

15.28.2 Epidemiology [63]

- Skin pseudoaneurysms are relatively rare and usually occur following trauma, such as penetrating injuries, surgical procedures, or needle punctures.
- They can occur at any age and are more common in individuals with underlying conditions that affect blood vessel integrity or healing, such as atherosclerosis or anticoagulant therapy.
- The incidence is higher in areas of the body where arteries are more superficial and vulnerable to injury.

15.28.3 Clinical Presentation (Fig. 15.96) [63]

- Pseudoaneurysms typically present as a pulsatile, tender mass beneath the skin. The overlying skin may appear normal, erythematous, or ecchymotic, depending on the extent of the trauma and the age of the lesion.
- Patients may experience pain, swelling, and a palpable thrill or bruit over the lesion. In some cases, the pseudoaneurysm may rupture, leading to sudden bleeding or the formation of a hematoma.
- Pseudoaneurysms can occur at any site of arterial injury, but they are most commonly found in areas such as the groin (following femoral artery catheterization), wrist, or areas of previous surgical intervention.

15.28.4 Histopathology [33]

- Histopathological examination of a pseudoaneurysm reveals:

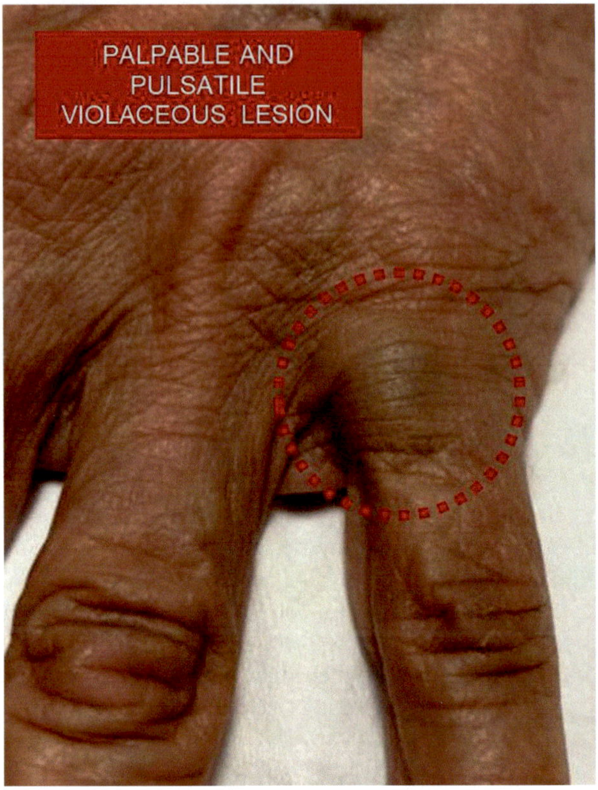

Fig. 15.96 Clinical photograph of patients with pseudoaneurysm

- The defining feature is the disruption of the arterial wall with extravasation of blood into the surrounding tissue.
- The extravasated blood is often surrounded by a fibrous capsule composed of fibrin and granulation tissue, which attempts to contain the hematoma.
- There may be a mild inflammatory response in the surrounding tissue, particularly if the pseudoaneurysm has been present for some time.

15.28.4.1 Ultrasonography (Fig. 15.97) [64, 65]

- A characteristic finding on power Doppler ultrasonography is the "yin-yang" sign, representing bidirectional blood flow within the pseudoaneurysm sac.
- Power Doppler studies may also show "to-and-fro" flow at the neck of the pseudoaneurysm, indicating blood movement into and out of the sac with each cardiac cycle.
- The pseudoaneurysm appears as a hypoechoic or anechoic sac adjacent to the artery, with turbulent flow patterns detected within.

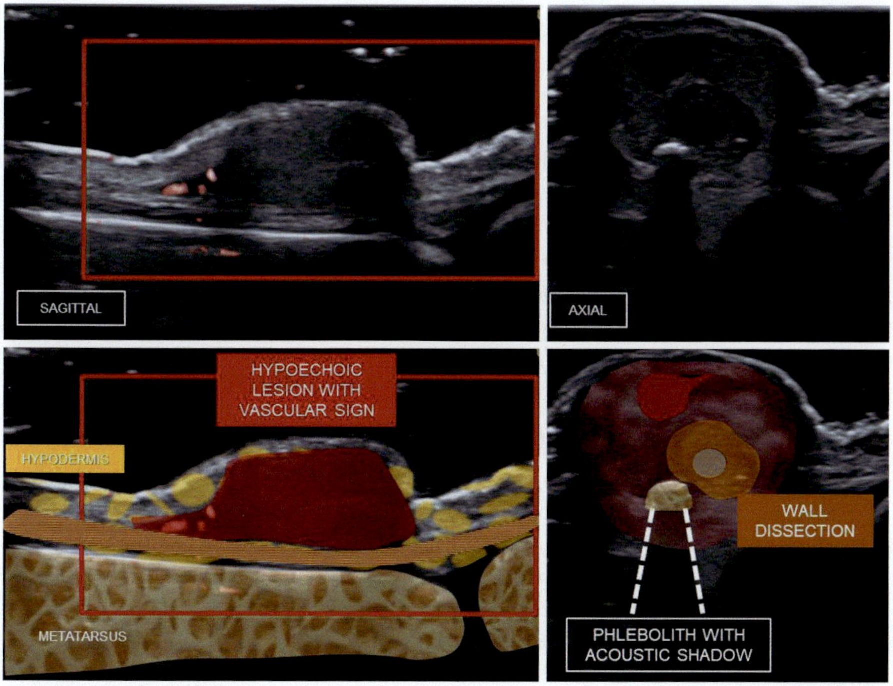

Fig. 15.97 Ultrasonographic findings of pseudoaneurysm with a 24 MHz probe (Aplio i800, Canon Medical Systems)

15.28.5 MRI

- MRI can provide detailed imaging of the pseudoaneurysm and surrounding structures:
  - The pseudoaneurysm sac typically appears as a hyperintense lesion on T1-weighted images due to the presence of subacute blood products (methemoglobin).
  - On T2-weighted images, the lesion may appear hyperintense, with a surrounding hypointense rim representing the fibrous capsule.
  - After gadolinium administration, the pseudoaneurysm sac may show peripheral enhancement, while the neck of the pseudoaneurysm may enhance due to the connection with the arterial lumen.

15.29 Angiokeratomas

15.29.1 Definition [66]

- The term angiokeratoma is derived from the Greek words "angeion" meaning vessel, "keras" meaning horn and "oma" meaning tumor.
- It is a benign skin condition characterized by the presence of small red or purple raised lesions on the skin, caused by dilated blood vessels.
- Typically, small lesion measuring few millimeters in diameter and can appear anywhere on the body, with a preference for the lower extremities.

15.29.2 Epidemiology [66]

- Epidemiologic information of angiokeratomas is scarce since they are often underreported.
- Their prevalence increases with age. It may affect all ages, with no gender predilection.
- While the precise cause is not fully understood, they are thought to be related to dilated blood vessels, genetic factors, or local trauma.
- Potential associations have been described: chronic venous insufficiency, varicose veins, and genetic disorders, like Fabry disease.

15.29.3 Clinical Presentation (Fig. 15.98) [66]

- Angiokeratomas may occur as isolated lesions or in clusters.

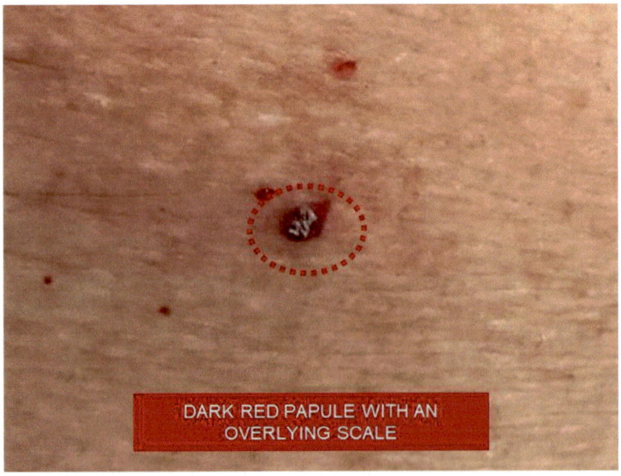

Fig. 15.98 Clinical photograph of patient with angiokeratoma

- Different forms of manifestation are described: solitary angiokeratomas, angiokeratomas of Fordyce (typically found in the genital region), and angiokeratoma corporis diffusum (widespread lesions, often associated with genetic disorders, like Fabry disease).

15.29.4 Dermoscopy (Fig. 15.99) [63, 66]

- Multiple dark red to violaceous, well-circumscribed papules.
- Vascular structures may be observed: dotted or linear vessels, globules, and milky-red areas.

15.29.5 Histopathology (Fig. 15.100) [33, 66]

- Superficial proliferation of small ecstatic venules, containing few or no red blood cells.
- Surrounded by the hyperplastic epidermis, giving an appearance of being falsely inside the epidermis; may present thrombosis occasionally.

15.29.6 Ultrasonography (Fig. 15.101) [67]

- Epidermal thickening and linear hyperechogenicity and a hypoechoic circumscribed lesion limited to the papillary dermis.
- There is no power Doppler signal.

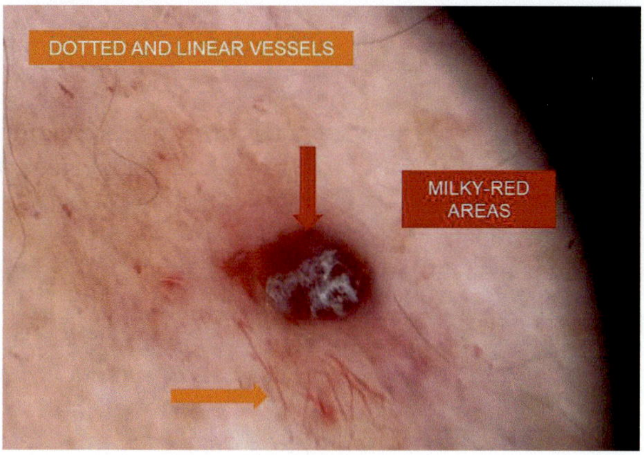

Fig. 15.99 Dermoscopic findings of patient angiokeratoma (x20)

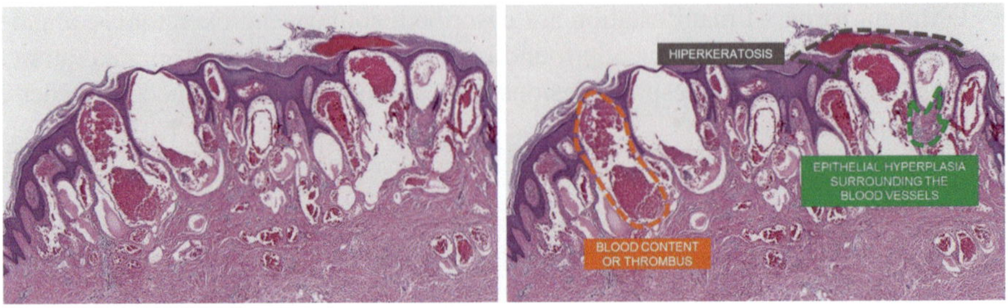

Fig. 15.100 Histological findings of angiokeratoma (H&E x4)

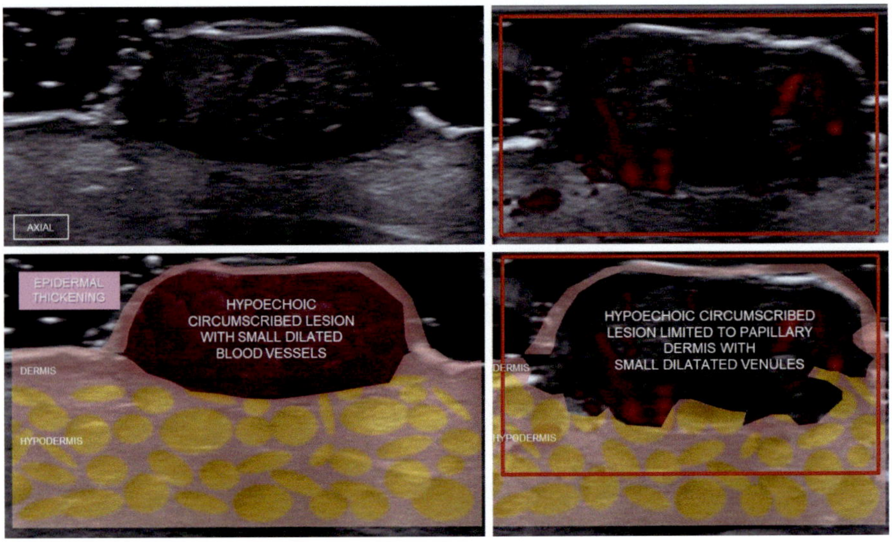

Fig. 15.101 Ultrasonographic findings of angiokeratoma with a 24 MHz probe (Aplio i800, Canon Medical Systems)

15.29.7 MRI [68]

- Angiokeratomas appear heterogeneous, presenting as hypo to isointense on T1-weighted images, hyperintense on T2-weighted and STIR sequences, and typically show a well-circumscribed soft tissue lesion with moderate contrast enhancement.
- Verrucous hemangiomas are often mistaken for angiokeratomas, differing primarily in their deeper tissue involvement. Only a deep tissue biopsy can reliably distinguish between them. If the biopsy does not include enough deep tissue, it may result in an incorrect diagnosis of superficial angiokeratoma.

15.30 Intravascular Papillary Endothelial Hyperplasia (Masson's Tumor)

15.30.1 Definition [69]

- Masson's tumor, also known as intravascular papillary endothelial hyperplasia (IPEH), is a rare, benign vascular lesion characterized by the proliferation of endothelial cells within blood vessels, typically veins, leading to the formation of papillary structures.
- It is not a true neoplasm but rather a reactive process, often occurring in response to vascular injury or thrombosis.

15.30.2 Epidemiology [69]

- Masson's tumor is an uncommon condition, representing less than 2% of all vascular tumors.
- It can occur at any age but is more commonly diagnosed in adults.
- There is no significant gender predilection.
- The lesion can develop in various locations, including the skin, subcutaneous tissues, and deep vascular structures, often in association with areas prone to trauma or venous stasis.

15.30.3 Clinical Presentation (Fig. 15.102) [69]

- Masson's tumor typically presents as a slowly growing, painless mass. It may appear as a firm, blue, or purple nodule or plaque, resembling a vascular lesion such as a hemangioma or thrombosed varix.
- The lesion is usually asymptomatic but may cause discomfort if located in an area subject to pressure or trauma. Rarely, it can ulcerate or become painful, particularly if complicated by thrombosis or hemorrhage.
- Common sites include the fingers, hands, forearms, head and neck, and lower extremities. The lesion can also occur in deeper tissues, including muscles and internal organs, where it may present as a more substantial mass.

15.30.4 Histopathology [33]

- Histopathological examination of Masson's tumor reveals:

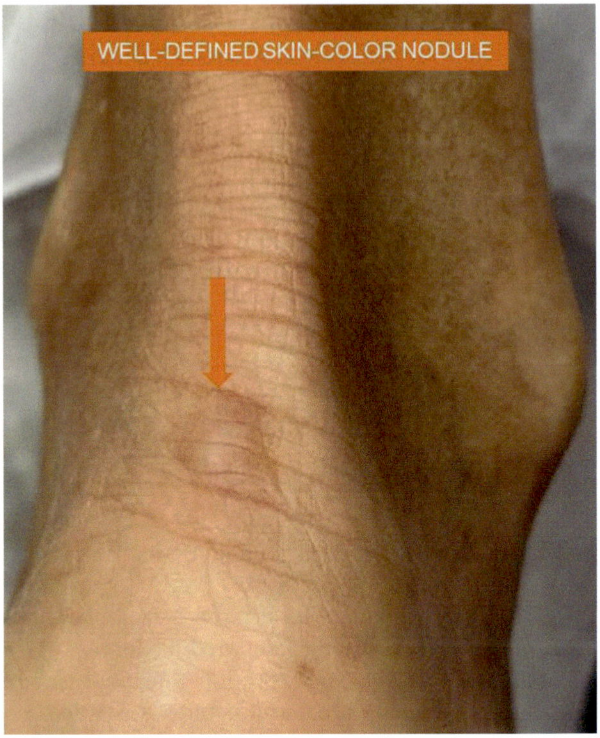

Fig. 15.102 Clinical photograph of patient with intravascular papillary endothelial hyperplasia

- The hallmark of Masson's tumor is the presence of papillary proliferations of endothelial cells within the lumen of a blood vessel. These papillae are often arranged around a central fibrin core.
- The lesion frequently contains an organized thrombus, with endothelial cell proliferation occurring in response to this thrombosis.
- The endothelial cells are typically bland and lack significant atypia or mitotic activity, distinguishing this lesion from malignant vascular tumors such as angiosarcoma.

15.30.5 Ultrasonography (Fig. 15.103)

- The lesion typically appears as a well-defined, hypoechoic mass within the dermis or subcutaneous tissue, often adjacent to or within a vessel.
- Power Doppler ultrasonography may reveal varying degrees of vascularity within the lesion, depending on the extent of endothelial proliferation and thrombosis. In some cases, flow may be absent, mimicking a thrombosed hemangioma.
- Ultrasonography is useful for assessing the lesion's size, depth, and relationship to adjacent structures, helping to guide biopsy or excision.

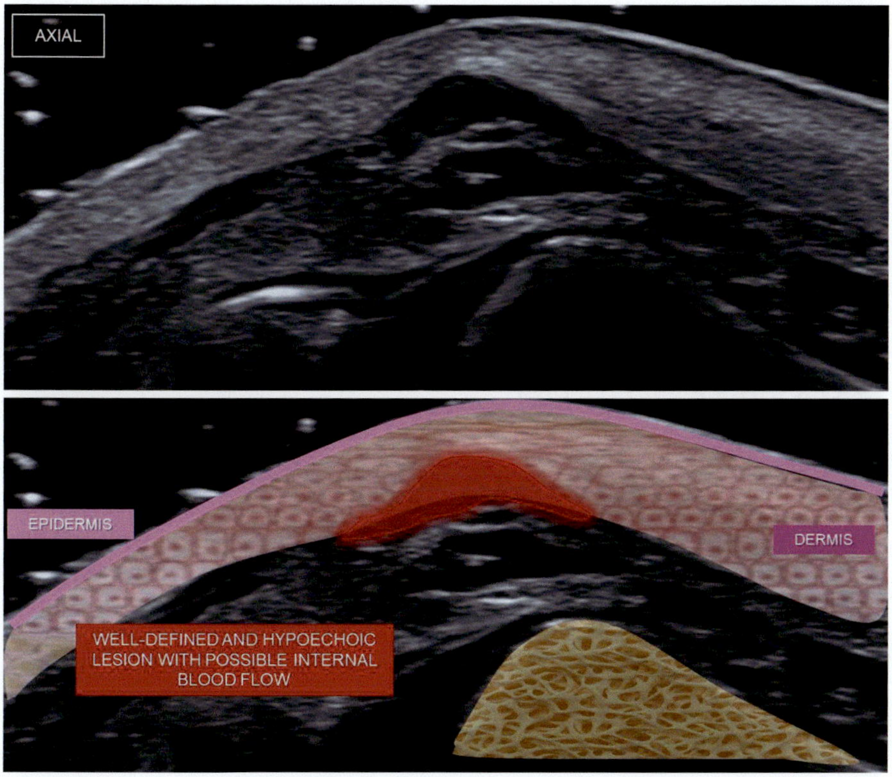

Fig. 15.103 Ultrasonographic findings of intravascular papillary endothelial hyperplasia with a 24 MHz probe (Aplio i800, Canon Medical Systems)

15.30.6 MRI

- The lesion may appear as a mass of intermediate signal intensity on T1-weighted images, reflecting its vascular nature and the presence of thrombus.
- On T2-weighted images, Masson's tumor typically shows high signal intensity due to the presence of fluid-filled spaces and proliferating vascular channels.
- Post-gadolinium, the lesion usually demonstrates marked enhancement, highlighting the proliferative endothelial component. The enhancement pattern may be nodular or diffuse, depending on the degree of vascular proliferation and organization.

15.31 Arteriovenous Malformation (AVM)

15.31.1 Definition [70]

- Abnormal connection between arteries and veins, bypassing the capillary system.
- Known as a "high-flow lesion" due to direct blood flow from the arterial to the venous system.
- Typically congenital.
- Can occur in various tissues (skin, soft tissue, and viscera).

15.31.2 Epidemiology [70]

- AVMs are relatively rare, with an estimated prevalence of 1 in 100,000 individuals.
- Occur sporadically or as part of genetic conditions (e.g., Hereditary Hemorrhagic Telangiectasia, Capillary Malformation-Arteriovenous Malformation syndrome).
- High-flow nature makes them potentially dangerous, leading to clinical complications like bleeding and tissue ischemia.

15.31.3 Clinical Presentation (Fig. 15.104) [70]

- Common Symptoms and Signs:
- Palpable, pulsating mass due to high blood flow.
- Pain is observed resulting from tissue ischemia or compression of surrounding structures.
- Potential bleeding for significant hemorrhage if AVMs rupture.

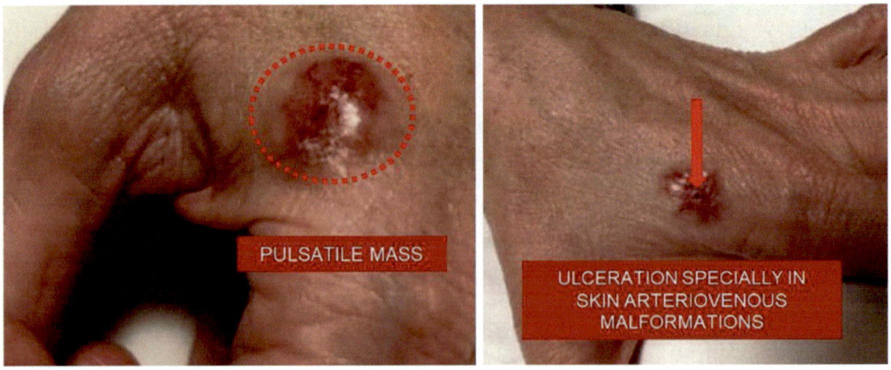

Fig. 15.104 Clinical photograph of patients with arteriovenous malformation

- Ulceration: is seen specially in skin AVMs where overlying tissue breaks down.
- Large AVMs can cause increased cardiac strain.
- Neurological symptoms such as headaches, seizures, or other deficits if AVM is near or in the brain.
- Schobinger clinical classification:
  - Stage I (Quiescence): Skin warmth and slight discoloration.
  - Stage II (Expansion): Enlargement, pulsation, and a bruit.
  - Stage III (Destruction): Pain, bleeding, ulceration, necrosis.
  - Stage IV (Decompensation): High-output cardiac failure due to arteriovenous shunting.

15.31.4 Dermoscopy [71]

- Port-wine stains (PWS):
  - Dermoscopic features include linear irregular vessels or linear serpentine vessels with variable diameters and sharp margins.
  - Vessels are arranged in parallel or haphazardly.
  - Lacunae are absent.
  - Red dots and globules are sparsely noted, mainly in early macules.
  - Advanced plaques show linear irregular vessels separated by white structureless areas.
  - Gray-whitish veils, brown dots, or purplish vessels are not observed.
- Hereditary hemorrhagic telangiectasia (HHT):
  - Dermoscopic features include small red clods and thick serpentine and linear vessels with a somewhat radial arrangement on a pinkish background.
- Unilateral nevoid telangiectasia:
  - Dermoscopic features mainly consist of red dots and globules, contrasting with prior descriptions of red tortuous capillaries with a reticulated appearance.
- Arteriovenous malformations (AS):
  - Dermoscopic features include short linear and linear irregular vessels of variable diameter with ill-defined/blurred margins.
  - Arranged in a haphazard arrangement.
  - Additional features described include hairpin-like and comma vessels.

15.31.5 Histopathology [33]

- Cutaneous vascular malformations are rare disorders representing errors in vascular development. These lesions occur much less commonly but are often confused with the common infantile hemangioma.
- Microscopically, different patterns of cutaneous hemangioma can be similar.
- They may present thrombosis at distinct stages of development.

15.31.6 Computed Tomography (Fig. 15.105) [72]

- Multiple dilated feeding arteries are observed.
- Early enhancement of draining veins is noted.
- No significant interposing mass is identified.

15.31.7 Ultrasonography (Fig. 15.106) [73]

- Presence of intralesional soft tissue:
  - Indicates vascular tumors, such as hemangiomas.

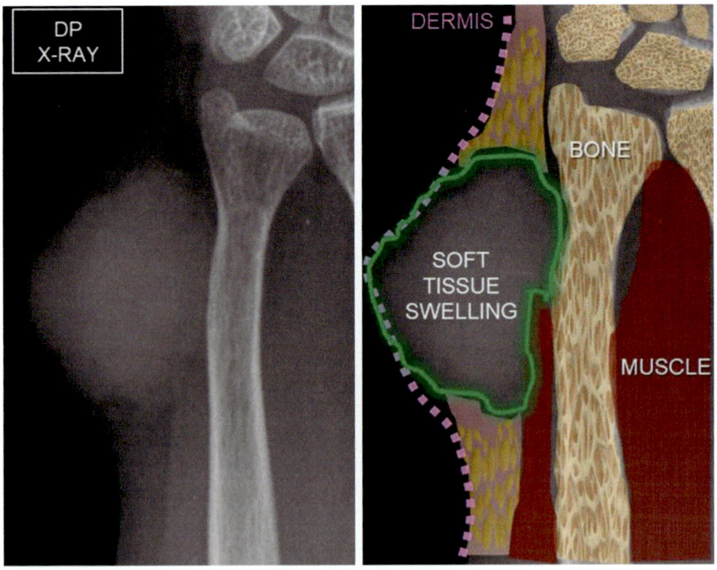

Fig. 15.105 Radiographic findings of arteriovenous malformation. Image kindly provided by Dr. Ciro Menna Barreto Duarte, Caxias do Sul—Brazil

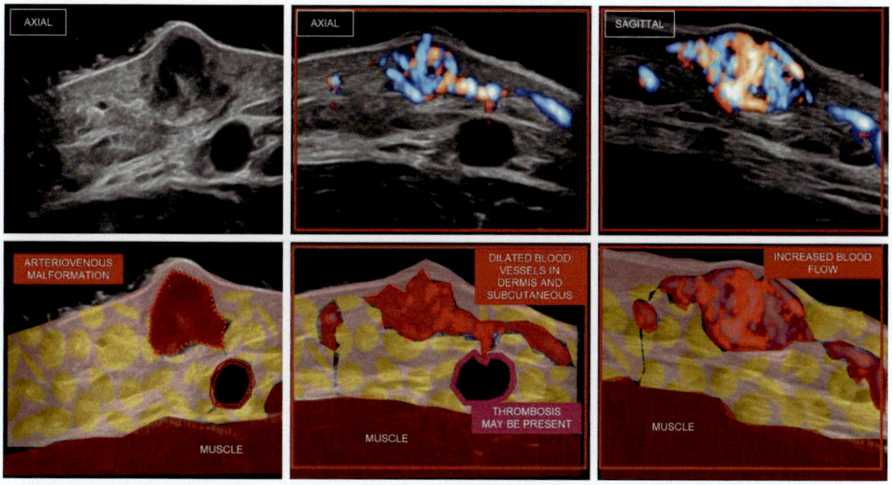

Fig. 15.106 Ultrasonographic findings of arteriovenous malformation with a 24 MHz probe (Aplio i800, Canon Medical Systems)

- Absence of soft-tissue components suggests high-flow malformations arteriovenous malformations (AVMs), arteriovenous fistulas (AVFs).
- Presence of soft-tissue mass is a reliable predictor for differentiating hemangiomas (or other vascular tumors) from AVMs.

- High-flow lesions without soft-tissue component:
  - Presence of arterial component.
  - Examples: Hemangiomas, arteriovenous malformations (AVMs), arteriovenous fistulas (AVFs).
- Low-flow lesions without soft-tissue component:
  - Absence of arterial component.
  - Examples: Capillary malformations, lymphatic malformations (LMs), venous malformations (VMs), and involuting hemangiomas.
- Step-by-step ultrasonographic approach for arteriovenous malformations:
  - Step 1: Assess arterial flow.

    Arterial flow suggests high-flow lesion; absence indicates low-flow lesion.

  - Step 2: Evaluate vessel density.

    Low density: < 2 vessels/cm^2.
    Moderate density: 2–4 vessels/cm^2.
    High density: = 5 vessels/cm^2.

  - Step 3: Measure peak arterial systolic velocity (PSV).
  - High PSV values are indicative of high-flow lesions.

- Arteriovenous malformations >1.5 cm:
  - Increased blood flow.
  - Dilated blood vessels.
  - Fast blood flow in the mid-lower dermis and subcutaneous tissue.
  - More pronounced findings in larger lesions with darker pink to red colors.
- Arteriovenous malformation 1–1.5 cm:
  - Typically shows one or two dilated blood vessels with fast flow in the underlying hypodermis.
- Arteriovenous malformation <1 cm:
  - No significant special ultrasonographic features observed.

15.31.8 MRI (Fig. 15.107) [74]

- Follow-up imaging to determine lesion extent and vascular supply, especially useful for high-flow lesions.
- T2-weigted and STIR images are helpful to map extent of lesions.
- Postcontrast 3D T1-weighted sequences evaluates vascularity.
- Dynamic 3D fast GRE indicates functional analysis and classification of lesions.
- T2 weighted GRE* detects calcification or hemorrhage.

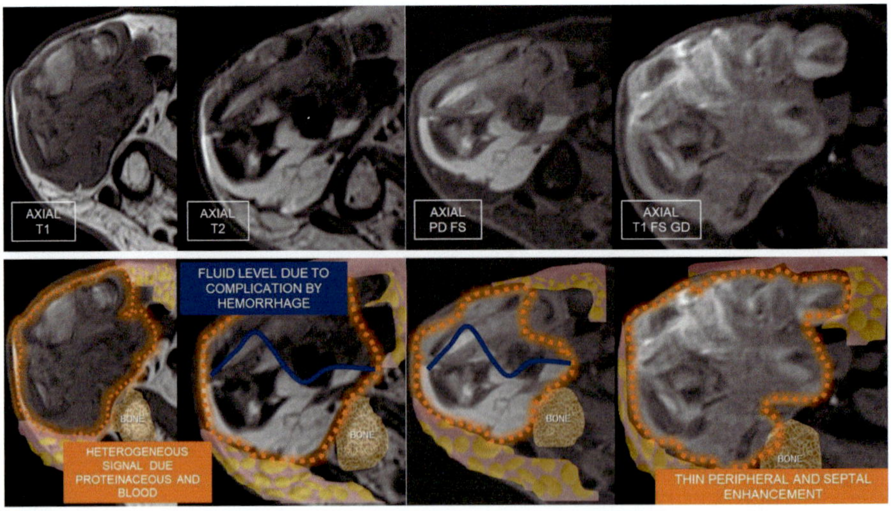

Fig. 15.107 MRI findings of arteriovenous malformation on T1, T2, DP FS, and T1 FS-weighted sequences after gadolinium administration. Image kindly provided by Dr. Ciro Menna Barreto Duarte, Caxias do Sul—Brazil

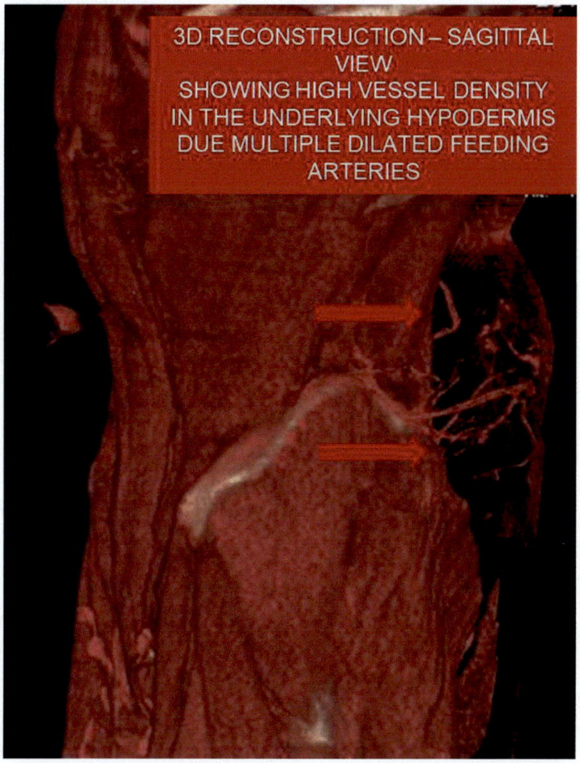

Fig. 15.108 3D images of arteriovenous malformation after segmentation of CT images for surgical planning

15.31.9 3D Images (Fig. 15.108, Video 15.5)

- Extremely beneficial for managing complex and persistent cases.
- Provides a detailed view of the lesion, including blood vessels and ramifications.
- Enhances the precision of surgical procedures.
- Biomodels can create physical replicas of the affected region, offering valuable information for surgical planning and patient education, especially in complex surgery.

15.32 Lymphangioma

15.32.1 Definition [75, 76]

- Lymphangiomas are uncommon, benign malformations of the lymphatic system that can occur anywhere on the skin and mucous membranes.

- They can be categorized as deep or superficial based on the depth and size of the abnormal lymphatic vessels, or as congenital or acquired.

15.32.2 Epidemiology [75]

- Lymphangiomas are rare in the United States, representing 4% of all vascular tumors and approximately 25% of all benign pediatric vascular tumors.
- There is no racial or gender predilection.
- Lymphangiomas typically present at birth or in the first few years of life, while the acquired form of cutaneous lymphangioma circumscriptum often presents in adulthood.

15.32.3 Clinical Presentation (Fig. 15.109) [75]

- Congenital lymphangiomas are present before the age of 5 years and are due to improper connection of lymphatic channels to the main lymphatic drainage duct.
- Acquired lymphangiomas occur as a sequela of any interruption of previously normal lymphatic drainage such as surgery, trauma, malignancy, and radiation therapy.
- Presentation includes papules or nodules of variable color, with a rare form restricted to the skin, predominantly in females and Asian populations.
- Diagnosis can be challenging due to clinical profile and histopathological characteristics.
- Surgical excision is an effective treatment for localized cutaneous lesions.

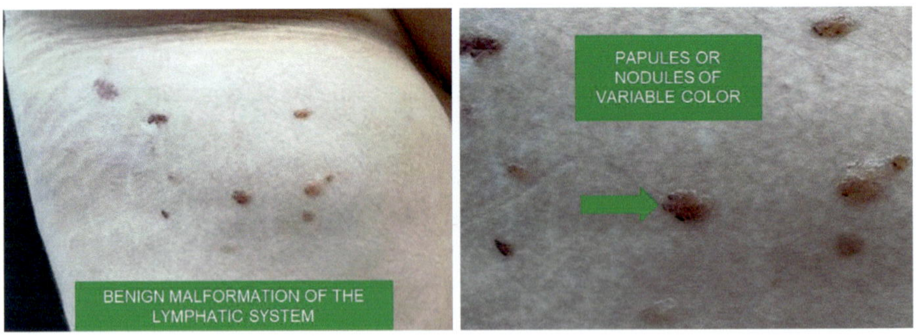

Fig. 15.109 Clinical photograph of patient with lymphangioma

15.32.4 Dermoscopy (Fig. 15.110) [77]

- Multiple white-yellowish well-circumscribed roundish lacunas surrounded by pale septa.
- Blood characteristically accumulated in the lowest part of the lacuna, resulting in an appearance similar to the so-called "hypopyon" of the eye.

15.32.5 Histopathology [33]

- Superficial form or circumscribed lymphangioma and deep form or cystic hygroma and cavernous lymphangioma.
- Regardless of the shape, the microscopic appearance is similar, changing only the location on the skin superficially or superficially and deeply.
- Presence of thin vessels with a thin anastomosing pattern, thin walls, and the nuclei are thicker than the walls, often without content or containing scarce amorphous hyaline material.
- Lesions in the late stages may have walls thickened by fibrosis.

15.32.6 Computed Tomography (Fig. 15.111) [72]

- Most appear homogeneous and cystic.
- Some may appear inhomogeneous due to the presence of proteinaceous, fluid, blood, or fat components.
- Intrinsic septations are rare, and there is minimal or no displacement or compression of adjacent structures.
- CT scans demonstrate masses with low attenuation, occasionally showing fluid levels, with minimal septal and peripheral enhancement.
- Angiography is not diagnostically valuable for this type of vascular malformation.

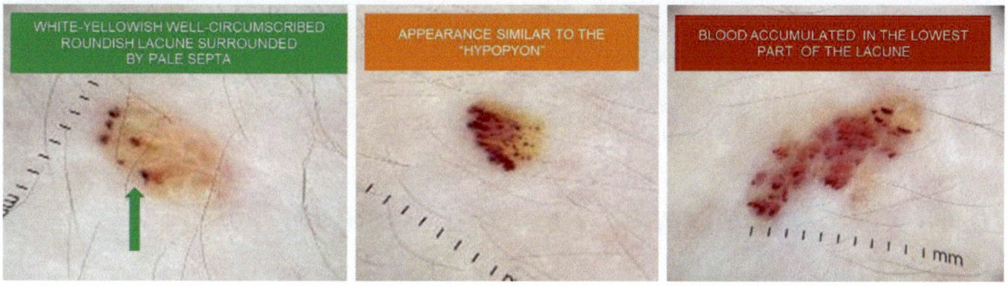

Fig. 15.110 Dermoscopic findings of patient with lymphangioma (x10)

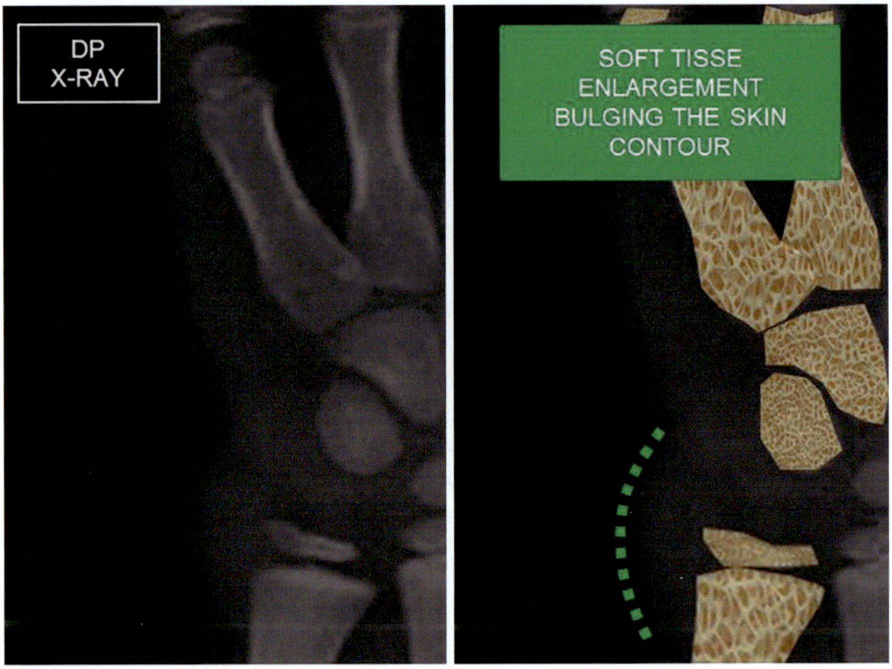

Fig. 15.111 Radiographic findings of lymphangioma (Philips Duo Diagnost R&F Room Digital RF and Tomo System)

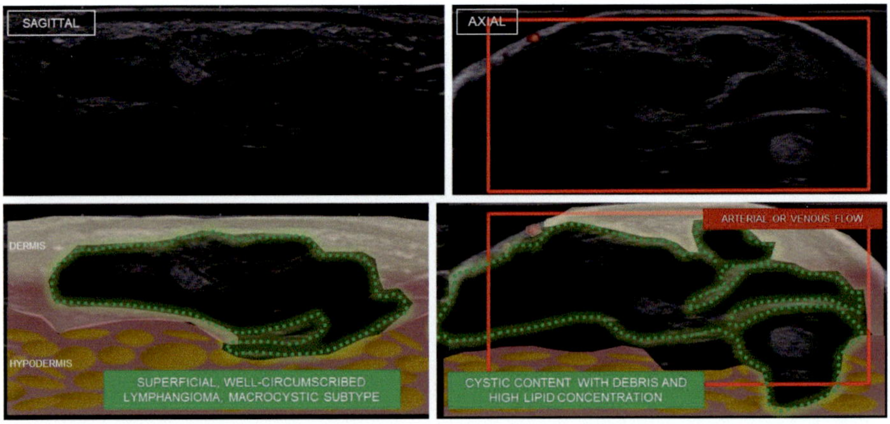

Fig. 15.112 Ultrasonographic findings of a well-defined lymphangioma with a 24 MHz probe (Aplio i800, Canon Medical Systems)

15.32.7 Ultrasonography (Figs. 15.112 and 15.113) [72]

- In ultrasonography, similar to other vascular malformations, it serves as a primary method for initial evaluation.

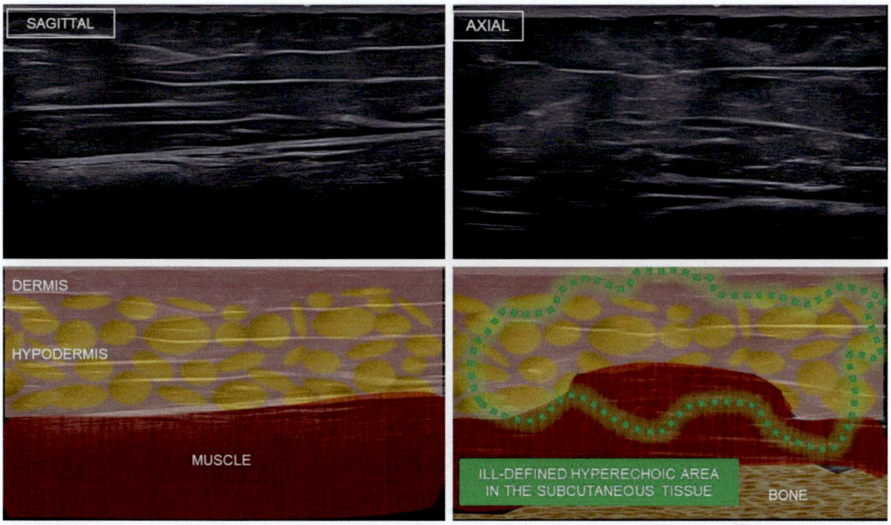

Fig. 15.113 Ultrasonographic findings of a ill-defined lymphangioma with a 24 MHz probe (Aplio i800, Canon Medical Systems)

- The macrocystic subtype is characterized by multilocular cystic masses without flow on power Doppler study, whereas the microcystic subtype appears hyperechoic.
- Multilocular cystic masses with internal septa of varying thickness.
- Cystic contents are usually anechoic but may be hyperechoic if containing debris, high lipid concentration, infection, or hemorrhage.
- Presence of solid areas or mostly solid masses with cystic foci.
- Power Doppler may show arterial or venous flow in the septa and often reveal the absence of significant vascularity within the lesion.

15.32.8 MRI (Fig. 15.114) [72]

- Fluid–fluid levels may be seen if complicated by hemorrhage.
- Signal characteristics on MRI:
  - Variable signal on T1-weighted sequences, especially dependent on protein content.
  - T2, STIR, and fat-saturated T2-weighted sequences demosntrate an hyperintense lesion.
  - No significant enhancement, some lesions show thin peripheral/septal enhancement.
- Mostly infiltrative and diffuse.

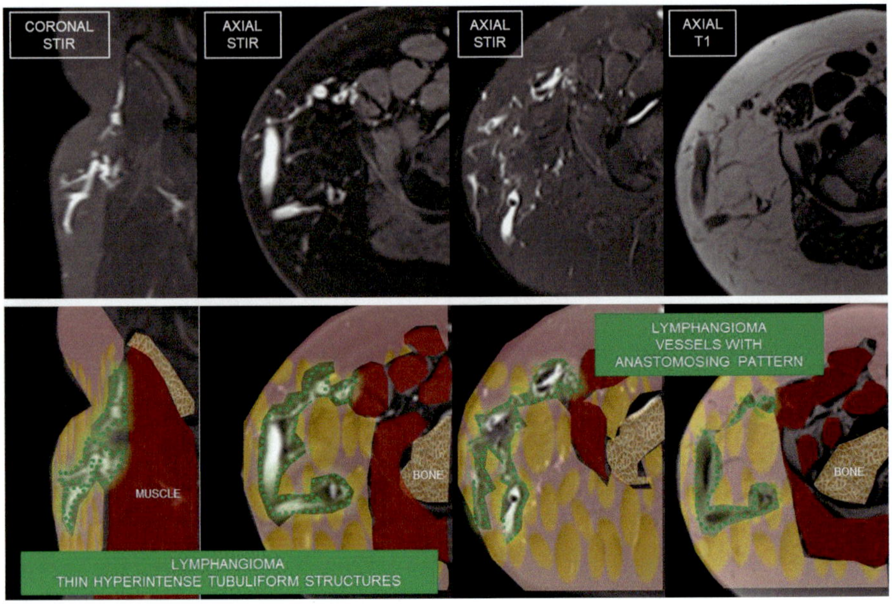

Fig. 15.114 MRI with surface coil findings of lymphangioma T1-weighted and STIR sequences (Magnetom Prisma 3T MRI, Siemens)

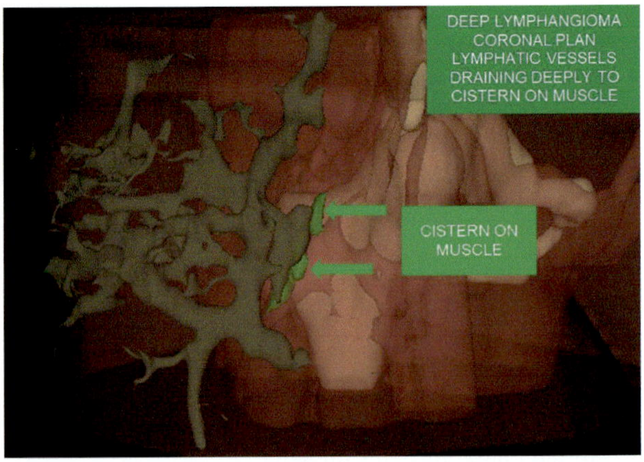

Fig. 15.115 3D images of lymphangioma after segmentation of MRI isotropic images for surgical planning

15.32.9 3D Images (Fig. 15.115, Video 15.6)

- Ideal for tackling challenging and ongoing cases.
- Allows for an in-depth examination of the lesion, aiding in the evaluation of its severity and its interaction with nearby tissues, especially in identifying the cisterne of the lesion.
- Improves the precision of surgical procedures, particularly in intricate areas.
- Physical replicas of the affected area, made from biomodels, can provide essential insights for both planning surgeries and educating patients.

15.33 Tumoral Lesions of the Tendon Sheath

15.33.1 Definition [78, 79]

- Tumoral lesions of the tendon sheath refer to abnormal growths that originate from the synovial tissue surrounding the tendons.
- These lesions are typically benign but can be locally aggressive.
- The most common type of tumoral lesion in this category is the giant cell tumor of the tendon sheath (GCTTS), also known as pigmented villonodular synovitis (PVNS) when occurring within the joint.

15.33.2 Epidemiology [79]

- Tumoral lesions of the tendon sheath, particularly GCTTS, are relatively uncommon but represent the second most common benign soft tissue tumor of the hand, following ganglion cysts.
- These lesions can occur in individuals of any age but are most frequently seen in adults between the ages of 30 and 50. There is a slight female predominance.
- While these lesions can occur in various locations, they are most commonly found in the fingers and hands, particularly around the flexor tendons.

15.33.3 Clinical Presentation (Fig. 15.116) [79]

- Patients typically present with a slowly growing, painless mass near a tendon, often in the fingers or hand. The mass may cause discomfort, reduced range of motion, or mechanical symptoms if it interferes with tendon function.
- On examination, the lesion is usually firm and well-circumscribed, with a tendency to adhere to the tendon. It may be slightly movable, depending on its relationship with surrounding structures.

15.33.4 Histopathology [33]

- Histopathologically, GCTTS is characterized by a mixture of mononuclear cells, multinucleated giant cells, foam cells, and hemosiderin-laden macrophages. The presence of hemosiderin gives the lesion its characteristic brownish color.
- The lesion typically shows a nodular growth pattern and is well-circumscribed, but it may infiltrate surrounding tissues, leading to local recurrence after excision.

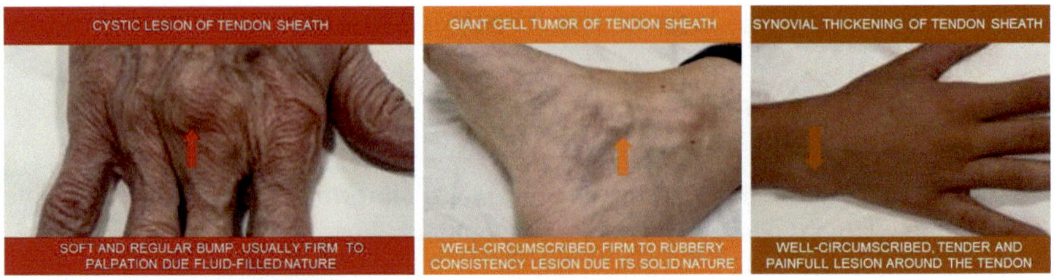

Fig. 15.116 Clinical photograph of patients with different types of tendon sheath lesions: cystic lesion, solid tumor, and synovial thickening

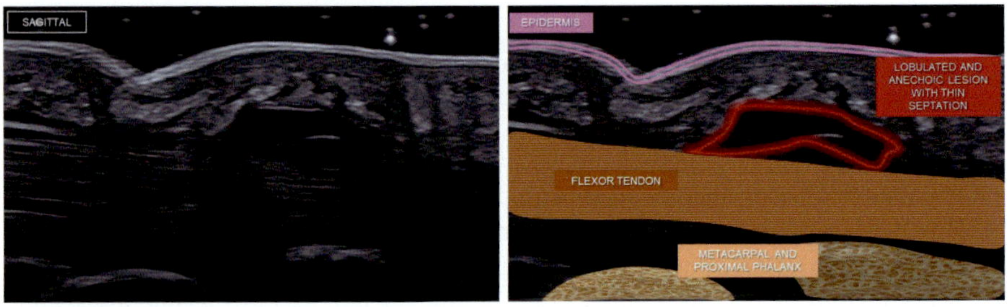

Fig. 15.117 Ultrasonographic findings of a cystic lesion of tendon sheath with a 24 MHz probe (Aplio i800, Canon Medical Systems)

15.33.5 Ultrasonography (Figs. 15.117, 15.118 and 15.119) [80]

- On ultrasonography, tumoral lesions of the tendon sheath, including GCTTS, typically appear as hypoechoic or mixed echogenicity masses adjacent to the tendon. They are usually well-defined and may exhibit posterior acoustic enhancement due to their solid nature.
- Power Doppler ultrasonography may show increased vascularity within the lesion, which can help differentiate it from other types of soft tissue masses or cysts.

15.33.6 MRI (Fig. 15.120)

- The lesion usually appears as a low to intermediate signal intensity mass on T1-weighted images due to the fibrous nature and hemosiderin content.
- On T2-weighted images, GCTTS may exhibit low to intermediate signal intensity, with areas of higher signal corresponding to the more cellular or edematous regions.

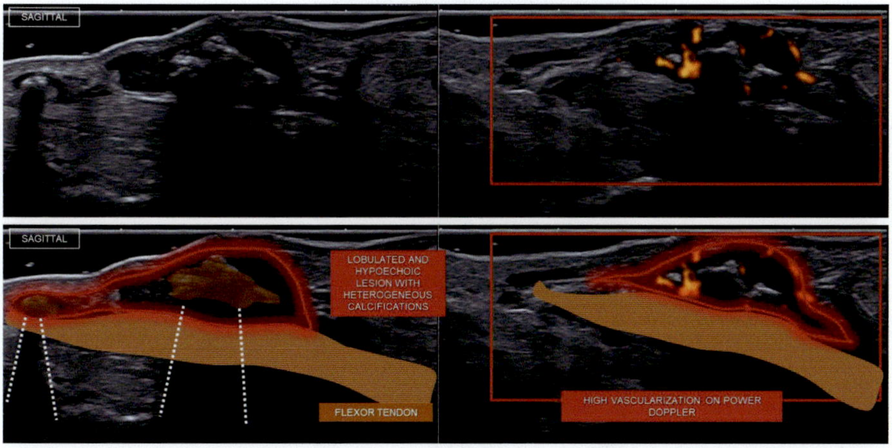

Fig. 15.118 Ultrasonographic findings of a solid tumor of tendon sheath (giant cell tumor) with a 24 MHz probe (Aplio i800, Canon Medical Systems)

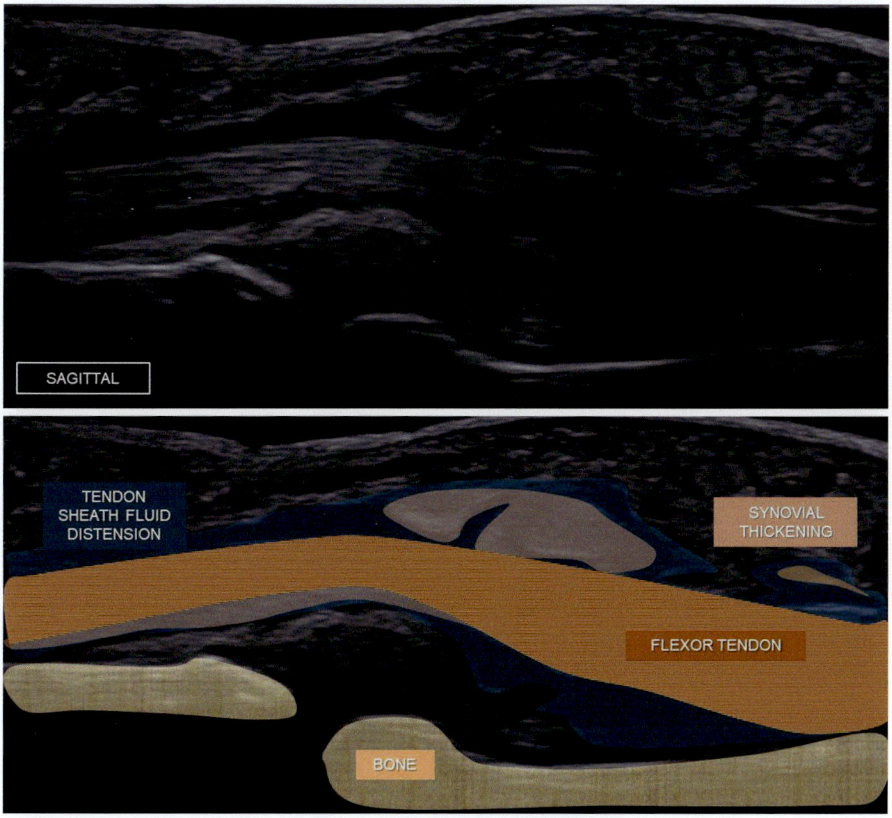

Fig. 15.119 Ultrasonographic findings of synovial thickening of tendon sheath lesions with a 24 MHz probe (Aplio i800, Canon Medical Systems)

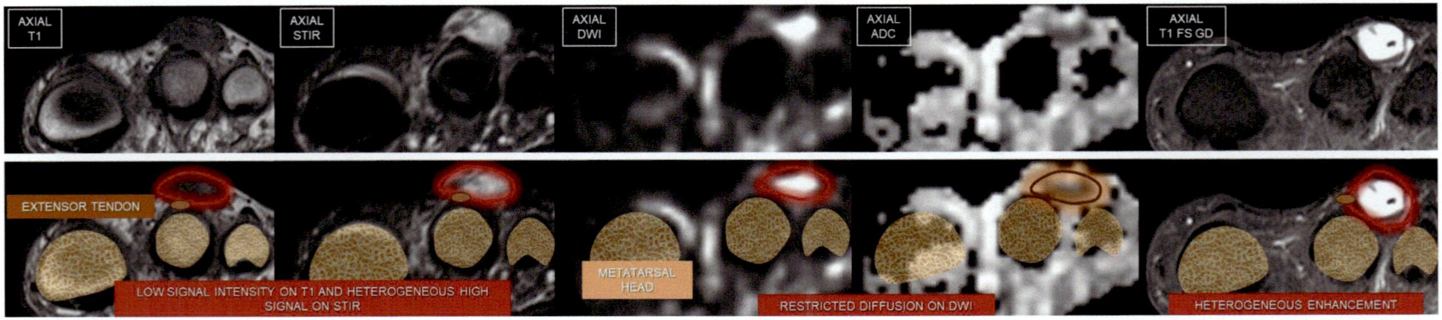

Fig. 15.120 MRI findings of giant cell tumor of tendon sheath on T1, DWI, T1 FS-weighted, and STIR sequences after gadolinium administration (Magnetom Avanto 1.5T MRI, Siemens)

- Gradient-echo sequences can highlight the presence of hemosiderin deposits, which appear as areas of low signal intensity, helping to confirm the diagnosis.
- After gadolinium administration, there is typically moderate to marked enhancement of the lesion, reflecting its vascularity and cellularity.

15.34 Plantar and Palmar Aponeurosis

15.34.1 Definition [81]

- The plantar and palmar aponeuroses are thick, fibrous connective tissue structures found in the sole of the foot and the palm of the hand, respectively.
- The plantar aponeurosis, also known as the plantar fascia, supports the arch of the foot and plays a crucial role in foot mechanics during walking.
- The palmar aponeurosis provides structural support to the palm and helps in gripping by anchoring the skin to underlying tissues.

15.34.2 Epidemiology [81]

- Conditions affecting the plantar and palmar aponeuroses, such as plantar fasciitis and Dupuytren's contracture, are relatively common:
  - Plantar Fasciitis: This is one of the most common causes of heel pain, particularly in middle-aged and older adults, affecting up to 10% of the population at some point in their lives.
  - Dupuytren's Contracture: Affects the palmar aponeurosis and is more prevalent in older adults, with a higher incidence in men. It is particularly common in individuals of Northern European descent.

15.34.3 Clinical Presentation (Fig. 15.121) [81, 82]

- Plantar aponeurosis (Plantar Fasciitis):
  - Patients typically present with heel pain, especially during the first steps in the morning or after periods of rest.
  - Pain is usually localized to the medial aspect of the heel but can extend along the arch of the foot.
  - Pain may be exacerbated by prolonged standing, walking, or activities that involve pushing off with the foot.
- Palmar aponeurosis (Dupuytren's Contracture):

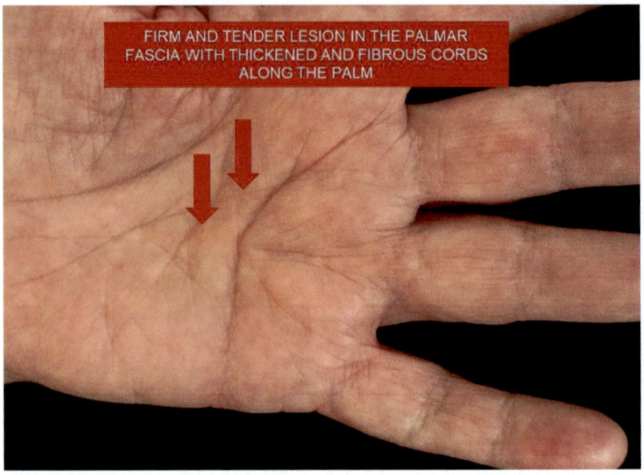

Fig. 15.121 Clinical photograph of patient with palmar fibromatosis

- Dupuytren's contracture presents with progressive thickening and shortening of the palmar aponeurosis, leading to flexion contractures of the fingers.
- The ring and little fingers are most commonly affected.
- Nodules and cords may develop in the palm, with patients eventually losing the ability to fully extend the affected fingers.

15.34.4 Histopathology [33]

- Plantar aponeurosis:
  - Histopathological examination of plantar fasciitis shows degenerative changes, including fragmentation of collagen fibers, increased fibroblastic activity, and occasionally, calcification.
  - There may be evidence of chronic inflammation with lymphocytic infiltration.
- Palmar aponeurosis:
  - In Dupuytren's contracture, histopathology reveals the proliferation of fibroblasts and myofibroblasts, leading to the thickening and shortening of collagen fibers within the palmar aponeurosis.
  - The tissue becomes dense and fibrotic, forming nodules and cords, which are responsible for the contractures.

15.34.5 Ultrasonography (Figs. 15.122 and 15.123) [33, 82]

- Plantar aponeurosis:

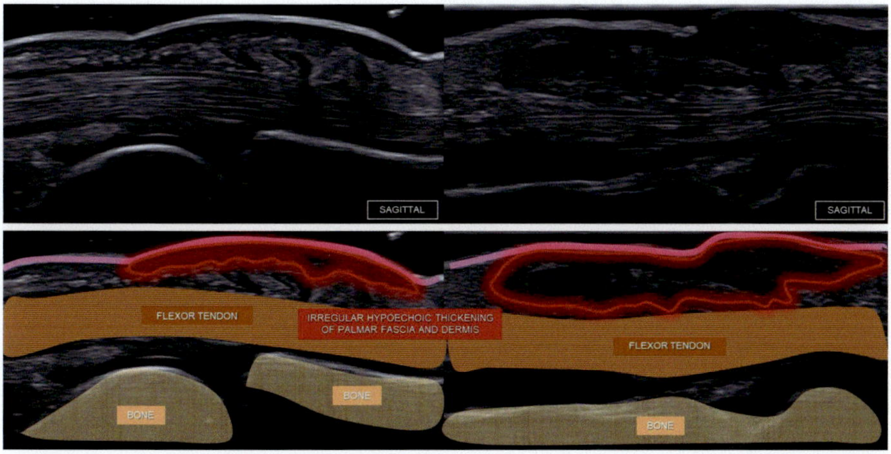

Fig. 15.122 Ultrasonographic findings of palmar fibromatosis with a 24 MHz probe (Aplio i800, Canon Medical Systems)

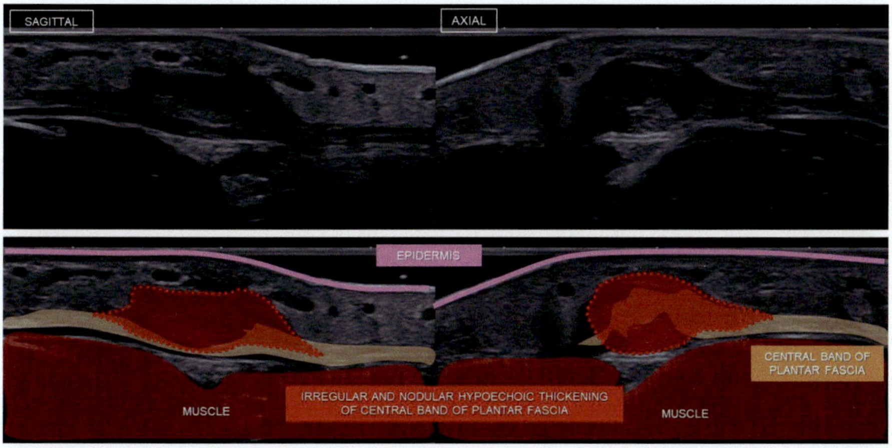

Fig. 15.123 Ultrasonographic findings of plantar fibromatosis with a 24 MHz probe (Aplio i800, Canon Medical Systems)

- Ultrasonography typically shows thickening of the plantar fascia, particularly near its insertion on the calcaneus, with normal thickness being less than 4 mm.
- There may be hypoechoic areas indicating degenerative changes or inflammation.
- Sometimes, calcifications can be detected within the fascia or at its insertion.

- Palmar aponeurosis:
  - Ultrasonography can identify the nodules and cords characteristic of Dupuytren's contracture. These appear as hypoechoic or mixed echogenicity structures within the palmar fascia.

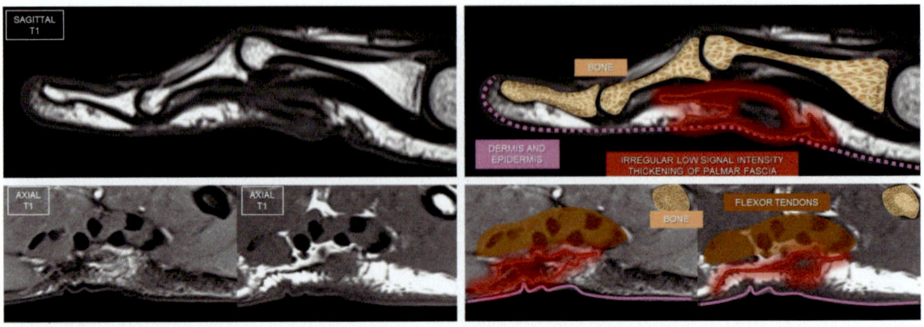

Fig. 15.124 MRI findings of palmar fibromatosis on T1-weighted sequences (Magnetom Avanto 1.5T MRI, Siemens)

- The degree of thickening and the extent of the disease can be assessed.

15.34.6 MRI (Fig. 15.124) [82]

- Plantar aponeurosis:
  - The plantar fascia typically appears as a low-signal-intensity structure on T1-weighted images. In plantar fasciitis, the fascia may appear thickened with intermediate signal intensity due to degeneration and inflammation.
  - Increased signal intensity may be seen on T2-weighted images, indicating inflammation, edema, or fluid accumulation in the surrounding tissues.
- Palmar aponeurosis:
  - In Dupuytren's contracture, MRI shows low-signal-intensity nodules and cords within the palmar fascia on T1-weighted sequences.
  - The nodules and cords usually have low to intermediate signal intensity on T2-weighted images, depending on the amount of fibrosis and cellularity.

15.35 Mycosis Fungoides (Patch and Tumoral)

15.35.1 Definition [83]

- Mycosis fungoid (MF) is the most common cutaneous T cell lymphoma (CTCL).
- It is caused by clonal proliferation of mature T cells, usually in the epidermis.
- It is a slow-growing lymphoma with well-defined clinicopathological features.
- In early stages, it involves the skin, but it can also spread to blood, lymph, and visceral organs.

15.35.2 Epidemiology [83]

- The incidence of MF is approximately 5.6 per million people.
- Although all ages can be affected, the average onset is between 50 and 60 years.
- It affects more men than women and the incidence is higher among black patients, who also have worse survival rates.

15.35.3 Clinical Presentation (Fig. 15.125) [83]

- Skin lesions may be patches, plaques, tumors, and/or generalized erythroderma, depending on the stage of the disease.
- Premycotic period precedes a definitive diagnosis of MF.
- It is characterized by pruritus and nonspecific, slightly scaling skin lesions.
- In the mycotic stage, there are infiltrative plaques that cover approximately 10% of the body.
- Tumor-stage lesions can be rounded or lobulated with varying sizes.
- In tumor d'emblee form, patients may develop large nodules without previous formation of plaques and patches.

15.35.4 Dermoscopy (Fig. 15.126) [84]

- Early stage mycosis fungoides (MF) typically presents with orange-yellowish patchy areas accompanied by dotted and linear vessels.
- A distinctive vascular pattern, termed "spermatozoa-like vessels," has been identified and is considered highly specific to MF.

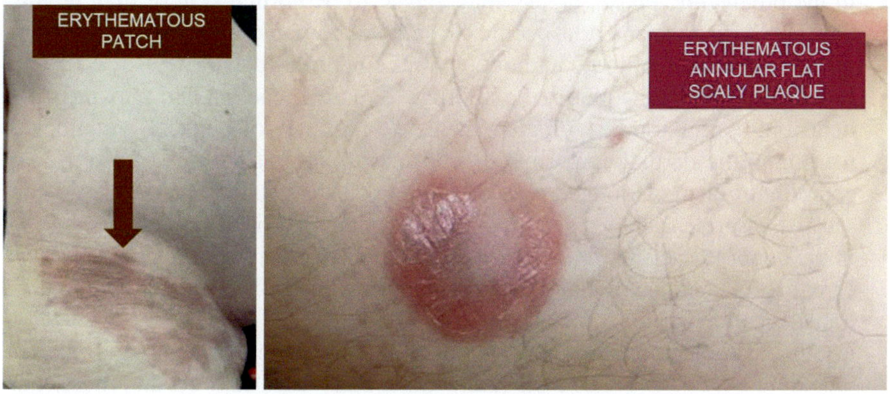

Fig. 15.125 Clinical photograph of patients with mycosis fungoides

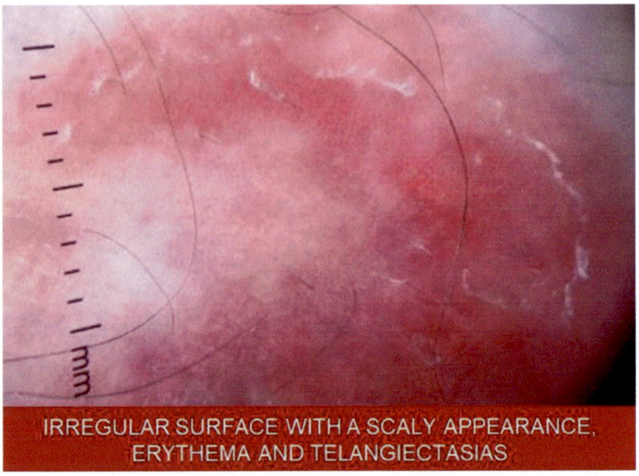

Fig. 15.126 Dermoscopic findings of patient with mycosis fungoides (x10)

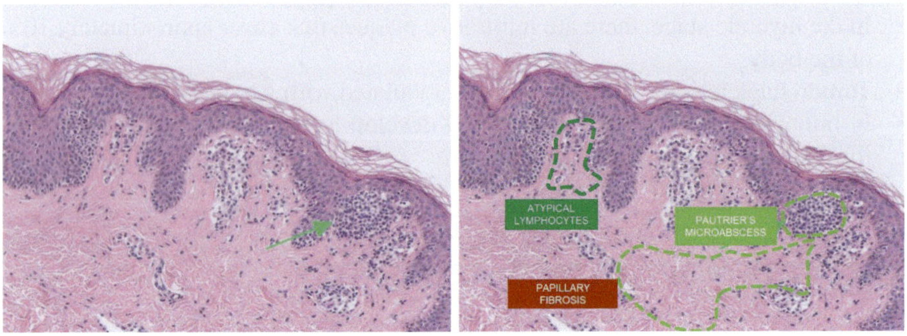

Fig. 15.127 Histological findings of mycosis fungoides (H&E x4)

15.35.5 Histopathology (Fig. 15.127) [33]

- In the premycotic phase, biopsy may appear to be normal skin or may be mistaken for a discrete and nonspecific chronic inflammatory process, as it presents mild lymphocytic infiltrate without obvious epidermotropism.
- In the patch or plaque phase, the infiltrate is more exuberant and may present a lichenoid-like or top-heavy pattern with the presence of atypical lymphocytes margining the dermal-epidermal junction, especially at the tips of rete ridges, epidermotropism of isolated cells or forming clusters called Pautrier's microabscesses, discrete acanthosis, hyperkeratosis, edema, or papillary fibrosis.
- In the tumor phase, the infiltrate is dense with relevant atypia, including classical cerebriform cells, there may be no more epidermotropic cells, and there may be transformation to the large cell pattern.
- Immunohistochemical profile: CD4 positive, in addition to other T cell markers, including CD2, CD3, CD5, CD7, and CD8; early CD7 loss occurs, most commonly and frequently mono or oligoclonal restriction; CD30 positive occurs on transformation to large cells.

15.35.6 Ultrasonography (Fig. 15.128) [85]

- Skin layer echo boundary (SLEB):
  - Clear boundaries.
  - Homogeneous echoes inside the lesions.
  - No changes in the posterior echoes.
- Patchy hypoechoic regions:
  - Around the hair follicles with unclear boundaries.
  - Extending upward to the epidermis and connected to the SLEB.
- Echogenic foci:
  - Detected in some regions.
- Power Doppler image shows rich blood flow.

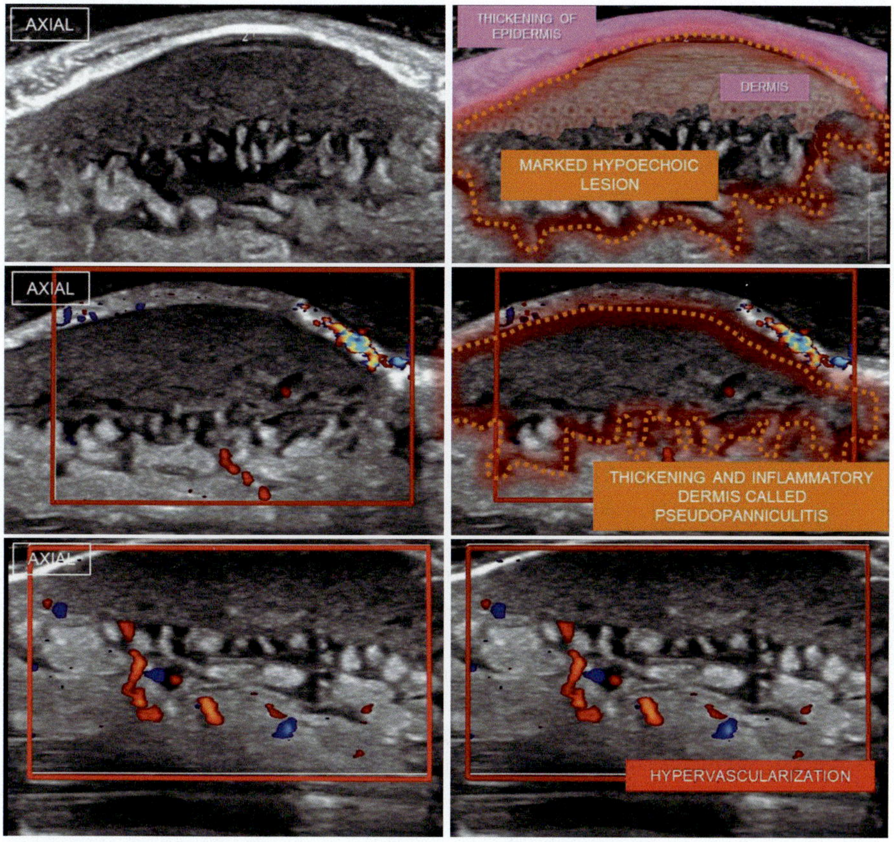

Fig. 15.128 Ultrasonographic findings of mycosis fungoides with a 24 MHz probe (Aplio i800, Canon Medical Systems)

15.36 Cutaneous Plasmocitoma

15.36.1 Definition [86]

- Cutaneous plasmacytoma can manifest as either a primary monoclonal B-cell proliferation in the skin without systemic involvement or as a secondary complication of multiple myeloma or systemic plasmacytoma.

15.36.2 Epidemiology [87]

- Primary cutaneous plasmacytoma is a rare subset of plasma cell neoplasms, accounting for approximately 3%–5% of cases.
- Typically occurs in individuals aged 55–60 years, with males being twice as likely as females to develop the condition.

15.36.3 Clinical Presentation (Fig. 15.129) [86, 87]

- Presents as cutaneous or subcutaneous nodules, typically ranging from 5 to 12 cm in diameter.
- Lesions are commonly erythematous-violaceous in color but can also appear normochromic.
- The surface of the nodules is smooth and raised, often presenting as multiple lesions predominantly on the trunk, extremities, and face.

15.36.4 Histopathology (Fig. 15.130) [33]

- Cutaneous plasmacytomas exhibit diffuse or nodular collections of plasma cells in the deep dermis and hypodermis.
- Cells show a well-differentiated pattern with mature plasma cells having small eccentric nuclei and spoke-wheel chromatin without nucleoli.
- Presence of Russell bodies and Dutch bodies may be observed due to immunoglobulin production.
- Immunohistochemistry typically reveals positivity for CD38, CD138, CD79, and MUM-1, with negativity for CD20 and occasional positivity for cyclin D1.
- Monoclonality for lambda or kappa chains confirms the neoplastic nature of the plasma cells.

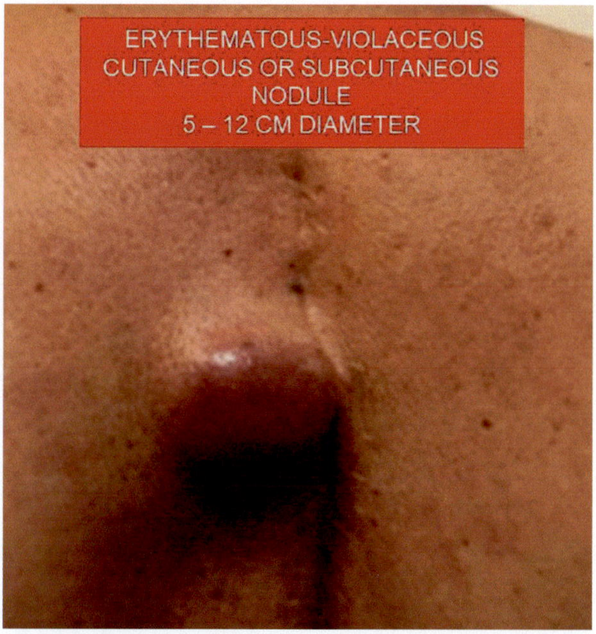

Fig. 15.129 Clinical photograph of patients with cutaneous plasmocitoma

15.36.5 Computed Tomography

- CT scans may reveal irregularly marginated soft-tissue density masses in the subcutaneous tissue, often contrast-enhanced without identifiable matrix.

15.36.6 Ultrasonography (Fig. 15.131)

- Cutaneous plasmacytomas typically appear as well-defined, hypoechoic lesions compared to surrounding tissues.
- The internal structure of the lesion often shows a homogeneous echogenicity, meaning the tissue inside the lesion is uniform.
- There might be posterior acoustic enhancement.
- Calcifications are generally not seen within the lesion.
- Power Doppler ultrasonography usually reveals minimal or no significant blood flow within the lesion.

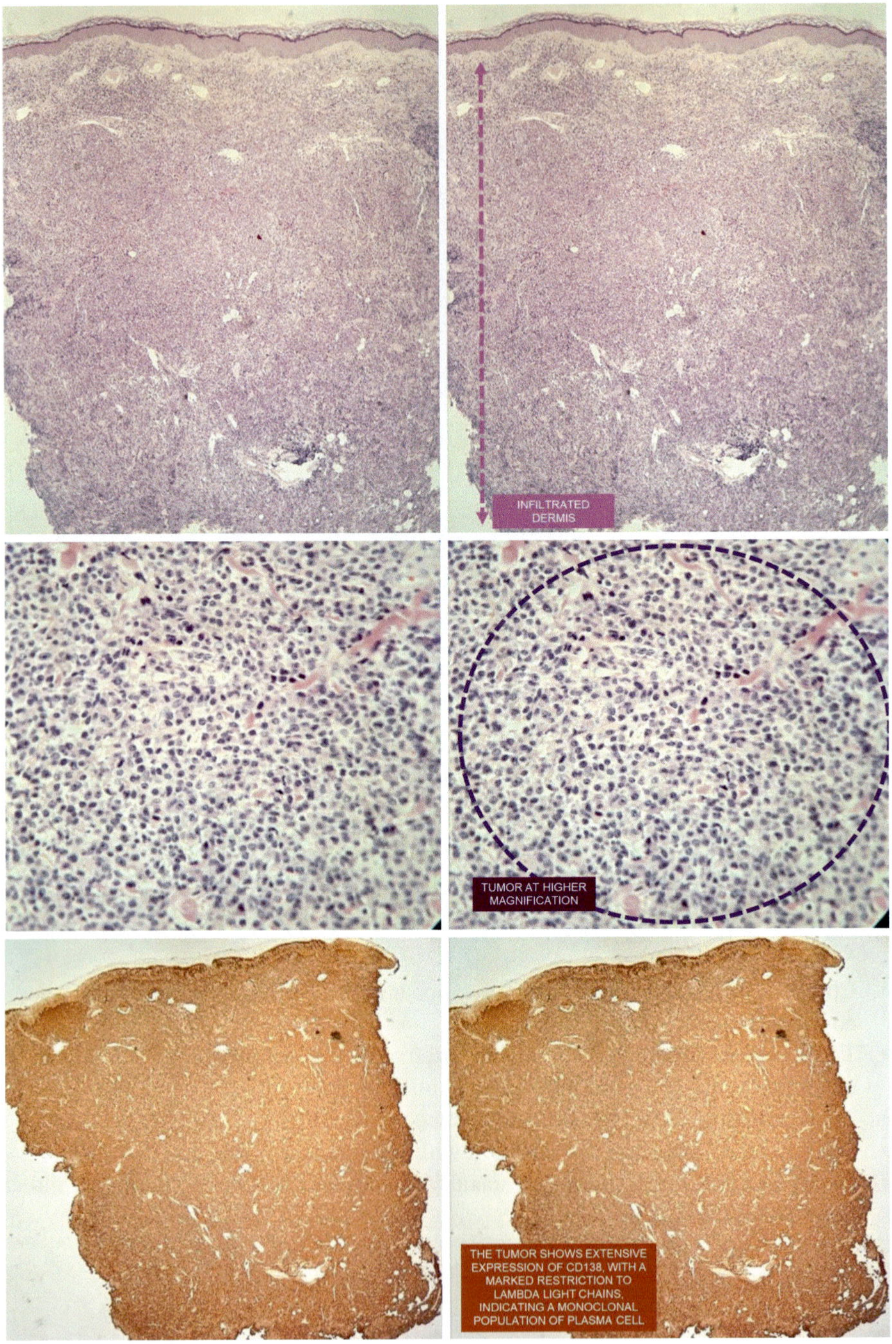

Fig. 15.130 Histological findings of cutaneous plasmocitoma (H&E x4, x10 and Congo red stain x4)

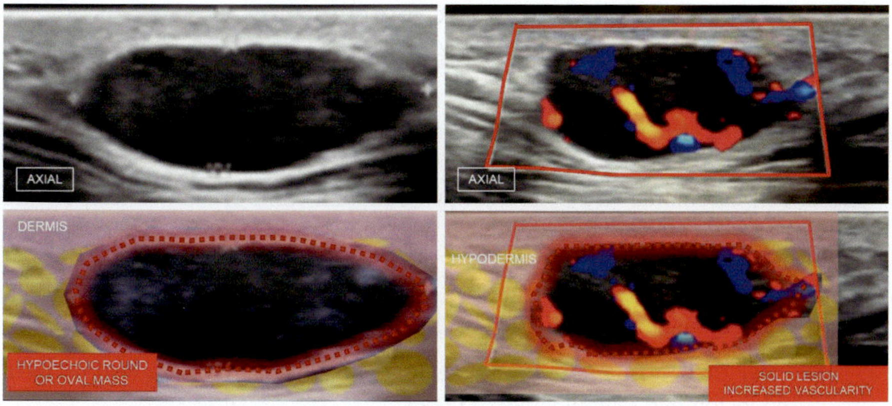

Fig. 15.131 Ultrasonographic findings of cutaneous plasmocitoma with a 24 MHz probe (Aplio i800, Canon Medical Systems)

15.36.7 MRI

- On T1-weighted MRI, cutaneous plasmacytomas typically appear as iso to hypointense lesions relative to surrounding soft tissues.
- On T2-weighted MRI, these lesions are usually hyperintense which helps in distinguishing them from surrounding tissues.
- The lesions often have well-defined margins, making them distinct from adjacent structures.
- After administration of contrast, cutaneous plasmacytomas often show moderate to marked enhancement, reflecting their vascularity and the presence of abnormal plasma cells.
- There is usually minimal surrounding edema or necrosis, distinguishing plasmacytomas from other types of tumors that may present with significant surrounding inflammatory or necrotic changes.

15.36.8 3D Images

- Provides a thorough analysis of the lesion, helping to assess its severity and how it interacts with adjacent tissues and blood vessels.
- Enhances the accuracy of surgical operations, especially in delicate or complicated regions.
- Creating physical models of the affected area using biomodels offers valuable information for surgical planning and patient education.

15.37 Basal Cell Carcinoma (BCC): Nodular, Micronodular, Sclerosing

15.37.1 Definition [88]

- Basal cell carcinoma (BCC) is the most common form of skin cancer, arising from the basal cells in the epidermis. It is a slow growing, locally invasive tumor that rarely metastasizes but can cause significant local tissue destruction if left untreated. BCC has several histologic subtypes, including nodular, micronodular, and sclerosing, each with distinct clinical and pathological characteristics.
  - Nodular BCC: The most common subtype, characterized by a well-defined, raised lesion that may ulcerate or bleed.
  - Micronodular BCC: A variant of BCC that is more aggressive and characterized by smaller, deeper nodules with poorly defined borders.
  - Sclerosing BCC: Also known as morpheaform BCC, this subtype presents as a scar-like, indurated plaque with ill-defined borders, often infiltrating deeper tissues.

15.37.2 Epidemiology

- BCC is the most frequently occurring form of skin cancer, with millions of new cases diagnosed globally each year. Nodular BCC is the most common subtype, while micronodular and sclerosing types are less common but more aggressive.
- Key risk factors include prolonged exposure to ultraviolet (UV) radiation, fair skin, age, a history of previous skin cancers, and genetic predispositions (e.g., Gorlin syndrome).
- BCC is most diagnosed in older adults, typically over the age of 50. There is a slight male predominance.
- Higher incidence rates are observed in regions with intense sunlight exposure, such as Australia and the southern United States.

15.37.3 Clinical Presentation [88]

- Nodular BCC: Presents as a pearly, flesh-colored or pink nodule, often with telangiectasia (visible small blood vessels) on the surface. The lesion may ulcerate, leading to a central depression or "rodent ulcer." Commonly found on sun-exposed areas like the face, particularly the nose.

- Micronodular BCC: Often appears as a smooth, firm, and slightly elevated lesion with less defined borders compared to nodular BCC. This subtype tends to infiltrate more deeply into the skin, making it more challenging to treat.
- Sclerosing BCC (Morpheaform BCC): Manifests as a firm, scar-like, yellowish or whitish plaque with poorly defined margins. The lesion may appear waxy or shiny, and the border is often difficult to distinguish from the surrounding skin. This subtype is more likely to invade surrounding tissues, including nerves and bones, making early detection and treatment crucial.

15.37.4 Dermoscopy (Figs. 15.132 and 15.133) [88]

- Ovoid nests in blue-gray, blue-gray globules, blue-gray dots. Maple leaf-like structures, cartwheel-like structures, concentric structures.
- Arborizing telangiectasias, fine and short telangiectasias.
- Ulceration, erosions, shiny white-red areas. Bright white structures (with polarized light).
- Specific patterns by histological subtype:
  - Superficial BCC: Maple leaf-like structures, fine telangiectasias.
  - Nodular BCC: Arborizing telangiectasias, bright white structures.
  - Morfeiform BCC: Hypopigmentation, scattered telangiectasias.
  - Infiltrative BCC: Arborizing telangiectasias, ulceration.

15.37.5 Histopathology (Fig. 15.134) [33]

- Presence of basaloid cells in nests or bundles, often related to hair follicles or epidermal layers.
- Collagen retraction and peripheral palisading of cell nuclei.
- Variable stromal characteristics such as fibrous or hyalinized tissue, and occasional pigmentation.

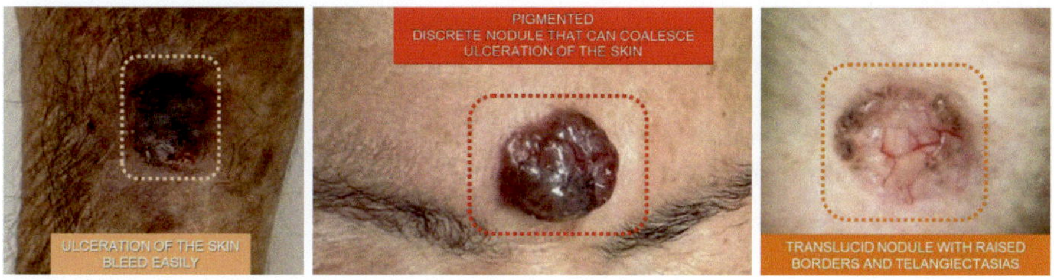

Fig. 15.132 Clinical photograph of patients with basal cell carcinoma (x20)

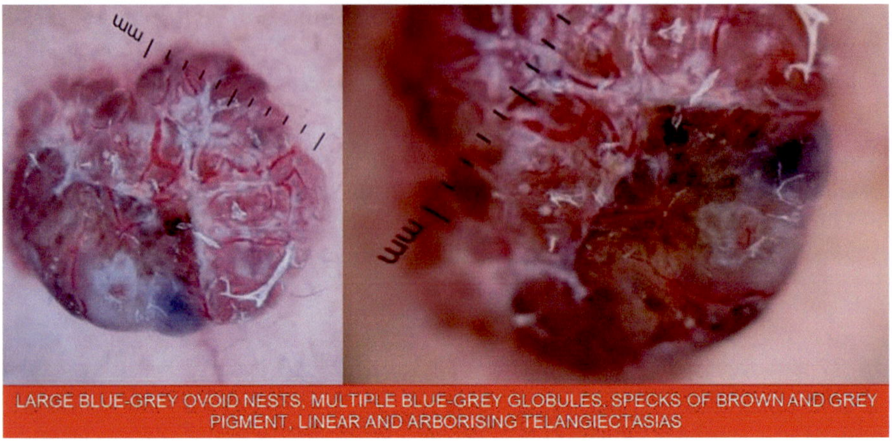

Fig. 15.133 Dermoscopic findings of patients with basal cell carcinoma (x20)

- Common inflammatory infiltrate, predominantly lymphocytic.
- *Microscopic forms:*
  - Nodular (60–80%): Well-demarcated with peripheral palisade, variants include adenoid and pigmented subtypes.
  - Micronodular: Small nodules resembling follicular bulbs, categorized as infiltrative despite clear borders.
  - Infiltrative (15%): Diffuse growth pattern with indistinct edges and variable stromal composition.
  - Sclerosing or morpheaform: Aggressive subtype with dense, sclerotic stroma.

15.37.6 Ultrasonography (Fig. 15.135) [89]

- Typically, hypoechoic or anechoic structures in the dermis, sometimes extending into subcutaneous layers. Also, hyperechoic spots can be visualized and correlate with worse prognosis if more than 7 spots.
- Generally well-defined borders but may appear irregular in infiltrative or sclerosing types.
- Often oval or round shape, occasionally irregular in aggressive forms.
- Increased blood flow is seen with power Doppler, indicative of angiogenesis.
- Types:
- Nodular BCC: Well-defined hypoechoic mass with possible internal vascularity, acoustic enhancement, and hyperechoic spots.

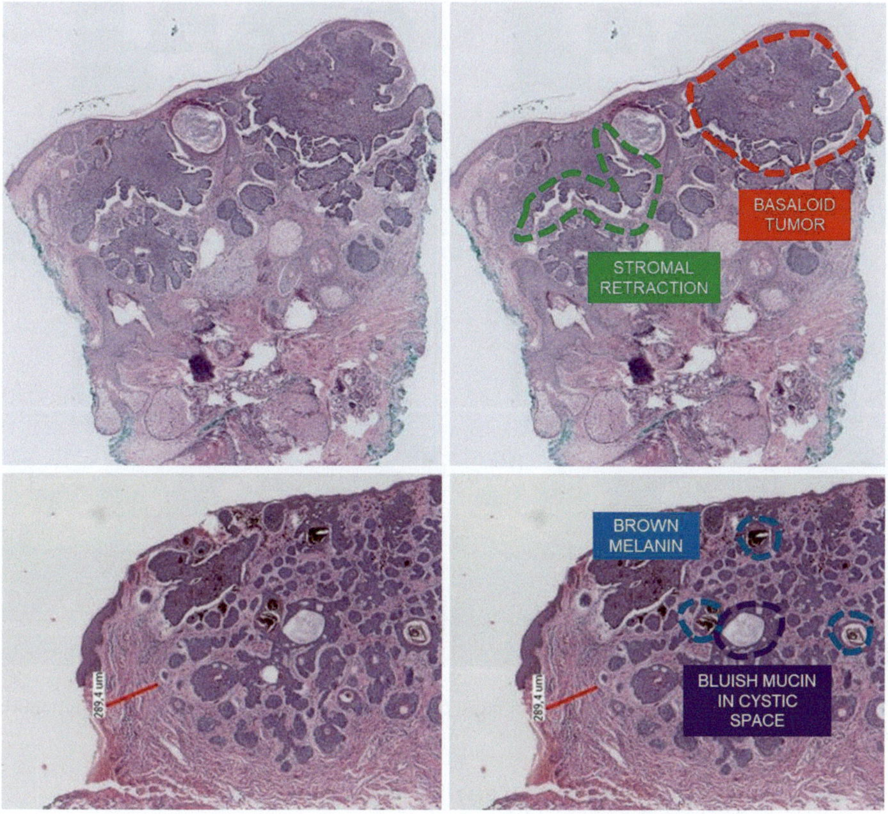

Fig. 15.134 Histological findings of basal cell carcinoma (H&E x4)

- Micronodular BCC: Multiple small hypoechoic nodules that can merge, with less distinct borders than nodular BCC.
- Sclerosing (Morpheaform) BCC: Poorly defined hypoechoic area blending into surrounding tissue, challenging to delineate due to infiltrative nature.
- Ultrasonography evaluation:
- High-frequency ultrasonography accurately measures invasion depth and lateral spread for surgical planning.
- Real-time ultrasonography assesses lesion mobility relative to underlying structures, aiding in extent determination.
- Contrasts lesion characteristics with adjacent normal tissue to differentiate BCC from other skin conditions.

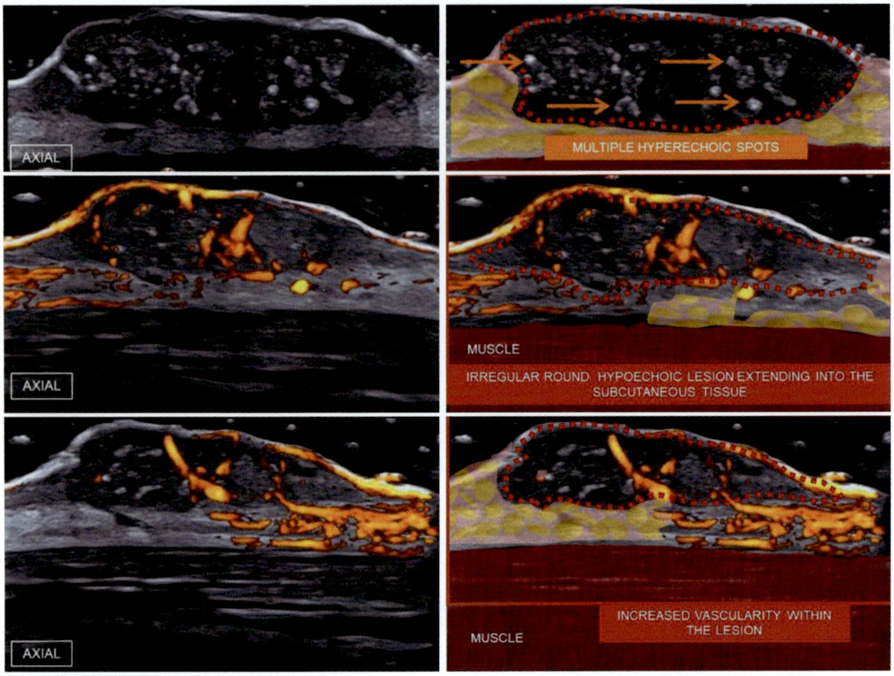

Fig. 15.135 Ultrasonographic findings of basal cell carcinoma with a 33 MHz probe (Aplio i800, Canon Medical Systems)

15.37.7 MRI (Fig. 15.136) [89]

- Basal cell carcinoma typically appears iso- to hypointense compared to the surrounding soft tissues on T1-weighted images. The lesion might be less conspicuous in this sequence, especially if it is small.
- On T2-weighted images, BCC often shows hyperintensity. This is due to the increased water content and cellularity within the tumor.
- After contrast administration, BCC usually demonstrates variable enhancement. The enhancement can range from mild to moderate, depending on the tumor's vascularity and the presence of fibrous stroma.
- Basal cell carcinoma typically has well-defined, irregular margins. The lesion might show an infiltrative pattern, where the borders are not entirely distinct from the surrounding tissue.
- There may be minimal surrounding edema or inflammatory changes, although this can vary. The surrounding tissues might show increased signal intensity on T2-weighted images if edema is present.
- In cases where BCC invades deeper, there might be adjacent bone involvement, especially in cases where the carcinoma is in areas like the nose or periocular regions.

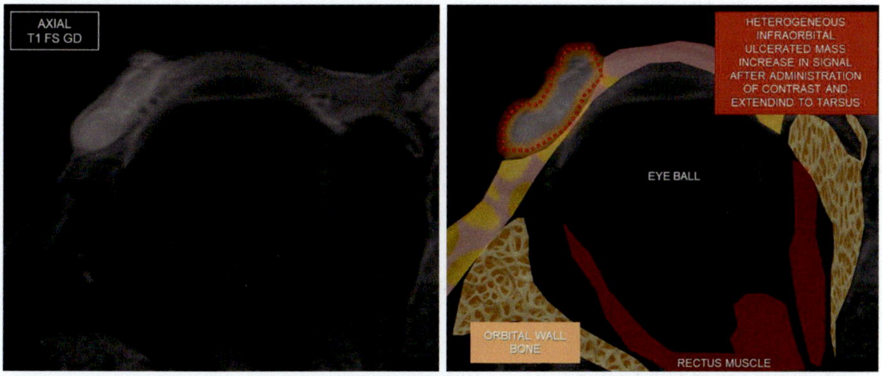

Fig. 15.136 MRI with surface coil findings of basal cell carcinoma on T1 FS-weighted sequences after gadolinium administration (Magnetom Prisma 3T MRI, Siemens)

15.37.8 3D Images

- Well-suited for addressing intricate and ongoing cases, especially in lesions on facial regions where surgery could be deforming.
- Enables a detailed assessment of the lesion, aiding in understanding its severity and its effects on nearby tissues and blood vessels.
- Refines the accuracy of surgical techniques, especially in complex areas.
- Using biomodels to produce physical replicas of the affected region provides crucial details for both surgical planning and patient instruction.

15.38 Squamous Cell Carcinoma: Actinic Keratosis, Hypertrophic Actinic Keratosis, Bowen's Disease, Keratoacanthoma, Invasive Squamous Cell Carcinoma

15.38.1 Definition [90]

- Actinic keratosis (AK) is a frequent premalignant skin lesion mainly caused by chronic sun exposure, which has the risk of progression to invasive squamous cell carcinoma.
- Cutaneous squamous cell carcinoma (cSCC) is caused by a malignant proliferation of keratinocytes originating from the epidermis and adnexal structures, including pilosebaceous units and eccrine glands and has several distinct in situ and invasive types.

15.38.2 Epidemiology [90]

- AK is influenced by various independent risk factors, which may include increased age, male gender, fair-skinned, immunosuppression, history of actinic keratosis or previous skin malignancy and excessive and chronic sun exposure. The prevalence varies, for example, in Australia is close to 60% due to its proximity to the Equator line (in addition to its sizable Causasian population). In contrast, in a non-equatorial location, such as the United States, is around 20%. Actinic keratoses represent the third reason for dermatological consultation, losing only to acne and dermatitis.
- cSCC is one of the most common cancers of the Caucasian population and accounts for 20% of all cutaneous tumors.

15.38.3 Clinical Presentation (Fig. 15.137) [90]

- AK presents as an erythematous, rough papule with scale and little to no induration on sun-exposed skin. Some variants of AKs are pigmented, cutaneous horn, atrophic, hypertrophic, Bowenoid, and lichen planus-like lesions.
- Cutaneous squamous cell carcinoma in situ (cSCCIS) or, commonly called, Bowen's disease appears as an erythematous scaly plaque, with the possibility of pigmentation, and may also present as hyperparakeratosis leading to the formation of a cutaneous horn.
- The keratoacanthoma (KA) is a low grade, rapidly growing, 1–2 cm dome-shaped skin tumor with a centralized keratinous plug.
- cSCC are solitary firm papules or erythematous nodules with significant scale, and the propensity for spontaneous bleeding.
- Although AKs are usually asymptomatic, they may be mildly painful and are more readily diagnosed on examination with palpation.

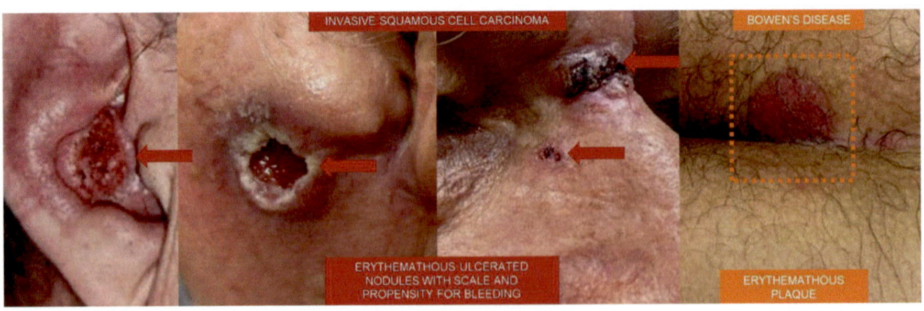

Fig. 15.137 Clinical photograph of patients with Bowen's disease and invasive squamous cell carcinoma

- Palpation is important. Suspicious lesions must be palpated to assess the degree of infiltration. Infiltrated lesions may be hypertrophic actinic keratoses, cSCCIS, or cSCC.

15.38.4 Dermoscopy (Fig. 15.138) [90]

- Coiled vessels are a strong clue to KA and SCC, actinic keratosis, and Bowen's disease.
- White circles are a specific feature of early SCC and actinic keratosis.
- The combination of clustered dotted and glomerular vascular patterns and hyperkeratosis, seen as discrete yellow scales are suggestive of cSCC.
- KA: central yellowish-whitish scaling (keratin); white circles (highest specificity); whitish structure within the circles; whitish lines and structureless areas and red globules within white area.
- cSCCIS: yellowish-white opaque scales and clusters of two types of roundish vascular pattern: small dotted vessels and glomerular or coiled vessels.
- cSCC: polymorphic vessels such as linear irregular, hairpin and grouped glomerular/dotted vessels over a whitish background with a central mass of keratin or ulceration. Such dermoscopic features reflect a dermal invasion.

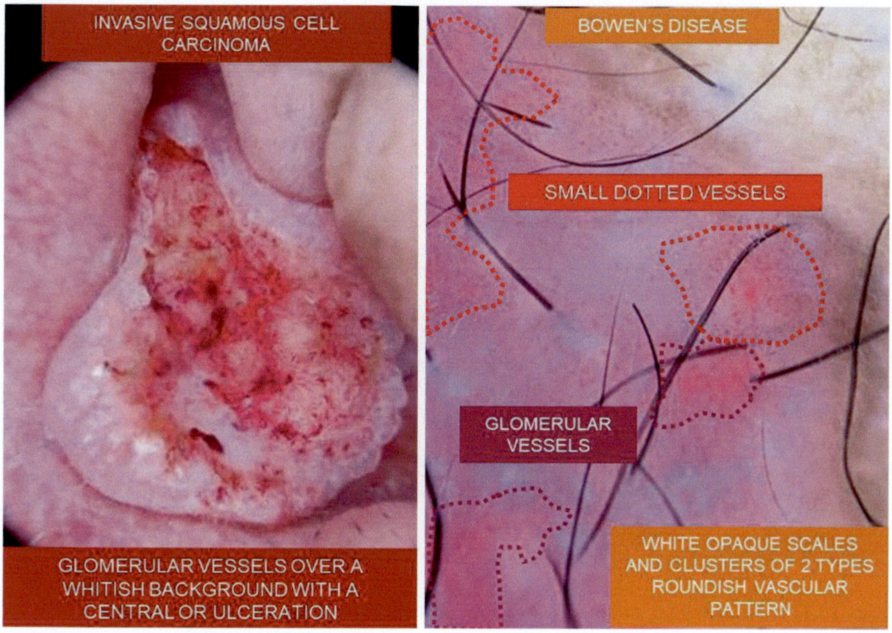

Fig. 15.138 Dermoscopic findings of patient with squamous cell carcinoma (x20)

15.38.5 Histopathology (Figs. 15.139 and 15.140) [33]

Actinic Keratosis

- Increasing atypia or dysplasia, loss of orderly maturation, and nuclear and cellular pleomorphism can be classified into different forms. The histological classification of the basal growth pattern (PRO) showed greater inter-rater reliability compared to the established classification of atypical keratinocytes along the epidermal layers. In addition, experienced dermatopathologists have considered basal proliferation to be more important in terms of progression risk than upward-directed growth patterns.
- -KIN 1, 2a, 2b, and 3—dysplasia by thirds, like that used in the uterine cervix; when the dysplasia occupies the entire thickness, the name bowenoid actinic keratosis can be used.
- -PRO 0, 1, 2, and 3—inward bulbous basilar proliferation.
- Dyskeratosis.
- Increased number of mitoses and mitoses in any stratum beyond the basal layer.

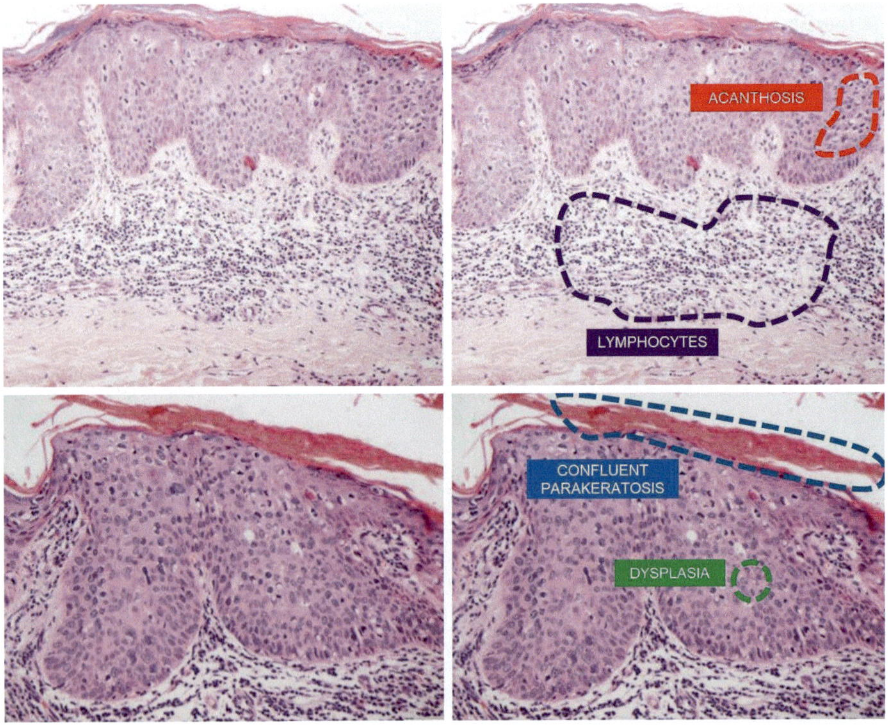

Fig. 15.139 Histological findings of squamous cell carcinoma (Bowen's disease) (H&E x4 and x10)

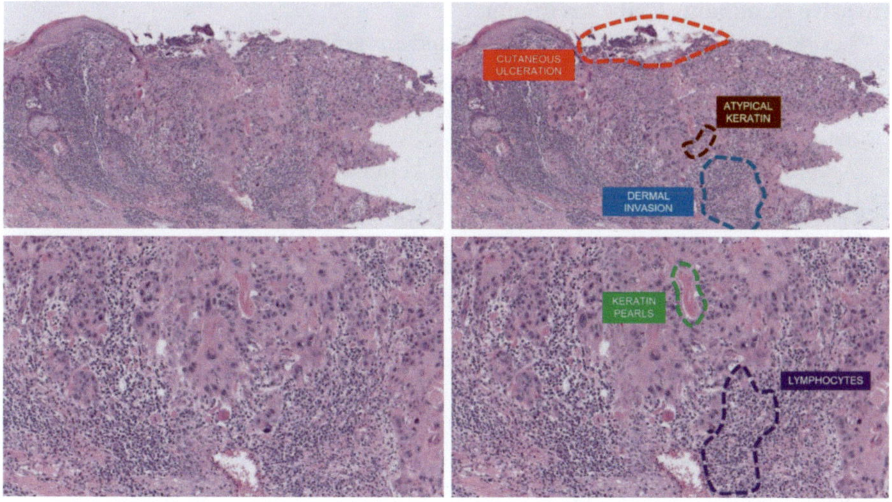

Fig. 15.140 Histological findings of invasive squamous cell carcinoma (H&E x4 and x10)

- Parakeratosis on the atypical keratinocytes between the appendages, called inter-adnexal epithelium, sparing the epiderma on the adnexal ostia, called alternate parakeratosis. This pattern is called hypertrophic, but hypertrophy does not occur, it is a disordered proliferation with dysplasia, and is better called hyperkeratotic by clinical impression.
- Tendency to erosion or ulceration with variable inflammatory.
- Infiltrate, variable solar elastosis, and other findings of chronic photodamage. Some authors list accentuated lymphocytic infiltration as a risk factor for microinvasion.
- It may also present with atrophy, erosion, pigmentation, and acantholysis.

Bowen's Disease

- It is an intraepithelial squamous cell carcinoma (in situ) without alternating parakeratosis, an important histopathological finding to differentiate from bowenoid actinic keratosis.
- It is present in the cutaneous appendages, spared in actinic keratosis.
- It can occur in covered areas—absence of underlying solar elastosis.
- 3 to 5% progress to invasive SCC.
- Differential diagnosis with Queyrat's erythroplakia and actinic cheilitis.
- Some authors refer to the importance of distinguishing Bowen's disease from AKs, as the latter points to non-actinic causes of squamous cell carcinoma (chromosomal or mutational) with an increased risk of internal squamous cell carcinoma when associated with chronic arsenicism, especially of the aerodigestive tract—esophagus and lungs.

Invasive Squamous Cell Carcinoma

- Lesion with asymmetric architecture and irregular and spiculated edges of the neoplasm.
- Extension inwards the dermis by irregular nests composed of atypical keratinocytes with an infiltrative aspect.
- Atypical, hyperchromatic, pleomorphic keratinocytes with nuclear aberrations, dyskeratosis, and increased number of mitoses, including atypical and off-basal mitosis.
- Hyperkeratosis with formation of atypical parakeratosis in varying amounts.
- Presence of well-expressed corneal pearls until total absence, related to the degree of the neoplasm.
- Tumor thickness can be used as an important risk factor.
- Tendency to erosion, ulceration of the epidermal surface.
- Broders classification—grades 1 to 4 or well, moderately, poorly differentiated, or undifferentiated.
- To assess the biological aggressiveness of the lesion, including risk of recurrence and metastases (Breuninger, 1992).
- Prognostic factors: ulceration greater than 3.0 mm, extension to the hypodermis or beyond, cartilage or bone invasion (face), perineural permeation, vascular invasion, acantholytic pattern, compromised surgical limit, multiple lesions, syndromes such as xeroderma pigmentosum, and immunosuppression.
- Subtypes: acantolytic, clear cells, fusiform cells (sarcomatoid), basaloid, keratoacanthoma-like and verrucous, including Buschke-Loewenstein tumor.

15.38.6 Computed Tomography

- Computed tomography scans primarily for the detection of extracapsular spread (ECS) in lymph nodes affected.
- SCC presents as a solid, nodular mass with irregular and poorly defined borders.
- Lesions enhance after the administration of contrast material, indicating their vascularity.
- Larger SCC lesions often display central areas of low attenuation, indicating necrosis.
- SCC can infiltrate surrounding structures such as subcutaneous tissues and muscles, leading to the loss of clear fat planes.
- Sometimes, SCC contains calcifications, which appear as hyperdense areas on CT scans.
- Regional lymph node metastasis is often detected, characterized by enlarged lymph nodes, sometimes with central necrosis and extracapsular spread.

15.38.7 Ultrasonography (Figs. 15.141 and 15.142) [91, 92]

- cSCC presents as a hypoechoic or irregular dermal or hypodermal structure.
- Generally, cSCC does not exhibit hyperechoic foci.
- Moderate increase in intralesional and peripheral blood flow detectable on power Doppler.
- Locoregional metastases of SCC can be detected and may involve the tumor's lymphatic drainage pathways.

15.38.8 MRI (Fig. 15.143) [93]

- T1-weighted images show hypointensity.
- T2-weighted images, generally exhibit iso-hyperintensity but may show heterogeneous signal intensities, especially when cystic necrosis occurs within the tumor.
- Protrusion into the subcutaneous tissue.
- Entrapment of peritumoral fat.
- Formation of superficial ulcers.
- Heterogeneous signal intensities in contrast-enhanced images due to cystic necrosis and aggressive invasion.

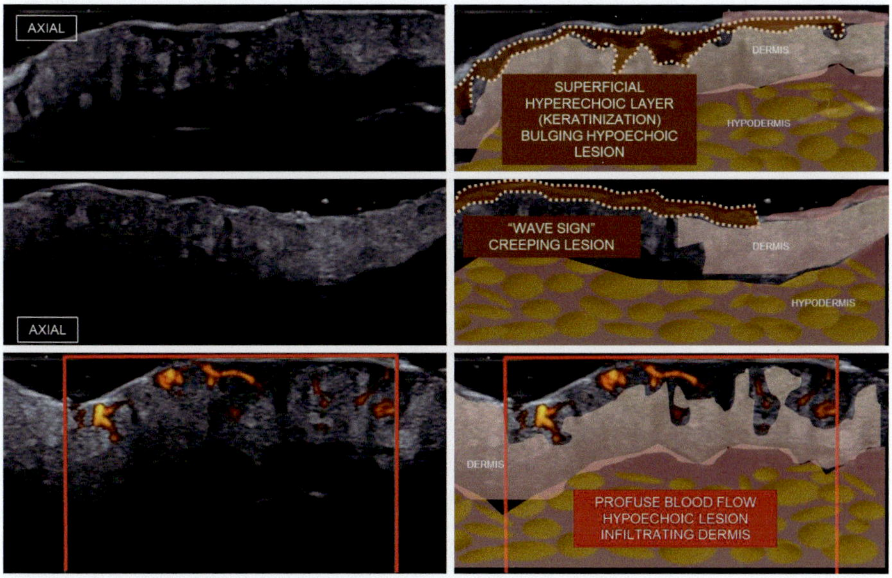

Fig. 15.141 Ultrasonographic findings of squamous cell carcinoma (Bowen's disease) with a 33 MHz probe (Aplio i800, Canon Medical Systems)

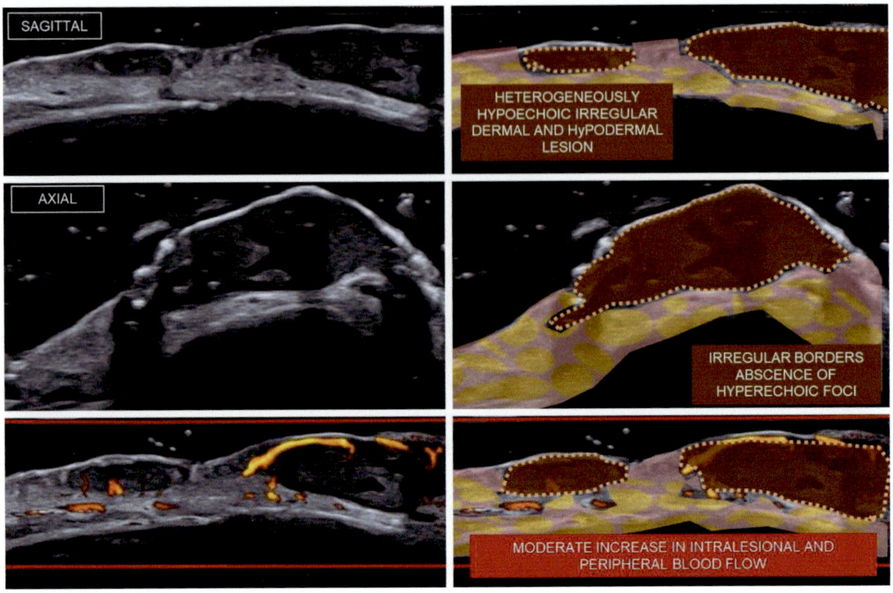

Fig. 15.142 Ultrasonographic findings of invasive squamous cell carcinoma with a 33 MHz probe (Aplio i800, Canon Medical Systems)

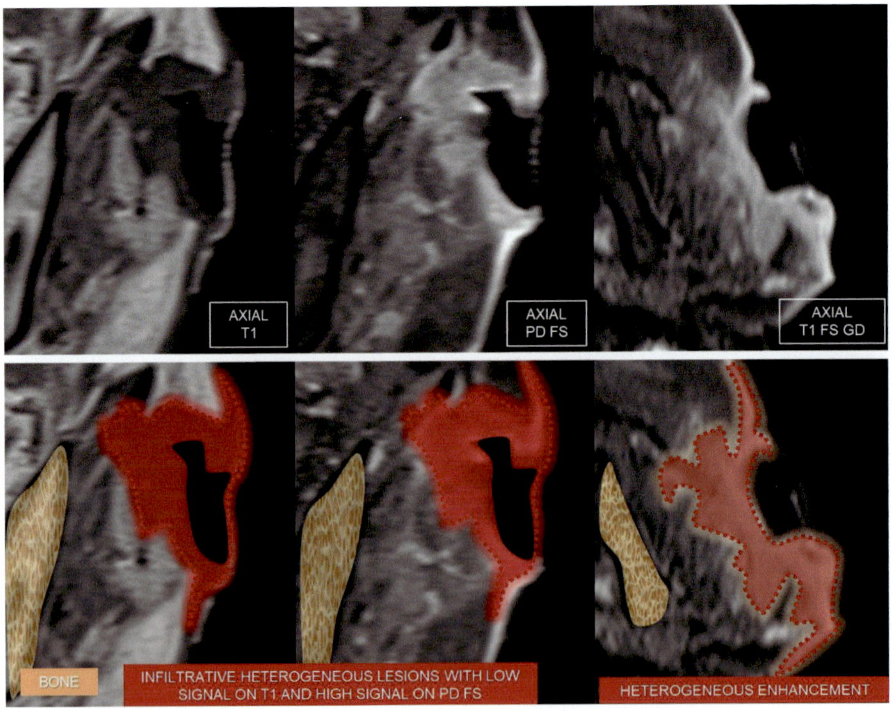

Fig. 15.143 MRI with surface coil findings of invasive squamous cell carcinoma on T1, DP FS, and T1 FS-weighted sequences after gadolinium administration (Magnetom Prisma 3T MRI, Siemens)

15.38.9 3D Images

- Ideal for managing complex and persistent cases, particularly in facial lesions where surgery may lead to significant cosmetic changes.
- Allows for a thorough evaluation of the lesion, helping to gauge its severity and its impact on surrounding tissues and blood vessels.
- Enhances the precision of surgical methods, especially in intricate areas.
- Creating physical models of the affected area with biomodels offers essential insights for both planning surgeries and educating patients.

15.39 Melanoma: Superficial Spreading and Nodular

15.39.1 Definition [94]

- Superficial spreading melanoma (SSM) is the most common subtype in fair-skinned individuals, corresponding to 70% of cases.
- SSM presents a radial growth phase, defined by growth limited to the epidermis or focused on the papillary dermis, followed by a phase of vertical growth with the presence of invasion.
- Nodular melanoma (NM) accounts for approximately 15–30% of melanoma diagnoses.
- NM are typically blue-black but may lack pigment.
- NM presents with greater thickness, a faster mitotic growth rate, and earlier metastasis to other vital organs than other subtypes of melanoma, which often results in a poor prognosis.
- Amelanotic melanomas are characterized by absence of pigment, being infrequent and corresponding in between 2% and 8% of all cases.

15.36.1. Epidemiology [94].

- The incidence of melanoma has increased 3–7% per year, faster than any other cancer, and is predicted to double every 10–20 years.

15.39.2 Clinical Presentation (Fig. 15.144) [94]

- SSM begins with an intraepidermal horizontal or radial growth phase, appearing first as a macular lesion that slowly evolves into a plaque, often with multiple colors and pale areas of regression.
- NM is a primarily nodular, exophytic brown–black, or red pink in amelanotic tumors, often eroded or bleeding tumor, which is characterized by a predominant aggressive vertical growth phase.

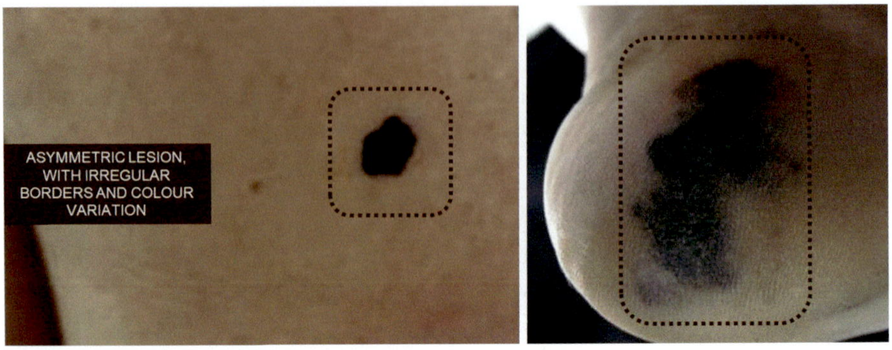

Fig. 15.144 Clinical photograph of patients with melanoma

15.39.3 Semiological Methodos [95]

- SSM: Asymmetry, Border irregularity, Colour variation, Diameter > 6 mm and Evolution of the lesions compose the mnemonic "ABCDE." Specifically, for SSM, it is a semiological tool to recognize melanoma in its early clinical presentation.
- NM: The mnemonic EFG: elevated, firm, growing can be useful to recognize the NM.

15.39.4 Dermoscopy (Fig. 15.145) [96]

- The dermoscopic characteristics most frequently found are asymmetry, three or more colors, atypical network, and atypical dots and globules.
- SSM: Atypical network, irregular dots, irregular globules, irregular streaks, and irregular blotch correspond to histopathologic alterations at the level of the junction, blue-white veil and atypical vessels suggest intradermal growth, whereas regression structures, negative network and white shiny streaks might reflect junctional or dermal alterations.
- NM: Nodular melanoma is typified by the coexistence of blue and black color, atypical vessels, and pink color.

15.39.5 Histopathology (Fig. 15.146) [33]

- The epidermis can present any type of alteration, including normal, atrophic, hyperplastic, erosive, or ulcerated.
- Compound asymmetric proliferation showing poorly demarcated intraepidermal lateral border.

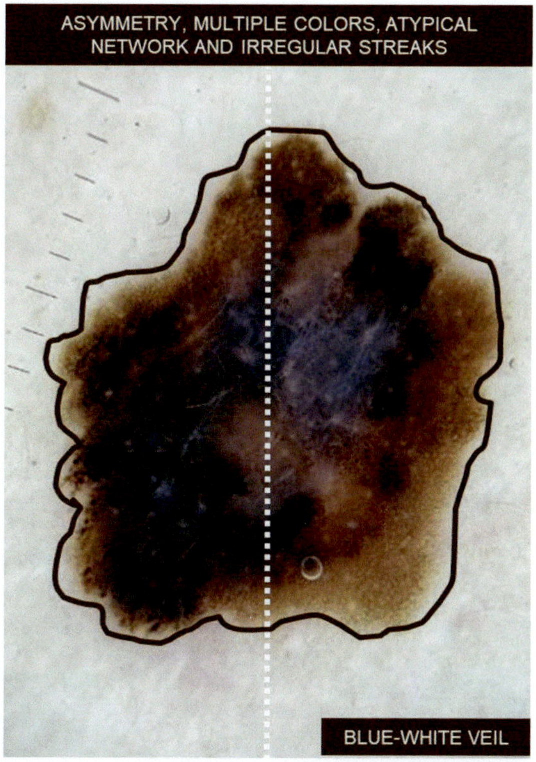
ASYMMETRY, MULTIPLE COLORS, ATYPICAL NETWORK AND IRREGULAR STREAKS
BLUE-WHITE VEIL

Fig. 15.145 Dermoscopic findings of patient with melanoma (x20)

- Atypical melanocytes with extreme variation in cell appearance from nevus melanocytic cell-like to epithelioid, basaloid, spindle-shaped, or giant cells resembling choriocarcinoma cells with total anaplasia; cellular atypia is not correlated with the degree of biological aggressiveness in malignant melanoma, as occurs with SCC in Broders grading. Cells exhibit nuclear pleomorphism, hyperchromatic, with prominent nucleoli, mitoses including atypical mitoses, and the presence of mitoses in the lower part of the tumor.
- Lack of maturation, and there may be pigmented cells at any level.
- Presence or absence of melanic pigmentation.
- Presence of variable lymphocytic infiltrate in the periphery of the lesion. The presence of plasma cells is characteristic of malignant melanoma.
- There may be intratumoral coagulation necrosis with neutrophils and hemorrhage.
- There may be vascular neoformation and neoplastic thrombi in the lymphatic vessels or perineural permeation.
- There may be an association with melanocytic nevus in 10–20% of cases. The risk is higher in congenital melanocytic nevi; Most cases occur "de novo," that is, it is malignant melanoma from the beginning.

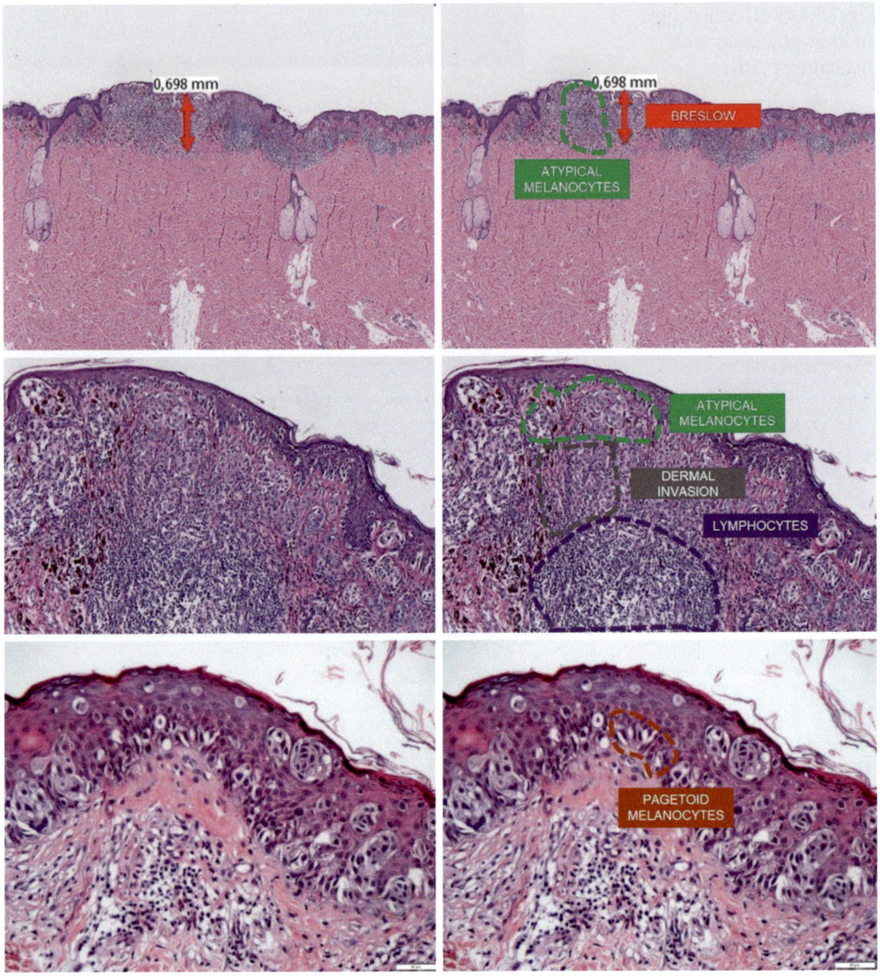

Fig. 15.146 Histological findings of melanoma (H&E x10)

- Expresses immunohistochemical markers of melanocytic differentiation; the most used are S100, HMB45, Melan-A, SOX 10 (positive), and PRAME (negative), as well as replicative index markers such as Ki67.
- Histogenetic classification of Clark:
  - Superficial spreading: Presence of pagetoid or horizontal or radial dissemination, intraepithelial, in addition to three interpapillary cones in relation to the tumor located in the dermis.
  - Nodular: Absence of relevant horizontal (radial) dissemination and tumor contact restricted to up to three interpapillary cones away from the dermal tumor component, in addition to the nodular silhouette.
  - Lentigo maligna: Absence of pagetoid nests, dissemination of cells usually restricted to the basal layer over the dermis with solar elastosis.

- Acral-lentiginous: Occurs in acral skin or nail apparatus with a pattern like lentigo maligna.

- Breslow index: is the measure of maximum tumor thickness and is related to the risk of metastases.

15.39.6 Ultrasonography (Fig. 15.147) [97, 98]

- Dermal and hypodermal lesion, hypoechoic and commonly fusiform.
- Appear as oval hypodermal structures, hypoechoic, commonly surrounded by hyperechoic hypodermal adipose tissue.
- On power Doppler, intralesional and peripheral hypervascularization is often detected.
- Satellite and in-transit metastases generally, follow the path of the lymphatic and venous drainage of the tumor.
- Melanoma metastases commonly exhibit hypervascularization on power Doppler.
- Staging and metastases detection:
  - Essential to perform locoregional staging
  - Detect satellite metastases (=2 cm from the primary tumor).
  - Detect in-transit metastases (<2 cm from the primary tumor).
  - Detect nodal metastases.

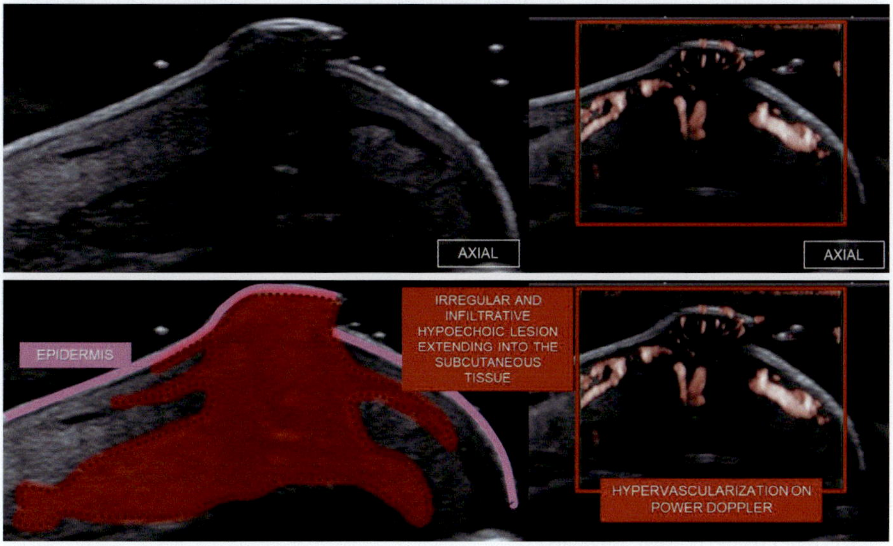

Fig. 15.147 Ultrasonographic findings of melanoma with a 33 MHz probe (Aplio i800, Canon Medical Systems)

15.39.7 MRI (Fig. 15.148) [99]

- Typically shows hyperintensity on T1-weighted images due to the paramagnetic effects of melanin on intratumoral hemorrhage.
- Typically shows hypointensity on T2-weighted images.
- Other MRI features include superficial depression and irregular superficial margins.

15.39.8 3D Images

- Perfect for handling complicated and ongoing cases, especially in facial lesions where surgical intervention could result in noticeable cosmetic changes.
- Facilitates a comprehensive assessment of the lesion, aiding in the determination of its severity and its effects on adjacent tissues and blood vessels.
- Improves the accuracy of surgical techniques, particularly in delicate and intricate regions.
- Developing physical replicas of the affected area using biomodels provides valuable information for surgical planning and patient education.

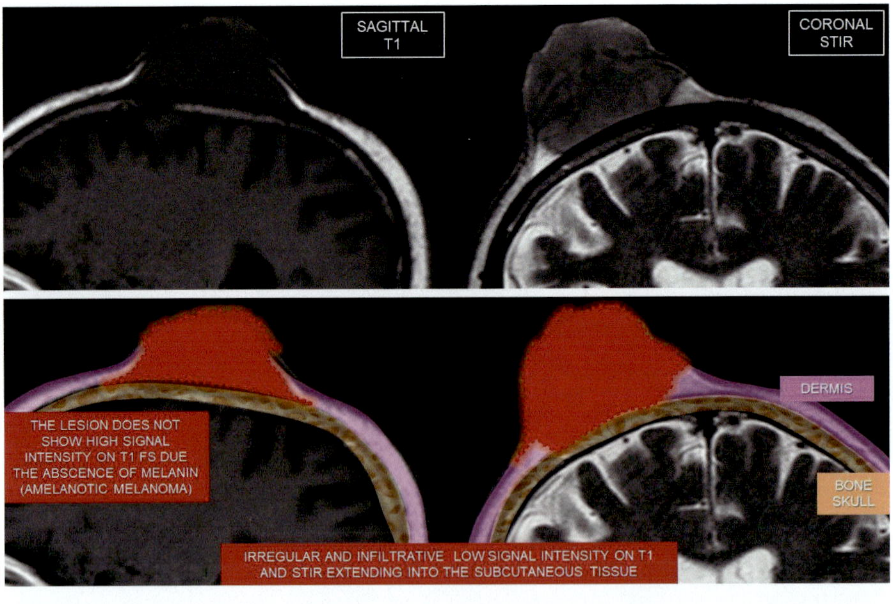

Fig. 15.148 MRI findings of amelanotic melanoma on T1-weighted and STIR sequences (Magnetom Prisma 3T MRI, Siemens)

15.40 Cutaneous Metastasis

15.40.1 Definition [100]

- Skin metastasis refers to the spread of cancer cells from a primary internal malignancy to the skin.
- These metastatic lesions can occur as a result of hematogenous or lymphatic spread and may present in various morphologies.

15.40.2 Epidemiology [100]

- Skin metastases are relatively rare, occurring in approximately 2–10% of all cancer patients. The incidence varies depending on the type of primary cancer.
- The most common cancers that metastasize to the skin are melanoma, breast cancer, lung cancer, colorectal cancer, and ovarian cancer. For men, lung cancer and melanoma are the most common sources, while in women, breast cancer is the predominant primary site.
- Skin metastases can occur in patients of any age, but they are more commonly seen in older adults due to the higher prevalence of primary cancers in this population.

15.40.3 Clinical Presentation (Figs. 15.149 and 15.150) [100]

- Skin metastases may present as nodules, plaques, ulcers, or erythematous patches. These lesions can vary in color from flesh-toned to red, purple, or even black, depending on the underlying cancer type and the degree of vascularization or hemorrhage.
- These lesions can appear anywhere on the body, but common sites include the chest, abdomen, and extremities. The location often correlates with the primary tumor's site of origin.
- Skin metastases are usually asymptomatic, but they can cause pain, tenderness, or itching if they ulcerate or become infected.

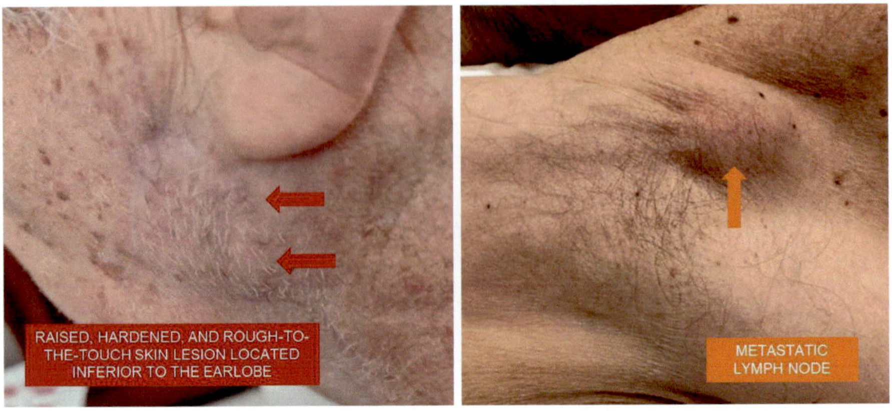

Fig. 15.149 Clinical photograph of patients with lymph node metastasis

Fig. 15.150 Clinical photograph of patients with cutaneous metastasis

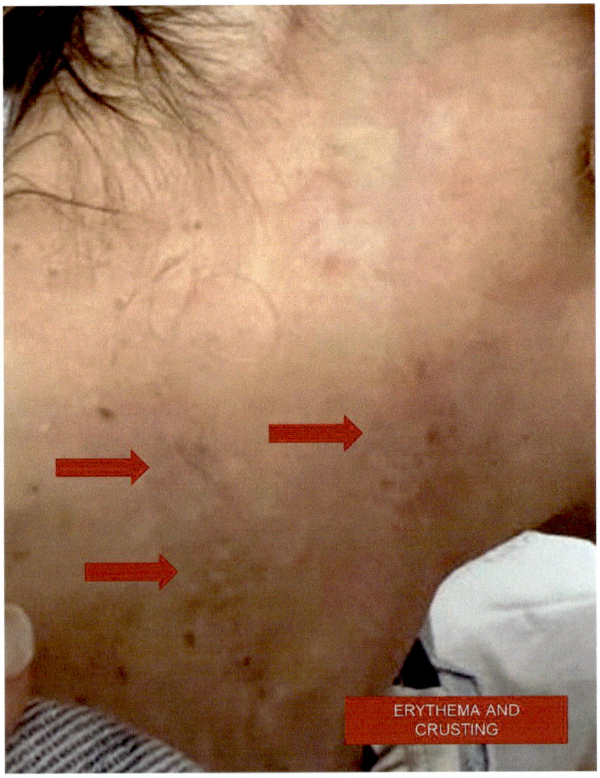

15.40.4 Histopathology [100]

- The histopathology of skin metastases reveals malignant cells similar to those of the primary tumor. These cells often infiltrate the dermis and may extend into the subcutaneous tissue. The arrangement of cells can vary, with patterns such as sheets, nests, or single cells dispersed within the dermis.
- Immunohistochemical staining is often necessary to confirm the diagnosis and to determine the origin of the metastatic cells, particularly when the primary site is unknown. Markers such as cytokeratin, S-100, or specific tumor markers can be used depending on the suspected primary tumor.

15.40.5 Ultrasonography (Figs. 15.151 and 15.152)

- On ultrasonography, skin metastases typically appear as hypoechoic or mixed echogenicity masses in the dermis or subcutaneous tissue. They may be well-circumscribed or poorly defined, depending on the degree of infiltration.
- Color Doppler ultrasonography may reveal increased vascularity within the lesion, which can help differentiate metastatic nodules from benign skin lesions.

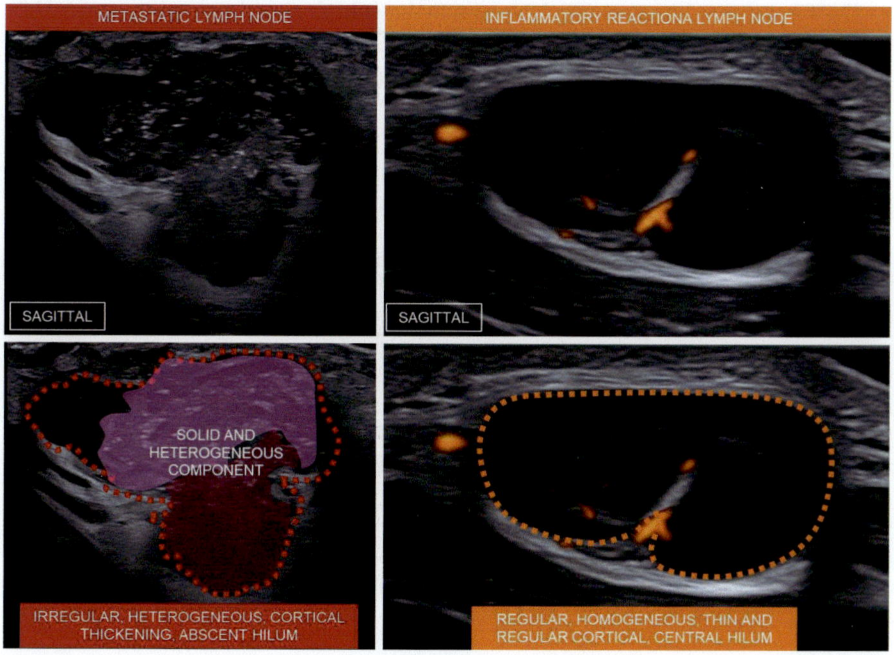

Fig. 15.151 Ultrasonographic findings of lymph node metastasis and an inflammatory reactional lymph node with a 24 MHz probe (Aplio i800, Canon Medical Systems)

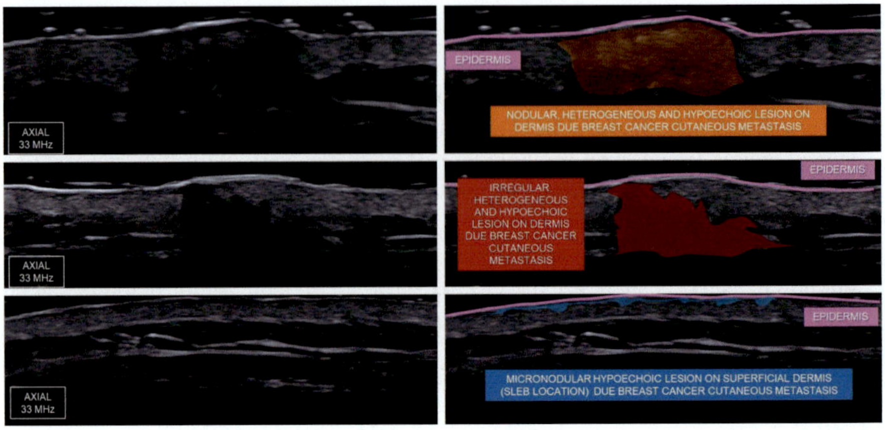

Fig. 15.152 Ultrasonographic findings of cutaneous metastasis of breast cancer with a 33 MHz probe (Aplio i800, Canon Medical Systems)

15.40.6 MRI (Figs. 15.153 and 15.154)

- Skin metastases typically appear as low to intermediate signal intensity lesions on T1-weighted images.
- On T2-weighted images, the lesions may have high signal intensity, particularly if there is associated edema or inflammation.
- After gadolinium administration, skin metastases usually show moderate to strong enhancement, reflecting their vascular nature.
- MRI can be particularly useful in assessing the extent of skin involvement, especially in cases where deeper structures or adjacent tissues are involved.

15.41 Spiradenocarcinoma Eccrine

15.41.1 Definition [101]

- Malignant spiradenoma, or spiradenocarcinoma, is an infrequent tumor characterized by the transformation of a benign spiradenoma, initially documented by Dabska in 1972.

15.41.2 Epidemiology [101]

- This tumor is exceedingly rare, predominantly documented through individual case reports and small case series.

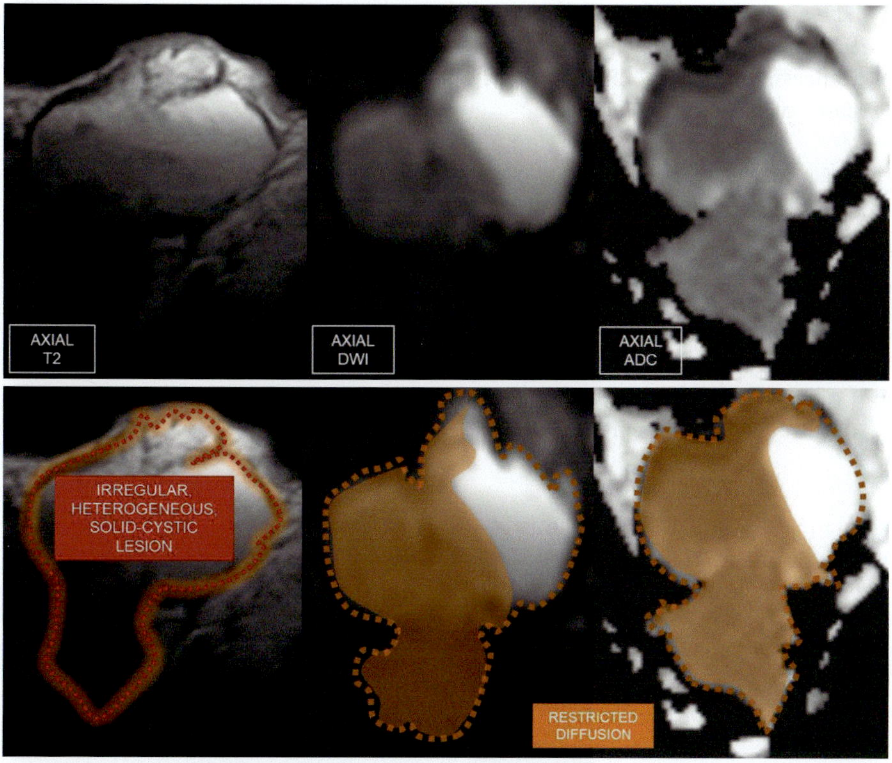

Fig. 15.153 MRI findings of lymph node metastasis of the axillae on T1-weighted and STIR sequences (Magnetom Avanto 1.5T MRI, Siemens)

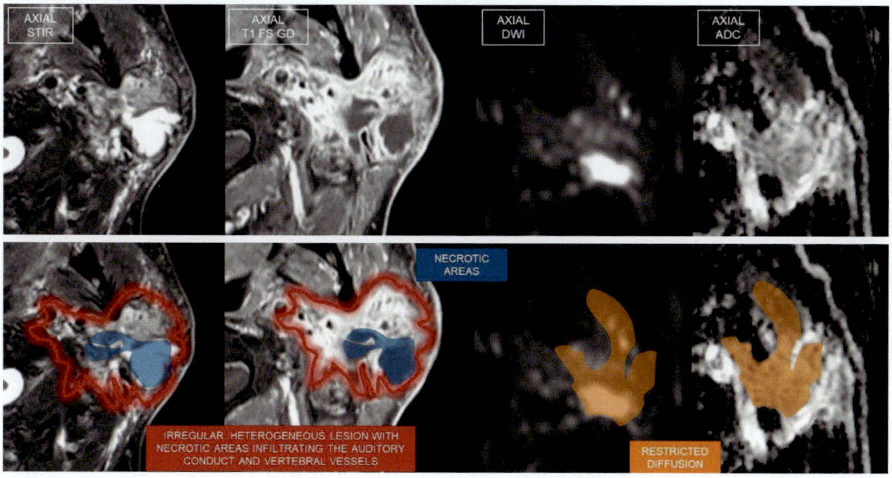

Fig. 15.154 MRI with surface coil findings of lymph node metastasis of the cervical region on T1-weighted and STIR sequences (Magnetom Prisma 3T MRI, Siemens)

- The average age at onset is around 50 years, ranging widely from 8 to 89 years.
- Females constitute a slight majority.
- Caucasians appear to be disproportionately affected, comprising almost 80% of cases where race was noted.

15.41.3 Clinical Presentation (Fig. 15.155) [101]

- Typically manifests as recent changes in a long-standing benign lesion.
- Common symptoms include noticeable growth of the lesion, associated pain, and sometimes ulceration.
- Primary sites of occurrence include the trunk, limbs, head and neck, with rare occurrences in the genital region.

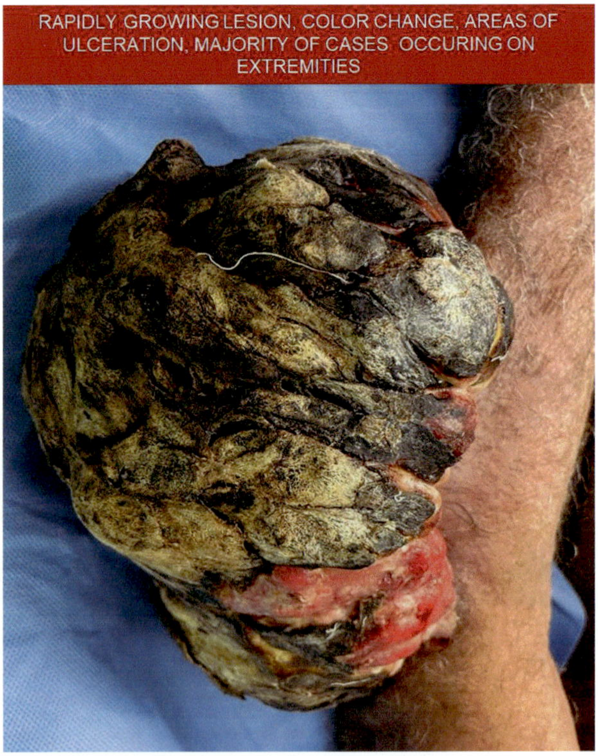

Fig. 15.155 Clinical photograph of patients with eccrine spiradenocarcinoma

15.41.4 Histopathology (Fig. 15.156) [102]

- Spiradenocarcinoma exhibits heterogeneous histology.
- Two main patterns include an abrupt transition from benign spiradenoma to high-grade carcinoma and a low-grade variant resembling benign spiradenoma, posing diagnostic challenges due to well-defined borders and uniform cell populations with mild to moderate atypia.
- High-grade tumors display features like pleomorphism, cytological atypia, mitotic activity, and necrosis.
- Immunohistochemical markers such as ER and p53 are relevant, with p53 overexpression noted specifically in the malignant component.

15.41.5 Ultrasonography

- Spiradenocarcinoma typically appears as a well-defined, hypoechoic mass on ultrasonography, reflecting fewer sound waves compared to surrounding tissues.
- The internal echogenicity may be heterogeneous, showing areas of varying echogenicity due to the tumor's cellularity and stroma.
- There might be posterior acoustic enhancement, where the area behind the lesion appears brighter due to increased sound wave transmission through the mass.
- Calcifications are generally not present in spiradenocarcinoma.
- On power Doppler ultrasonography, there is often minimal or no significant blood flow within the lesion.

15.41.6 MRI (Fig. 15.157)

- On T1-weighted MRI, spiradenocarcinoma usually appears iso- to hypointense relative to the surrounding soft tissues.
- On T2-weighted MRI, the lesion typically shows hyperintensity, reflecting its higher water content and cellularity.
- After contrast administration, spiradenocarcinoma often demonstrates intense enhancement.
- The lesion may have irregular and ill-defined margins, which can help differentiate it from other types of skin tumors.
- There might be surrounding edema or inflammatory changes, which can appear as increased signal intensity on T2-weighted images.

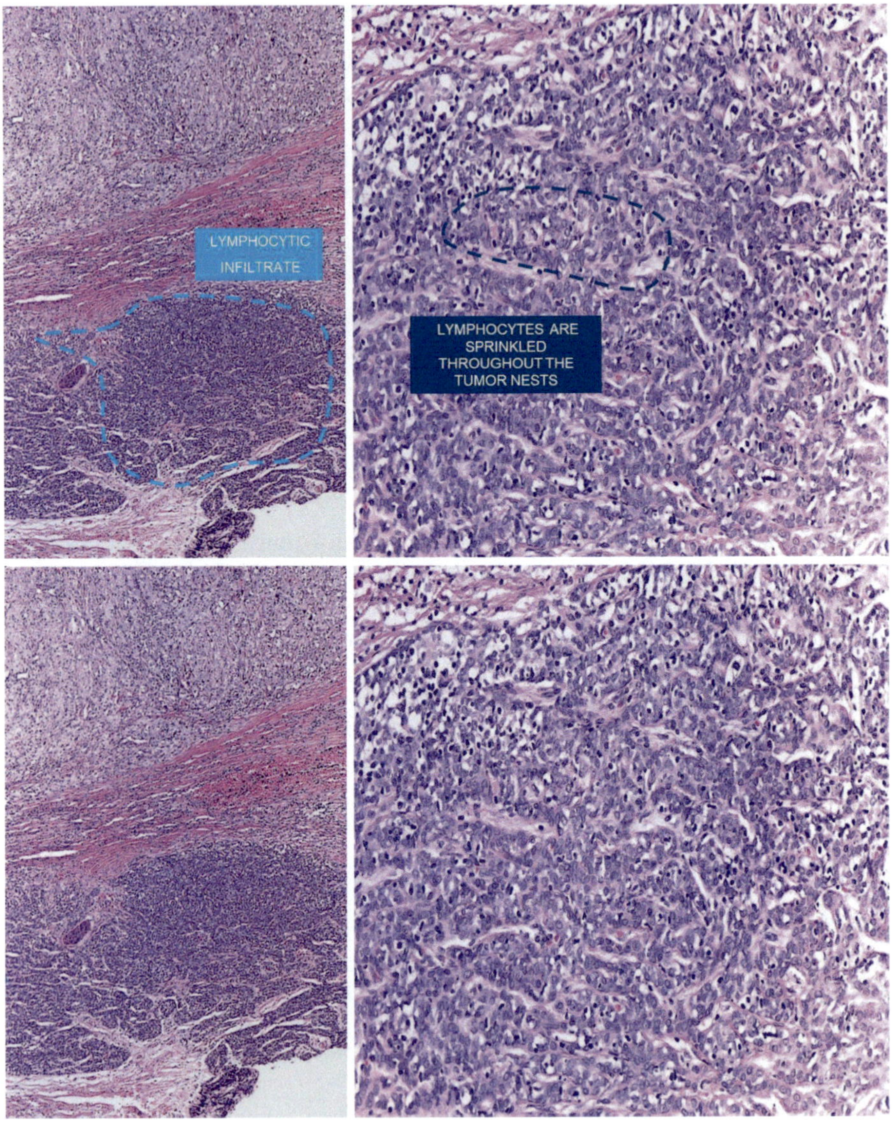

Fig. 15.156 Histological findings of eccrine spiradenocarcinoma (H&E x10 and x20)

15.41.7 3D Images

- Facilitates a detailed evaluation of the lesion, assisting in understanding its severity and impact on nearby tissues and blood vessels.
- Enhances the accuracy of surgical procedures, particularly in delicate and complex areas.

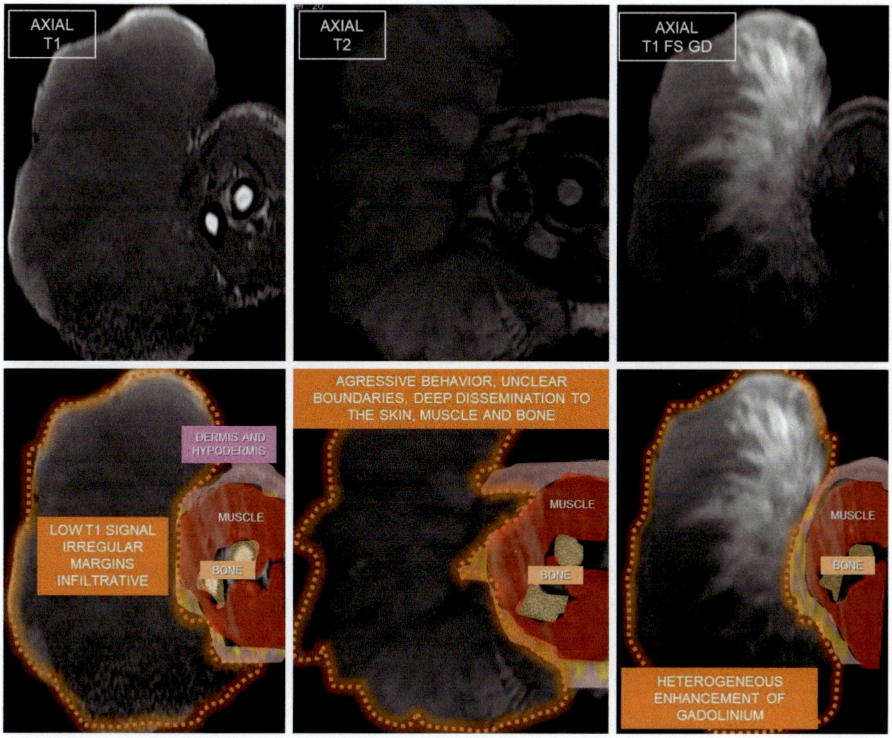

Fig. 15.157 MRI findings of eccrine spiradenocarcinoma on T1, T2, and T1 FS-weighted sequences after gadolinium administration

- Provides essential information for surgical planning and patient education by creating physical replicas of the affected area using biomodels.

15.42 Dermatofibrosarcoma Protuberans

15.42.1 Definition [103]

- Dermatofibrosarcoma protuberans is a rare mesenchymal tumor, a soft tissue sarcoma, of intermediate malignancy, that arises in the dermis and invades deeper tissue.
- Occurs more frequently on the trunk and proximal extremities, and nearly 15% on the head and neck.
- Can be often associated with a t(17;22) (q22;q13) translocation, generating the fusion protein COL1A1-PDGFB.

15.42.2 Epidemiology

- Represents 1–6% of all soft tissue sarcomas and 18% of cutaneous soft tissue sarcomas.
- The highest incidence is between 30 and 50 years old but can occur at any age.
- The frequency is similar in genders, but some studies show a slight male predominance.

15.42.3 Clinical Presentation (Fig. 15.158) [103]

- Appears as a slowly developing, robust plaque, exhibiting shades of pink or violet, underscoring the challenge of timely diagnosis.
- Dermatofibrosarcoma protuberans is a slow-growing and rare tumor, which generally delays the diagnosis of this tumor.
- The lesion may exhibit accelerated growth during pregnancy.
- The pigmented variant often presents with irregular brown pigmentation.
- The atrophic variant appears as a violaceous plaque resembling morphea or scar tissue.
- It is possible to arise from preexisting scars or tattoos.

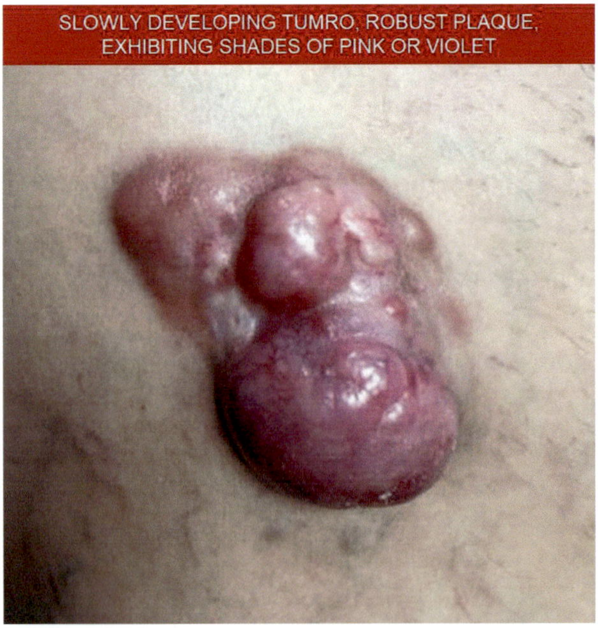

Fig. 15.158 Clinical photograph of patients with dermatofibrosarcoma protuberans

- Some lesions can ulcerate and become painful when expanded.
- The tumor is locally aggressive and has a high rate of recurrence, but metastasizes is not common.

15.42.4 Dermoscopy

- Some dermoscopic characteristics are delicate pigmented network, vessels, structureless light brown areas, shiny white streaks, pink background coloration, and structureless hypo- or depigmented areas.
- Dermoscopic pattern frequently shows the coexistence of reticular pigmentation and unfocused and/or focused arborizing vessels.
- Arborizing vessels were the most prevalent vascular structure.
- A high number of dermoscopic features per lesion (around 4) is called a multicomponent pattern and is suggestive of malignant tumors.

15.42.5 Histopathology (Fig. 15.159) [33]

- Dermatofibrosarcoma protuberans (DFSP), the most common dermal sarcoma, is a malignant fibroblastic tumor most frequently arising in middle-aged adults. It is typically a low-grade sarcoma that grows slowly but has a high rate of local recurrence with low metastatic potential.
- The epidermis overlying DFSP shows thinning and may be separated from the neoplasm by a Grenz zone.
- Melanin hyperpigmentation may occur in the basal layer.
- Dermatofibrosarcoma protuberans are typically an ill-defined neoplasm that forms a nodule or ill-defined dermal plaque that infiltrates the subcutis or sometimes skeletal muscle with a characteristic "honeycomb" pattern.
- The neoplasm is composed of prominent storiform fascicles of uniform spindle cells showing little atypia or mitotic activity. Presence of atypia, necrosis, and/or hemorrhage occurs in the least differentiated forms.
- Although clinically they seem circumscribed, histologically they can be very infiltrative, which is the reason for frequent recurrences.
- Tumoral hemorrhage and cystic degeneration may be present, but necrosis is rare and suggests the possibility of a higher-grade neoplasm.
- Dermatofibrosarcoma has morphologic variants that share similar clinical, histologic, and immunohistochemical features, including myxoid, pigmented forms (Bednar's tumor), giant cell fibroblastoma (GCF), and progression to fibrosarcomatous change.
- In immunohistochemistry, the main marker is strong and diffuse CD34 positivity and smooth muscle actin (SMA) negativity.

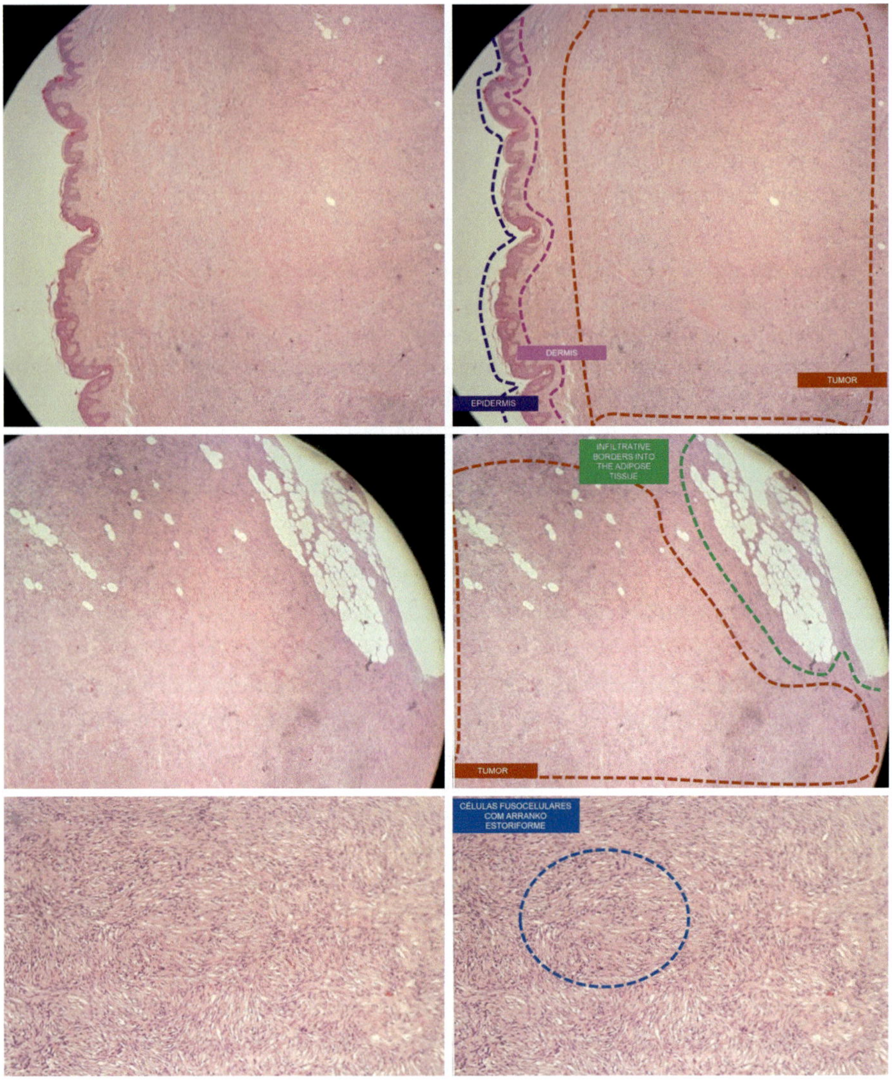

Fig. 15.159 Histological findings of dermatofibrosarcoma protuberans (H&E x10)

15.42.6 Radiography [103]

- Radiography usually shows a nodular soft-tissue mass or soft-tissue swelling without bone involvement or calcification.

15.42.7 Computed Tomography [103]

- On CT images, this tumor usually appears as a well-defined, homogenous isodense lesion, without calcification. After contrast administration often shows intermediate and marked heterogeneous enhancement but rarely can present intermediate homogeneous or a mild heterogeneous enhancement.
- Lesions that present more than 5 cm may show intratumoral non-enhancement areas, which could indicate intratumoral necrotic and cystic degeneration.
- Bony destruction is uncommon.

15.42.8 Ultrasonography (Fig. 15.160) [103]

- Dermatofibrosarcoma Protuberans is usually small and superficial, so high-frequency ultrasonography is superior in the assessment of superficial soft-tissue masses due to their high-resolution images.
- Generally, is a single lesion located in the dermis and hypodermis, but can involve deeper structures, such as fascia and muscle.
- The lesion is typically ill defined, nodular or ovoid, that exhibits a mixed echogenicity, with hyper and hypoechoic echotexture and tentacle-like projections or a "claw" sign.
- Was described that this lesion can also present as a well-defined hypoechogenic solid nodule, hypoechogenic infiltrate with ill-defined borders, an ill-defined plaque lesion, or a pseudonodular inflammatory lesion.
- Most tumors show intralesional hypervascularization on Color Doppler image, with arterial and venous vessels, that tends to be more profound peripherally.
- Furthermore, satellite metastasis, around 2 cm of the primary tumor, can be observed as hypoechogenic nodules.

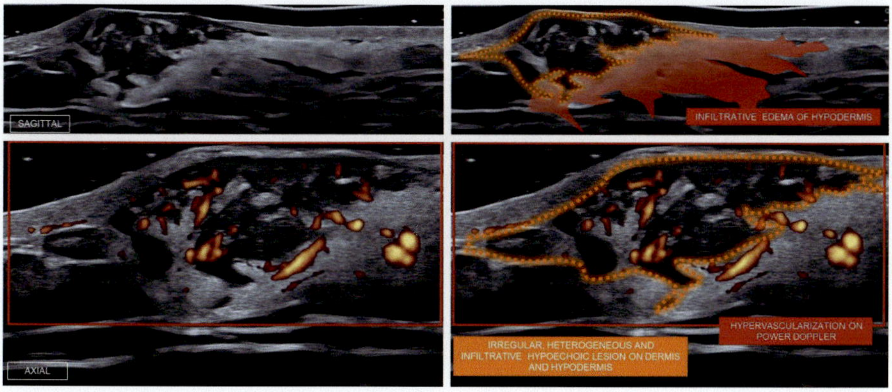

Fig. 15.160 Ultrasonographic findings of dermatofibrosarcoma protuberans with a 24 MHz probe (Aplio i800, Canon Medical Systems)

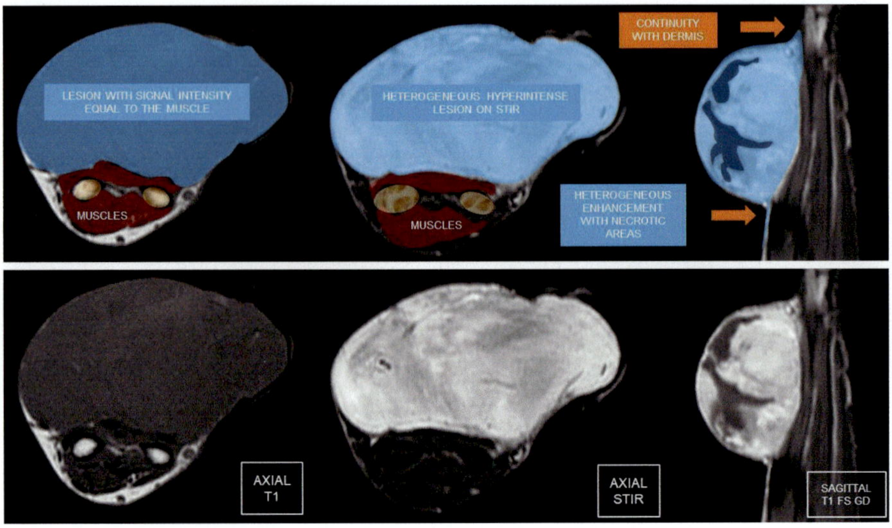

Fig. 15.161 MRI findings of dermatofibrosarcoma protuberans on T1, STIR, and T1 FS-weighted sequences after gadolinium administration (Magnetom Prisma 3T MRI, Siemens)

15.42.9 MRI (Fig. 15.161) [103]

- On MRI is typically T1-isointense and T2-hyperintense to muscle.
- T1 post-contrast sequence usually shows a moderate or marked enhancement that usually is homogeneous, but can be heterogeneous in some cases.
- Necrotic and hemorrhagic signals can be present.

15.42.10 3D Images (Fig. 15.162, Video 15.7)

- Enables thorough assessment of the lesion, helping to gauge its severity and how it affects surrounding tissues and blood vessels.
- Improves surgical precision, especially in sensitive and complex areas.
- Offers valuable insights for both surgical planning and patient education through the creation of physical models of the affected area with biomodels.

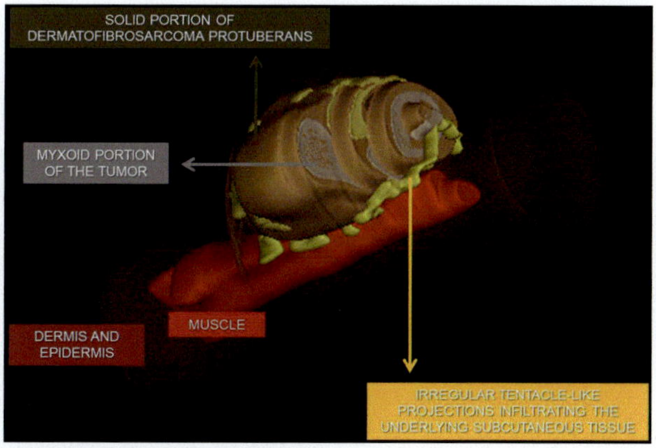

Fig. 15.162 3D images of dermatofibrosarcoma protuberans after segmentation of MRI isotropic images for surgical planning

15.43 Skin Invasive Breast Carcinoma

15.43.1 Definition [104]

- Also called Inflammatory Breast Carcinoma (IBC) is classified as a T4d tumor according to the American Joint Committee on Cancer criteria.
- It is characterized by diffuse erythema and edema of the skin (peau d'orange), often presenting without a discrete mass.

15.43.2 Epidemiology [104]

- The incidence of IBC varies widely, reported to be between less than 1% and 10%, depending on diagnostic criteria.
- It constitutes a rare subset, accounting for approximately 2–4% of breast cancer cases in the United States, yet significantly contributing to breast cancer mortality due to its aggressive nature.

15.43.3 Clinical Presentation (Fig. 15.163) [104]

- IBC typically manifests with diffuse skin thickening, trabecular or stromal alterations, and nipple retraction. Clinical examination reveals inflammatory changes in the skin.
- The rapid onset of symptoms such as breast erythema, edema, and characteristic skin changes (peau d'orange) can mimic conditions like mastitis or cellulitis, often leading to diagnostic delays.

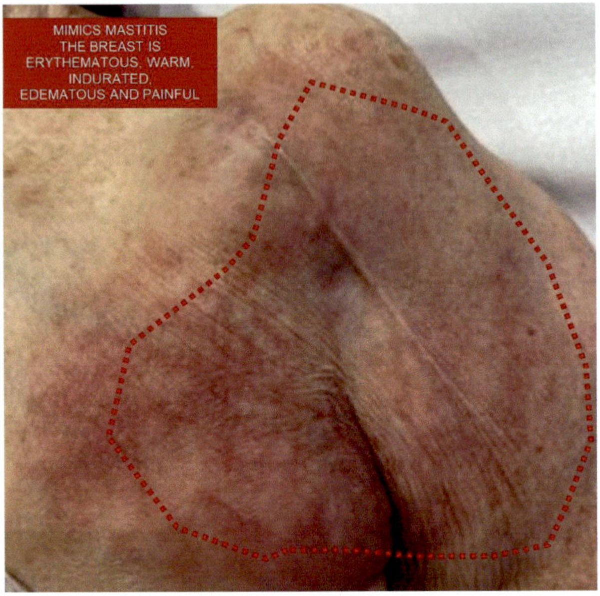

Fig. 15.163 Clinical photograph of patient with cutaneous invasive breast cancer

15.43.4 Dermatoscopy [104]

- Widespread erythema of the skin, which can be more intense and diffuse than typical inflammatory reactions. This is often one of the primary signs.
- Increased swelling and edema of the breast skin, which can appear as a thickened and puffy texture on dermoscopy.
- The presence of prominent, dilated blood vessels (telangiectasia) may be visible, indicating increased blood flow to the area.
- The skin surface may show a rough or uneven texture, with possible scaling or peeling in some areas.
- Small, palpable nodules or masses may be observed, often due to underlying tumor infiltration.
- Unlike benign conditions, inflammatory breast carcinoma may not exhibit the regular patterns seen in other skin conditions. The findings are often more diffuse and irregular.
- The normal demarcation between skin structures may be blurred, reflecting the invasive nature of the carcinoma.

15.43.5 Histopathology (Fig. 15.164) [104]

- Histologically, IBC is characterized by tumor cell infiltration into dermal lymphatics, resulting in skin thickening and edema.

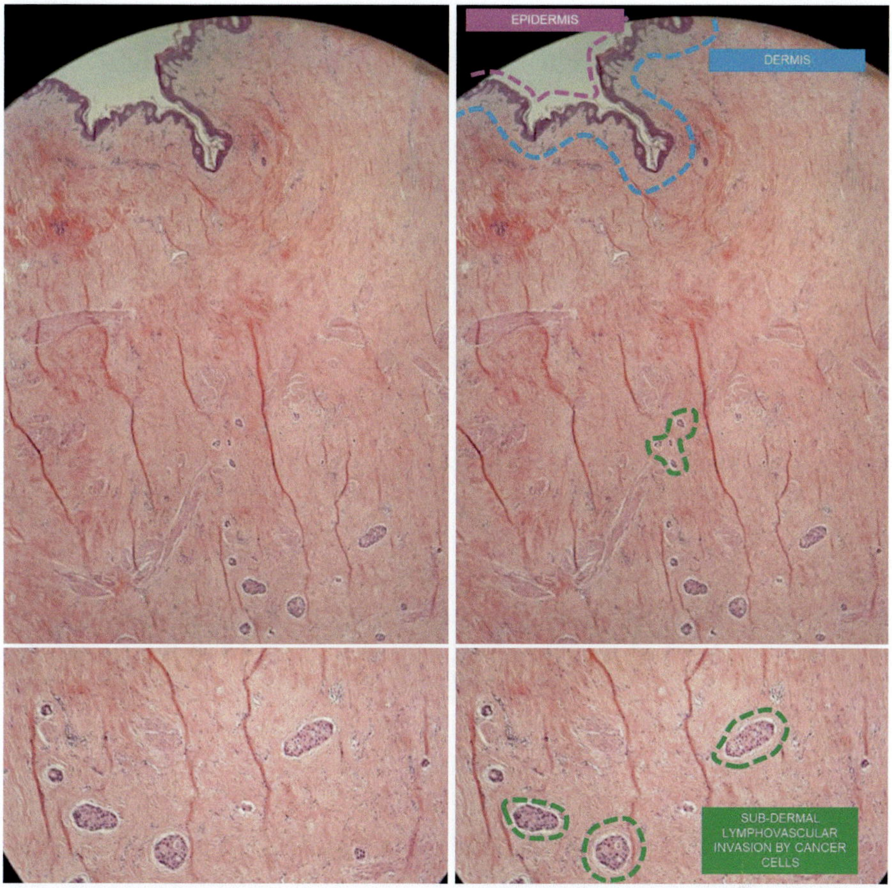

Fig. 15.164 Histological findings of cutaneous invasive breast cancer (H&E x4)

- Key findings include scattered tumor emboli and invasion of dermal lymphatics.
- Molecular subtypes frequently associated with IBC include HER2-positive and triple-negative breast cancer, which tend to exhibit more aggressive behavior compared to non-IBC forms.

15.43.6 Mammography (Fig. 15.165) [105]

- Mammography typically reveals skin thickening, trabecular thickening, and diffuse density changes.
- The presence of malignant microcalcifications is a specific finding when visible.

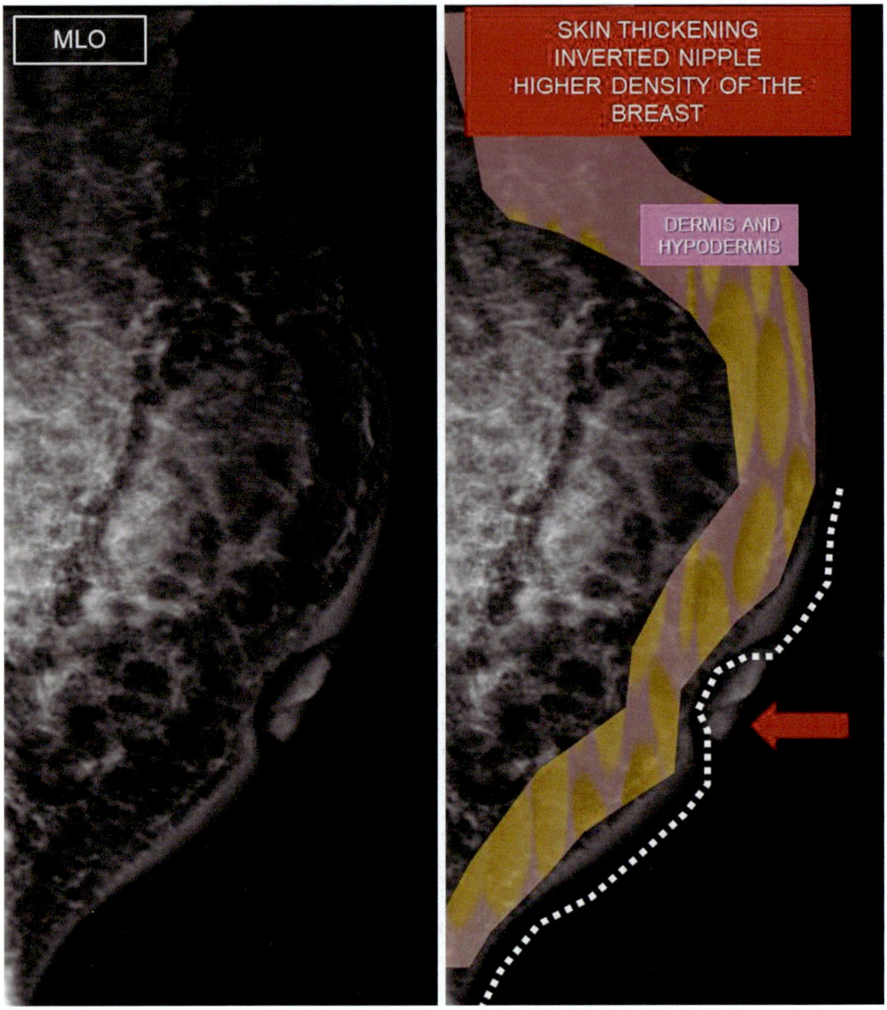

Fig. 15.165 Mammographic findings of cutaneous invasive breast cancer

15.43.7 Computed Tomography [105]

- CT imaging demonstrates increased skin thickness and may occasionally reveal diffuse calcifications, aiding in staging and ongoing monitoring of the disease.

15.43.8 Ultrasonography (Fig. 15.166) [105]

- Ultrasonography is valuable for localizing masses and assessing axillary lymph nodes.
- It typically shows irregular and heterogeneous skin thickeninhg, hypoechoic masses and disrupted echogenic lines within affected tissues. Usually, hypervascularization on power Doppler imaging.

15.43.9 MRI (Fig. 15.167) [105]

- MRI is highly sensitive for detecting skin involvement and evaluating tumor extent and response to treatment.
- It often reveals enhancing tendrils extending toward the skin and may demonstrate axillary adenopathy.

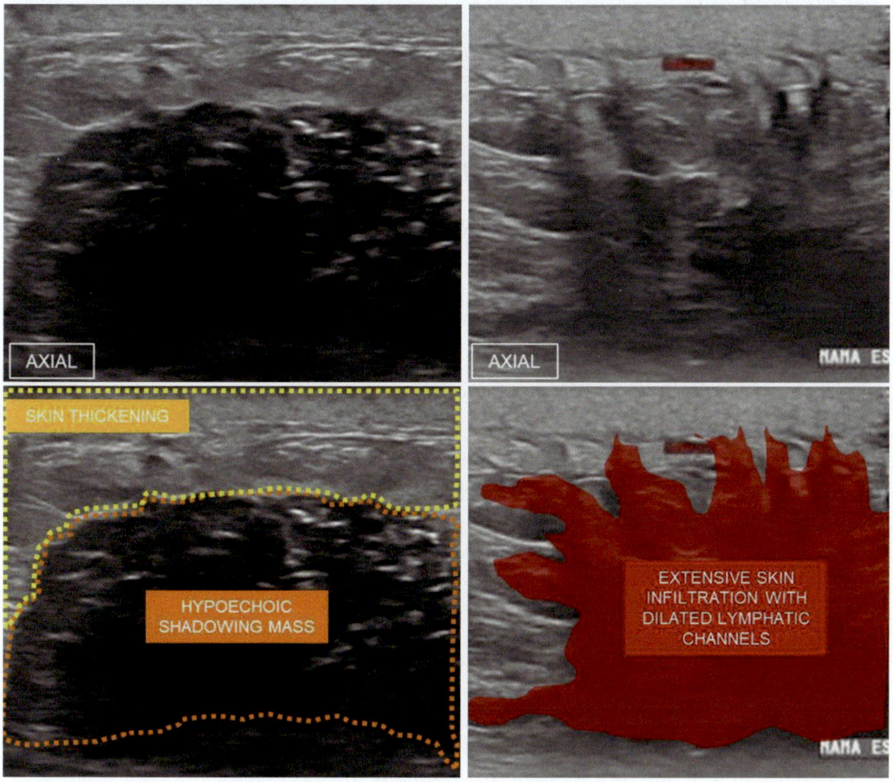

Fig. 15.166 Ultrasonographic findings of cutaneous invasive breast cancer with 16 MHz probe

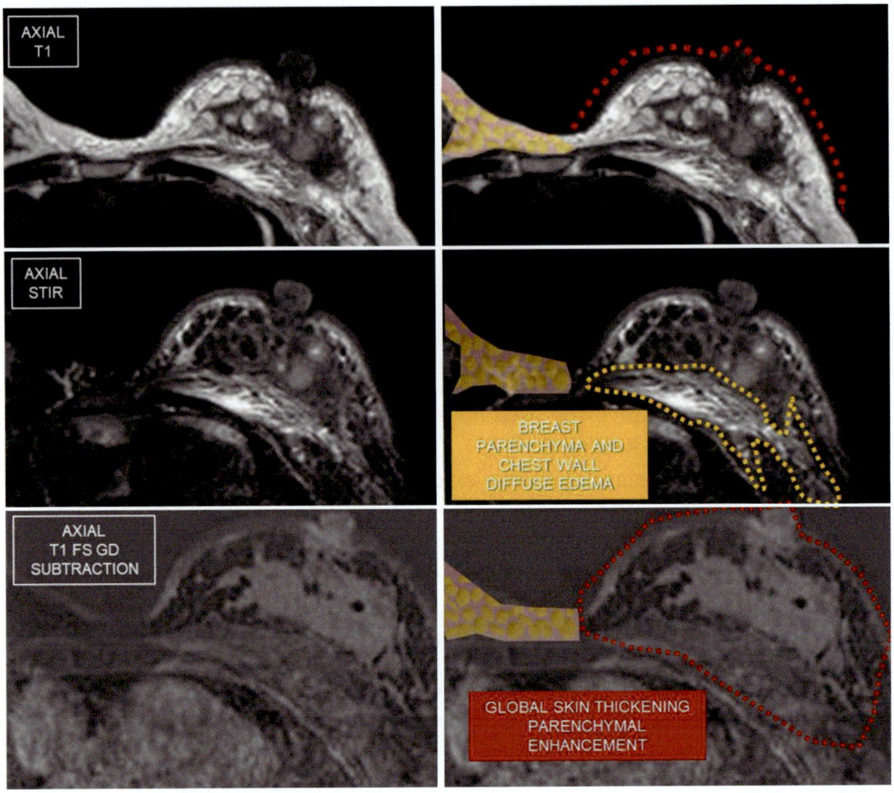

Fig. 15.167 MRI findings of cutaneous invasive breast cancer on T1, STIR, and T1 FS-weighted sequences after gadolinium administration

15.44 Mammary Paget's Disease

15.44.1 Definition [106]

- Mammary Paget disease is an uncommon intraepithelial malignancy characterized by the proliferation of large epidermal adenocarcinoma cells, called Paget's cells, within the nipple, that can extend to the areola and adjacent skin.
- It is often associated with intraductal cancer especially in postmenopausal women.

15.44.2 Epidemiology [106]

- Rare condition accounts for 1–4% of all breast cancers.
- It can affect any age, but its peak incidence is after 60 years.
- Although it is much more common in women, men can also have the disease.

15.44.3 Clinical Presentation (Fig. 15.168) [106]

- It starts with unilateral eczematoid, erythematous lesions, with fine scaling.
- More established cases present with thickened, infiltrated, lesions.
- Advanced cases can be accompanied by bloody or serous papillary discharge, ulceration, and nipple invagination.
- Pigmented lesions, similar to superficial melanoma, have also been described.

15.44.4 Dermoscopy (Fig. 15.169) [107]

- Classic mammary paget disease presents dotted and a few short linear vessels over pink structureless areas, with fine white scales.
- Pigmented paget disease can mimic melanoma. It presents brown structureless areas with pigmented granules, resembling regressive lesions.

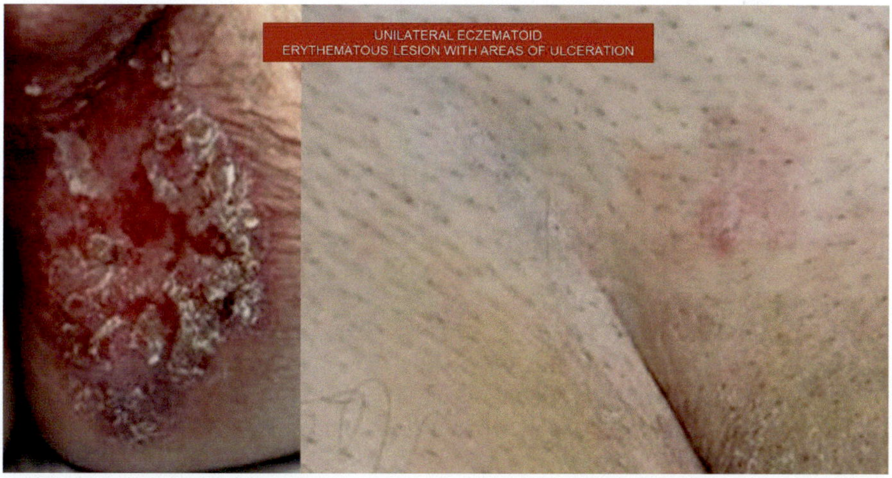

Fig. 15.168 Clinical photograph of patient with Paget's disease of the breast

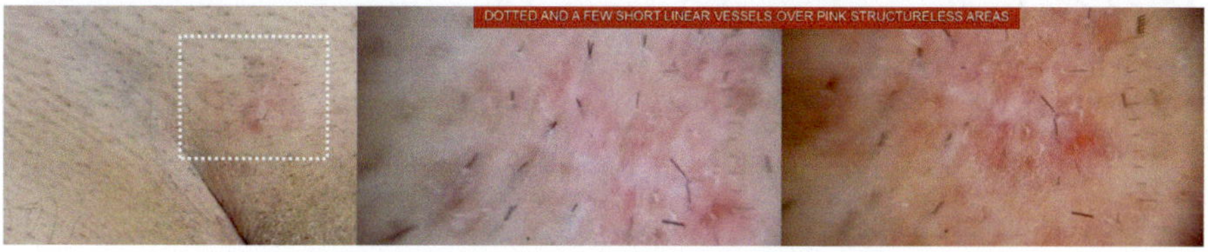

Fig. 15.169 Dermoscopic findings of patient with Paget's disease of the breast (x10)

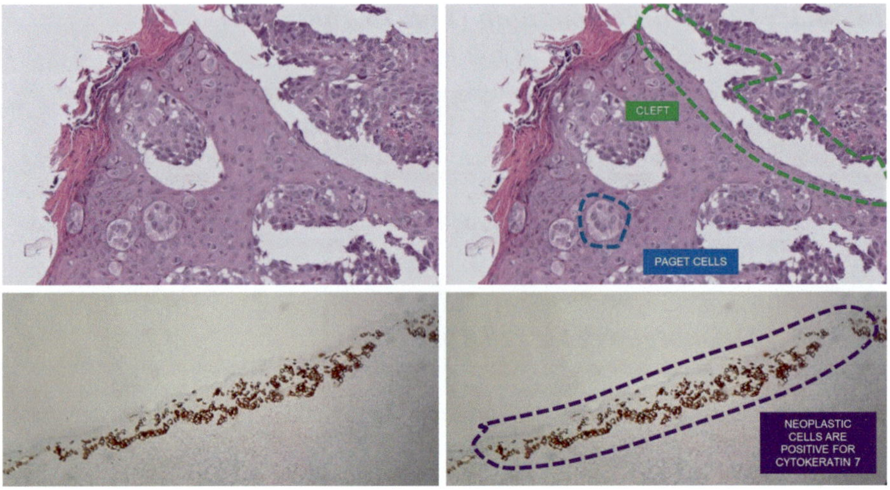

Fig. 15.170 Histological findings of Paget's disease of the breast (H&E x4 and Immunohistochemistry x4)

15.44.5 Histopathology (Fig. 15.170) [106]

- Presence of clear cells, called pagetoid cells, large and polygonal, with atypical nuclei, diffusely distributed throughout the epiderma, which may form groups that compress the basal cells and may present permeation of the adnexal structures (hair follicle and eccrine ducts); often presents with underlying chronic inflammatory infiltrate; erosion may occur and may eventually express melanin; may be differential diagnosis with melanoma superficial scattering, requiring immunohistochemical evaluation; Paget's cells stain with resistant PAS, diastase, and mucicarmine.
- Immunohistochemical profile: CEA, EMA, CAM 5.2, and CK7 (Ber-EP4); CK20 indicates a gastro-intestinal origin in the extra-mammary Paget; GFCD15 and Her-2/neu are also less positive in extramammary, 85.5% vs. 35.5%, aiming at the use of trastuzumab.

15.44.6 Radiography and Computed Tomography (Fig. 15.171) [106]

- Mammary Paget disease can be undetectable on mammography in approximately 50% of cases.

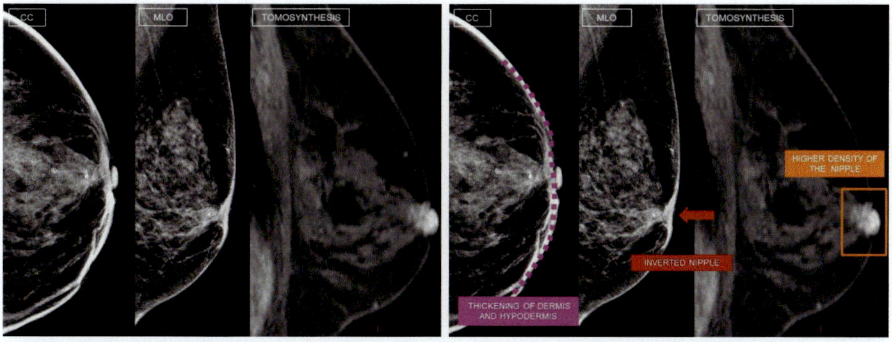

Fig. 15.171 Mammographic findings of Paget's disease of the breast

- Visible features:
- Increased thickness of the skin over the nipple-areolar complex.
- Pulling back of the nipple into the breast due retraction.
- Presence of discrete subareolar masses beneath the areola.
- Malignant microcalcifications that are subareolar or more diffusely spread within the breast.

15.44.7 Ultrasonography (Fig. 15.172) [106]

- Lobulated or irregular masses without posterior acoustic shadowing.
- Nipple-areolar complex presenting flattening, asymmetry, and thickening.
- Ductal ectasia by dilation of the milk ducts.
- Parenchymal heterogeneity.

15.44.8 MRI (Fig. 15.173) [106]

- MRI may show abnormal nipple enhancement, thickening, and enhancement of the nipple-areolar complex.
- There are usually clear asymmetries between the affected and unaffected sides in the characteristics of the nipple-areolar complex.
- MRI has a higher sensitivity than mammography for detecting tumors of the nipple and retroareolar area, showing involvement even when clinically unsuspected.

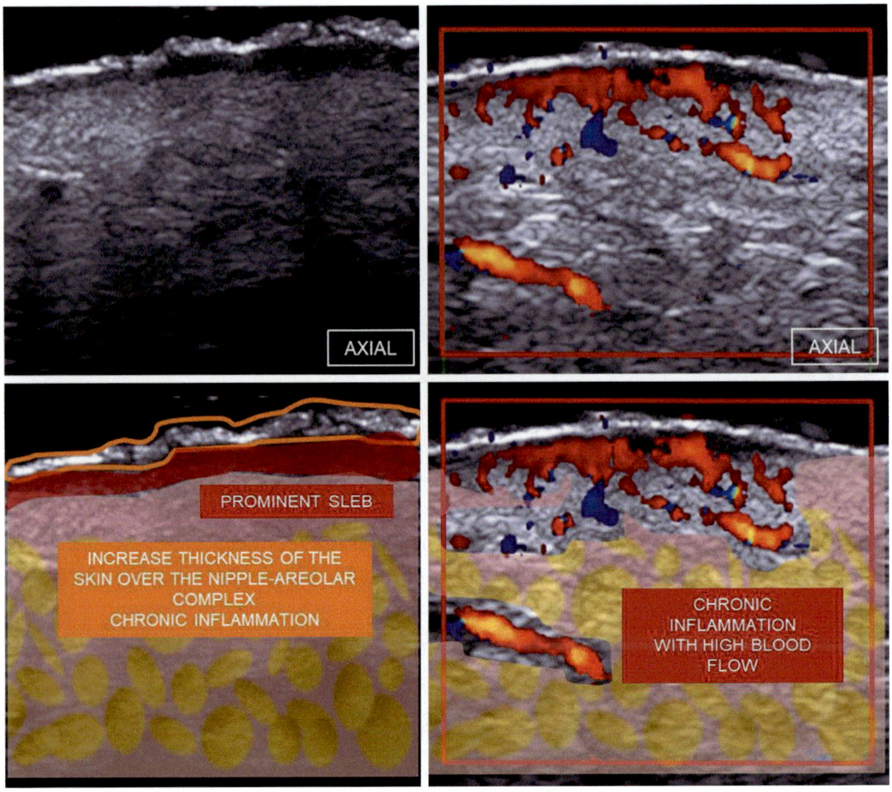

Fig. 15.172 Ultrasonographic findings of Paget's disease of the breast 16 MHz probe (Aplio i800, Canon Medical Systems)

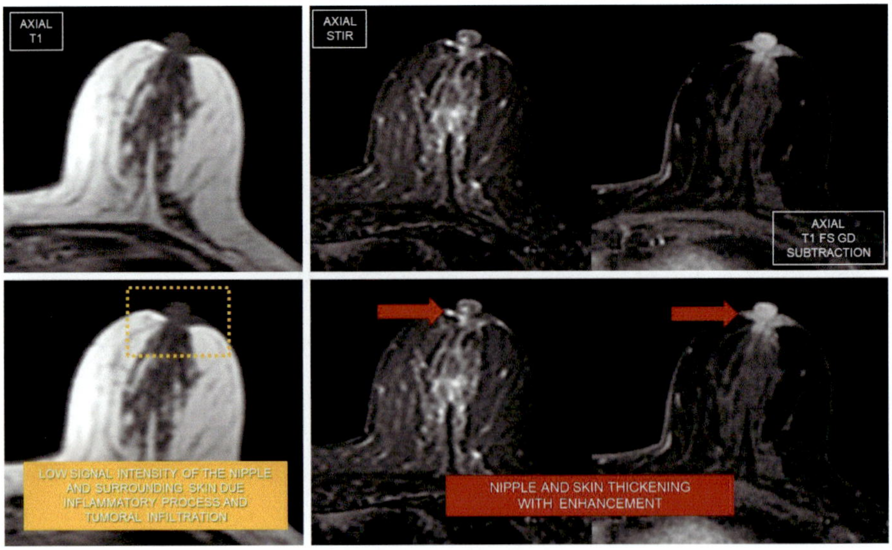

Fig. 15.173 MRI findings of Paget's disease of the breast on T1, STIR, and T1 FS-weighted sequences after gadolinium administration (Magnetom Avanto 1.5T MRI, Siemens)

15.45 Liposarcoma

15.45.1 Definition [6]

- Liposarcoma is a malignant tumor derived from adipocytes.

15.45.2 Epidemiology [6]

- Liposarcomas are the most common soft tissue sarcomas in adults, representing about 15–20% of all soft tissue sarcomas.
- They typically occur in adults aged 50–70 years.

15.45.3 Clinical Presentation (Fig. 15.174) [6]

- Liposarcomas often present as large, painless masses.

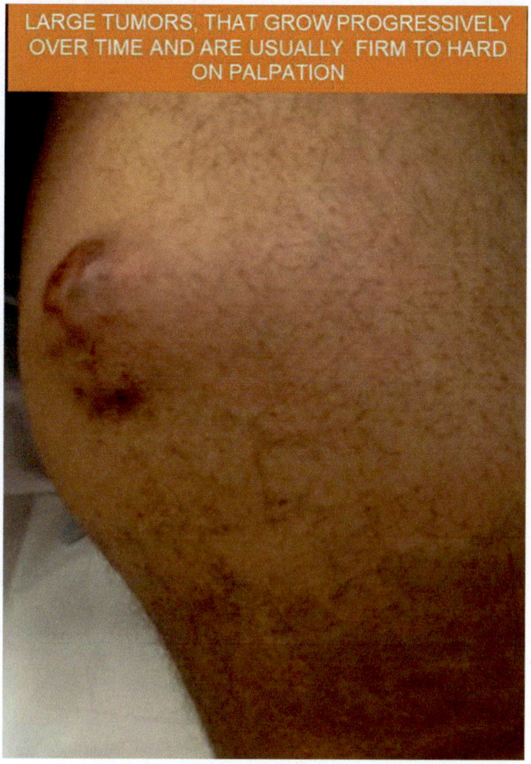

Fig. 15.174 Clinical photograph of patient with liposarcoma

15.45.4 Histopathology (Fig. 15.175) [6]

- Liposarcomas are classified into several subtypes: well-differentiated, myxoid, round cell, pleomorphic, and dedifferentiated.
- They contain varying amounts of lipoblasts, which are indicative of malignancy.

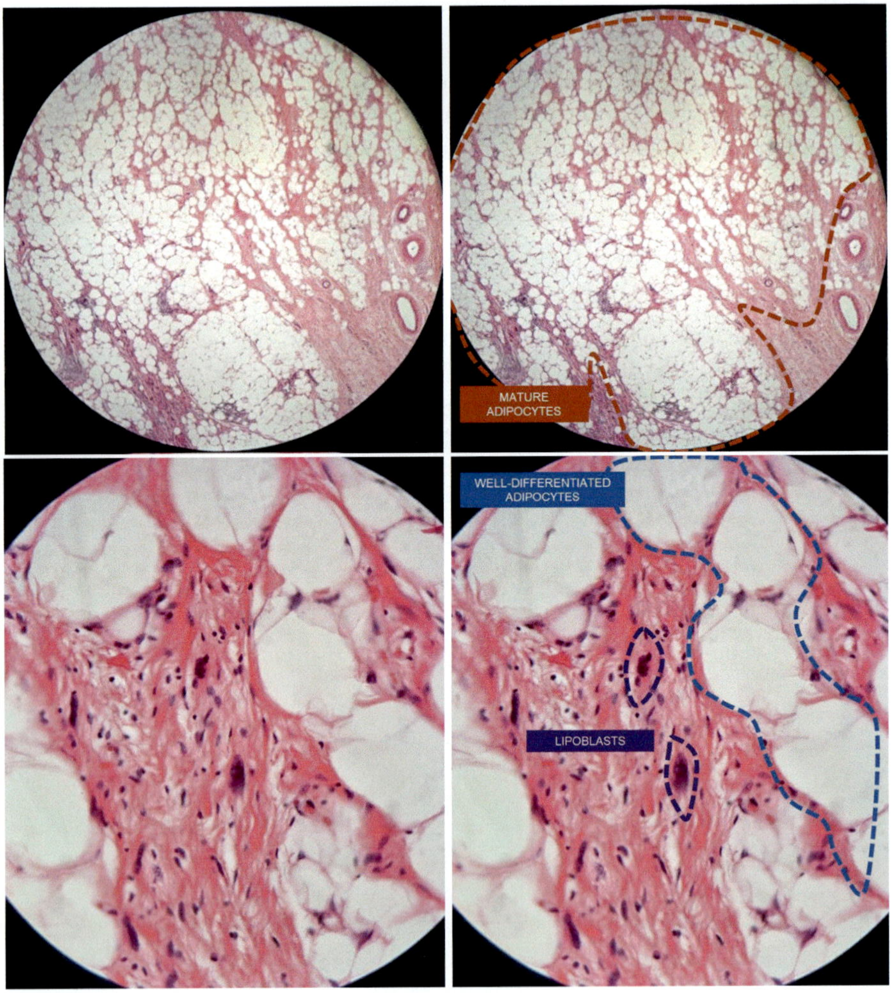

Fig. 15.175 Histological findings of liposarcoma (H&E x10 and x40)

15.45.5 Radiography [108]

- Radiographs of liposarcomas are nonspecific but may show a large soft tissue mass. Calcifications are uncommon but can be present in myxoid and dedifferentiated subtypes.

15.45.6 Computed Tomography [108]

- CT scans show liposarcomas as heterogeneous masses with areas of fat density.
- Well-differentiated liposarcomas can be difficult to distinguish from benign lipomas on CT alone.

15.45.7 Ultrasonography [108]

- Ultrasonography images of liposarcomas show large masses with heterogeneous echogenicity.
- Well-differentiated liposarcomas may appear similar to lipomas but often have thicker septa and high vascularization on power Doppler imaging. Usually present intramuscular location.

15.45.8 MRI (Fig. 15.176) [108]

- MRI is crucial for liposarcoma diagnosis and staging.
- Liposarcomas appear as heterogeneous masses with both high and low signal intensity on T1-weighted and T2-weighted images.
- They often show enhancement with gadolinium contrast.
- Characteristics indicative of well-differentiated liposarcoma include:
  - Tumor size greater than 10 cm.
  - Fat content less than 75%.
  - Septa that are thick or nodular (greater than 2 mm).
  - Presence of nodular or globular areas.
  - Prominent regions of high signal intensity on T2-weighted images.
  - Significant enhancement after contrast administration.
  - Associated nonfatty mass.
  - Location in the lower limb.
  - Intramuscular location.

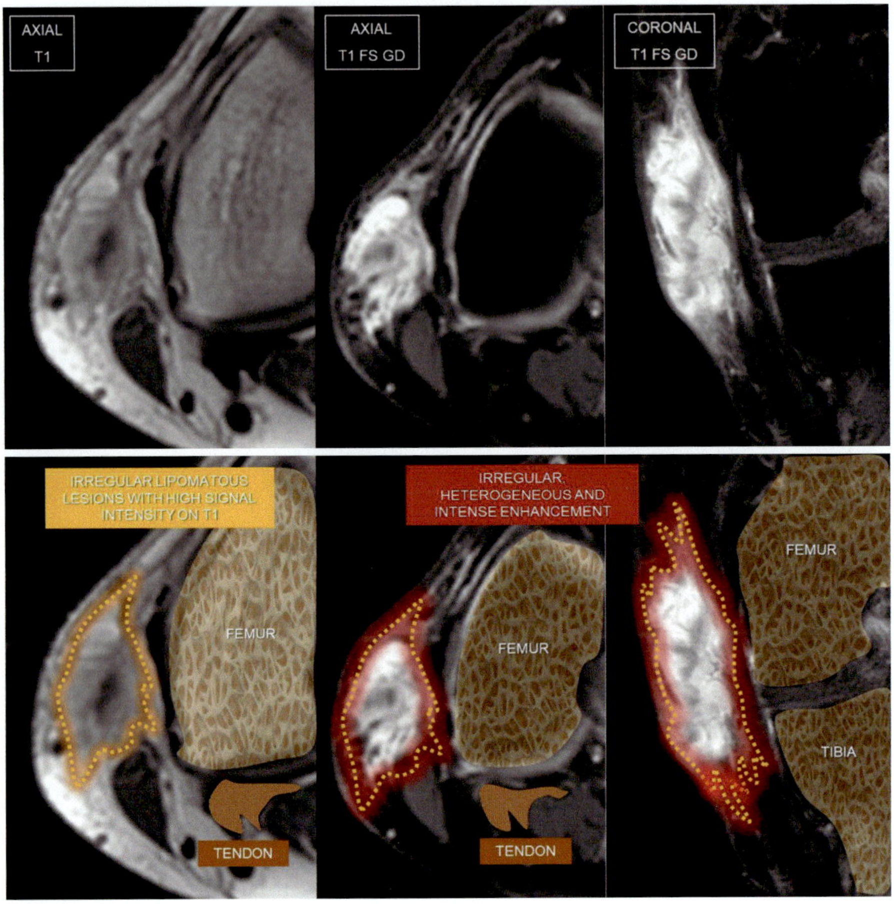

Fig. 15.176 MRI findings of liposarcoma on T1 and T1 FS weighted sequences after gadolinium administration (Magnetom Avanto 1.5T MRI, Siemens)

15.45.9 3D Imaging

- Enables thorough assessment of the lesion, helping to gauge its severity and how it affects surrounding tissues and blood vessels.
- Improves surgical precision, especially in sensitive and complex areas, especially in large tumors.
- Offers valuable insights for both surgical planning and patient education through the creation of physical models of the affected area with biomodels.

15.46 Fibrosarcoma

15.46.1 Definition [109]

- Skin fibrosarcoma is a rare malignant tumor of mesenchymal origin that arises from fibroblasts within the dermis or subcutaneous tissue.
- It is characterized by the proliferation of spindle-shaped cells that produce collagen and other extracellular matrix components.

15.46.2 Epidemiology [109]

- Fibrosarcomas of the skin are rare, accounting for a small percentage of soft tissue sarcomas. They are more commonly found in deeper soft tissues, with cutaneous forms being less frequent.
- These tumors can occur at any age but are more commonly seen in adults, with a slight male predominance.
- There are no well-defined risk factors for skin fibrosarcoma, but previous radiation therapy, chronic lymphedema, and certain genetic conditions may increase the risk.

15.46.3 Clinical Presentation (Fig. 15.177, Video 15.8) [109]

- Skin fibrosarcomas typically present as firm, painless nodules or masses. The overlying skin may be normal or exhibit erythema or ulceration.
- These tumors can vary in size and often grow slowly, though they can be locally aggressive and infiltrative.
- Commonly affected areas include the extremities, particularly the lower legs, but they can occur anywhere on the body.
- They are often asymptomatic until they reach a larger size, at which point they may cause discomfort or functional impairment depending on their location.

15.46.4 Histopathology (Fig. 15.178) [109]

- Histologically, fibrosarcomas are composed of interlacing bundles of spindle-shaped cells with a high degree of cellularity. The cells have elongated nuclei and variable amounts of collagenous stroma. The tumors often show a "herringbone" pattern, which is characteristic but not pathognomonic.
- Fibrosarcomas are graded based on cellularity, mitotic activity, and necrosis. High-grade tumors have a higher likelihood of metastasis and poorer prognosis.

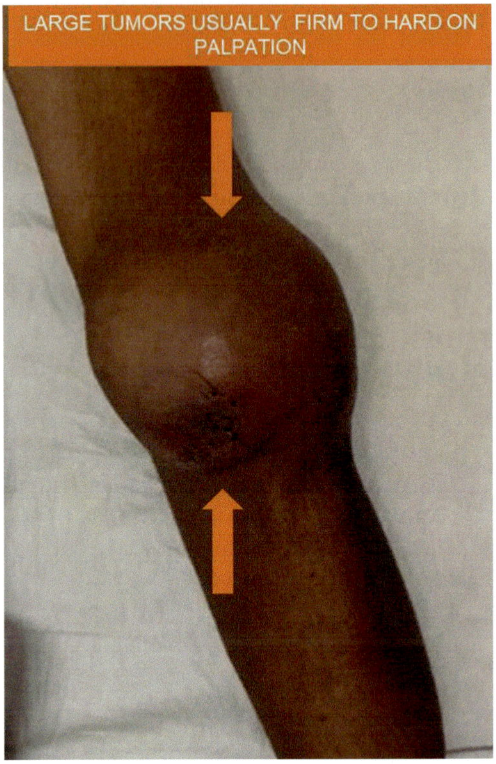

Fig. 15.177 Clinical photograph of patient with fibrosarcoma

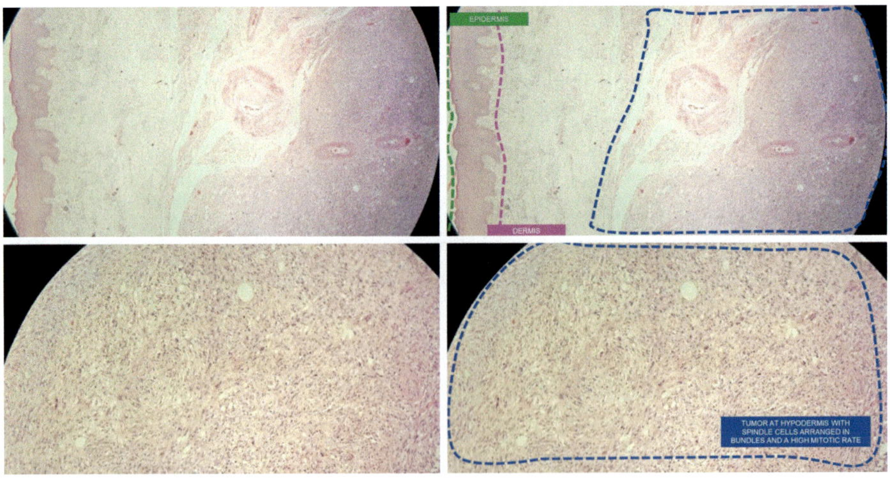

Fig. 15.178 Histological findings of fibrosarcoma (H&E x10)

- These tumors are typically positive for vimentin and may express smooth muscle actin (SMA) but are usually negative for markers of epithelial, neural, or melanocytic differentiation.

15.46.5 Ultrasonography [110]

- On ultrasonography, skin fibrosarcomas usually appear as hypoechoic or mixed echogenicity masses. They may have irregular margins and may show posterior acoustic enhancement due to their solid nature.
- Power Doppler ultrasonography can reveal varying degrees of vascularity within the tumor, which may help differentiate it from benign soft tissue masses.

15.46.6 MRI (Fig. 15.179) [110]

- Fibrosarcomas generally appear as low to intermediate signal intensity lesions on T1-weighted images.
- On T2-weighted images, these tumors typically exhibit high signal intensity, although the degree of signal heterogeneity can vary depending on the tumor's collagen content and cellularity.
- After gadolinium administration, fibrosarcomas usually show heterogeneous enhancement, reflecting their variable cellularity and vascularity.

15.46.7 3D Images (Fig. 15.180 and Video 15.8)

- Facilitates comprehensive imaging evaluation of the lesion, allowing for accurate assessment of its severity and impact on adjacent tissues and vascular structures.
- Enhances surgical accuracy, particularly in delicate or anatomically complex regions, and is especially beneficial when managing large tumors.

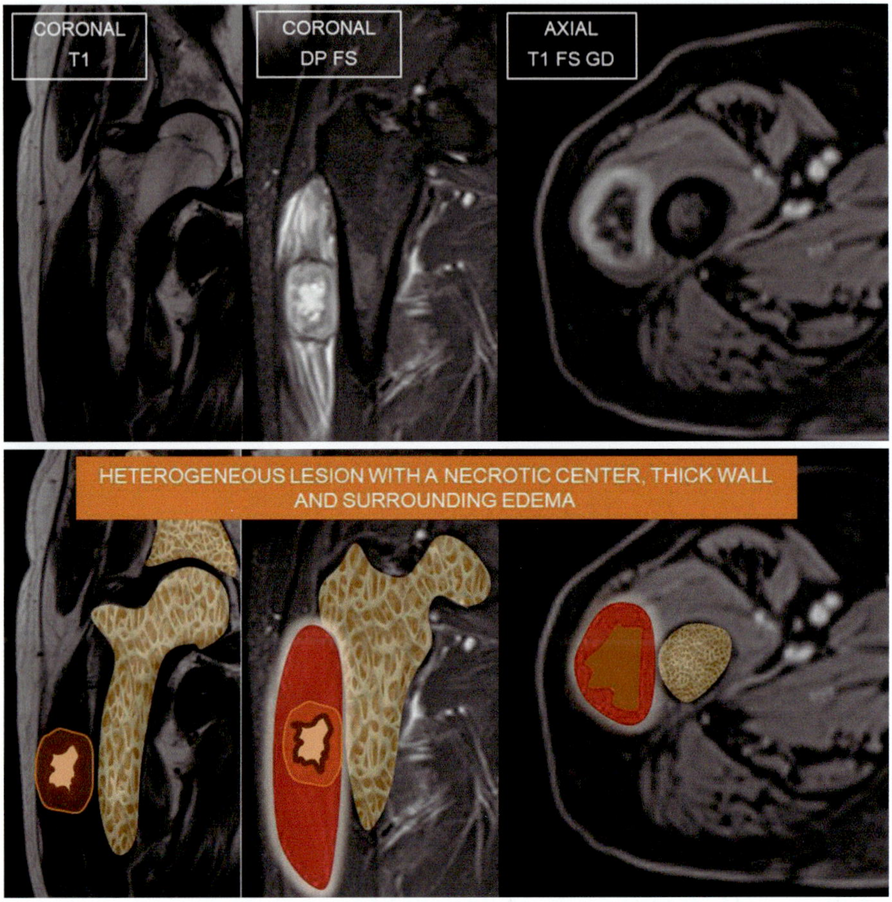

Fig. 15.179 MRI findings of fibrosarcoma on T1, PD FS, and T1 FS-weighted sequences after gadolinium administration (Magnetom Avanto 1.5T MRI, Siemens)

Fig. 15.180 3D images of fibrosarcoma after segmentation of MRI isotropic images used for surgical planning

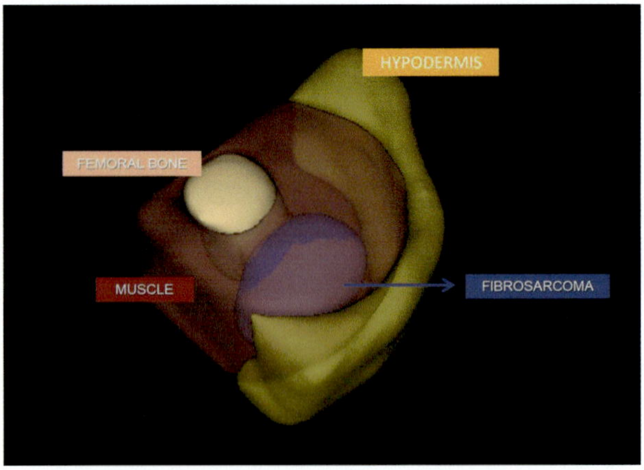

15.47 Synovial Sarcoma

15.47.1 Definition [111]

- Synovial sarcoma is a rare, malignant soft tissue tumor that typically arises near joint capsules, tendons, and bursae.
- Despite its name, it does not originate from synovial tissue but rather from mesenchymal stem cells capable of differentiating into both epithelial and spindle cell components.

15.47.2 Epidemiology [111]

- Synovial sarcoma accounts for approximately 5–10% of all soft tissue sarcomas.
- It primarily affects young adults, with the highest incidence in individuals aged 15–40 years.
- There is a slight male predominance.
- Commonly occurs in the extremities, particularly around the knee and ankle. However, it can also be found in the head and neck, thorax, and abdominal cavity.

15.47.3 Clinical Presentation (Fig. 15.181, Video 15.9) [111]

- Patients often present with a slow-growing, painless mass near a joint. Pain and tenderness may develop as the tumor enlarges.
- The mass is usually firm and may be fixed to deeper tissues. It can vary in size, with larger tumors potentially causing symptoms due to compression of nearby structures.
- Although typically located near joints, synovial sarcomas rarely invade the joint itself. When near a joint, it may cause restricted movement or discomfort.
- Rarely, patients may present with systemic symptoms such as weight loss or fatigue, particularly in advanced cases.

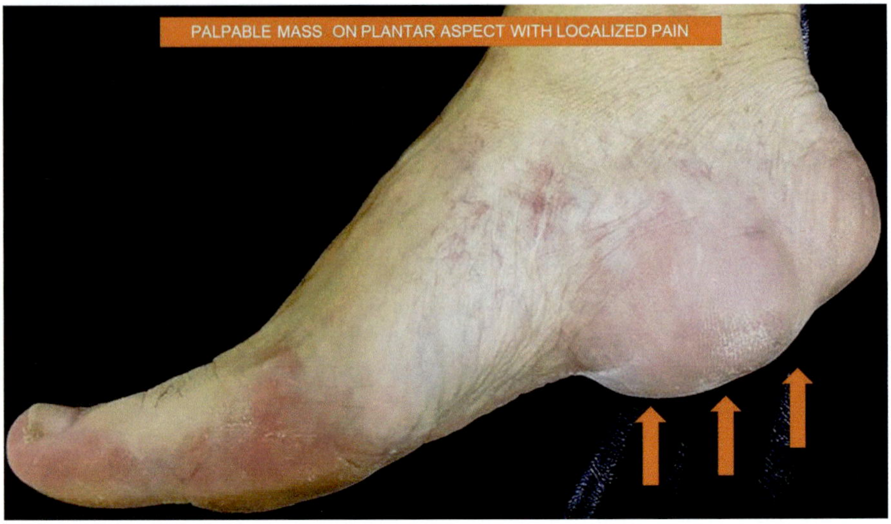

Fig. 15.181 Clinical photograph of patient with synovial sarcoma

15.47.4 Histopathology (Fig. 15.182) [111]

- Synovial sarcomas are characterized by a biphasic pattern, with both spindle cells (mesenchymal component) and epithelial cells. The epithelial component forms gland-like structures, while the spindle cells form dense, intersecting fascicles.
- Some synovial sarcomas may show a predominantly spindle cell (monophasic) or poorly differentiated pattern, making diagnosis challenging.
- A defining feature of synovial sarcoma is the presence of the t(X;18) translocation, which results in the SS18-SSX fusion gene. This translocation is found in over 90% of cases.
- Typically positive for markers such as TLE1, cytokeratins, and epithelial membrane antigen (EMA).

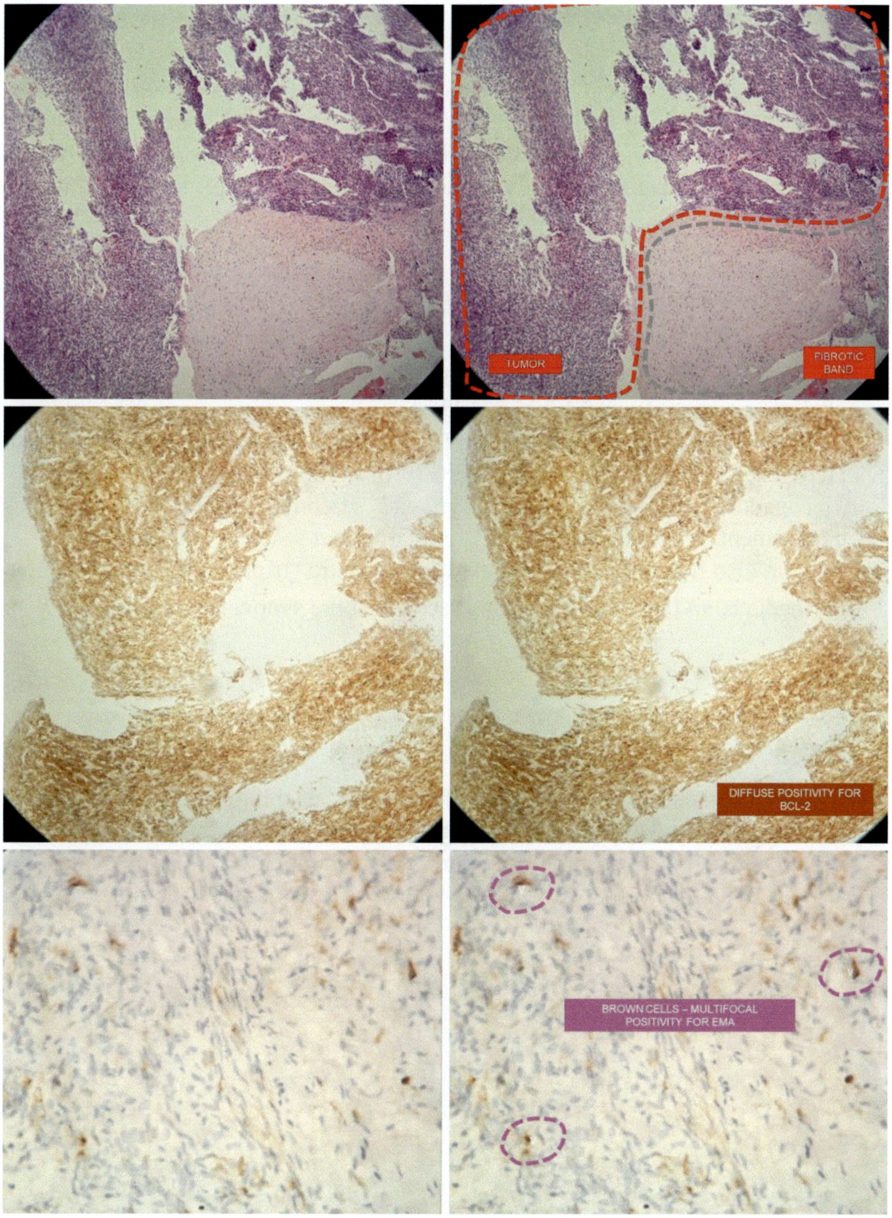

Fig. 15.182 Histological findings of synovial sarcoma (H&E x10 and Immunohistochemistry x10)

15.47.5 *Ultrasonography [112]*

- Synovial sarcomas appear as heterogeneous, hypoechoic masses on ultrasonography. They may have areas of calcification and can be well-defined or irregular.
- Increased vascularity is often seen on power Doppler ultrasonography, which may help in differentiating synovial sarcoma from benign soft tissue lesions.

15.47.6 MRI (Fig. 15.183) [112]

- Synovial sarcomas typically present with isointense or slightly hyperintense signal relative to muscle on T1-weighted images.
- They show high signal intensity on T2-weighted images, often with areas of heterogeneity due to hemorrhage, necrosis, or cystic changes.
- After gadolinium administration, synovial sarcomas exhibit heterogeneous enhancement, reflecting their mixed cellularity and vascular components.
- MRI can also help in identifying the characteristic "triple sign" (areas of high, intermediate, and low sgnal intensity) seen in some synovial sarcomas.

15.47.7 3D Images (Fig. 15.184 and Video 15.9)

- Provides a detailed imaging analysis of the lesion, enabling precise evaluation of its extent and its relationship with surrounding tissues and blood vessels.
- Supports greater surgical precision, particularly in intricate or sensitive anatomical areas, and proves especially useful in the treatment of large or complex tumors.

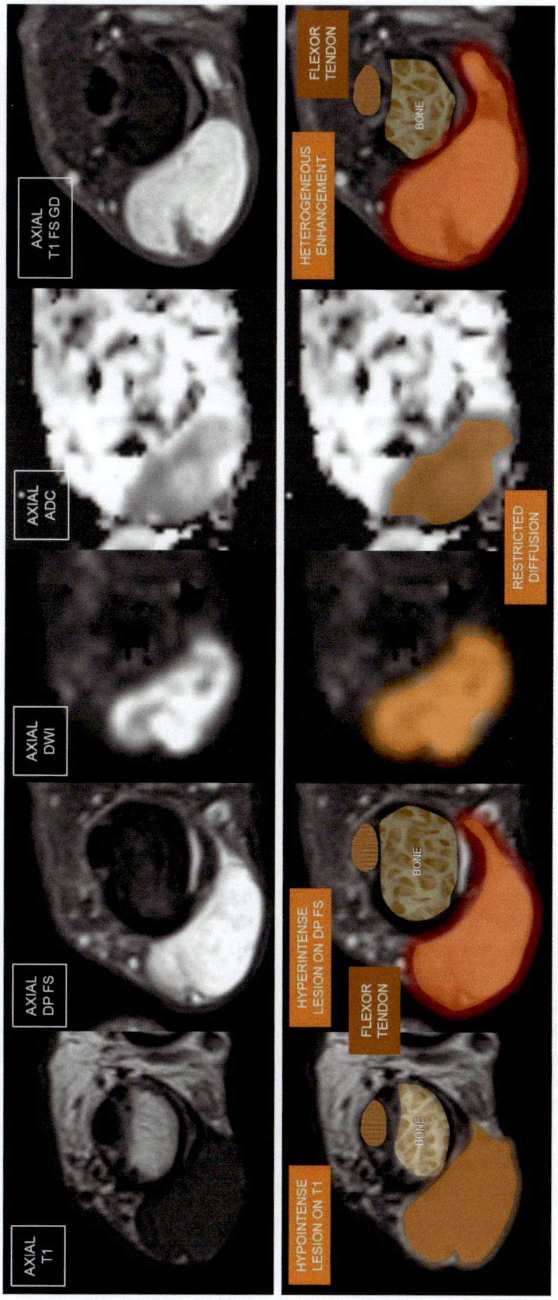

Fig. 15.183 MRI findings of synovial sarcoma on T1, PD FS, DWI, and T1 FS-weighted sequences after gadolinium administration (Magnetom Avanto 1.5T MRI, Siemens)

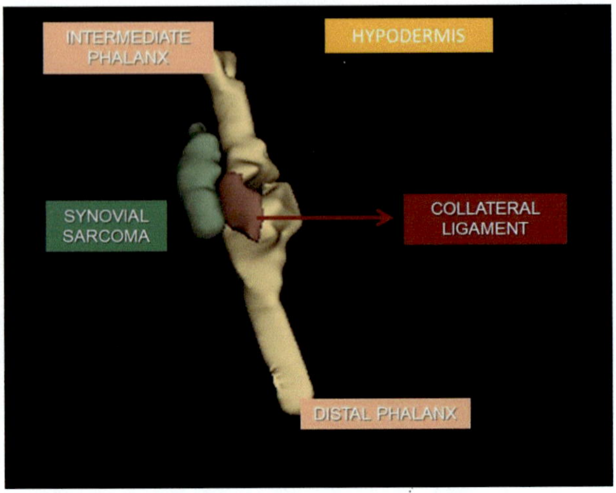

Fig. 15.184 3D images of synovial sarcoma after segmentation of MRI isotropic images used for surgical planning

References

1. Sellami K, Fourati M. Epidermal cyst of unusual localization. Skinmed. 2022;20:291.
2. Ghigliotti G, Cinotti E, Parodi A. Usefulness of dermoscopy for the diagnosis of epidermal cyst: the 'pore' sign. Clin Exp Dermatol. 2014;39:649–50. https://academic.oup.com/ced/article/39/5/649/6621040.
3. López-Ríos F, Rodríguez-Peralto JL, Castaño E, Benito A. Squamous cell carcinoma arising in a cutaneous epidermal cyst. Am J Dermatopathol. 1999;21:174–7.
4. Park JW, Shin SH, Kim BJ, Li K. Usefulness of ultrasound in diagnosis of plantar epidermal cyst. Indian J Dermatol Venereol Leprol. 2021;87:872.
5. Hong SH, Chung HW, Choi J-Y, Koh YH, Choi J-A, Kang HS. MRI findings of subcutaneous epidermal cysts: emphasis on the presence of rupture. Am J Roentgenol. 2006;186:961–6.
6. Kransdorf MJ, Bancroft LW, Peterson JJ, Murphey MD, Foster WC, Temple HT. Imaging of fatty tumors: distinction of lipoma and well-differentiated Liposarcoma. Radiology. 2002;224:99–104.
7. Kolb L, Naga Yarrarapu SS, Atif Ameer M, Rosario-Collazo JA. Lipoma. 2023. https://www.ncbi.nlm.nih.gov/books/NBK507906/?report=printable.
8. Johnson CN, Ha AS, Chen E, Davidson D. Lipomatous soft-tissue tumors. J Am Acad Orthop Surg. 2018;26:779–88. https://journals.lww.com/00124635-201811150-00001.
9. Burt AM, Huang BK. Imaging review of lipomatous musculoskeletal lesions. SICOT J. 2017;3:34. https://doi.org/10.1051/sicotj/2017015.
10. Ferrari A, Argenziano G, Buccini P, Cota C, Sperduti I, De Simone P, et al. Typical and atypical dermoscopic presentations of dermatofibroma. J Eur Acad Dermatol Venereol. 2013;27:1375–80.
11. Han TY, Chang HS, Lee JHK, Lee W-M, Son S-J. A clinical and histopathological study of 122 cases of dermatofibroma (benign fibrous histiocytoma). Ann Dermatol. 2011;23:185.
12. Zaballos P, Puig S, Llambrich A, Malvehy J. Dermoscopy of dermatofibromas: a prospective morphological study of 412 cases. Arch Dermatol. 2008;144:75–83.
13. Li D, Yang F, Zhao Y, Wang Q, Ren W, Sun L, et al. High-frequency ultrasound imaging to distinguish high-risk and low-risk dermatofibromas. Diagnostics. 2023;13:3305.
14. Sawaya JL, Khachemoune A. Poroma: a review of eccrine, apocrine, and malignant forms. Int J Dermatol. 2014;53:1053–61. https://doi.org/10.1111/ijd.12448.
15. McCoskey M, Neerukonda VK, Hatton MP, Wolkow N. Eccrine poroma of the eyelid. Orbit. 2021;43:1–1. https://doi.org/10.1080/01676830.2021.1939732.
16. Kyrmanidou E, Fotiadou C, Kemanetzi C, Trakatelli M-G, Trigoni A, Patsatsi A, et al. Eccrine Poroma: pathogenesis, new diagnostic tools and association with Porocarcinoma—a review. Diagnostics. 2023;13:2689. https://www.mdpi.com/2075-4418/13/16/2689.

17. Takada T. Diagnostic features of a non-pigmented eccrine poroma with a collarette: histopathological and dermoscopic correlation. Clin Case Rep. 2021;9:1601–4. https://doi.org/10.1002/ccr3.3848.
18. Maciel MG, Enokihara MMSES, Seize MBDMP, Marcassi AP, Piazza CADD, Cestari SDCP. Elastoma: clinical and histopathological aspects of a rare disease. An Bras Dermatol. 2016;91:39–41.
19. Klevos G, Jose J, Pretell-Mazzini J, Conway S. Imaging series hibernoma. Am J Orthop. 2015;44(6):284–7. www.amjorthopedics.com.
20. Santos MA, Foulke G. Koebnerization and eruptive xanthomas. J Gen Intern Med. 2019;34:1947–8.
21. Marogi EP, Ohiomoba RO, Stone NJ. Eruptive xanthomas: importance of recognition to reduce delay of effective triglyceride reduction. Am J Med. 2022;135:444–7.
22. Lee JY, Kang BS, Shim HS, Song IH, Kim M, Lee SH, et al. Clear cell hidradenoma: characteristic imaging features on ultrasonography, computed tomography, and magnetic resonance imaging. J Ultrasound Med. 2018;37:1993–2000.
23. Belgam Syed SY, Lipoff JB, Acrochordon CK. StatPearls. 2024. http://www.ncbi.nlm.nih.gov/pubmed/22345761.
24. Nath MC, Torbenson MS, Erickson LA. Desmoid Tumor. Mayo Clin Proc. 2018;93:549–50.
25. Milos RI, Moritz T, Bernathova M, Amann G, Panotopoulos J, Huhmann IMN, et al. Superficial desmoid tumors: MRI and ultrasound imaging characteristics. Eur J Radiol. 2015;84:2194–201.
26. Luna A, Molinari L, Bollea Garlatti LA, Ferrario D, Volonteri V, Roitman P, et al. Nodular fasciitis, a forgotten entity. Int J Dermatol. 2019;58:190–3.
27. Yen H-H, Chiou H-J, Chou Y-H, Chen C-H, Guo W-Y. Nodular Fasciitis: Sonographic–Pathologic Correlation. Ultrasound Med Biol. 2017;43:860–7.
28. Dinauer PA, Brixey CJ, Moncur JT, Fanburg-Smith JC, Murphey MD. Pathologic and MR imaging features of benign fibrous soft-tissue tumors in adults. Radiographics. 2007;27:173–87.
29. Helm T, Bir C, Chilstrom M, Claudius I. Ultrasound characteristics of bruises and their correlation to cutaneous appearance. Forensic Sci Int. 2016;266:160–3.
30. Shelly MJ, Hodnett PA, MacMahon PJ, Moynagh MR, Kavanagh EC, Eustace SJ. MR imaging of muscle injury. Magn Reson Imaging Clin N Am. 2009;17:757–73.
31. Behzad B, Dianat S. Magnetic resonance imaging of nerve tumors. Semin Musculoskelet Radiol. 2022;26:172–81.
32. Woertler K. Tumors and tumor-like lesions of peripheral nerves. Semin Musculoskelet Radiol. 2010;14:547–58.
33. Barnhill RL, Neil Crowson A, Magro CM, Piepkorn MW, Kutzner H, Desman GT. Barnhill's Dermatopathology. 4th ed. New York: McGraw Hill/Medical; 2019. https://dermatology.mhmedical.com/content.aspx?bookid=2802&sectionid=238125236.
34. Raffin D, Zaragoza J, Georgescou G, Mourtada Y, Maruani A, Ossant F, et al. High-frequency ultrasound imaging for cutaneous neurofibroma in patients with neurofibromatosis type I. Eur J Dermatol. 2017;27:260–5.
35. Sieratzki JS. Traumatic neuroma. Hum Pathol. 1986;17:866.
36. Whitehouse HJ, Urwin R, Stables G. Traumatic subungual neuroma. Clin Exp Dermatol. 2018;43:65–6.
37. Forte AJ, Boczar D, Oliver JD, Sisti A, Clendenen SR. Ultra-high-frequency ultrasound to assess nerve fascicles in median nerve traumatic neuroma. Cureus. 2019;11:e4871.
38. Majbar A, Hrora A, Jahid A, Ahallat M, Raiss M. Perineal schwannoma. BMC Res Notes. 2016;9:304.
39. Ghosh BC, Ghosh L, Huvos AG, Fortner JG. Malignant schwannoma. A clinicopathologic study. Cancer. 1973;31:184–90.
40. Yuan Y, Gao J, Xiong G, Guo L. Diagnostic accuracy of multiparametric ultrasound for peripheral nerve schwannoma. Acta Radiol. 2023;64:1608–14.
41. Pfeiffer J, White CL. Large, presacral schwannoma: imaging and treatment. PM&R. 2021;13:427–8.
42. Muradia I, Khullar G, Pareek V. Porokeratosis. JAMA Dermatol. 2023;159:209.

43. Vargas-Mora P, Morgado-Carrasco D, Fustà-Novell X. Poroqueratosis. Revisión de su etiopatogenia, manifestaciones clínicas, diagnóstico y tratamiento. Actas Dermosifiliogr. 2020;111:545–60.
44. Nicola A, Magliano J. Dermoscopy of disseminated superficial actinic Porokeratosis. Actas Dermosifiliogr. 2017;108:e33–7.
45. Sharma A, Agrawal S, Dhurat R, Shukla D, Vishwanath T. An unusual case of facial steatocystoma multiplex: a clinicopathologic and dermoscopic report. Dermatopathology. 2018;5:58–63.
46. Sonnenblick EB, Buchness MR, Austin JHM. CT demonstration of Steatocystoma multiplex. J Comput Assist Tomogr. 1986;10:357–9. http://journals.lww.com/00004728-198603000-00043.
47. Arceu M, Martinez G, Alfaro D, Wortsman X. Ultrasound morphologic features of Steatocystoma multiplex with clinical correlation. J Ultrasound Med. 2020;39:2255–60.
48. Nepal P, Alam SI, Rodrigue P, Sajid S, Taha NM. Imaging findings of rare plantar eccrine spiradenoma. Foot Ankle Surg Tech Rep Cases. 2021;1:100014. https://linkinghub.elsevier.com/retrieve/pii/S2667396721000148.
49. Lugowska-Umer H, Czarny J, Rydz A, Nowicki RJ, Lange M. Current challenges in the diagnosis of pediatric cutaneous mastocytosis. Diagnostics. 2023;13:3583.
50. Baba A, Okuyama Y, Yakabe H, Yamazoe S, Kobashi Y, Mogami T. Surfers' knots in the anterior chest. Clin Case Rep. 2019;7:597–8.
51. McManus LJ, Thomson A, Whan A. The magnetic resonance appearance of surfers' knots: a case report. Radiol Case Rep. 2016;11:201–6.
52. Rupert J, Honeycutt JD, Odom MR. Foreign bodies in the skin: evaluation and management. Am Fam Physician. 2020;101:740–7. http://www.ncbi.nlm.nih.gov/pubmed/32538598.
53. del Cura JL, Aza I, Zabala RM, Sarabia M, Korta I. US-guided localization and removal of soft-tissue foreign bodies. RadioGraphics. 2020;40:1188–95. https://doi.org/10.1148/rg.2020200001.
54. Molina-Ruiz AM, Requena L. Foreign body granulomas. Dermatol Clin. 2015;33:497–523.
55. Brown F, Cook C. Piezogenic Pedal Papule Continuing Education Activity. https://www.ncbi.nlm.nih.gov/books/NBK482153/?report=printable.
56. Clinite KL, Wyble A, Sugarman JL. Tibialis anterior muscle herniation in adolescents: a case series and review of the literature. Pediatr Dermatol. 2019;36:664–7.
57. Matei A-M, Draghici-Ionescu A-M, Cioplea M, Zurac S, Boda D, Serban I, et al. Skin endometriosis: a case report and review of the literature. Exp Ther Med. 2021;21:532. https://doi.org/10.3892/etm.2021.9964.
58. Tognetti L, Cinotti E, Tonini G, Habougit C, Cambazard F, Rubegni P, et al. New findings in non-invasive imaging of cutaneous endometriosis: dermoscopy, high-frequency ultrasound and reflectance confocal microscopy. Skin Res Technol. 2018;24:309–12. https://doi.org/10.1111/srt.12431.
59. Raffi L, Suresh R, McCalmont TH, Twigg AR. Cutaneous endometriosis. Int J Womens Dermatol. 2019;5:384–6.
60. Quirós-Roldán E, Pan A, Moretti F, Casari S, Carosi G. Lipodistrofia periférica. Rev Clin Esp. 2002;202:622.
61. Giovannini I, Zandonella Callegher S, Errichetti E, De Vita S, Zabotti A. Knuckle pads mimic early psoriatic arthritis. Reumatismo. 2021;73:67–9.
62. Qadeer HA, Singal A, Patel BC. Cherry Hemangioma. 2024.
63. Deborah Rachelle Shatzkes. Vascular anomalies: description, classification and nomenclature. Appl Radiol. 2018;18:4. https://www.appliedradiology.com/articles/vascular-anomalies-description-classification-and-nomenclature.
64. Alfageme Roldán F, Salgüero Fernández I, Zamanta Muñoz Garza F, Roustán Gullón G. Update on the use of ultrasound in vascular anomalies. Actas Dermo-Sifiliográficas (English Edition). 2016;107:284–93.
65. Mittal A, Anand R, Gauba R, Choudhury SR, Abbey P. A step-by-step sonographic approach to vascular anomalies in the pediatric population: a pictorial essay. Indian J Radiol Imaging. 2021;31:157–71.
66. Assiri A, Perier-Muzet M, Dalle S. Angiokératome. Ann Dermatol Venereol. 2020;147:575–6.

67. Amat-Samaranch V, Morales-Múnera C, Puig L, Roé E. Diagnostic value of cutaneous ultrasound in verrucous venous malformation. Actas Dermosifiliogr (Engl Ed). 2021;112:958–61.
68. Nagarajan K, Banushree C. Usefulness of MRI in delineation of dermal and subcutaneous verrucous hemangioma. Indian J Dermatol. 2015;60:525.
69. Sasso SE, Naspolini AP, de Milanez TB, Suchard G. Masson's tumor (intravascular papillary endothelial hyperplasia). An Bras Dermatol. 2019;94:620–1.
70. Utami AM, Azahaf S, de Boer OJ, van der Horst CMAM, Meijer-Jorna LB, van der Wal AC. A literature review of microvascular proliferation in arteriovenous malformations of skin and soft tissue. J Clin Transl Res. 2021;7:540–57.
71. Viswan P, Behera B, Sethy M, Dash S, Palit A, Ayyanar P. Dermoscopic analysis of vascular malformations and tumors based upon dominant vascular dermoscopic features: a retrospective analysis from a tertiary care center of East India. Cureus. 2022;14:1.
72. Monsignore LM, Nakiri GS, Dos SD, Giansante Abud T, Abud DG. Peripheral vascular malformations Radiol Bras Mai. 2010.
73. Rodríguez Bandera AI, Feito Rodríguez M, Chiloeches Fernández C, Stewart N, Valdivielso-Ramos M. Role of colour-Doppler high-frequency ultrasonography in capillary malformation-arteriovenous malformation syndrome: a case series. Australas J Dermatol. 2020;61:349–52.
74. Dhagat PK, Jain M, Farooq A. MRI evaluation of soft tissue vascular malformations. Indian J Radiol Imaging. 2020;30:184–9.
75. Sen I, Agarwal S. Cutaneous lesions from lymphangioma circumscriptum. ANZ J Surg. 2017;87:E20.
76. Miceli A, Stewart KM. Lymphangioma. In: StatPearls. Treasure Island, FL: StatPearls Publishing; 2024.
77. Jha AK, Lallas A, Sonthalia S. Dermoscopy of cutaneous lymphangioma circumscriptum. Dermatol Pract Concept. 2017;7:37.
78. Minotto R, Rodrigues CB, Grill AB, Furian R. Giant cell tumor of the tendon sheath: a rare periungual location simulating myxoid cyst. An Bras Dermatol. 2017;92:121–3.
79. Di Grazia S. Giant cell tumor of tendon sheath: study of 64 cases and review of literature. G Chir. 2013;34:284.
80. Wan JMC, Magarelli N, Peh WCG, Guglielmi G, Shek TWH. Imaging of giant cell tumour of the tendon sheath. Radiol Med. 2010;115:141–51.
81. Stewart BD, Nascimento AF. Palmar and plantar fibromatosis: a review. J Pathol Transl Med. 2021;55:265–70.
82. Walker EA, Petscavage JM, Brian PL, Logie CI, Montini KM, Murphey MD. Imaging features of superficial and deep fibromatoses in the adult population. Sarcoma. 2012;2012:1–17.
83. Larocca C, Kupper T. Mycosis Fungoides and Sézary syndrome. Hematol Oncol Clin North Am. 2019;33:103–20.
84. Piccolo V, Russo T, Agozzino M, Vitiello P, Caccavale S, Alfano R, et al. Dermoscopy of cutaneous lymphoproliferative disorders: where are we now? Dermatology. 2018;234:131–6.
85. Wang Y, Niu Z, Liu J, Zhu Q, Liu Z, Liu Y, et al. Value of high-frequency ultrasound in accurate staging of mycosis Fungoides/Sézary syndrome. J Ultrasound Med. 2020;39:1927–37.
86. Ortín X, Llorente A, Martínez S, Ugarriza A. Plasmocitoma cutáneo en el curso del tratamiento del mieloma múltiple inmunoglobulina A-kappa. Med Clin (Barc). 2004;123:597–8.
87. Koletsa T, Patsatsi A, Kostopoulos I, Kartsios C, Korantzis I, Sotiriadis D. A case of a primary cutaneous Plasmacytoma presenting in adolescence. Am J Dermatopathol. 2012;34:537–40.
88. Kim DP, Kus KJB, Ruiz E. Basal Cell Carcinoma Review. Hematol Oncol Clin North Am. 2019;33:13–24.
89. Parashar K, Torres AE, Boothby-Shoemaker W, Kohli I, Veenstra J, Neel V, et al. Imaging technologies for presurgical margin assessment of basal cell carcinoma. J Am Acad Dermatol. 2023;88:144–51.
90. Majores M, Bierhoff E. Aktinische Keratose, Morbus Bowen, Keratoakanthom und Plattenepithelkarzinom der Haut. Pathologe. 2015;36:16–29.
91. Dinnes J, Bamber J, Chuchu N, Bayliss SE, Takwoingi Y, Davenport C, et al. High-frequency ultrasound for diagnosing skin cancer in adults. Cochrane Database Syst Rev. 2018;12:CD013188.

92. Catalano O, Corvino A. Ultrasound of skin cancer: what we need to know. Semin Ultrasound CT MRI. 2024;45:216–32.
93. Kawaguchi M, Kato H, Noda Y, Kobayashi K, Miyazaki T, Hyodo F, et al. Imaging findings of malignant skin tumors: radiological–pathological correlation. Insights Imaging. 2022;13:52.
94. Rastrelli M, Tropea S, Rossi CR, Alaibac M. Melanoma: epidemiology, risk factors, pathogenesis, diagnosis and classification. In Vivo. 2014;28:1005–11.
95. Levit EK, Kagen MH, Scher RK, Grossman M, Altman E. The ABC rule for clinical detection of subungual melanoma. J Am Acad Dermatol. 2000;42:269–74.
96. Lallas A, Paschou E, Manoli S-M, Papageorgiou C, Spyridis I, Liopyris K, et al. Dermatoscopy of melanoma according to type, anatomic site and stage. Italian J Dermatol Venereol. 2021;156:156.
97. Guitera P, Li LX, Crotty K, Fitzgerald P, Mellenbergh R, Pellacani G, et al. Melanoma histological Breslow thickness predicted by 75-MHz ultrasonography. Br J Dermatol. 2008;159:364–9.
98. Hayashi K, Koga H, Uhara H, Saida T. High-frequency 30-MHz sonography in preoperative assessment of tumor thickness of primary melanoma: usefulness in determination of surgical margin and indication for sentinel lymph node biopsy. Int J Clin Oncol. 2009;14:426–30.
99. Kawaguchi M, Kato H, Tomita H, Hara A, Suzui N, Miyazaki T, et al. MR imaging findings for differentiating cutaneous malignant melanoma from squamous cell carcinoma. Eur J Radiol. 2020;132:109212.
100. Vernemmen AIP, Li X, Roemen GMJM, Speel EM, Kubat B, Zur HA, et al. Cutaneous metastases of internal malignancies: a single-institution experience. Histopathology. 2022;81:329–41.
101. Wagner K, Jassal K, Lee JC, Ban E, Cameron R, Serpell J. Challenges in diagnosis and management of a spiradenocarcinoma: a comprehensive literature review. ANZ J Surg. 2021;91:1996–2001.
102. Cardoso JC, Calonje E. Malignant sweat gland tumours: an update. Histopathology. 2015;67:589–606.
103. Torreggiani WC, Al-Ismail K, Munk PL, Nicolaou S, O'Connell JX, Knowling MA. Dermatofibrosarcoma Protuberans. Am J Roentgenol. 2002;178:989–93.
104. Menta A, Fouad TM, Lucci A, Le-Petross H, Stauder MC, Woodward WA, et al. Inflammatory breast cancer. Surg Clin N Am. 2018;98:787–800.
105. Alunni J-P. Imaging inflammatory breast cancer. Diagn Interv Imaging. 2012;93:95–103.
106. Lim HS, Jeong SJ, Lee JS, Park MH, Kim JW, Shin SS, et al. Paget disease of the breast: mammographic, US, and MR imaging findings with pathologic correlation. Radiographics. 2011;31:1973–87.
107. Apalla Z, Errichetti E, Kyrgidis A, Stolz W, Puig S, Malvehy J, et al. Dermoscopic features of mammary Paget's disease: a retrospective case-control study by the international dermoscopy society. J Eur Acad Dermatol Venereol. 2019;33:1892–8.
108. O'Regan KN, Jagannathan J, Krajewski K, Zukotynski K, Souza F, Wagner AJ, et al. Imaging of liposarcoma: classification, patterns of tumor recurrence, and response to treatment. Am J Roentgenol. 2011;197:W37–43.
109. Folpe AL. Fibrosarcoma: a review and update. Histopathology. 2014;64:12–25.
110. Ainsworth KE, Chavhan GB, Gupta AA, Hopyan S, Taylor G. Congenital infantile fibrosarcoma: review of imaging features. Pediatr Radiol. 2014;44:1124–9.
111. Gazendam AM, Popovic S, Munir S, Parasu N, Wilson D, Ghert M. Synovial sarcoma: a clinical review. Curr Oncol. 2021;28:1909–20.
112. Bakri A, Shinagare AB, Krajewski KM, Howard SA, Jagannathan JP, Hornick JL, et al. Synovial sarcoma: imaging features of common and uncommon primary sites, metastatic patterns, and treatment response. Am J Roentgenol. 2012;199:W208–15.
113. Kawaguchi M, Kato H, Imada H, Miyazaki T, Matsuyama K, Seishima M, Matsuo M. Magnetic resonance imaging characteristics of poroma and porocarcinoma. J Comput Assist Tomogr. 2021;45(3):447–51.
114. Chotai N, Lim SK. Imaging features of steatocystoma multiplex back to basics. Breast J. 2021;27:389–90.

Part V
Nail and Periungual Region

Chapter 16
Clinical, Imaging, and Histological Findings in Inflammatory Lesions of the Nail and Periungual Region

Robertha Nakamura, Andreia Pizarro Leverone, Nathália Matos, Renata Brandão Villa Verde, André da Silva Cartell, Philippe Alcântara Gonçalves Martins, Carolina Ávila de Almeida, Ana Paula Kunning Casqueiro, Tatiana de Almeida Gonçalves Secco, and Clarissa Canella Moraes do Carmo

In dermatology, imaging plays a pivotal role in diagnosing inflammatory conditions affecting the nail and surrounding areas. This chapter focuses on the use of advanced imaging techniques to examine common yet often difficult-to-diagnose inflammatory issues, including psoriasis, lichen planus, and ingrown nails. Each condition has its own distinct imaging characteristics that can complicate diagnosis and treatment. By examining how these imaging technologies can reveal the specific features

R. Nakamura
Institute of Dermatology Professor Rubem David Azulay, Rio de Janeiro, RJ, Brazil

Dermatology by the Brazilian Society of Dermatology, Rio de Janeiro, RJ, Brazil

Dermatology from the Federal University of Medicine at Rio de Janeiro, Rio de Janeiro, RJ, Brazil

Nail Study Center—Institute of Dermatology Professor Ruben David Azulay, Santa Casa da Misericórdia do Rio de Janeiro, Rio de Janeiro, RJ, Brazil

A. P. Leverone
Nail Study Center—Institute of Dermatology Professor Ruben David Azulay, Santa Casa da Misericórdia do Rio de Janeiro, Rio de Janeiro, RJ, Brazil

N. Matos
Dermatology Department of Fundação de Medicina Tropical Doutor Heitor Vieira Dourado, Manaus, Brazil

R. B. V. Verde
Marcilio Dias Naval Hospital, Lins de Vasconcelos, Rio de Janeiro, RJ, Brazil

A. da Silva Cartell
Adjunct Professor at Faculdade de Medicina da Universidade Federal do Rio Grande do Sul, Rio de Janeiro, Brazil

Dermatologist and Dermatopathologist in Private Practice, Rio de Janeiro, Brazil

© The Author(s), under exclusive license to Springer Nature Switzerland AG 2025

C. Canella Moraes do Carmo (ed.), *Atlas of Diagnostic Imaging in Dermatology*, https://doi.org/10.1007/978-3-031-77987-9_16

of these conditions, we aim to improve diagnostic accuracy and treatment strategies. This chapter provides essential knowledge for clinicians to better understand and manage the diverse presentations of nail and periungual inflammatory disorders.

16.1 Nail Psoriasis

16.1.1 Definition [1–4]

- Psoriasis is a chronic inflammatory disease that is common and debilitating, significantly impacting patients both functionally and psychologically.
- Nail psoriasis manifests as various changes in the nails, often causing discomfort and aesthetic concerns.
- Inflammation in nail psoriasis is typically found around the enthesis of the distal interphalangeal joints and extends from the supporting fascia of the nail.
- The association with psoriatic arthritis suggests a shared underlying pathophysiological mechanism.
- Disruption of the nail barrier due to psoriasis makes the nails more prone to secondary infections, commonly fungal.

P. A. G. Martins
Bronstein DASA—Tijuca, Rio de Janeiro, RJ, Brazil

Américas Medical City, Barra da Tijuca, Rio de Janeiro, RJ, Brazil

C. Á. de Almeida
Faculty of Medicine of Valença—UniFaa, Valença, Brazil

Federal University of Rio de Janeiro—UFRJ, Rio de Janeiro, Brazil

A. P. K. Casqueiro
Clinica Multi-Imagem Ipanema—RJ, Rio de Janeiro, RJ, Brazil

Musculoskeletal Imaging at DASA—RJ, Rio de Janeiro, RJ, Brazil

T. de Almeida Gonçalves Secco
Musculoskeletal Imaging at DASA—RJ, Rio de Janeiro, RJ, Brazil

Fleury Group—RJ, Rio de Janeiro, RJ, Brazil

C. Canella Moraes do Carmo (✉)
Fluminense Federal University—UFF, Rio de Janeiro, Brazil

Federal University of Rio de Janeiro—UFRJ, Rio de Janeiro, Brazil

Diagnóstico das Américas—DASA—RJ, Rio de Janeiro, Brazil

Biodesign Laboratory, DASA-PUC, Rio de Janeiro, Brazil

16.1.2 Epidemiology [2, 3, 5, 6]

- The prevalence of nail involvement in psoriasis patients ranges from 7% to 56%, with a lifetime incidence reaching 80–90%.
- Nail psoriasis occurring without associated skin lesions or arthritis is relatively rare, with a prevalence estimated between 0% and 6%.
- The severity of nail psoriasis does not always correspond to the severity of skin psoriasis. Patients with nail psoriasis tend to be older and experienced nail symptoms later than skin symptoms.

16.1.3 Clinical Presentation (Fig. 16.1) [3, 7]

- Nail psoriasis more commonly affects fingernails than toenails, and involvement of multiple nails is frequent. This condition arises from changes in the nail matrix, nail bed, and periungual region, leading to several distinct clinical features.
  - Changes in the nail matrix:

    Nail pitting: Small depressions on the nail plate caused by focal and transient disorder in the proximal matrix, resulting in parakeratosis islands that create pits when the nail grows out.
    Trachyonychia: A rough, dull surface on the nail due to permanent or transient alterations in the proximal matrix.
    Crumbling: Nails become brittle and may easily crumble.
    Leukonychia (White Spots): Partial whitish discoloration of the nail plate caused by disease in the intermediate matrix.
    Red lunulae: Red spots at the lunulae, resulting from disease in the distal matrix.
    Beau's lines: Deep or shallow transverse grooves spanning the width of the nail, resulting from temporary interruptions in nail matrix growth.
    Onychomadesis: Transverse separation of the proximal nail plate, which can lead to complete loss of the nail plate in severe cases.

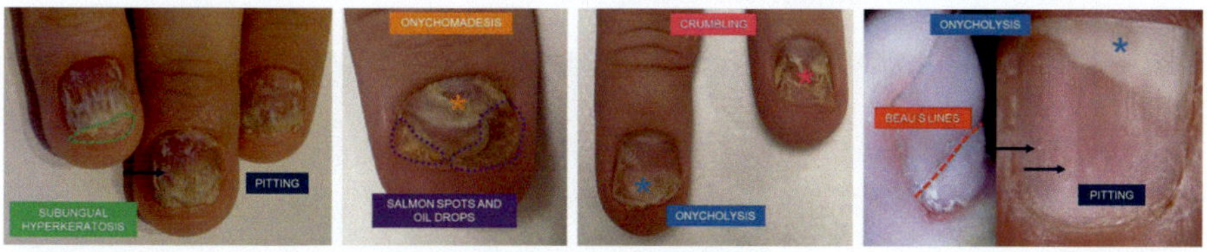

Fig. 16.1 Clinical photograph of patient with nail psoriasis

- Changes in the nail bed:

  Onycholysis: Separation of the nail plate from the nail bed.
  Subungual hyperkeratosis: Thickening of the stratum corneum in the hyponychium and nail bed, with the accumulation of keratinocytes and debris.
  Nail discoloration: Color changes in the nails, often appearing as yellow-brown spots, known as "oil drops" or "salmon spots."
  Splinter hemorrhages: Small, elongated blood spots under the nail, caused by the rupture of small capillaries in the nail bed.

- Changes in the periungual region:

  Psoriatic paronychia: A common manifestation of psoriasis characterized by erythematous, scaly lesions affecting the proximal and/or lateral edges of the nail, often associated with changes in the nail matrix or plate.

16.1.4 Onychoscopy (Fig. 16.2) [8, 9]

• Onychoscopy is a valuable tool for improving the accuracy of diagnosis of nail lesions, even before clinical signs become evident. It is particularly useful for detecting early nail involvement in nail psoriasis and monitoring treatment and disease progression.

  - Nail matrix characteristics:

    Pitting: Small depressions on the nail surface.
    Longitudinal ridging: Vertical lines running along the length of the nail.
    Fuzzy lunula: An irregular, wide white lunula observed under dermoscopy.
    Leukonychia: White discoloration of the nail plate.
    Nail plate thickening: Increased thickness of the nail plate.
    Crumbling: Brittleness and fragmentation of the nail.
    Red lunula: Red coloration at the lunula area.

  - Nail bed findings:

    Onycholysis: Separation of the nail plate from the nail bed.
    Oil Spots and Salmon Patches: Yellow-brown discolorations appearing as oil drops and salmon-colored spots.

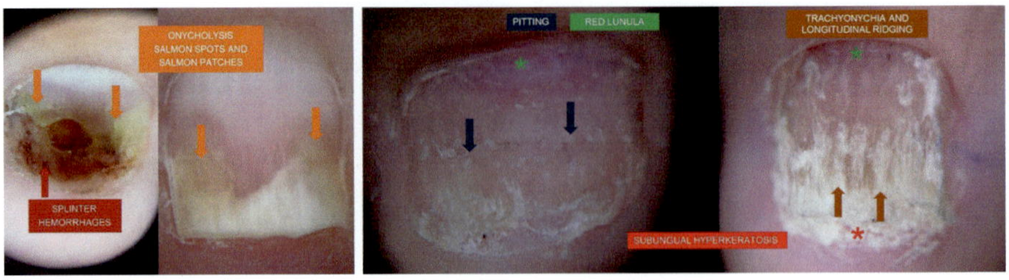

Fig. 16.2 Dermoscopic findings of patient with nail psoriasis (x20)

Scaling: Accumulation of flaky skin or debris.
Splinter Hemorrhages: Elongated blood spots under the nail.
Dilated Nail Bed Capillaries: Enlarged blood vessels in the nail bed.
Subungual Hyperkeratosis: Thickening of the nail bed and hyponychium with keratin accumulation.

- Nail fold examination:

  Dotted capillaries: Small, pinpoint blood vessels observed in the proximal and lateral nail folds and in the hyponychium region.
  Dilated capillaries: Enlarged blood vessels found in the proximal and lateral nail folds and in the hyponychium region.

16.1.5 Histopathology (Fig. 16.3) [7]

- Characterized by a psoriasiform onychitis with spongiform pustulation.
- The most common microscopic feature:
  - Parakeratosis (78% of biopsies).
  - Neutrophilic infiltration of the nail bed epithelium (63%).
  - Hypergranulosis (58%).
- PAS staining is especially important to exclude onychomycosis that can clinically and histologically mimic nail psoriasis, especially in clipping biopsies.

16.1.6 Radiography and Computed Tomography [10]

16.1.6.1 Nail Involvement

- Unique nail involvement is not detected by radiography or computed tomography.

16.1.6.2 Involvement of Surrounding Tissues

- Most commonly identified at interphalangeal joints.
- Central and marginal erosions at enthesis.
- Pseudo-enlargement of joint space.
- Reactive osseous proliferation at enthesis.
- Ankylosis, subluxation, and deformities:
  - Pencil in cup deformity: periarticular erosions and bone resorption of phalanx and metacarpal heads.
  - Ivory phalanx: result of bony proliferation as an exaggerated healing response to injured bone.

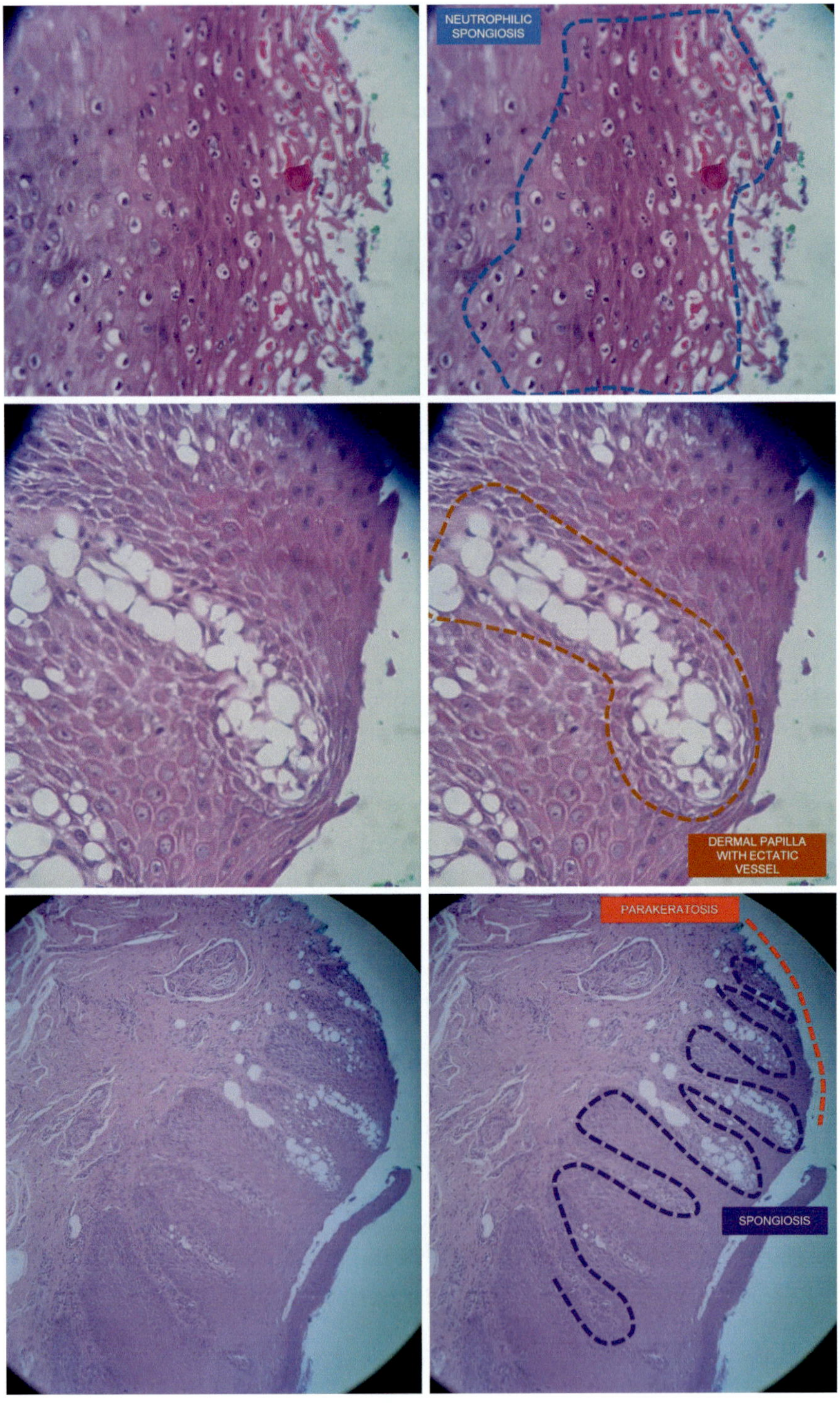

Fig. 16.3 Histological findings of nail psoriasis (H&E x10)

16.1.7 Ultrasonography (Figs. 16.4, 16.5, 16.6, 16.7 and 16.8) [11–15]

16.1.7.1 Nail Involvement

- Thickening of the nail bed.
- Hypervascularity of the nail bed on power Doppler.
- Loss of definition of the volar plate at early phases.
- Hyperechoic focal thickening of the volar plate.
- Diffuse thickening, loss of definition, and irregularities of both dorsal and volar plates.
- Wavy-shaped nail plates and posterior acoustic shadowing in the nail bed.
- Thickening and rounded shape of the proximal nail fold caused by inflammatory changes.
- Onychomadesis—the shedding of nail plaques, beginning at the proximal end, with loss of continuity of the plates.
- Beau's lines deep, horizontal grooves that appear as nails without disrupting the continuity of the nail plates.

16.1.7.2 Involvement of Surrounding Tissues

- Most commonly identified at interphalangeal joints.
- Marginal erosions at enthesis.
- Reactive osseous proliferation at enthesis.
- Reactive mild synovitis.
- Extensive and multiple tenosynovitis and hypervascularity on power Doppler imaging.
- Perienthesis bursitis and hypervascularity on power Doppler imaging.

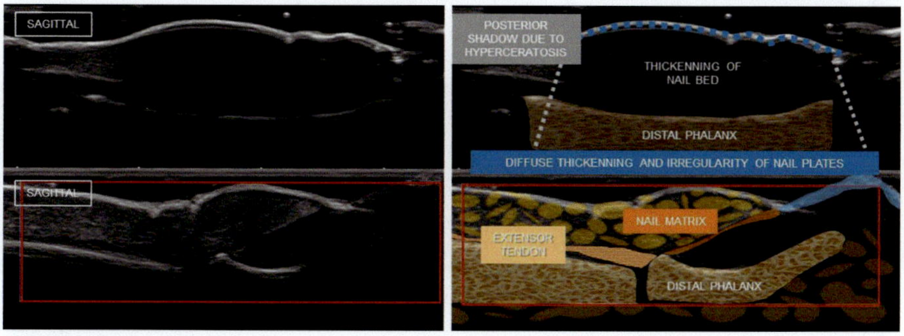

Fig. 16.4 Ultrasonographic findings of nail psoriasis with a 24 MHz probe (Aplio i800, Canon Medical Systems)

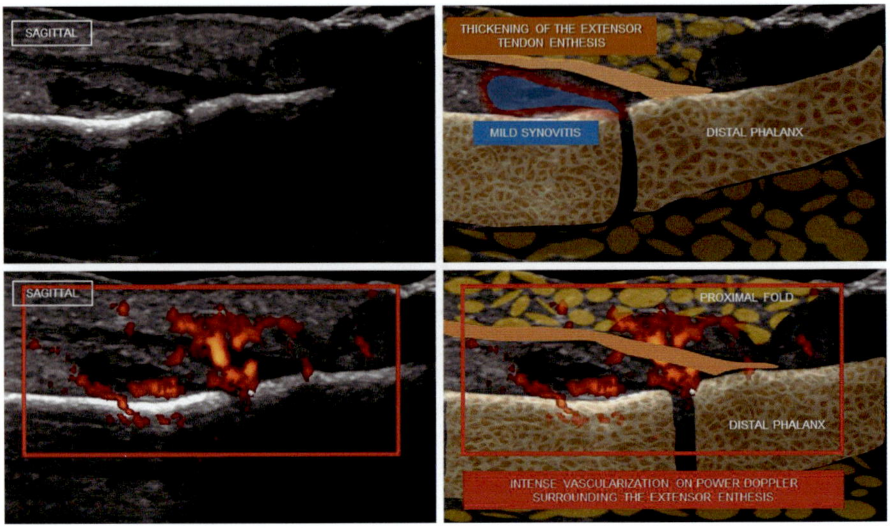

Fig. 16.5 Ultrasonographic findings of enthesitis due nail psoriasis with a 24 MHz probe (Aplio i800, Canon Medical Systems)

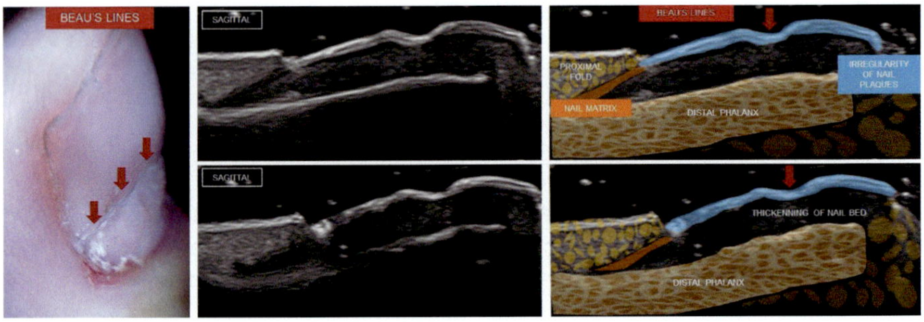

Fig. 16.6 Ultrasonographic findings of Beau's lines due nail psoriasis with a 24 MHz probe (Aplio i800, Canon Medical Systems)

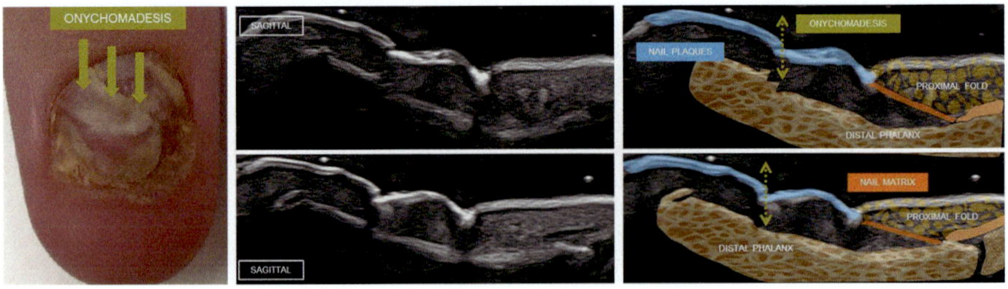

Fig. 16.7 Ultrasonographic findings of onychomadesis due nail psoriasis with a 24 MHz probe (Aplio i800, Canon Medical Systems)

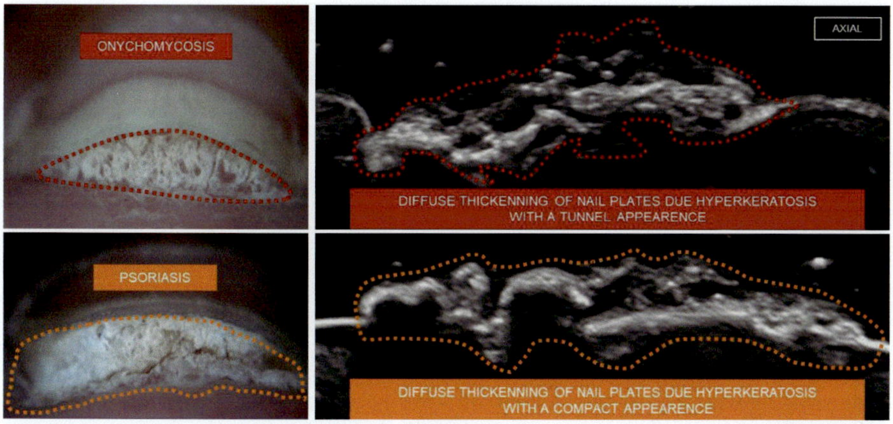

Fig. 16.8 Ultrasonographic findings of nail plaques in nail psoriasis and onychomycosis with a 33 MHz probe (Aplio i800, Canon Medical Systems)

16.1.8 MRI (Fig. 16.9) [10]

16.1.8.1 Nail Involvement

- Thickening of the nail bed.
- High signal intensity of the nail bed on STIR images and contrast enhancement on T1 FS, suggesting hypervascularization.
- Irregularities and wavy shape at nail bed surface.
- Thickening, high signal intensity, and rounded shape of the proximal nail fold on STIR images and contrast enhancement on T1 FS caused by inflammatory changes.

16.1.8.2 Involvement of Surrounding Tissues

- Most commonly identified at interphalangeal joints.
- Bone marrow edema at site of enthesis.
- Central and marginal erosions.
- Pseudo-enlargement of joint space.
- Reactive osseous proliferation and periostitis.
- Ankylosis, subluxation, and deformities.
- Reactive mild synovitis and arthritis.
- Extensive and multiple tenosynovitis associated with thickening of the tendon sheath with contrast enhancement on STIR and T1 FS images.

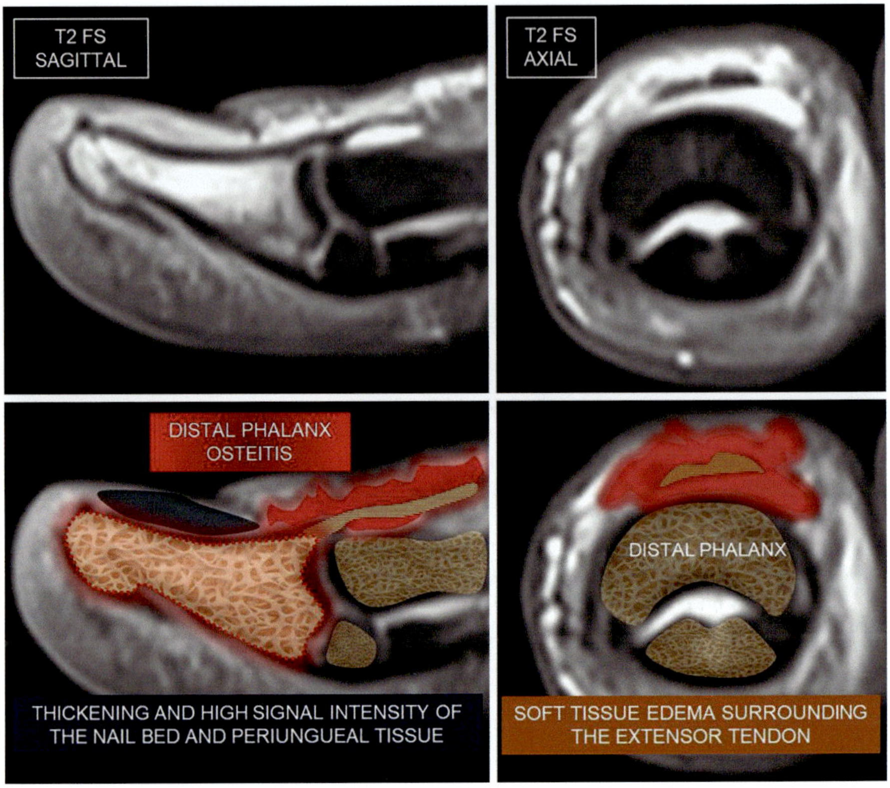

Fig. 16.9 MRI with surface coil findings of nail psoriasis on T2 FS weighted sequence after gadolinium administration (Magnetom Prisma 3T MRI, Siemens)

- Periarticular and periosseous edema suggesting dactilitis with contrast enhancement on STIR and T1 FS images.
- Perienthesis bursitis with thickening of the bursae wall with contrast enhancement on STIR and T1 FS images.

16.2 Acrodermatitis Continua of Hallopeaux

16.2.1 Definition [16, 17]

- Acrodermatitis continua of Hallopeau is a rare chronic inflammatory disease characterized by a sterile pustular eruption on one or more fingers.
- This condition is considered a variant of pustular psoriasis.
- It is known for its painful nature and recurrent course.

16.2.2 Epidemiology [16–18]

- Acrodermatitis continua of Hallopeau is most commonly seen in middle-aged females and often starts after localized trauma or infection on a single digit.
- Various other potential causes have been identified, including infectious, neural, inflammatory, and genetic factors.
- Due to the rarity of the disease, epidemiological data is limited to case reports.

16.2.3 Clinical Presentation (Fig. 16.10) [18, 19]

- Acrodermatitis continua of Hallopeau is characterized by multiple pustules and scalling on an erythematous base, typically confined to the distal parts of one or two fingers.
- The pustules may merge to form larger pus-filled areas and can progressively spread to the dorsum of the hands, forearms, and feet.
- When pustules involve the nail bed and nail matrix, they are often associated with onychodystrophy and, in some cases, complete loss of the nail on the affected fingers.
- Over time, some patients may develop osteolysis of the distal phalanx beneath the lesions.

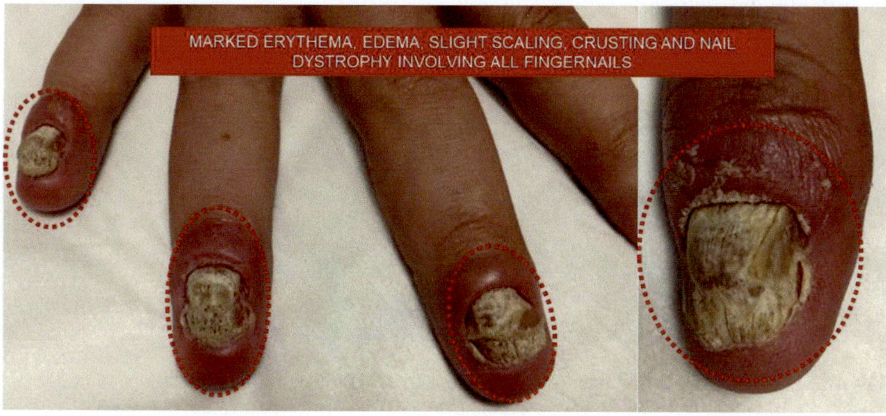

Fig. 16.10 Clinical photograph of patient with acrodermatitis continua of Hallopeau

16.2.4 Onychoscopy (Fig. 16.11) [20, 21]

- The diagnosis of acrodermatitis continua of Hallopeau can be established through clinical evaluation and dermoscopic findings.
- In the early stages, onychoscopy of the nail plate typically reveals distal onycholysis with a proximal erythematous border, longitudinal nail striations, occasional subungual hemorrhage, and minimal subungual hyperkeratosis.
- Dermoscopy of the pustular lesions may show regularly distributed yellow globules, punctate vessels, and hemorrhagic spots.
- Dermoscopy of the tips of the affected fingers often reveals yellowish-white hyperkeratosis or scaling, along with punctate and linear vessels, and shiny hemorrhagic spots.

16.2.5 Histopathology [22, 23]

- Display of more spongiform pustulation.
- Overlap with the findings of Reactive Arthritis Syndrome, which should be characterized by the clinical aspects.

16.2.6 Radiography and Computed Tomography (Fig. 16.12)

- Findings resembling nail psoriasis but with more pronounced structural and inflammatory alterations.

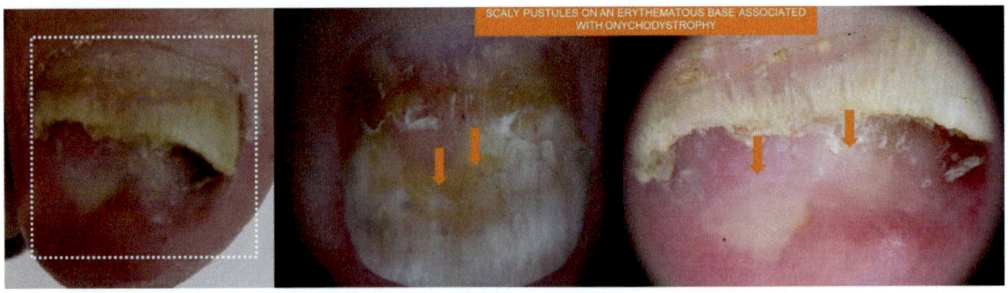

Fig. 16.11 Dermoscopic findings of patient with acrodermatitis continua of Hallopeau (x20)

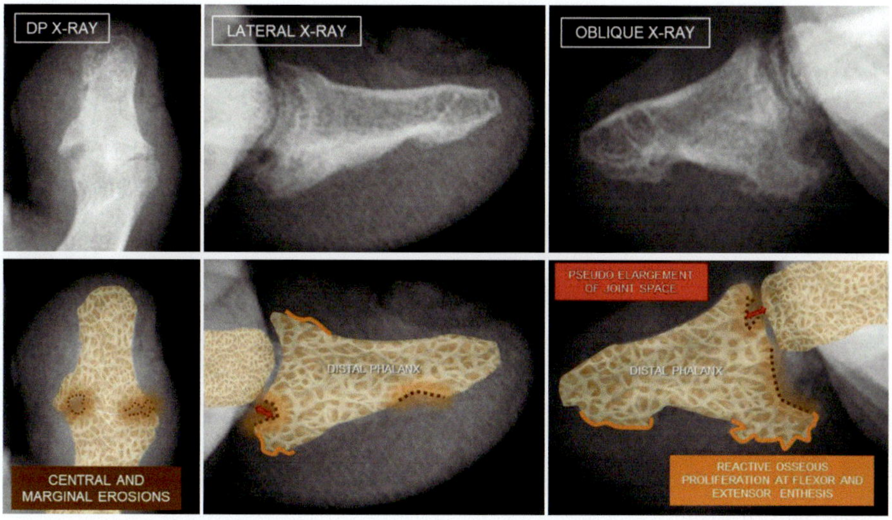

Fig. 16.12 Radiographic findings of acrodermatitis continua of Hallopeau (Philips Duo Diagnost R&F Room Digital RF and Tomo System)

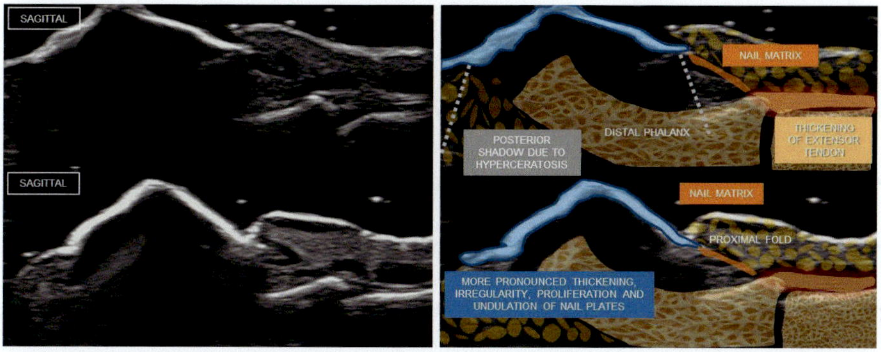

Fig. 16.13 Ultrasonographic findings of acrodermatitis continua of Hallopeau with a 24 MHz probe (Aplio i800, Canon Medical Systems)

16.2.7 Ultrasonography (Fig. 16.13)

- Findings resembling nail psoriasis but with more pronounced structural and inflammatory alterations.
- More pronounced thickening, irregularity, proliferation, and undulation of nail plates.
- Occasionally, heterogeneous collections at periungual tissues.

16.2.8 MRI

- Findings resembling nail psoriasis but with more pronounced structural and inflammatory alterations.
- More pronounced thickening, high signal intensity, irregularities and wavy shape of the nail bed.
- Occasionally, pustulae collections at periungual tissues.

16.3 Psoriatic Onychopachydermoperiostitis (POPP)

16.3.1 Definition [24–26]

- Psoriatic onychopachydermoperiostitis (POPP) syndrome is a rare variant of psoriatic arthritis.
- It is characterized by psoriatic onychodystrophy, painful swelling of the soft tissue near the distal phalanx, and specific radiologic changes.
- Radiologic findings include periosteal reactions and bone erosions in the distal phalanges.

16.3.2 Epidemiology [24, 25, 27]

- A limited number of cases of psoriatic onychopachydermoperiostitis (POPP) have been documented in the literature.
- The majority of affected patients are male and typically over 30 years old, with a mean age of 44.9 years.
- The duration of symptoms varies from 2 months to 20 years, with the big toe being involved in most cases.
- Distal interphalangeal joint involvement occurs in approximately half of the cases.
- Like other forms of psoriatic arthritis, POPP is associated with a higher frequency of the HLA-B27 antigen.
- One potential pathogenic mechanism involves inflammation starting in the subungual structures and spreading between the tendons and bones of the terminal phalanx.
- Patients often experience functional impairment as a result of the condition.

16.3.3 Clinical Presentation (Fig. 16.14) [25, 27]

- Patients with Psoriatic Onychopachydermoperiostitis (POPP) syndrome typically present with painful, swollen, and tender fingers or toes. The condition is often associated with severe psoriasis, which can lead to significant functional disability. The involvement is usually asymmetrical and features prominent and distressing nail changes.
  - Nail changes: The big toenail is more frequently affected than the fingernails. Common nail changes include thickening of the nail plate, subungual hyperkeratosis, onycholysis, and periungual erosions. When the fingernails are affected, typical onychodystrophies seen in psoriasis may include pitting, nail plate crumbling, onycholysis, nail discoloration, and splinter hemorrhages.
  - Skin thickening (Pachydermia): Patients exhibit thickening of the skin and erosion around the nails and distal phalanges. This results in the affected fingers or toes appearing swollen and inflamed.
  - Bone and periosteal changes (Periostitis): Inflammation of the periosteum leads to periosteal bone formation and specific radiographic changes. These changes include new bone formation and periosteal reaction, which can result in digit deformities, pain, and functional impairment.

16.3.4 Onychoscopy [27]

- The dermoscopic characteristics are similar to the changes observed in isolated nail psoriasis, with greater intensity in lesions that affect the nail bed due to the aggressiveness of the disease.

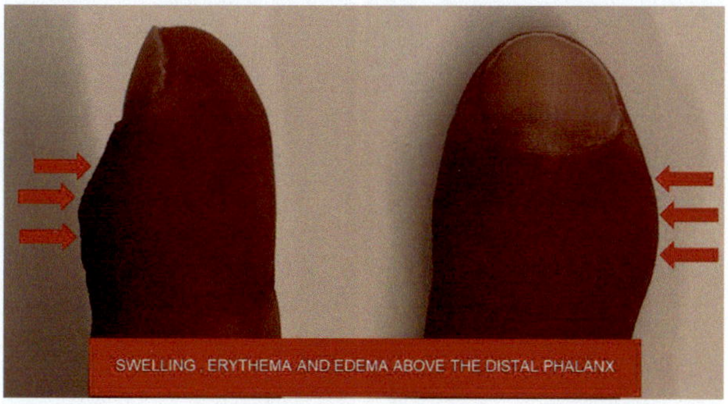

Fig. 16.14 Clinical photograph of patient with psoriatic onychopachydermoperiostitis

16.3.5 Histopathology [24, 28]

- The histopathologic appearance is similar to those observed in isolated nail psoriasis but with greater intensity in lesions affecting the nail bed due to the disease's aggressiveness.

16.3.6 Radiography and Computed Tomography (Fig. 16.15)

- Findings resembling nail psoriasis but with more pronounced structural and inflammatory alterations at nail surrounding tissues.

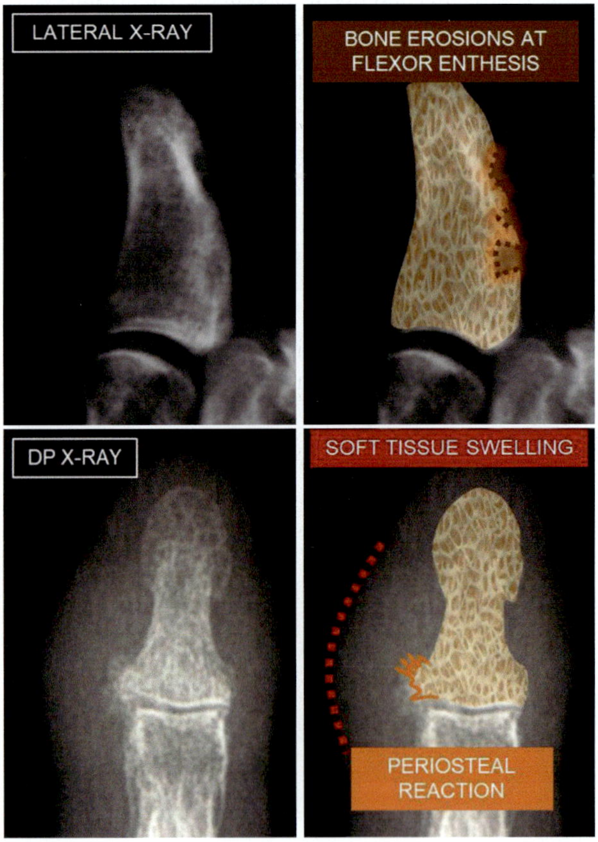

Fig. 16.15 Radiographic findings of psoriatic onychopachydermoperiostitis (Philips Duo Diagnost R&F Room Digital RF and Tomo System)

16.3.7 *Ultrasonography (Figs. 16.16 and 16.17)*

- Findings resembling nail psoriasis but with more pronounced structural and inflammatory alterations at nail surrounding tissues.

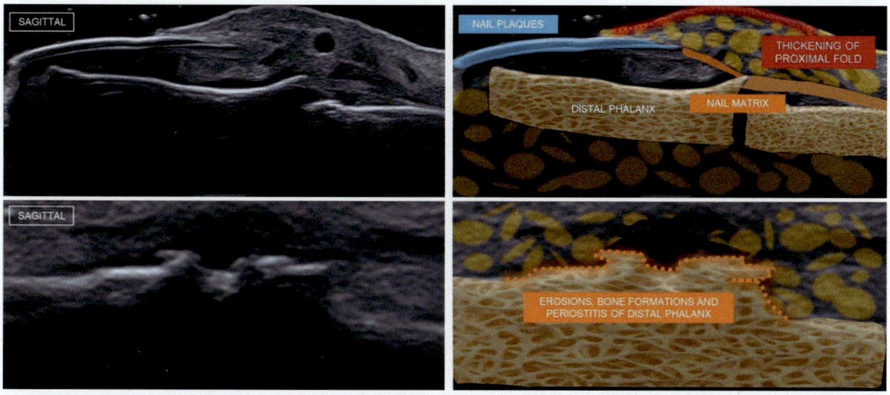

Fig. 16.16 Ultrasonographic findings of psoriatic onychopachydermoperiostitis with a 24 MHz probe (Aplio i800, Canon Medical Systems)

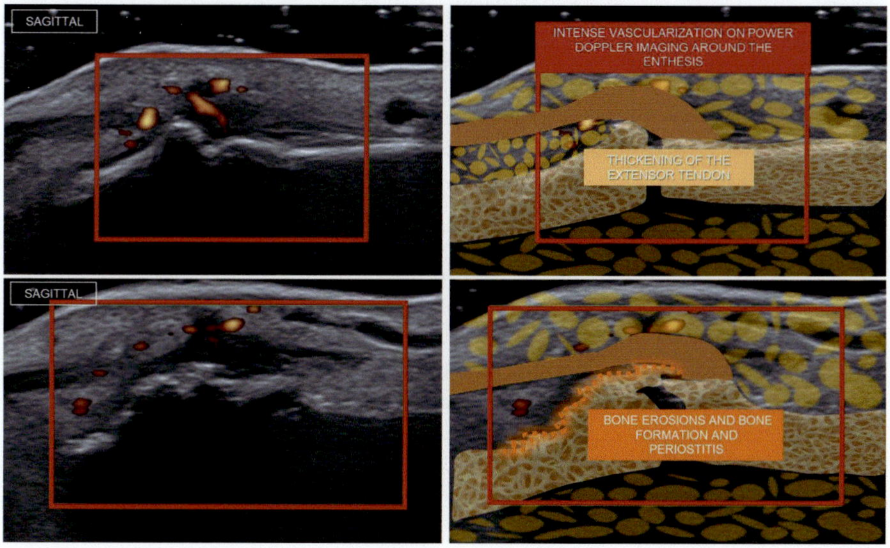

Fig. 16.17 Ultrasonographic findings of enthesitis due psoriatic onychopachydermoperiostitis with a 24 MHz probe (Aplio i800, Canon Medical Systems)

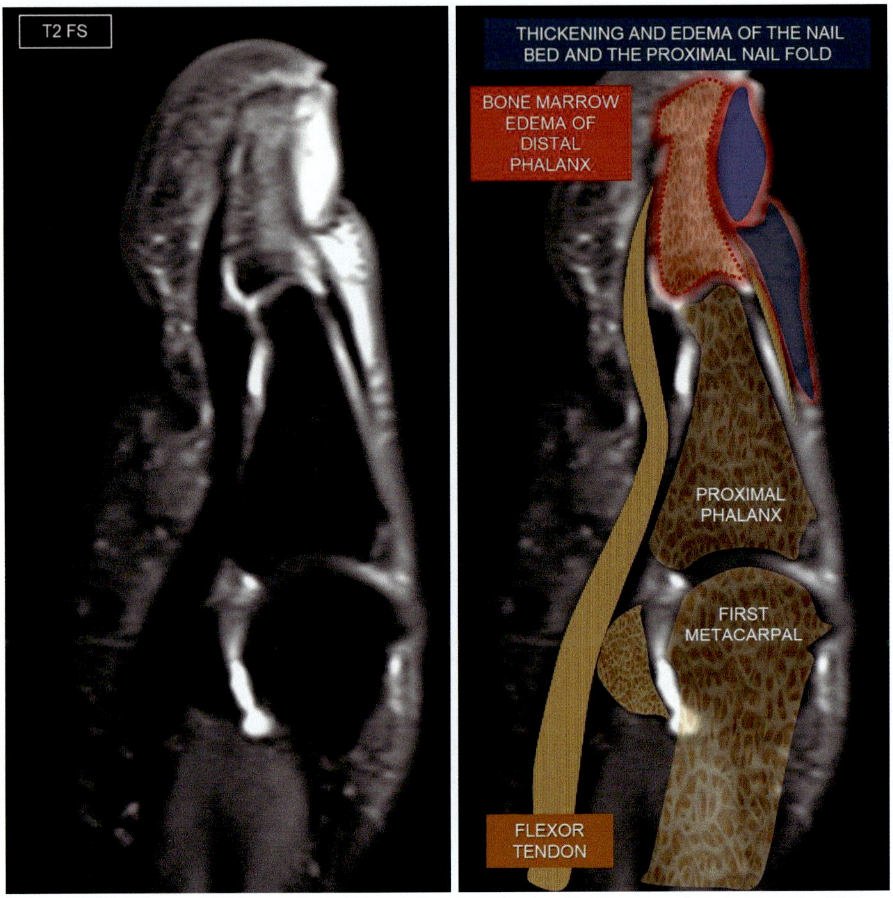

Fig. 16.18 MRI with surface coil findings of psoriatic onychopachydermoperiostitis on T2 FS weighted sequence (Magnetom Avanto 1.5T MRI, Siemens)

16.3.8 MRI (Fig. 16.18)

- Findings resembling nail psoriasis but with more pronounced structural and inflammatory alterations at nail surrounding tissues.

16.4 Lichen Planus

16.4.1 Definition [29, 30]

- Chronic inflammatory disease that causes alterations in the matrix, bed, and perionychium.

- Irreversible damage can occur if diagnosis and treatment are delayed and may arise as the first manifestation of the disease.

16.4.2 Epidemiology [29–31]

- Low and variable prevalence, reported between 0.5% and 1% of the population.
- Affects 10% of patients with involvement of the skin, scalp, or mucosa, being the isolated nail form quite uncommon.
- Usually affected the third decade of life, but can be seen in children and the elderly.
- Nails of the hands are more affected than those of the feet.
- Without gender predominance.

16.4.3 Clinical Presentation (Fig. 16.19) [29–33]

- Clinical characteristics of nail lichen are not specific, especially in the early stages of the disease. Clinical manifestations depend of the affected area:
  - Nail folds: violaceous papule and diffuse red-blue discoloration [4].
  - Matrix: thinning of the plate, onychorrhexis, distal fissure, crumbling, discoloration of the reddish lunula, leukonychia, pitting, trachyonychia, onychomadesis, red dots, diffuse redness, flame-shaped or yellowish lunula [4, 5].
  - Nail Bed: onycholysis, hemorrhagic splinters, melanonychia, erythronychia, and mild subungual hiperkeratosis [4, 6].

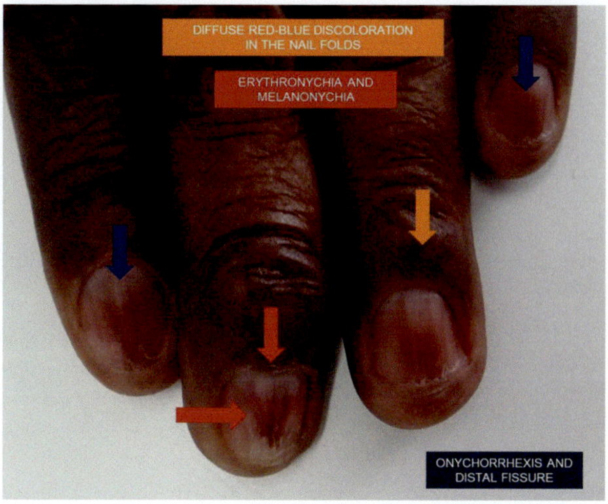

Fig. 16.19 Clinical photograph of patient with nail lichen planus

- Matrix and bed: dorsal pterygium, anonychia [2, 6].
- Perionychium changes: paronychia.

- The most recent classification defines stages [7]:
  - Mild: thinning, longitudinal ridges, distal splitting less than 3 mm in length, onycholysis less than 25%, without hyperkeratosis on the nail bed;
  - Moderate: partial fissure, longitudinal grooves, distal splitting between 3 and 5 mm, onycholysis between 25% and 50%, erythematous spots on the lunula, and subungual keratosis.
  - Severe: complete fissures, deep longitudinal ridges, fissures greater than 5 mm, onycholysis greater than 50%, diffuse erythema of the lunula.

16.4.4 Onychoscopy (Fig. 16.20) [34, 35]

- In addition to the onychodystrophies seen during physical examination, onychoscopy shows the convergence of longitudinal striae to the center of the nail unit, indicating a worst prognosis, leading to atrophy and even anonychia [8].

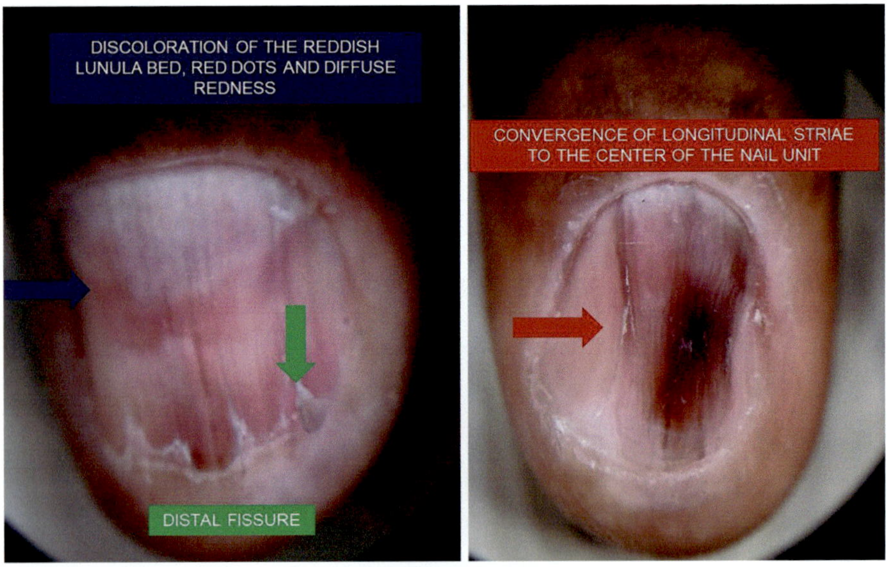

Fig. 16.20 Dermoscopic findings of patient with nail lichen planus (x20)

16.4.5 Histopathology (Fig. 16.21) [33, 36]

- In half of the cases where the nail was biopsied, there were no sufficient diagnostic criteria and the diagnosis depends on the clinical characteristics.
- Bandlike lymphocytic infiltrate and basal damage to the nail matrix, characteristic of lichenoid interface dermatitis.
- Sometimes hyperkeratosis, hypergranulosis, and the presence of plasma cells.

16.4.6 Ultrasonography (Fig. 16.22)

- Nail bed involvement:
  - Thickening of the nail bed.
  - Reduced echogenicity of the nail bed.
  - Hypervascularization on power Doppler of the nail bed.
- Periungual involvement:
  - Thickening of periungual parts.
  - Reduced echogenicity of the proximal dermis.
  - Hypervascularization on power Doppler periungually.
- Plaques involvement:
  - Hypoechoic halo surrounding the matrix.
  - Thickening.
  - Irregularity.
  - Loss of definition.
  - Undulation.
  - Superior displacement.
  - Hyperechoic "spots" within the plaques.

16.4.7 MRI (Fig. 16.23)

- Thickening of the nail bed.
- High signal intensity of the nail bed on STIR images and enhancement after contrast administration on T1 FS sequences.
- Thickening of the proximal fold.
- High signal intensity of the nail fold on STIR images and enhancement after contrast administration on T1 FS sequences.
- Absence of articular, osseous, or enthesis involvement.

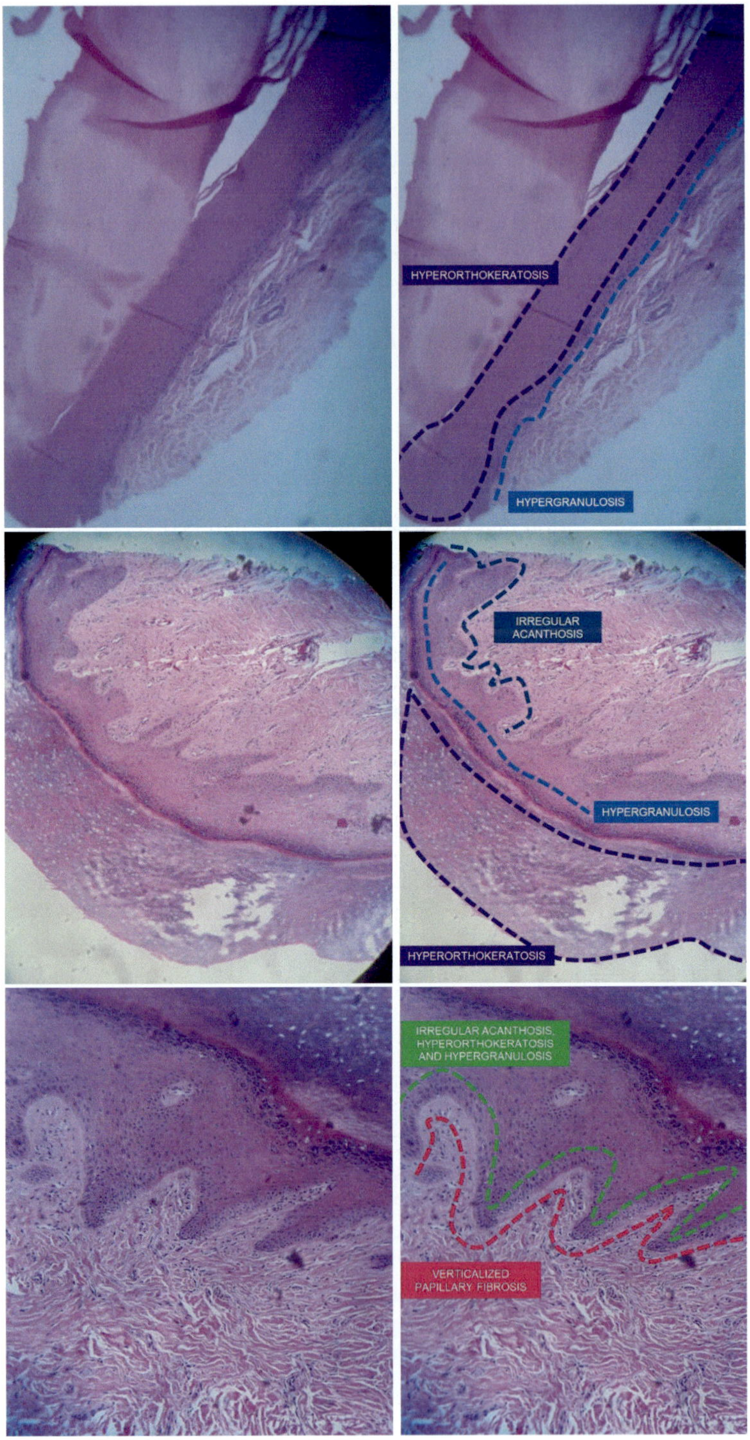

Fig. 16.21 Histological findings of nail lichen planus (H&E x4)

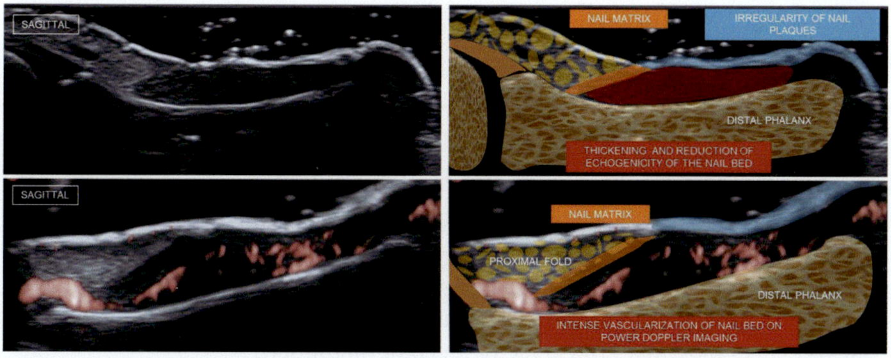

Fig. 16.22 Ultrasonographic findings of nail lichen planus with a 24 MHz probe (Aplio i800, Canon Medical Systems)

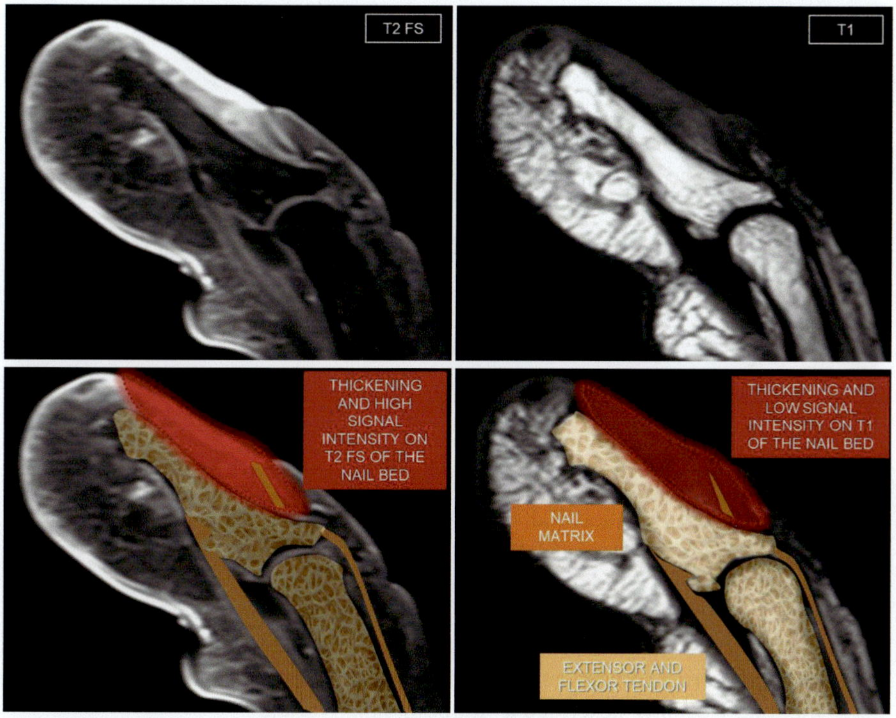

Fig. 16.23 MRI with surface coil findings of nail lichen planus on T1 and T2 FS weighted sequence (Magnetom Prisma 3T MRI, Siemens)

16.5 Ingrown Toenail

16.5.1 Definition [37–39]

- Common, multifactorial, and painful inflammatory condition with significant morbidity that can interfere with daily activities [1].
- Represents a nail spicule that traumatizes the adjacent soft tissues, causing inflammation and sometimes secondary infection.
- Predisposing factors: improper nail cutting (most common etiology), tight shoes, poor foot hygiene, hyperhidrosis, trauma, and the use of certain medications (especially epidermal growth factor receptor inhibitors).
- Pinched nail deformity, wide nail plates, congenital misalignment of the toenails, and thickening of the nail plate are possible risk factors for ingrown toenails [2, 3].

16.5.2 Epidemiology [37]

- Prevalence around 2.5–5%.
- Male 2:1 Female.
- Affects all age groups, but adolescents, children, and obese individuals are most affected.
- Hallux more commonly affected and the involvement of the lateral fold of the toe occurs twice as often as the medial.

16.5.3 Clinical Presentation (Fig. 16.24) [37]

- Five clinical types:
  - Type 1 —Ingrown toenail due to hypertrophy of the nail fold: Total or partial absence of the nail plate after surgical procedures (nail excision, trauma, overly short cuts), the folds project upward, causing a hypertrophic reaction.
  - Type 2 —Subcutaneous onychocryptosis or juvenile ingrown toenail: Lateral cutting of the nail plate, followed by lateral spicule formation, with the lateral folds projecting forward of the spicule leading to local trauma, exacerbated by walking. Recently described a "harpoon nail" variant.
  - Type 3 —Increased transverse curvature of the nail: Divided into three clinical types: Pinched nail, tile nail, and plicated nail.
  - Type 4 —Pediatric ingrown toenail: when present in neonatal age, the hallux nail may not have grown completely to the distal edge. When present in infantile age, it can occur due to congenital misalignment of the hallux or hypertrophy of the lateral fold.

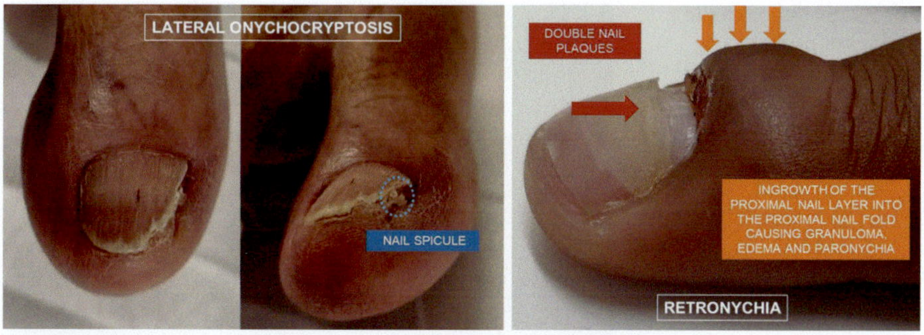

Fig. 16.24 Clinical photograph of patients with lateral onychocryptosis and retronychia

- Type 5 —Retronychia is a disorder caused by the ingrowth of the proximal nail plate into the proximal nail fold. This condition is often suspected when persistent paronychia occurs, especially following trauma.

16.5.4 Onychoscopy (Fig. 16.25) [37, 40]

- In the presence of secondary a pyogenic granuloma, few vessels are observed on its surface.3.

16.5.5 Histopathology [40, 41]

- Ingrown squamous epithelium, either of the matrix or the hyponychium.
- Chronic inflammation that is rich in plasma cells with granulation tissue and fibrosis.
- More pronounced lesions may present pseudoepitheliomatous epithelial hyperplasia.

16.5.6 Radiography and Computed Tomography

- Soft tissue swelling due to granulation tissue and loss of the normal fat planes at affected nail fold.

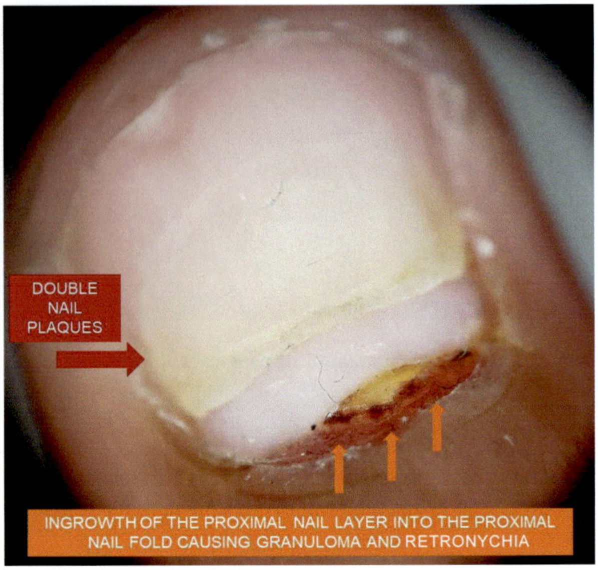

Fig. 16.25 Dermoscopic findings of patient with lateral ingrown nail (x20)

16.5.7 Ultrasonography (Figs. 16.26 and 16.27) [40, 42]

- Ingrown nail and onychocryptosis:
  - Billaminar hyperechoic fragment of the nail plates embedded in the nail fold surrounded by hypoechoic inflammatory tissue.
  - Thickening, reduction of echogenicity, and hypervascularization of the nail fold surrounding the nail fragment.
  - Prominence of SLEB (hypoechogenic subepidermal stripe) from the nail fold.
  - Absence of involvement of nail bed.
- Retronychia.
  - Matrix aspect:

    Hypoechoic halo surrounding the origin of the nail plate.
    Matrix dystrophy.
  - Nail plate-phalanx distance:

    Distance between the origin of the nail plate and the base of the distal phalanx is less than or equal to 5.1 mm in the big toe and thumbs.
    Difference of greater than or equal to 0.5 mm between the affected nail and the healthy contralateral nail.

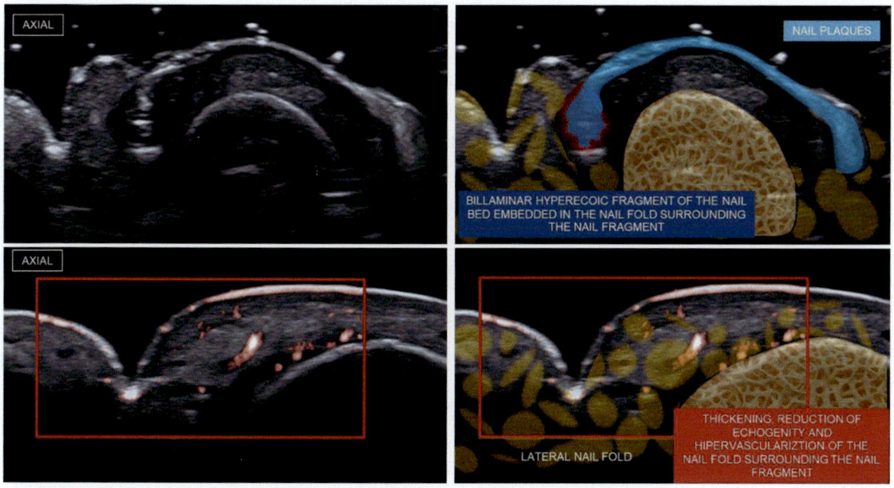

Fig. 16.26 Ultrasonographic findings of lateral ingrown nail with a 24 MHz probe (Aplio i800, Canon Medical Systems)

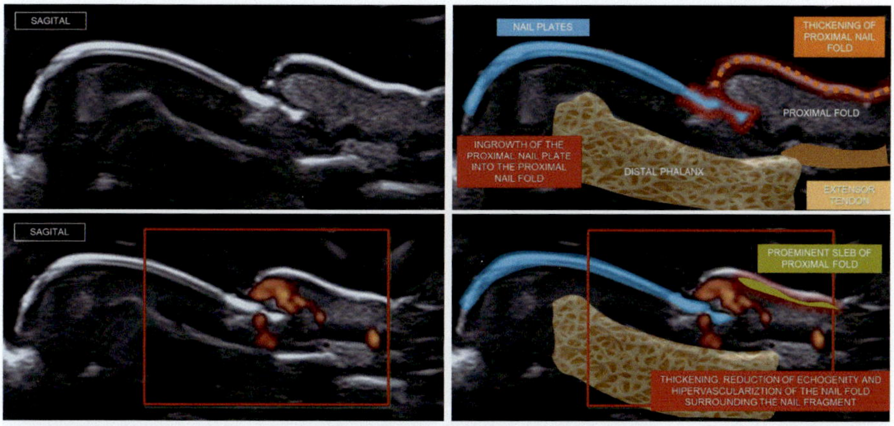

Fig. 16.27 Ultrasonographic findings of retronychia with a 24 MHz probe (Aplio i800, Canon Medical Systems)

– Proximal fold:

Proximal fold thickness greater than or equal to 2.2 mm for male patients. Proximal fold thickness greater than or equal to 1.9 mm for female patients. Difference of greater than or equal to 0.3 mm in the proximal fold thickness between the affected nail and the healthy contralateral nail.

16.5.8 MRI (Figs. 16.28 and 16.29)

- Ingrown nail and onychocryptosis:
  - Low signal intensity in all sequences of the nail fragment embedded in the nail fold.
  - Thickening of the nail fold surrounded by high signal intensity inflammatory tissue.
  - Thickening of the dermis of the nail fold, specially identified on T1 sequences.
  - Contrast enhancement on T1 FS of the nail fold.
  - Absence of involvement of nail bed.
  - Reactive bone marrow edema of distal phalanx.
- Retronychia.
  - Matrix aspect:

    Matrix dystrophy.
    Inflammatory tissue surrounding the origin of the nail plate with high signal intensity on T2-weighted images and low signal intensity on T1-weighted images.

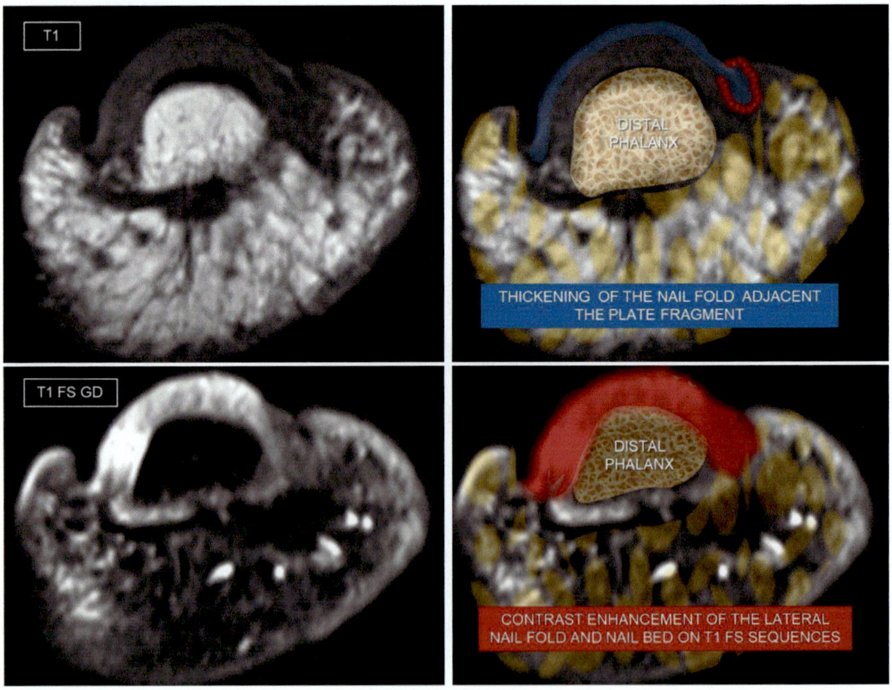

Fig. 16.28 MRI with surface coil findings of lateral ingrown nail on T1 and T1 FS weighted sequences after gadolinium administration (Magnetom Prisma 3T MRI, Siemens)

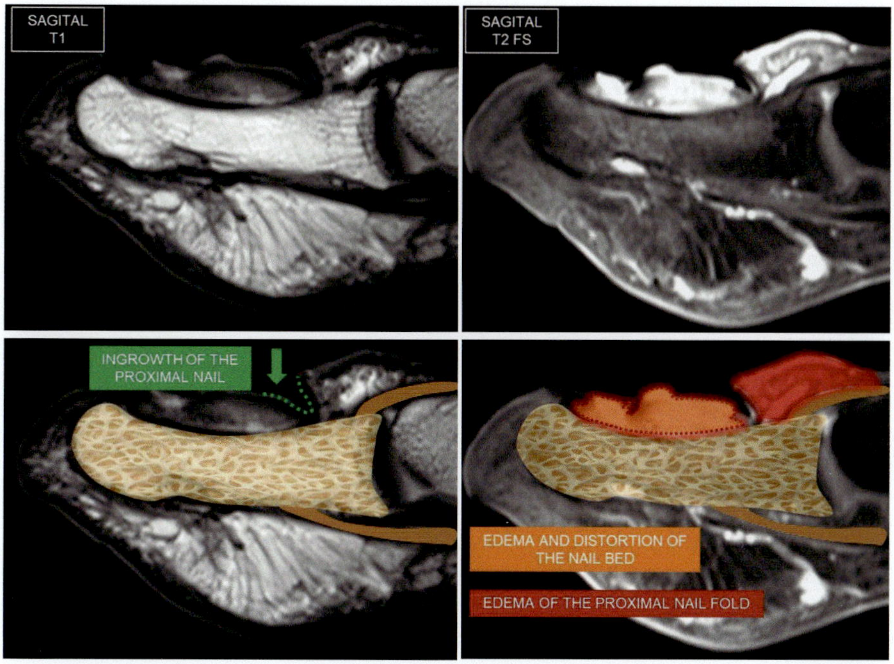

Fig. 16.29 MRI with surface coil findings of retronychia on T1 and T2 FS weighted sequence (Magnetom Prisma 3T MRI, Siemens)

– Nail plate-phalanx distance:

  Reduction in the distance between the origin of the nail plate and the base of the distal phalanx.

– Proximal fold:

  Thickening of the proximal fold and high signal intensity on T2-weighted images and low signal intensity on T1-weighted images.

16.5.9 3D Images

- Allow the visualization of the affected area, especially the exact location of the nail plaque fragment, enabling to assess the severity of the ingrown nail and its underlying causes.
- Contribute to more precise surgical interventions, minimizing the risk of complications and optimizing outcomes.
- Biomodels can be used and allow the creation of physical replicas of the affected area, offering representations that aid in surgical planning and patient education.

16.6 Inflammatory Paronychia

16.6.1 Definition [43, 44]

- Inflammatory irritative dermatitis of nail folds caused by the break of the protective barrier of the nails.
- Repeated exposure to irritants can lead to chronic inflammation, if the process is longer than 6 weeks.

16.6.2 Epidemiology [43]

- Woman 3:1 Man.
- Caused by contact with irritants, moisture, drug reaction, manicures, artificial nails, onychocryptosis.
- Usually limited to one nail; however, if induced by drugs, it can involve many nails.
- Diabetic and immunocompromised patients are at higher risk of developing chronic paronychia that can be classified into the following types:
  - Contact allergy (topical medication ingredients and rubber).
  - Food hypersensitivity.
  - Candida hypersensitivity.
  - Irritative reaction.

16.6.3 Clinical Presentation (Fig. 16.30) [43, 45]

- Acute paronychia:
  - Rapid onset of erythema and edema., less than six weeks
  - Discomfort and pain in the proximal or lateral fold.
- Chronic paronychia:
  - Persist more than 6 weeks. Absence of the cuticle.
  - Nail fold may appear cloudy and hypertrophied, sometimes presenting retraction and nail dystrophy.
  - Nail plate thickened and discolored [5].

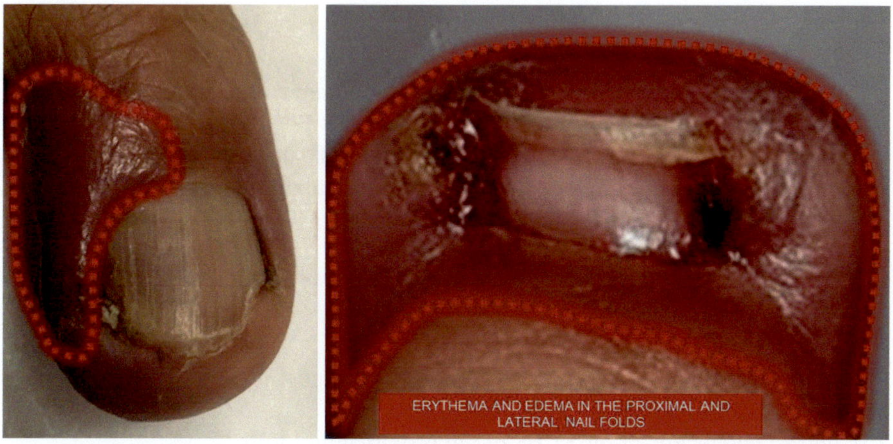

Fig. 16.30 Clinical photograph of a patient with lateral ingrown toenail and consequent paronychia

16.6.4 Onychoscopy [43]

- Periungual region: erythema, edema, scaling, occasional purulent exudate when caused by infection.
- Nail plaques: chromonychia, Beau's lines, fragmented surface, onychomadesis.

16.6.5 Histopathology [23]

- Acute paronychia: neutrophilic and fibrinous exudate is present at the nail border, which may be organized with the formation of granulation tissue.
- Chronic paronychia: chronic inflammatory infiltrate and fibrosis. Infectious causal agents can be visualized.

16.6.6 Radiography and Computed Tomography

- Soft tissue swelling due to granulation tissue adjacent to distal phalanx with loss of the normal fat planes.
- Focal soft tissue swelling of the dorsal aspect of the finger, due to inflammatory tissue on proximal nail fold giving an appearance of "step."

16.6.7 Ultrasonography (Fig. 16.31) [46]

- Thickening, reduction of echogenity, and heterogenicity of the proximal nail fold.
- Hypervascularization of the proximal nail fold.
- Prominence of SLEB (hypoechogenic subepidermal stripe) from the nail fold.
- Thickening and reduction of echogenicity of the subungual space.

16.6.8 MRI (Fig. 16.32) [46]

- Swelling and high signal intensity on STIR images involving the soft tissues proximal nail fold.
- Contrast enhancement on T1 FS of the proximal nail fold.
- Thickening of the dermis of the proximal nail fold.
- Reactive bone marrow edema of distal phalanx.

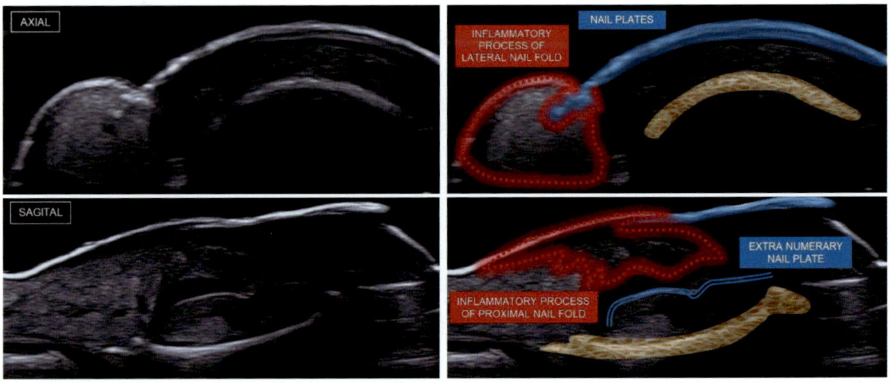

Fig. 16.31 Ultrasonographic findings of paronychia with a 24 MHz probe (Aplio i800, Canon Medical Systems)

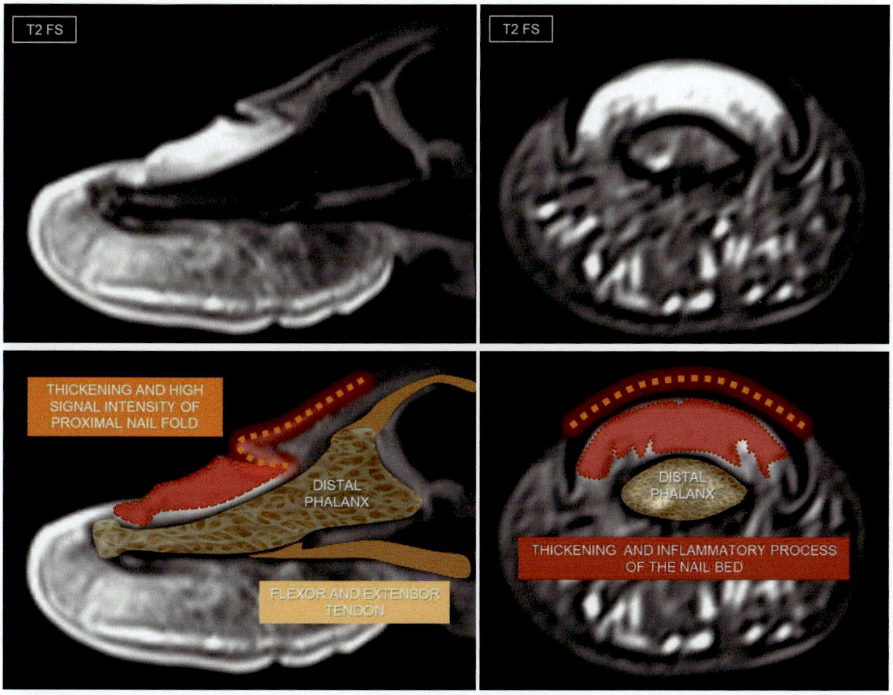

Fig. 16.32 MRI with surface coil findings of paronychia on T1 and T2 FS weighted sequence (Magnetom Prisma 3T MRI, Siemens)

References

1. Sánchez-Regaña M, Umbert P. Diagnosis and management of nail psoriasis. Actas Dermosifiliogr. 2008;99:34–43.
2. Ricardo JW, Lipner SR. Nail psoriasis in older adults. Dermatol Clin. 2021;39:183–93.
3. Schons KRR, Knob CF, Murussi N, Beber AAC, Neumaier W, Monticielo OA. Nail psoriasis: a review of the literature. An Bras Dermatol. 2014;89:312–7.
4. Canal-García E, Bosch-Amate X, Belinchón I, Puig L. Psoriasis ungueal. Actas Dermosifiliogr. 2022;113:481–90.
5. Armesto S, Esteve A, Coto-Segura P, Drake M, Galache C, Martínez-Borra J, et al. Psoriasis ungueal: estudio en 661 pacientes con psoriasis vulgar. Actas Dermosifiliogr. 2011;102:365–72.
6. Castelino M, Eyre S, Barton A. Psoriasis and psoriatic arthritis. In: The microbiome in rheumatic diseases and infection; 2018. p. 239–50.
7. Kaul S, Singal A, Grover C, Sharma S. Clinical and histological spectrum of nail psoriasis: a cross-sectional study. J Cutan Pathol. 2018;45:824–30.
8. Mashal ZR, Elgamal EEA, Zaky MS, Elsaie ML. Dermoscopic features of psoriatic nails and their correlation to disease severity. Dermatol Res Pract. 2023;2023:1–6.
9. Chauhan A, Singal A, Grover C, Sharma S. Dermoscopic features of nail psoriasis: an observational, analytical study. Skin Appendage Disord. 2020;6:207–15.

10. Ortner VK, Mandel VD, Bertugno S, Philipsen PA, Haedersdal M. Imaging of the nail unit in psoriatic patients: a systematic scoping review of techniques and terminology. Exp Dermatol. 2022;31:828–40.
11. Cunha JS, Qureshi AA, Reginato AM. Nail enthesis ultrasound in psoriasis and psoriatic arthritis: a report from the 2016 GRAPPA annual meeting. J Rheumatol. 2017;44:688–90.
12. Ally Essayed SM, Al-Shatouri MA, Nasr Allah YS, Atwa MA. Ultrasonographic characterization of the nails in patients with psoriasis and onychomycosis. Egypt J Radiol Nucl Med. 2015;46:733–9. https://doi.org/10.1016/j.ejrnm.2015.04.009.
13. Krajewska-Wlodarczyk M, Owczarczyk-Saczonek A. Usefulness of ultrasound examination in the assessment of the nail apparatus in psoriasis. Int J Environ Res Public Health. 2022;19:5611.
14. Zhang Y-K, Li W-J, Chen W. Evaluation of nail psoriasis with ultrasound enhanced blood flow imaging (eflow) and power Doppler (PD). Eur Rev Med Pharmacol Sci. 2023;27:2881–7.
15. Mondal S, Dutta S, Lahiri D, Sinha D, Sircar G, Mandal AK, et al. Assessment of nail unit structures by ultrasound in patients with psoriatic arthritis and their correlations with disease activity indices: a case–control study. Rheumatol Int. 2018;38:2087–93. https://doi.org/10.1007/s00296-018-4160-8.
16. Mengesha YM, Bennett ML. Pustular Skin Disorders. Am J Clin Dermatol. 2002;3:389–400.
17. Mansouri B, Benjegerdes K, Hyde K, Kivelevitch D. Pustular psoriasis: pathophysiology and current treatment perspectives. Psoriasis. 2016;6:131–44.
18. Sehgal VN, Verma P, Sharma S, Srivastava G, Aggarwal AK, Rasool F, et al. Acrodermatitis continua of Hallopeau: evolution of treatment options. Int J Dermatol. 2011;50:1195–211.
19. Smith MP, Ly K, Thibodeaux Q, Bhutani T, Liao W, Beck KM. Acrodermatitis continua of Hallopeau: clinical perspectives. Psoriasis. 2019;9:65–72.
20. Mittal S, Muralitharan A, Shanmugasekar C. Dermoscopy of Acrodermatitis continua of Hallopeau. Indian Dermatol Online J. 2023;14:301–2.
21. Errichetti E, Stinco G. Dermoscopy in facilitating the recognition of acrodermatitis continua of Hallopeau. J Dermatol. 2017;44:e286.
22. Baran R, de Berker D, Holzberg M, Piraccini BM, Richert B, Thomas L, editors. Baran & Dawber's diseases of the nails and their management. Chichester: Wiley; 2019. https://doi.org/10.1002/9781119323396.
23. Barnhill RL, Neil Crowson A, Magro CM, Piepkorn MW, Kutzner H, Desman GT. Barnhill's dermatopathology. 4th ed. New York: McGraw Hill/Medical; 2019. https://dermatology.mhmedical.com/content.aspx?bookid=2802&sectionid=238125236. Accessed 3 Aug 2024.
24. Mahoney JM, Scott R. Psoriatic Onychopachydermoperiostitis (POPP). J Am Podiatr Med Assoc. 2009;99:140–3.
25. Vasudevan B, Pragasam V, Verma R, Dabbas D. Unilateral psoriatic onychopachydermoperiostitis. Indian J Dermatol Venereol Leprol. 2012;78:499.
26. Süzen ÖS. A rapidly progressive variant of psoriatic arthritis: psoriatic Onycho-Pachydermo-Periostitis. Arch Rheumatol. 2016;31:94–7.
27. Sakellariou GT, Tsifountoudis I, Vounotrypidis P. Psoriatic onycho-pachydermo periostitis (POPP): a case report treated successfully with IL-17 blockade and a literature review on characteristics, pathogenesis, and treatment. Clin Rheumatol. 2021;40:4749–57.
28. Patterson JW. Weedon's skin pathology. 6th ed. Amsterdam: Elsevier; 2024.
29. Gupta MK, Lipner SR. Review of nail lichen planus. Dermatol Clin. 2021;39:221–30.
30. Yesudian PD, Berker DAR. Inflammatory nail conditions. Part 2: nail changes in lichen planus and alopecia areata. Clin Exp Dermatol. 2021;46:16–20. https://doi.org/10.1111/ced.14352.
31. Iorizzo M, Tosti A, Starace M, Baran R, Daniel CR, Di Chiacchio N, et al. Isolated nail lichen planus: an expert consensus on treatment of the classical form. J Am Acad Dermatol. 2020;83:1717–23.
32. Richert B, Iorizzo M, Tosti A, André J. Nail bed lichen planus associated with onychopapilloma. Br J Dermatol. 2007;156:1071–2.

33. Ceccarelli MA, Gavilanes-Coloma MC, D'almeida L, Azulay D, Iorizzo M, Starace M, et al. Description of the most severe signs in nail lichen planus: a strategy to contribute to the diagnosis of the severe stage. Int J Dermatol. 2022;61:1124–30.
34. Nakamura R, Broce AAA, Palencia DPC, Ortiz NIA, Leverone A. Dermatoscopy of nail lichen planus. Int J Dermatol. 2013;52:684–7.
35. Kharghoria G, Grover C, Bhattacharya SN. Nail dermatoscopic (onychoscopic) features of nail lichen planus: a cross-sectional study. Australas J Dermatol. 2021;62:62.
36. Kharghoria G, Grover C, Bhattacharya SN, Sharma S. Histopathological evaluation of nail lichen planus: a cross-sectional study. J Cutan Pathol. 2021;48:11–7.
37. Chabchoub I, Litaiem N. Ingrown toenails. Treasure Island, FL: StatPearls; 2023. http://www.ncbi.nlm.nih.gov/pubmed/25770573.
38. de Mello CDBF, da Souza M, Noriega LF, di Chiacchio N. Retronychia. An Bras Dermatol. 2018;93:707–11.
39. Nakamura R, Baran R, da Unha D. Do Diagnostico ao Tratamento. 2nd ed. Rio de Janeiro: Elsevier; 2018.
40. Liu Z. A preliminary study on high-frequency ultrasonography and dermoscopy for grade 3 ingrown toenail. Skin Res Technol. 2020;26:762–5.
41. Fernandez-Flores A, Martínez-Nova A, Salgado-Fernandez S. Ingrown toenail: histopathologic and Immunohistochemical study. Am J Dermatopathol. 2009;31:439–45.
42. Wortsman X, Wortsman J, Guerrero R, Soto R, Baran R. Anatomical changes in Retronychia and Onychomadesis detected using ultrasound. Dermatol Surg. 2010;36:1615–20. https://journals.lww.com/00042728-201010000-00024.
43. Leggit JC. Acute and chronic paronychia [internet]. Am Fam Physician. 2017;96:44. www.aafp.org/afp.
44. Wollina U. Systemic drug-induced chronic paronychia and periungual pyogenic granuloma. Indian Dermatol Online J. 2018;9:293.
45. Hay RJ, Elewski B, Piraccini BM, Sullivan N, Wang C, Baran R. Fungal (onychomycosis) and other infections involving the nail apparatus. In: Baran & Dawber's diseases of the nails and their management. Chichester: Wiley; 2018. p. 349–89.
46. de Almeida CÁ, Nakamura R, Leverone A, Costa F, Estrada BD, Haui P, et al. Imaging features for the evaluation of skin and nail infections. Skeletal Radiol. 2024;53:2051. https://doi.org/10.1007/s00256-023-04557-4.

Chapter 17
Clinical, Imaging, and Histological Findings in Infectious Lesions of the Nail and Periungual Region

Robertha Nakamura, Andreia Pizarro Leverone, Nathália Matos, Renata Brandão Villa Verde, André da Silva Cartell, Simone Guarçoni, Miguel Angel Ceccarelli, Philippe Alcântara Gonçalves Martins, Carolina Ávila de Almeida, Tatiana de Almeida Gonçalves Secco, and Clarissa Canella Moraes do Carmo

Infectious lesions of the nail and periungual region present unique diagnostic challenges that are increasingly addressed through advanced imaging techniques. This chapter explores the application of diagnostic imaging in identifying and managing three prevalent infectious conditions: onychomycosis, viral warts, and cellulitis.

Supplementary Information The online version contains supplementary material available at https://doi.org/10.1007/978-3-031-77987-9_17.

R. Nakamura
Institute of Dermatology Professor Rubem David Azulay, Rio de Janeiro, RJ, Brazil

Dermatology by the Brazilian Society of Dermatology, Rio de Janeiro, RJ, Brazil

Dermatology from the Federal University of Medicine at Rio de Janeiro, Rio de Janeiro, RJ, Brazil

Nail Study Center—Institute of Dermatology Professor Ruben David Azulay, Santa Casa da Misericórdia do Rio de Janeiro, Rio de Janeiro, RJ, Brazil

A. P. Leverone
Nail Study Center—Institute of Dermatology Professor Ruben David Azulay, Santa Casa da Misericórdia do Rio de Janeiro, Centro, Rio de Janeiro, RJ, Brazil

N. Matos
Dermatology Department of Fundação de Medicina Tropical Doutor Heitor Vieira Dourado, Manaus, Brazil

R. B. V. Verde
Marcilio Dias Naval Hospital, Rio de Janeiro, Brazil

A. da Silva Cartell
Adjunct Professor at Faculdade de Medicina da Universidade Federal do Rio Grande do Sul, Rio de Janeiro, Brazil

Dermatologist and Dermatopathologist in Private Practice, Rio de Janeiro, Brazil

© The Author(s), under exclusive license to Springer Nature Switzerland AG 2025

C. Canella Moraes do Carmo (ed.), *Atlas of Diagnostic Imaging in Dermatology*,
https://doi.org/10.1007/978-3-031-77987-9_17

Each of these infections affects the nail and surrounding tissues in distinct ways, requiring precise imaging to differentiate between them and guide effective treatment. By examining the role of various imaging modalities in detecting these infections, this chapter aims to enhance the understanding of their clinical manifestations and improve diagnostic accuracy. Clinicians will find valuable insights into how imaging can support the diagnosis and management of these common yet complex infectious conditions.

17.1 Nail Apparatus-Originated Infections

17.1.1 Onychomycosis

17.1.1.1 Definition [1–3]

- Infection that affects the nail bed is caused by dermatophyte fungi, yeasts, and non-dermatophyte filamentous fungi (FFND).
- Can also affect the adjacent skin [1–3].

17.1.1.2 Epidemiology [1–3]

- Distribution is worldwide and more prevalent in temperate regions [3].
- Global prevalence is approximately 5.5%.

S. Guarçoni
Clinica ALTA – Rio de Janeiro, Botafogo, Brazil

M. A. Ceccarelli
Nail Diseases Outpatient Clinic at Dermatology Department, Hospital Universitário Pedro Ernesto – Universidade Estadual do Rio de Janeiro – UERJ, Maracanã, Rio de Janeiro, Brazil

P. A. G. Martins
Bronstein DASA – Tijuca, Rio de Janeiro, Brazil

Américas Medical City, Barra da Tijuca, Rio de Janeiro, Brazil

C. Á. de Almeida
Faculty of Medicine of Valença—UniFaa, Valença, Brazil

Federal University of Rio de Janeiro—UFRJ, Rio de Janeiro, Brazil

T. de Almeida Gonçalves Secco
Fleury Group – RJ, Barra da Tijuca, Rio de Janeiro, Brazil

Musculoskeletal Imaging at DASA – RJ, Barra da Tijuca, Rio de Janeiro, Brazil

C. Canella Moraes do Carmo (✉)
Fluminense Federal University—UFF, Rio de Janeiro, Brazil

Federal University of Rio de Janeiro—UFRJ, Rio de Janeiro, Brazil

Diagnóstico das Américas—DASA—RJ, Rio de Janeiro, Brazil

Biodesign Laboratory, DASA-PUC, Rio de Janeiro, Brazil

- Occurs at any age, although the elderly are most affected. Prevalence is lower in children [4].
- Persistent nail trauma, psoriasis, diabetes, poor peripheral circulation, HIV, immunosuppression, and smokers are factors that favor the development of the disease.
- Plantar tinea and interdigital tinea pedis are risk factors for nail infections and may occur concomitantly with onychomycosis [3].
- Onychomycosis most commonly affects the feet, with the hallux being the most frequently impacted [5].
- Male predisposition.

17.1.1.3 Clinical Presentation (Fig. 17.1) [1, 2, 4, 5]

- Most common clinical findings:
  - Chromonychia (yellow, white, brown).
  - Onycholysis, nail plate fragility, and thickening.
  - Subungual hyperkeratosis.
  - Streaks and onychocryptosis in severe cases.
  - Dermatophytomas and fungal abscesses can also be observed in chronic cases.
  - Pseudomonas bacterial infections may be present and cause greenish chromonychia.
- Fungal nail infections are classified by the pattern of nail apparatus invasion:
  - Distal and lateral subungual onychomycosis (DLSO): Infection affects the onychodermal band and lower nail parts, including the hyponychium, nail bed, or lateral nail fold, with dermatophyte tunnels or gaps causing opaque streaks. Treatment is challenging due to poor drug penetration, leading to friable, eroded nails.
  - White superficial onychomycosis (WSO): affects toenails with initial invasion of the nail plate's upper surface, forming small white spots that coalesce into leukonychia trichophytica.
  - Endonyx (EO): superficial invasion by dermatophytes occurs primarily in the distal portion between the nail plates, resulting in less thickening of the nail plate and erosion.

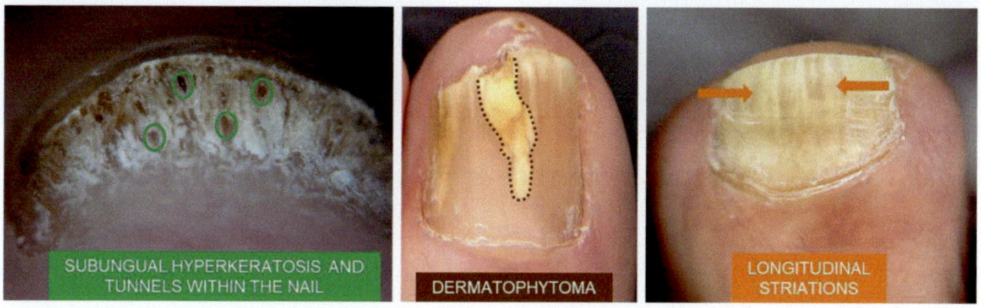

Fig. 17.1 Clinical photograph of patient with onychomycosis

- Proximal subungual onychomycosis (PSO): is also known as proximal white subungual onychomycosis (PWSO), affects fingernails and toenails with a white spot under the proximal nail fold spreading distally, and is associated with paronychia.
- Total dystrophic onychomycosis (TDO): advanced form, caused by Candida in immunocompromised individuals, with diffusely thickened, destroyed nails and inflamed periungual tissues.
- Mixed onychomycosis: concurrent clinical forms or fungal species in the same patient.

17.1.1.4 Onychoscopy (Fig. 17.2) [6]

- Different types of onychomycosis have particular characteristics in dermoscopy and this method can also be used to choose the best location to collect a mycological sample when using abrasion.
- Jagged edge of the proximal margin of onycholysis, which shows pointed structures toward the proximal fold, called "spikes", which are the subungual streaks. They indicate the progression of infection.

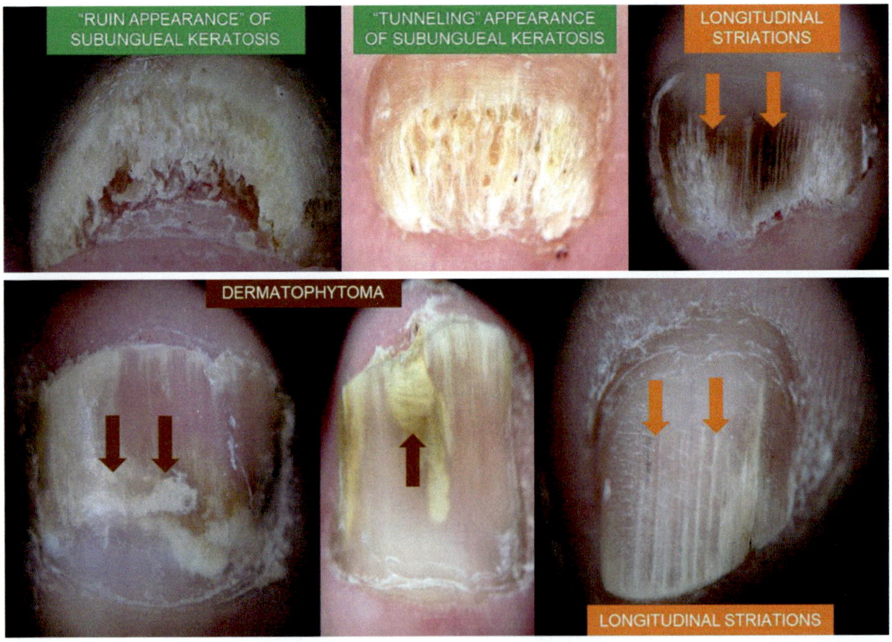

Fig. 17.2 Dermoscopic findings of patient with onychomycosis (x20)

- Longitudinal striations in the nail plate, with colors ranging from white to yellow, orange, and brown, are often not detectable with the naked eye.
- Yellow-orange-brown discoloration of the plate, arranged in parallel bands of faded color, similar to the aurora borealis, indicative of dermatophytoma.
- "Ruin appearance" of subungual keratosis attached to the ventral part of the plate, consisting of scales and hyphae, more evident at the distal margin of the nail, and irregular distal termination, due to the extreme fragility and fragmentation of the nail plate after fungal invasion. Occurs also in total dystrophic onychomycosis.
- "Dermatophytoma" shows an irregular, round, discolored area under the plaque, yellow-orange in color, homogeneous, matte, connected to the distal margin by a yellowish-white longitudinal band. In fungal melanonychia, dermoscopy allows differentiation from other causes of darkened nail pigmentation, including subungual hematoma and melanonychia.
- White and matte shadows.
- Transverse streak pattern.
- Homogeneous opacity.
- Micro-lamellar division.

17.1.1.5 Histopathology (Fig. 17.3) [1]

- Microscopic alterations resemble nail psoriasis with the presence of spongiform pustulation, parakeratosis, and the presence of neutrophils.
- PAS and silver stains show the causal agent.

17.1.1.6 Ultrasonography (Fig. 17.4)

- Thickening and hypervascularization of the nail bed and proximal nail folds.
- Loss of the trilaminar appearance, loosely compact thickening of the nail plates, areas of dermatophytoma.
- Complications:
  - Narrow, dark channels in ultrasonography images that extend irregularly, often indicative of abnormal pathways due to inflammation or infection with peripheral hypervascularization.
  - Poorly defined anechoic areas with posterior acoustic enhancement (collections and abscesses), that appear brighter on ultrasonography due to signal enhancement with peripheral hypervascularization.
  - Regions of high echogenicity causing reverberation patterns on ultrasonography images, often due to the presence of gas.

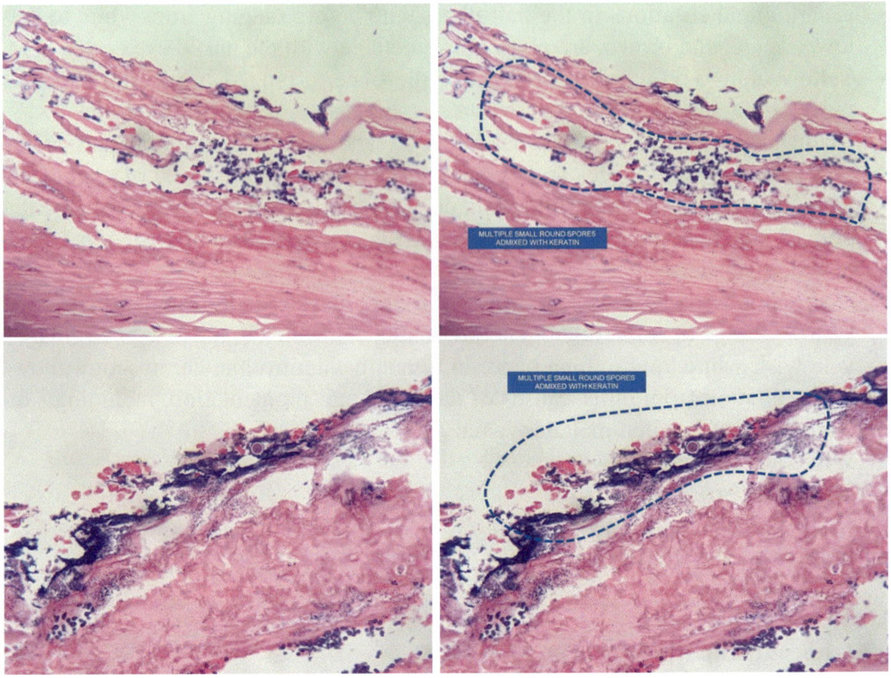

Fig. 17.3 Histological findings of onychomycosis (H&E x4)

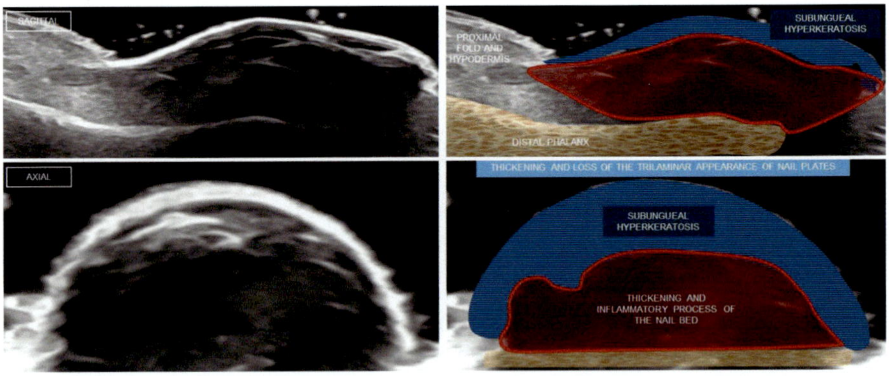

Fig. 17.4 Ultrasonographic findings of onychomycosis with a 24 MHz probe (Aplio i800, Canon Medical Systems)

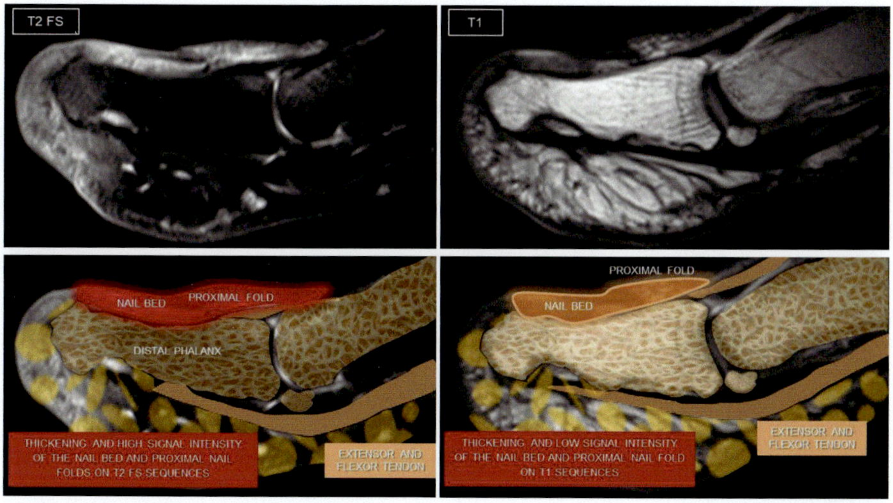

Fig. 17.5 MRI with surface coil findings of onychomycosis on T2 FS and T1-weighted sequences (Magnetom Prisma 3T MRI, Siemens)

17.1.1.7 MRI (Fig. 17.5)

- Thickening and high signal intensity of the nail bed and proximal nail folds on T2-weighted images.
- Enhancement of the nail bed and proximal nail folds after gadolinium administration.
- Complications:
  - Irregular fistulae with edema and with peripheral inflammation.
  - Periungual collections and abscesses with peripheral enhancement after gadolinium administration.

17.1.2 Viral Warts

17.1.2.1 Definition [1, 7, 8]

- Benign fibroepithelial tumors, periungual and subungual, caused by different genotypes of the human papillomavirus, usually HPV types 1, 2, 4, 27, and 57.
- Biting, picking, and tearing the nails and nail walls are common habits in individuals with periungual warts. This type of trauma can also result in disease spreading to the face and lips.
- Usually grow slowly from the hyponychium toward the nail bed, affecting the nail matrix and causing a secondary upward displacement and dystrophy of the nail plates.

17.1.2.2 Epidemiology [7–9]

- Any age group can be affected, but they are more common in children and adolescents [1].
- Affect the nails of the hands more often on the lateral aspect of the proximal nail fold [2].
- Nail biting is a significant predisposing factor because it causes repeated trauma and facilitates virus installation [1].

17.1.2.3 Clinical Presentation (Fig. 17.6) [7–9]

- Periungual warts are generally asymptomatic, although fissures may cause pain [2].
- Single or multiple papules, keratotic surface, with blackened spots (thrombosed capillaries) that initially affect the hyponychium.
- Slowly grow toward the nail bed, and eventually raise the plate.
- Warts in the proximal nail fold produce periungual hyperkeratosis, resembling hyperkeratotic cuticle.

17.1.2.4 Onychoscopy (Fig. 17.7) [1, 7]

- Keratotic papule.
- Thrombosed vessels.
- Onycholysis and depression in the nail plate.

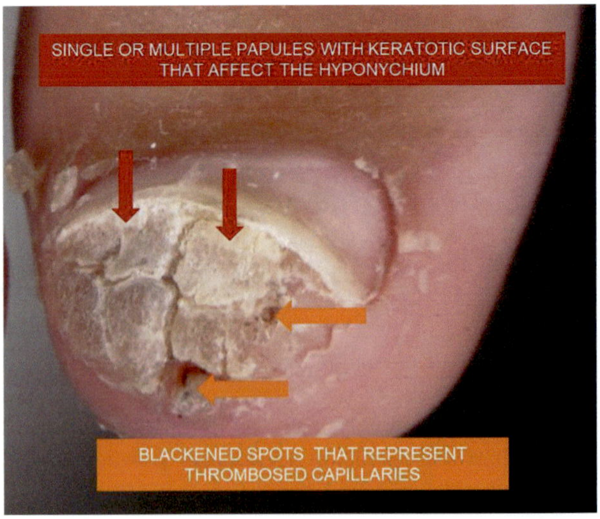

Fig. 17.6 Clinical photograph of patient with periungual viral wart

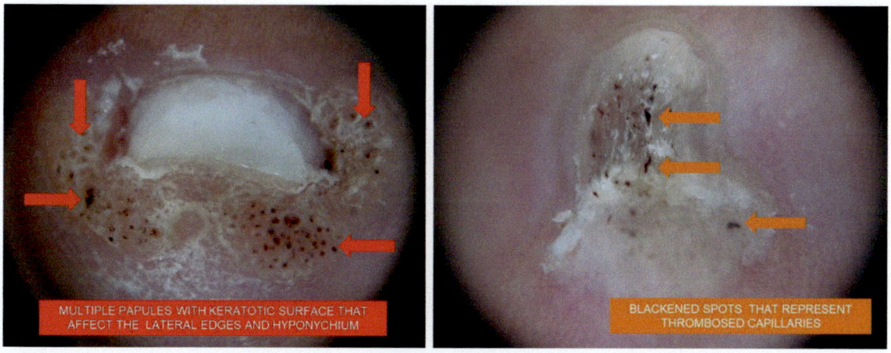

Fig. 17.7 Dermoscopic findings of patient with periungual viral wart (x20)

17.1.2.5 Histopathology (Fig. 17.8) [7, 10]

- Quite similar to cutaneous viral warts.
- Digitated epithelial hyperplasia with the presence of koilocytes in the upper epidermis.
- Hyperkeratosis.
- Chronic inflammatory changes.

17.1.2.6 Ultrasonography (Fig. 17.9) [11]

- Eccentric hypoechoic fusiform and nodular lesions usually at hyponychium or lateral folds.
- Hyperkeratosis, irregularity, and erosion in the skin surface can be observed.
- Thickening of the nail plates and interplate spaces.
- Hypovascular on power Doppler ultrasound but may occasionally present hypervascularity in the underlying or surrounding dermis.

17.1.2.7 MRI (Fig. 17.10)

- Eccentric nodular lesions with low signal intensity on T1 weighted images and high signal intensity in T2 and STIE weighted images, usually at hyponychium or lateral folds.
- Irregularity and erosion in the skin surface.
- Mild enhancement after gadolinium administration.
- Irregular thickening of the dermis and epidermis.

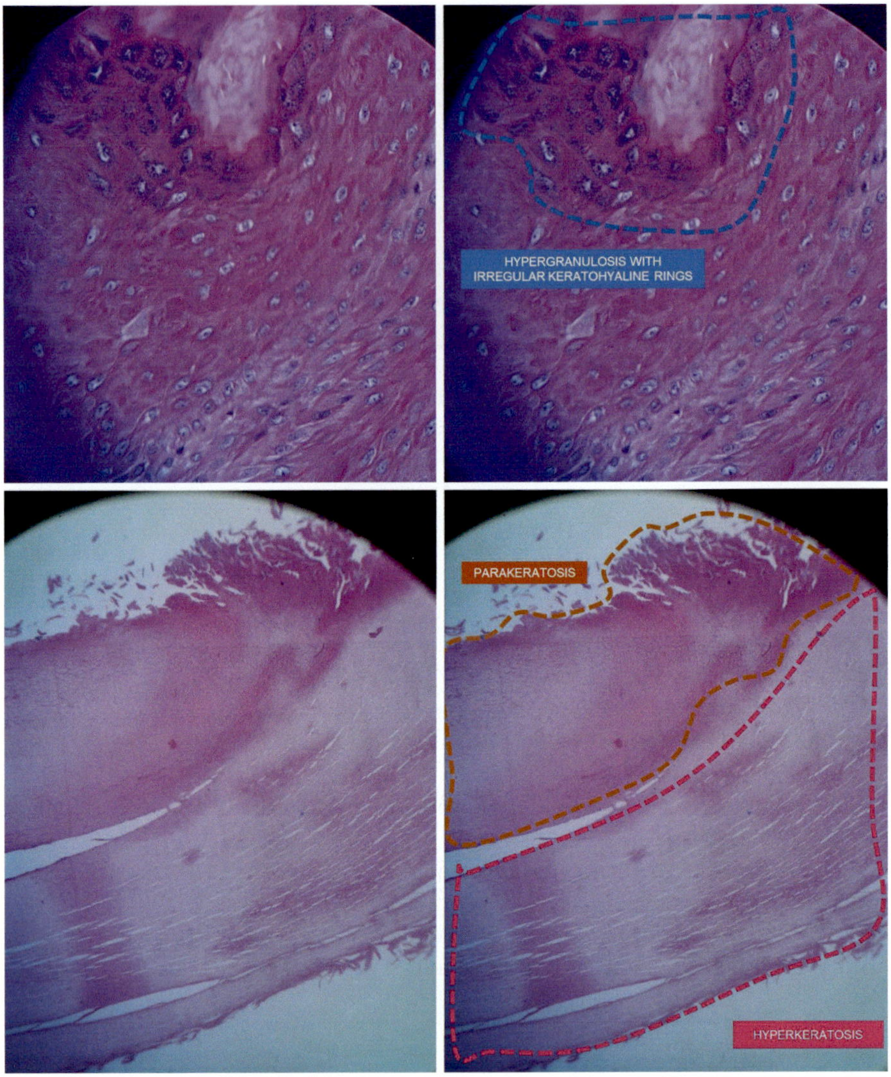

Fig. 17.8 Histological findings of periungual viral wart (H&E x4 and x10)

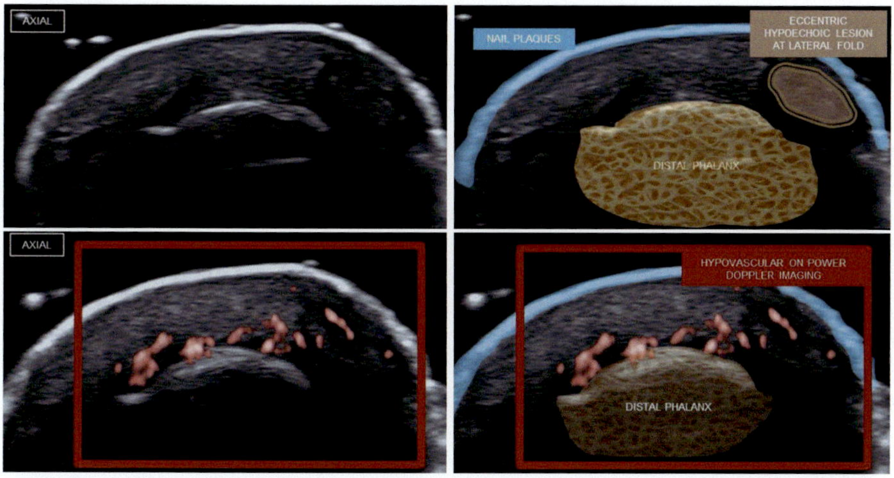

Fig. 17.9 Ultrasonographic findings of periungual viral wart with a 24 MHz probe (Aplio i800, Canon Medical Systems)

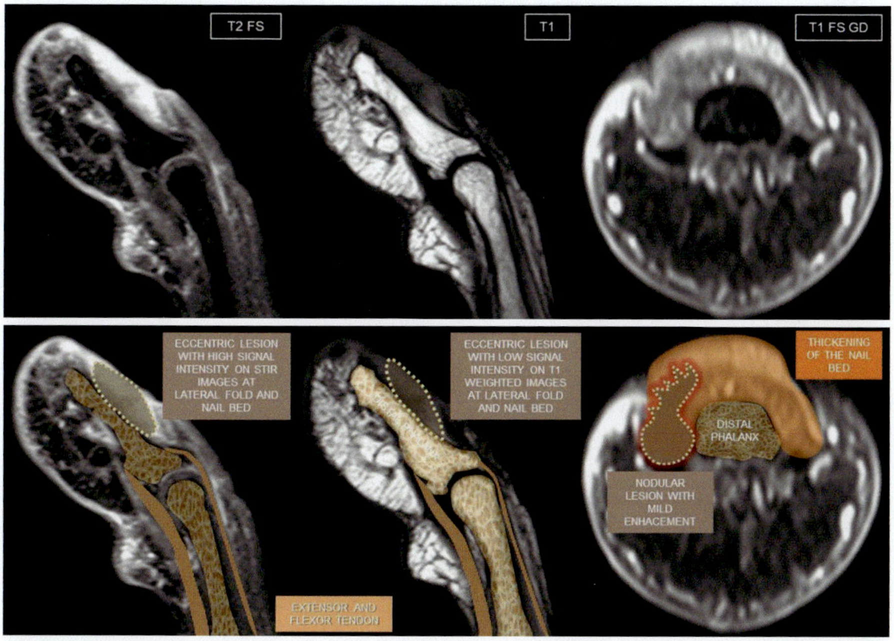

Fig. 17.10 MRI with surface coil findings of periungual viral wart on T2 FS, T1, and T1 FS weighted sequences after gadolinium administration (Magnetom Prisma 3T MRI, Siemens)

17.2 Infections Affecting the Nail Apparatus by Contiguity

17.2.1 Typical Infectious Paronychia

17.2.1.1 Definition [1, 12]

- Paronychia is an inflammatory process of the periungual tissue that usually occurs after trauma or manipulation [1].
- Disruption of the cuticular seal allows entry of irritants, allergens, and infectious agents.
- The principal etiological agent of infectious acute paronychia is Staphylococcus aureus.
- Candida albicans is the most commonly associated pathogen with chronic paronychia [2].

17.2.1.2 Epidemiology [12]

- More common in women than men, with a ratio of 3:1.
- Affects patients who frequently expose their hands to excessive moisture, irritants, starches, or trauma to the cuticle.
- Middle-aged women are at higher risk of infection.

17.2.1.3 Clinical Presentation (Fig. 17.11) [12]

- Acute paronychia:
  - Initial phase: Inflammation of the proximal nail fold without pus formation.
  - Progression: Development of abscesses of varying degrees, absence of the cuticle, onycholysis, and chromonychia (yellowish or greenish discoloration), Beau's lines, or onychomadesis.

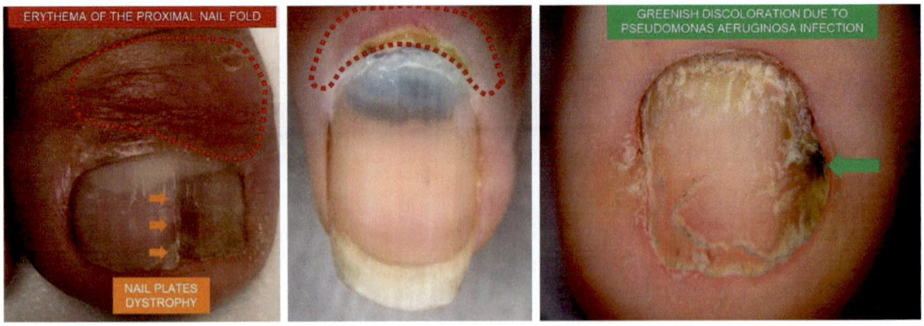

Fig. 17.11 Clinical photograph of patient with infectious paronychia

- Chronic paronychia:
  - Repeated episodes of subacute infection by opportunistic organisms lead to chronicity, usually lasting more than 6 weeks.
  - The proximal nail fold may be swollen and resistant, and the nail plate may be thickened and discolored.
  - May present with retraction of the proximal nail fold, nail dystrophy, and loss of the cuticle.
- Chloronychia:
  - Considered an occupational disease.
  - Generally caused by frequent exposure to water, creating ideal conditions for the growth of Pseudomonas aeruginosa.
  - Clinical presentation includes green discoloration of the nail plate, onycholysis, and chronic proximal paronychia.

17.2.1.4 Onychoscopy [12]

- Acute paronychia:
  - Onycholysis.
  - Chromonychia (yellowish or greenish).
  - Irregular transverse grooves.
  - Onychomadesis.
- Chronic paronychia:
  - Chromonychia.
  - Beau's lines.
  - Fragmented nail surface.
  - Onychomadesis.

17.2.1.5 Histopathology [10, 12]

- In acute paronychia, a neutrophilic and fibrinous exudate is present at the nail border.
- This exudate may become organized with the formation of granulation tissue, leading to chronic inflammatory infiltrate and fibrosis in the chronic phase.
- Infectious causal agents can often be visualized in these cases.

17.2.1.6 Radiography and Computed Tomography [11]

- Soft tissue swelling due to granulation tissue adjacent to distal phalanx with loss of the normal fat planes.

- Focal soft tissue swelling of the dorsal aspect of the finger, due to inflammatory tissue on proximal nail fold giving an appearance of "step."
- Periungual collections are visualized especially by CT.
- Erosion, fragmentation, or destruction of the distal phalanx when osseous involvement.

17.2.1.7 Ultrasonography (Fig. 17.12) [13, 14]

- Thickening of the subungual space.
- Thickening, reduction of echogenicity, and heterogenicity of the proximal nail fold.
- Hypervascularization of the proximal nail fold.
- Prominence of SLEB (hypoechogenic subepidermal stripe) from the nail fold.
- Fluid collections, abscesses, and fistulous tracts.
- Bubbles generate a hyperechoic band with reverberation and posterior acoustic shadowing.

17.2.1.8 MRI (Fig. 17.13)

- Swelling and high signal intensity on STIR images involving the soft tissues proximal nail fold.
- Thickening and contrast enhancement on T1 FS weighted images of the proximal nail fold.
- Fluid collections, abscesses, and fistulous tracts at periungual soft tissue.
- Bone marrow edema, irregularity and erosion of distal phalanx.
- Reactive articular effusion of the distal interphalangeal joint.

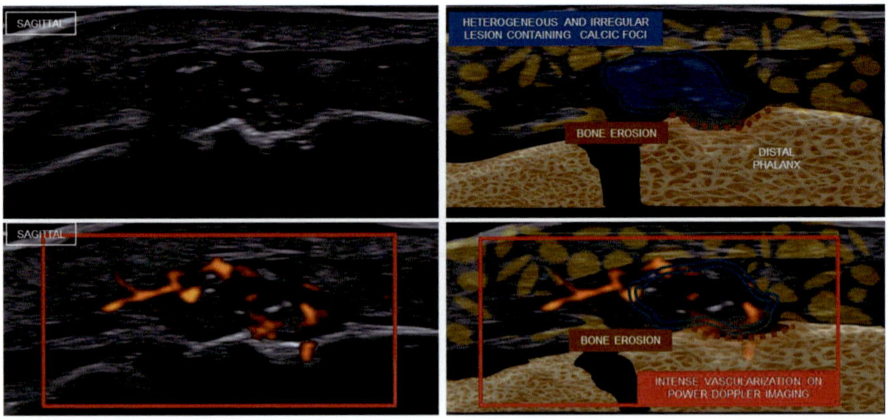

Fig. 17.12 Ultrasonographic findings of infectious paronychia with a 24 MHz probe (Aplio i800, Canon Medical Systems)

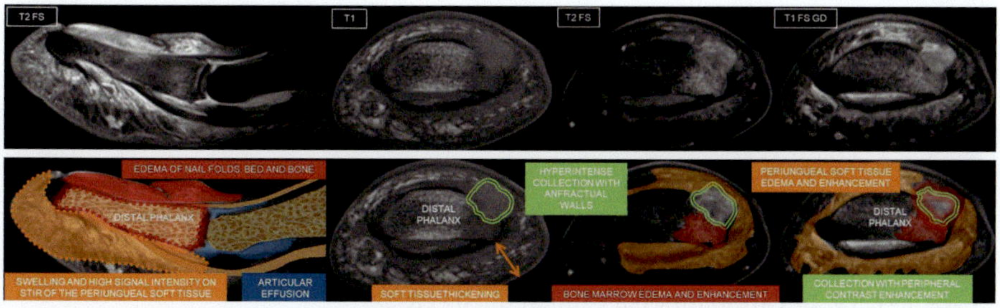

Fig. 17.13 MRI with surface coil findings of infectious paronychia on T2 FS, T1, and T1 FS weighted sequences after gadolinium administration (Magnetom Prisma 3T MRI, Siemens)

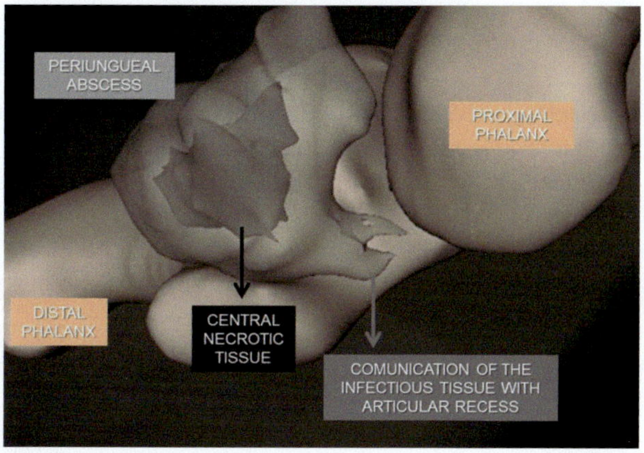

Fig. 17.14 3D virtual images of infectious paronychia after segmentation of isotropic MRI images

17.2.1.9 3D Images (Fig. 17.14; Video 17.1)

- Highly beneficial for treating recurrent cases with fluid collections, abscesses, and fistulous tracts.
- Facilitates visualization of the lesion's extent, aiding in the assessment of its relationship with adjacent structures.
- Enhances precision in surgical interventions.
- Biomodels can be utilized to create physical replicas of the affected area, providing representations that support surgical planning and patient education.

17.2.2 Atypical Infectious Paronychia

17.2.2.1 Definition [12, 15, 16]

- Involves nonstandard infectious agents and presents with unusual clinical features, often requiring specialized diagnostic and treatment approaches.

- The most common causative agent of atypical infectious paronychia is Mycobacterium avium-intracellular complex and contiguous involvement of the nail by an underlying tuberculous focus must also be considered.

17.2.2.2 Epidemiology [12, 15, 16]

- Cutaneous tuberculosis, also called scrofuloderma, is a rare condition accounting for 1–1.5% of extrapulmonary tuberculosis cases.
- In cases of contiguous involvement of the ungual complex, dactylitis is commonly seen in association.

17.2.2.3 Clinical Presentation (Figs. 17.15 and 17.16) [12, 15, 16]

- Swelling, redness, and pain in periungual soft tissues can be associated with nodules, ulcers, or sinus tracts near the nail.
- Thickening and deformity of the nail plates associated with onycholysis.

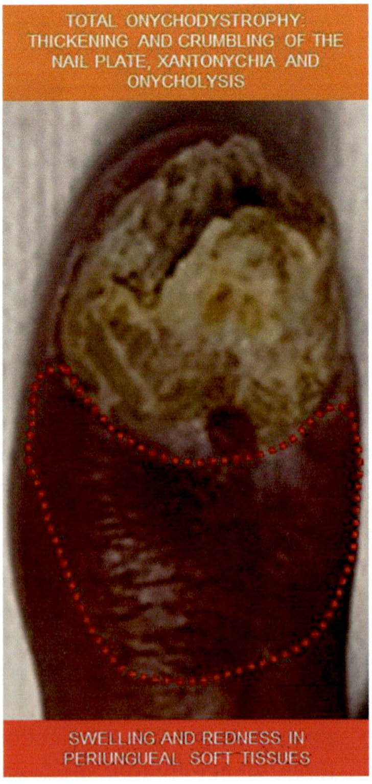

Fig. 17.15 Clinical photograph of patient with infectious paronychia due to tuberculosis

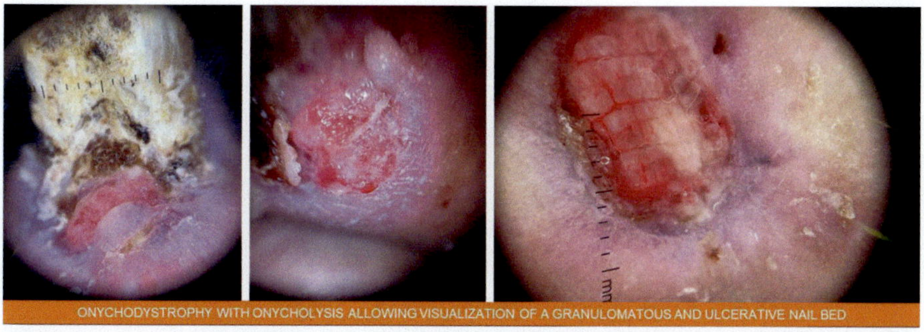

Fig. 17.16 Dermoscopic findings of patient with infectious paronychia due to tuberculosis (x20)

- Often associated with dactylitis:
  - Trabecular destruction and cortical thinning involve the small tubular bones of the hands and feet.
  - Occurs in children under 6 years old.
- Possible systemic signs of tuberculosis, such as fever, weight loss, and night sweats, if associated with active pulmonary or disseminated tuberculosis.

17.2.2.4 Histopathology [12, 15, 16]

- The hallmark of tuberculosis is the presence of caseating granulomas. These granulomas are organized aggregates of macrophages that have transformed into epithelioid cells, often with a central area of necrosis that appears cheesy or caseous under the microscope.
- In the granulomas, Langerhans cells (a type of dendritic cell) may be present. These cells are important in the immune response to Mycobacterium tuberculosis.
- Acid-fast bacilli, which are the causative agents of tuberculosis, can sometimes be seen within the granulomas when special stains, such as Ziehl-Neelsen or auramine-rhodamine, are used. However, they may not always be visible in all cases.
- Surrounding the granulomas, there is often significant edema and a mixed inflammatory infiltrate that may include lymphocytes, plasma cells, and neutrophils.
- The nail matrix or nail bed can show hyperkeratosis (thickening of the outer layer of the skin) and acanthosis (thickening of the stratum spinosum), although these changes are less specific and more related to the chronicity of the infection.
- In advanced cases, there may be destruction of nail structures, including the nail matrix and nail bed, leading to nail dystrophy or loss.
- The inflammatory infiltrate may also be observed around blood vessels and appendages within the nail bed and matrix.

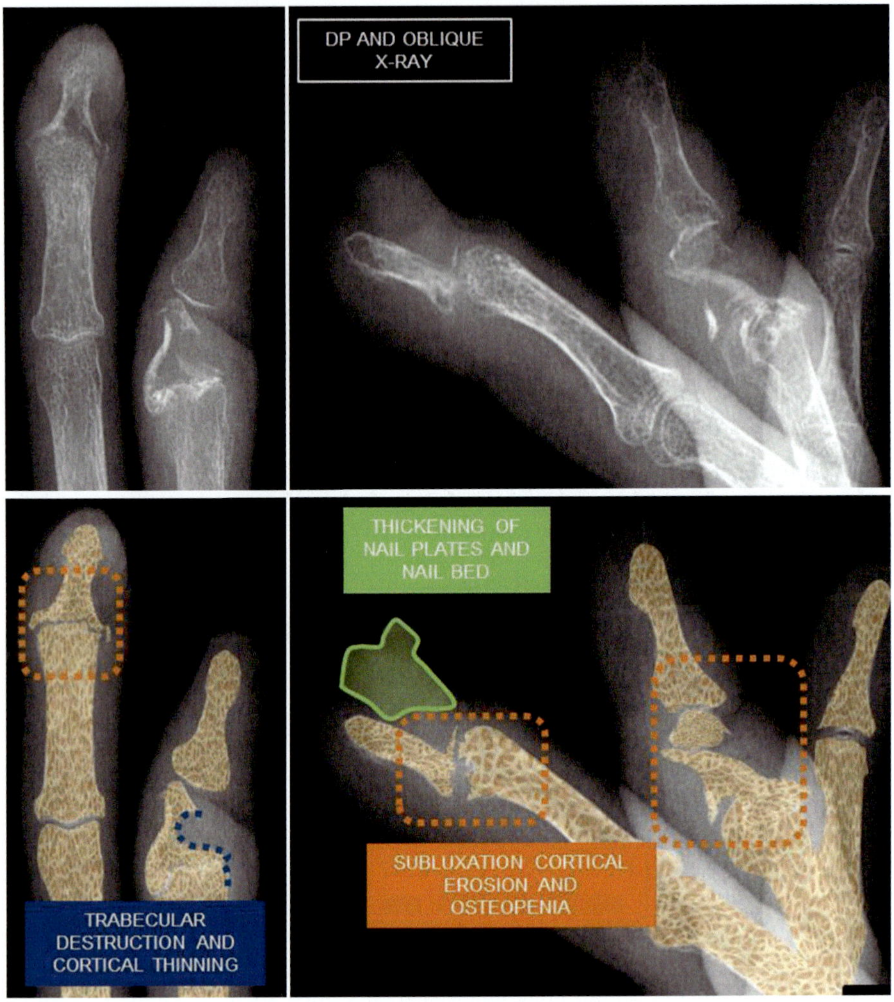

Fig. 17.17 Radiographic findings of infectious paronychia due to tuberculosis (Philips Duo Diagnost R&F Room Digital RF and Tomo System)

17.2.2.5 Radiography and Computed Tomography (Fig. 17.17) [12, 15]

- Usually demonstrated only the bone involvement of tuberculosis:
  - Lytic lesion of the distal phalanx associated with bone expansion.
  - Cortical erosion, irregularity, and osteopenia.
  - Trabecular destruction and cortical thinning.
  - Resembles an inflated balloon, known as "spina ventosa."

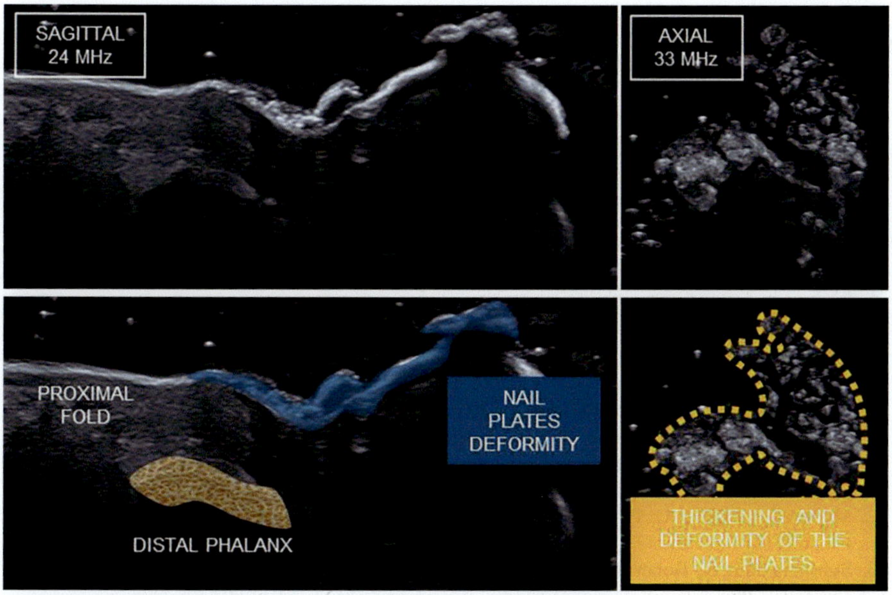

Fig. 17.18 Ultrasonographic findings of infectious paronychia due to tuberculosis with a 24 MHz and 33 MHz probes (Aplio i800, Canon Medical Systems)

- Radiography is useful for excluding differential diagnoses affecting the nail bed and matrix, such as tumors, and can show thickening of the nail bed with increased vascularity, indicating inflammation.

17.2.2.6 Ultrasonography (Fig. 17.18) [14, 17–19]

- Increased thickness in the nail bed and surrounding nail folds.
- Poorly defined hypoechoic lesions that indicate fluid collections, abscesses, or fistulous tracts on periungual soft tissues.
- Presence of areas with increased vascularity suggests granulation tissue formation.
- Signs of bone involvement, especially in dactylitis, present as cortical erosion, irregularity, and destruction.

References

1. Nakamura R, Baran R. Doenças da Unha. Do Diagnostico ao Tratamento, 2a edição. Rio de Janeiro: Elsevier; 2018.
2. Vlahovic TC. Onychomycosis. Clin Podiatr Med Surg. 2016;33:305–18.

3. Gupta AK, Stec N, Summerbell RC, Shear NH, Piguet V, Tosti A, Piraccini BM. Onychomycosis: a review. J Eur Acad Dermatol Venereol. 2020;34:1972–90.
4. Hay RJ, Baran R. Onychomycosis: a proposed revision of the clinical classification. J Am Acad Dermatol. 2011;65:1219–27.
5. Lipner SR, Scher RK. Onychomycosis. J Am Acad Dermatol. 2019;80:835–51.
6. De Crignis G, Valgas N, Rezende P, Leverone A, Nakamura R. Dermatoscopy of onychomycosis. Int J Dermatol. 2014; https://doi.org/10.1111/ijd.12104.
7. Herschthal J, McLeod MP, Zaiac M. Management of ungual warts. Dermatol Ther. 2012;25:545–50.
8. Lynch MD, Cliffe J, Morris-Jones R. Management of cutaneous viral warts. BMJ. 2014;348:g3339.
9. Ball SLR, Winder DM, Vaughan K, Hanna N, Levy J, Sterling JC, Stanley MA, Goon PKC. Analyses of human papillomavirus genotypes and viral loads in anogenital warts. J Med Virol. 2011;83:1345–50.
10. Barnhill RL, Neil Crowson A, Magro CM, Piepkorn MW, Kutzner H, Desman GT. Barnhill's Dermatopathology. 4th ed. McGraw Hill/Medical; 2019.
11. de Almeida CÁ, Nakamura R, Leverone A, Costa F, Estrada BD, Haui P, Luz F, Yamada AF, Werner H, Canella C. Imaging features for the evaluation of skin and nail infections. Skeletal Radiol. 2024; https://doi.org/10.1007/s00256-023-04557-4.
12. Macneal P, Milroy C. Paronychia Drainage. 2023 Jun 5. In: StatPearls [Internet]. Treasure Island (FL): StatPearls Publishing; 2025 Jan–. PMID: 32644572.
13. Subramaniam S, Bober J, Chao J, Zehtabchi S. Point-of-care ultrasound for diagnosis of abscess in skin and soft tissue infections. Acad Emerg Med. 2016;23:1298–306.
14. Wortsman X. Sonography of dermatologic emergencies. J Ultrasound Med. 2017;36:1905–14.
15. Khanna D, Chakravarty P, Agarwal A, Gupta R. Tuberculous dactylitis presenting as paronychia with pseudopterygium and nail dystrophy. Pediatr Dermatol. 2013; https://doi.org/10.1111/j.1525-1470.2012.01843.x.
16. Wollina U. Systemic drug-induced chronic paronychia and periungual pyogenic granuloma. Indian Dermatol Online J. 2018;9:293.
17. Wortsman X. Role of color Doppler ultrasound in cutaneous inflammatory conditions. Seminars in Ultrasound, CT and MRI. 2023 https://doi.org/10.1053/j.sult.2023.12.001.
18. Wortsman X (2018) Atlas of dermatologic ultrasound. Atlas of Dermatologic Ultrasound. https://doi.org/10.1007/978-3-319-89614-4.
19. Wortsman X. Sonography of cutaneous and ungual lumps and bumps. Ultrasound Clin. 2012;7:505–23.

Chapter 18
Clinical, Imaging, and Histological Findings in Tumoral Lesions of the Nail and Periungual Region

Robertha Nakamura, Andreia Pizarro Leverone, Renata Brandão Villa Verde, Nathália Matos, André da Silva Cartell, Flavia Martins Costa, Heron Werner, Philippe Alcântara Gonçalves Martins, Carolina Ávila de Almeida, Gerson Ribeiro, Vinicius Arcoverde, Weydler Hottz, Matilde Iorizzo, and Clarissa Canella Moraes do Carmo

Accurate diagnosis of tumoral lesions in the nail and periungual region requires a nuanced understanding of advanced imaging techniques. This chapter explores the essential roles of magnetic resonance imaging with surface coil, computed tomography, and ultrasonography in identifying and assessing these complex lesions. Each imaging modality offers unique benefits: MRI provides superior soft tissue

---

Supplementary Information The online version contains supplementary material available at https://doi.org/10.1007/978-3-031-77987-9_18.

R. Nakamura
Institute of Dermatology Professor Rubem David Azulay, Rio de Janeiro, RJ, Brazil

Dermatology by the Brazilian Society of Dermatology, Rio de Janeiro, RJ, Brazil

Dermatology from the Federal University of Medicine at Rio de Janeiro, Rio de Janeiro, RJ, Brazil

Nail Study Center—Institute of Dermatology Professor Ruben David Azulay, Santa Casa da Misericórdia do Rio de Janeiro, Rio de Janeiro, RJ, Brazil

A. P. Leverone
Nail Study Center—Institute of Dermatology Professor Ruben David Azulay, Santa Casa da Misericórdia do Rio de Janeiro, Rio de Janeiro, RJ, Brazil

R. B. V. Verde
Marcilio Dias Naval Hospital, Rio de Janeiro, RJ, Brazil

N. Matos
Dermatology Department of Fundação de Medicina Tropical Doutor Heitor Vieira Dourado, Manaus, Brazil

A. da Silva Cartell
Adjunct Professor at Faculdade de Medicina da Universidade Federal do Rio Grande do Sul, Rio de Janeiro, Brazil

Dermatologist and Dermatopathologist in Private Practice, Rio de Janeiro, Brazil

© The Author(s), under exclusive license to Springer Nature Switzerland AG 2025

C. Canella Moraes do Carmo (ed.), *Atlas of Diagnostic Imaging in Dermatology*, https://doi.org/10.1007/978-3-031-77987-9_18

contrast, CT delivers detailed images of bone structures, and USG allows for dynamic, real-time evaluation of lesions with more resolution. By examining these imaging methods, this chapter aims to equip clinicians with the knowledge needed to effectively diagnose and manage tumoral conditions in the nail and periungual regions, leading to better patient care and outcomes.

18.1 Glomus Tumor

18.1.1 Definition [1–4]

- Benign vascular hamartoma, originating from the neuromyoarterial apparatus or glomus body (Sucquet–Hoyer canal).
- Hyperplasia of any of the components of the glomus body can lead to the development of a glomus tumor: glomus cells, the vascular system, and smooth muscle cells.
- It includes the glomus tumor, glomangioma, and glomangiomyoma, clinically referred to as glomus tumors.

F. M. Costa
Clinica ALTA—DASA—Rio de Janeiro, Rio de Janeiro, RJ, Brazil

Universidade Federal do Rio de Janeiro—UFRJ, Rio de Janeiro, RJ, Brazil

H. Werner
Clinica ALTA—DASA—Rio de Janeiro, Rio de Janeiro, RJ, Brazil

Universidade Federal do Rio de Janeiro—UFRJ, Rio de Janeiro, RJ, Brazil

Biodesign Lab DASA—PUC—Rio de Janeiro, Rio de Janeiro, RJ, Brazil

P. A. G. Martins
Bronstein DASA—Tijuca, Rio de Janeiro, RJ, Brazil

Américas Medical City, Barra da Tijuca, Rio de Janeiro, RJ, Brazil

C. Á. de Almeida
Faculty of Medicine of Valença—UniFaa, Valença, Brazil

Federal University of Rio de Janeiro—UFRJ, Rio de Janeiro, Brazil

G. Ribeiro · V. Arcoverde
Biodesign Lab DASA—PUC—Rio de Janeiro, Rio de Janeiro, RJ, Brazil

W. Hottz
Clinica CDPI—DASA—Rio de Janeiro, Rio de Janeiro, RJ, Brazil

M. Iorizzo
Private Dermatology Practice, Bellinzona, Switzerland

C. Canella Moraes do Carmo (✉)
Fluminense Federal University—UFF, Rio de Janeiro, Brazil

Federal University of Rio de Janeiro—UFRJ, Rio de Janeiro, Brazil

Diagnóstico das Américas—DASA—RJ, Rio de Janeiro, Brazil

Biodesign Laboratory, DASA-PUC, Rio de Janeiro, Brazil

18.1.2 Epidemiology [4–8]

- More common in the young and middle-aged population (around 40–50 years).
- Female predisposition.
- Usually a solitary lesion (multiple in 10% of cases).
- Usually seen in the hands (75%), on the fingertips, and subungual space.
- Accounts for 1–2% of all hand tumors.

18.1.3 Clinical Presentation (Fig. 18.1) [4, 7–10]

- Intense pain, often pulsating, spontaneous, or caused by minor trauma, cold, or touch.
- Classic triad: hypersensitivity to cold, paroxysmal pain, and precise pain localization (present in 75% of patients).
- Small painful blue-red spot a few millimeters (<1 cm) in diameter was seen through the nail plate.
- Erythematous focus often visible on the lunula that does not completely blanch with pressure.
- Longitudinal groove of the nail plate.
- Longitudinal erythronychia with superimposed distal notch or longitudinal fissure.
- The sign of Love: localized pain when applying the tip of a needle to the nail plate that reliefs after removing needle pressure.
- The ice test: exacerbation of pain when the injured finger is placed in a container with ice cubes.
- Hildreth sign: relief of pain following the application of a tourniquet proximally.
- Fingertip transillumination: bluish area within the nail bed allowing demarcation of the lesion.

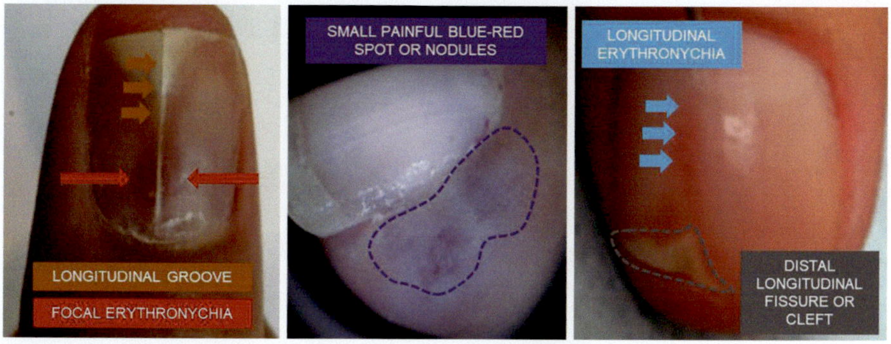

Fig. 18.1 Clinical photograph of a patient with a glomus tumor

18.1.4 Onychoscopy (Fig. 18.2) [11–14]

- Branched vascular structures in the bluish patches (not observed clinically).
- Dermoscopic patterns observed in a large series of subungual glomus tumors:
  - Pattern S1: subungual spot without structure, purplish to reddish, with or without vessels.
  - Pattern S2: subungual spot without structure, purplish to reddish and longitudinal erythronychia.
  - Pattern S3 (single bed glomus tumor pattern): structureless purplish subungual spot, longitudinal erythronychia, and V-shaped distal notch.
  - Pattern S4 pattern (single bed glomus tumor pattern): structureless purplish subungual redness and onycholysis.

18.1.5 Histopathology (Fig. 18.3) [11, 15, 16]

- Well-circumscribed nonencapsulated nodules, composed of perivascular clusters, round or oval, forming some layers, can be multifocal, composed of round cells in a concentric arrangement, resembling umbrellas around a lake, referred to as a punch-out pattern, arranged around vessels of varying sizes.
- Cells are extensively monomorphic in the glomus tumor itself, with large vesicular nuclei and scant eosinophilic cytoplasm, derived from vascular smooth muscle cells.
- Hyalinized and myxoid tumor stroma.
- Absence of necrosis, cellular pleomorphism, or mitotic activity.

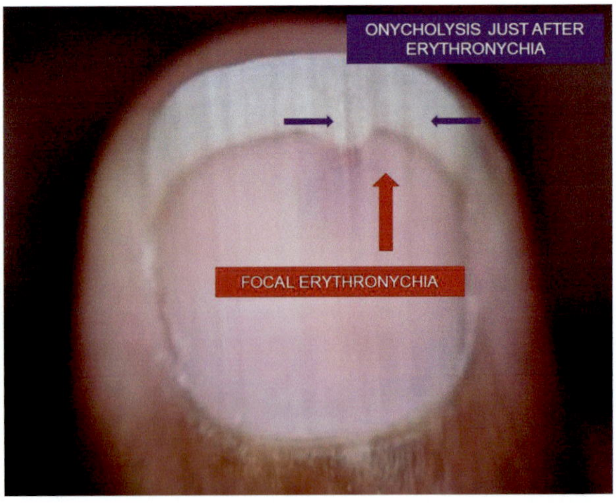

Fig. 18.2 Dermoscopy of a patient with a glomus tumor (x20)

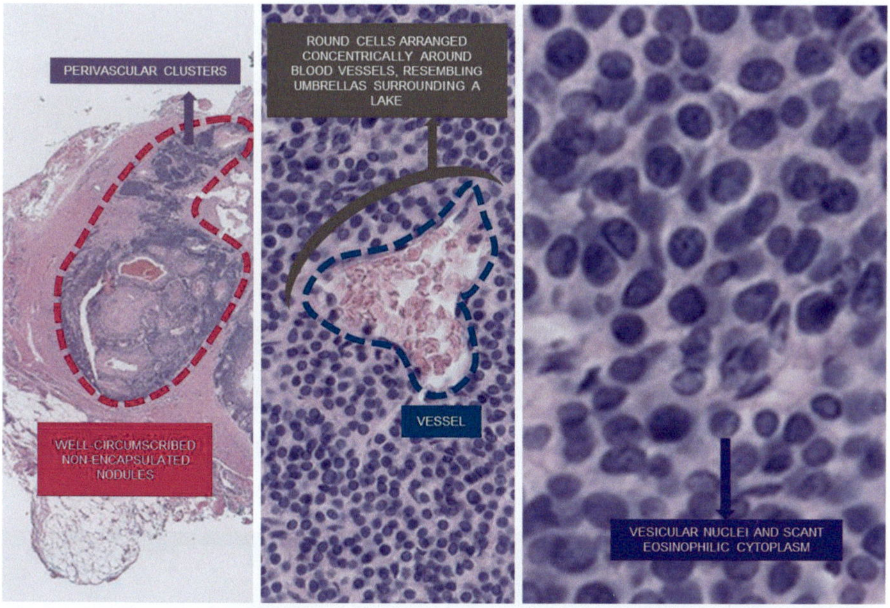

Fig. 18.3 Histological findings of a glomus tumor (H&E x4, x10 and x40)

- The amount of smooth muscle determines the classification of the group, less muscle in the glomus tumor, more in the glomangiomyoma.
- Immunohistochemistry: positive for smooth muscle actin and caldesmon and negative for desmin, S100, cytokeratins, and synaptophysin.
- Histopathological differential diagnoses: myopericytoma, benign adnexal tumors, especially eccrine spiradenoma, melanocytic nevus, and paraganglioma.

18.1.6 Radiography and Computed Tomography (Fig. 18.4) [17, 18]

- Difficult to identify by radiography and computed tomography.
- Well-defined osseous erosion or cortical bone thinning (bone remodeling).

18.1.7 Ultrasonography (Figs. 18.5 and 18.6) [19, 20]

- Solid hypoechoic lesions with well-defined margins (88% of the tumors are homogeneous and hypoechoic).
- Central location at nail bed.

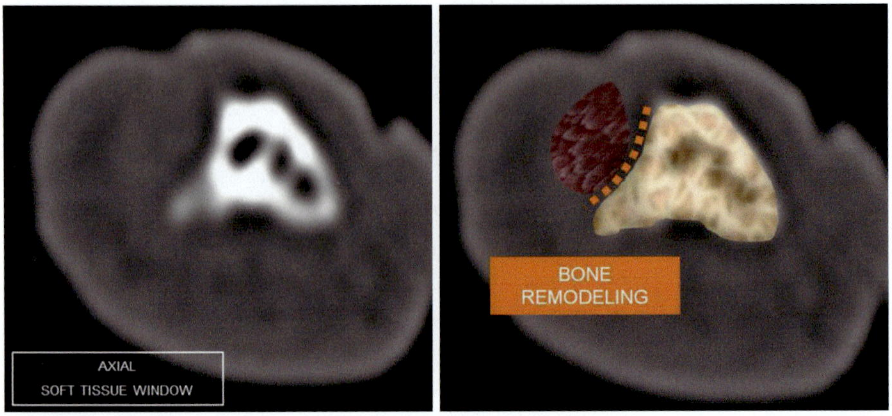

Fig. 18.4 Computed tomography of a glomus tumor on axial plane (Philips Brilliance CT 64-slice)

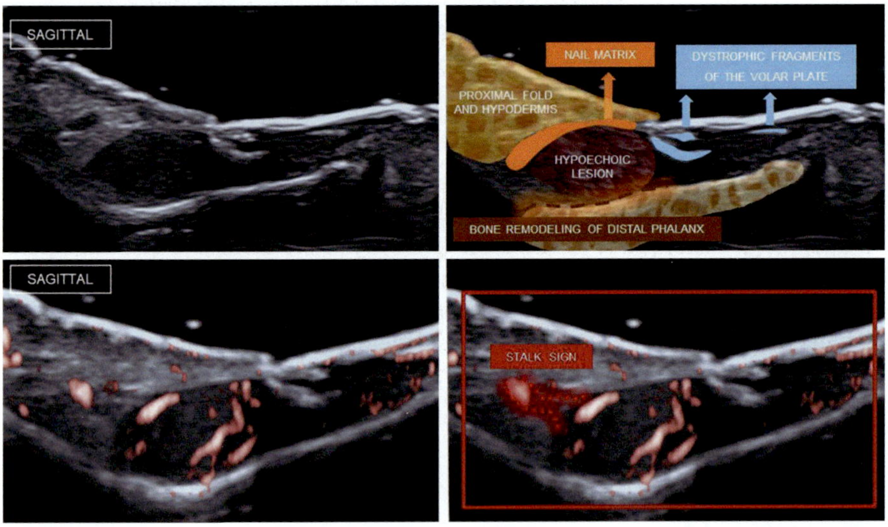

Fig. 18.5 Ultrasonographic findings of a glomus tumor with a 24 MHz probe on sagittal plane (Aplio i800, Canon Medical Systems)

- Intense vascularization on power Doppler imaging (55.8% Intense Vascularity on power Doppler).
- Stalk sign represents intense vascular flow connecting the lesion to the adjacent tissue (70.5% of cases).
- Bone remodeling without erosion (85% Distal Phalanx Bone Remodeling).
- Loss of physiological sphericity of the distal phalanx on axial images.

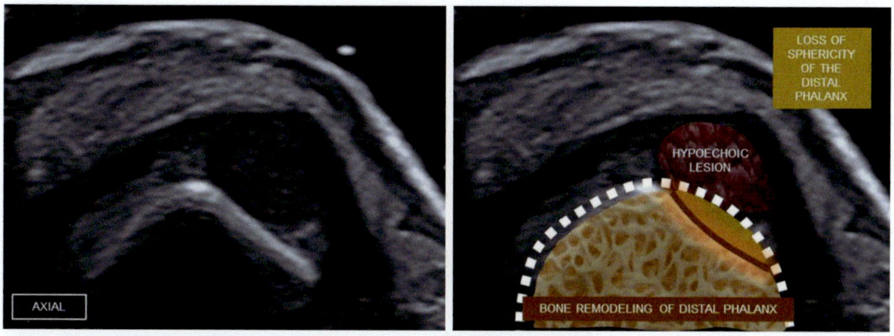

Fig. 18.6 Ultrasonographic findings of a glomus tumor with a 24 MHz probe on axial plane (Aplio i800, Canon Medical Systems)

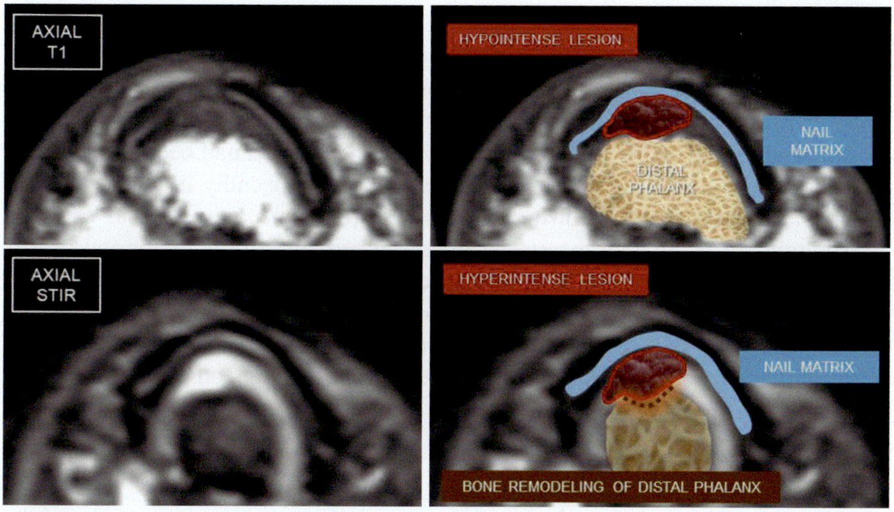

Fig. 18.7 MRI with surface coil findings of a glomus tumor on T1-weighted and STIR sequences (Magnetom Prisma 3T MRI, Siemens)

18.1.8 MRI (Fig. 18.7) [21]

- Well-defined oval or round lesion, hypointense on T1-weighted and hyperintense on T2-weighted sequences.
- Enhances markedly after gadolinium administration due to high vascularity.
- Stalk signs can also be observed.
- Angiography MRI sequences also reveal dilation of the adjacent blood vessels supplying the tumor.
- Bone remodeling and edema, usually without irregularity.

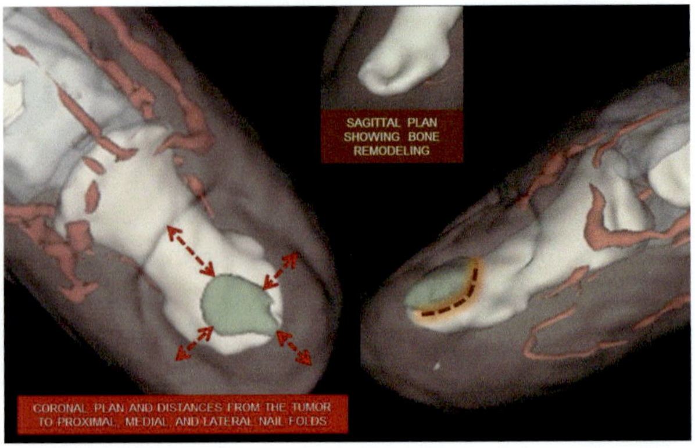

Fig. 18.8 3D virtual findings of a glomus tumor after image segmentation of MRI isotropic sequences for surgical planning

18.1.9 3D Images (Fig. 18.8, Video 18.1)

- Most useful on small lesions or recurrent difficult cases.
- Allow the visualization of the extension of the lesion, enabling to assess the severity and relation with adjacent structures, especially the vascular dilatation surrounding the tumor and relashiopship with matrix and nail bed.
- Contribute to more precise surgical interventions, especially in recurrent cases where anatomy is often distorted due to fibrosis and post-surgical changes. Additionally, accurately measuring the distance between the tumor and nearby structures, such as the nail folds, helps in precisely locating the lesion and planning a more targeted and conservative excision.
- Biomodels can be used and allow the creation of physical replicas of the affected area, offering representations that aid in surgical planning and patient education.

18.2 Digital Fibrokeratoma and Koenen Tumor

18.2.1 Definition [22–25]

- Acquired tumor of fibrous tissue of the distal extremities.
- Major related factors are trauma and infection.
- Patients with tuberous sclerosis have multiple periungual fibromas (Koenen tumors) that represent major diagnostic criteria of tuberous sclerosis complex.

18.2.2 Epidemiology [23, 26]

- Digital fibrokeratoma:

- Commonly located on the fingers.
- Solitary lesion.
- Usually in adults.
- Generally, affects men.

- Koenen tumor:
  - Age of 12–14 years and increase progressively in size and number with age.
  - Develop in 50% of cases of tuberous sclerosis.
  - More frequently on toes.
  - Female predilection.

18.2.3 Clinical Presentation (Fig. 18.9) [13, 22]

- Fibrokeratoma:
  - Asymptomatic.
  - Small, single papule surrounded by a collar of slightly raised skin.
  - Emerge from the most proximal part of the nail sulcus, causing a sharp longitudinal depression.
  - When emerging from the nail bed can cause onycholysis.
- Koenen tumor:
  - Asymptomatic.
  - Firm, smooth, skin-colored, or reddish papules around or under the nail.
  - Longitudinal erythronychia.
  - Depending on the location can cause longitudinal depressions in the nail plate.

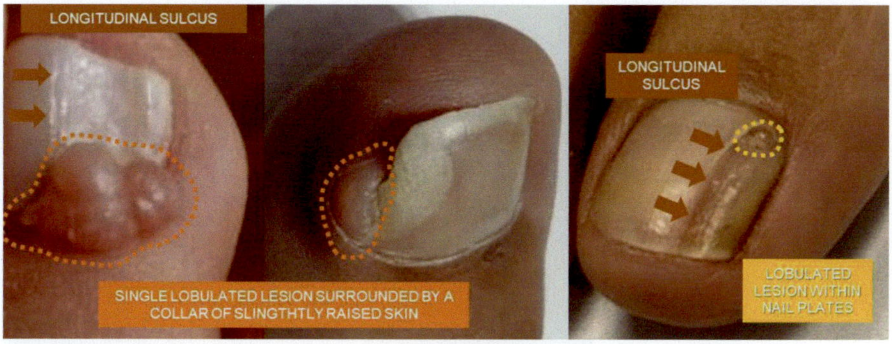

Fig. 18.9 Clinical photograph of a patient with a fibrokeratoma

18.2.4 Onychoscopy (Fig. 18.10) [13, 22]

- Shows a central homogeneous pale-yellow area surrounded by a hyperkeratotic white scaly collarette.
- Whitish-yellow area with dotted vessels peripherally.
- Clumps of homogeneous red lacunae divided by a white meshwork-like keratotic septi. 6, 7.

18.2.5 Histopathology (Fig. 18.11) [22, 27]

- Hyperkeratotic and acanthotic epidermis, accompanied by thick bundles of collagen oriented vertically in the dermis.
- The dermal nucleus of an ADFK presents histological variants [2]:
  - Type I is the most common variant, which presents as a dome-shaped lesion and consists of a dermal core of thick, densely packed collagen bundles with thin elastic fibers.
  - Type II is a tall, hyperkeratotic tumor with more fibroblasts arranged in the skin than in the first type. It also exhibits reduced elastic fibers.
  - Type III is the less common variant, presents as a flat to dome lesion with a poorly cellular dermal nucleus, edematous structures, and absence of elastic fibers.

18.2.6 Ultrasonography (Fig. 18.12) [28–30]

- Round, fusiform, or polypoid lesion.

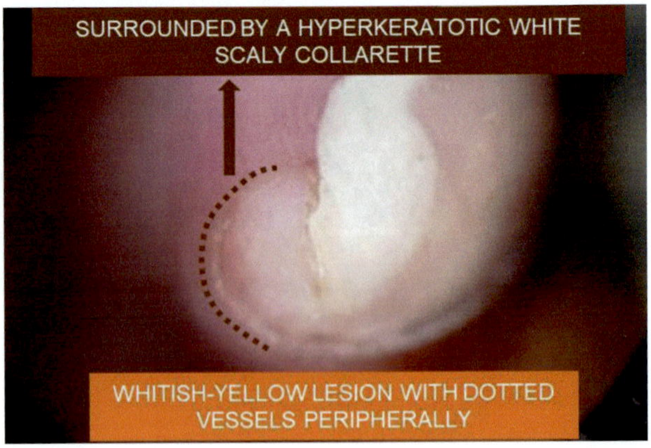

Fig. 18.10 Dermoscopy of a patient with a fibrokeratoma (x20)

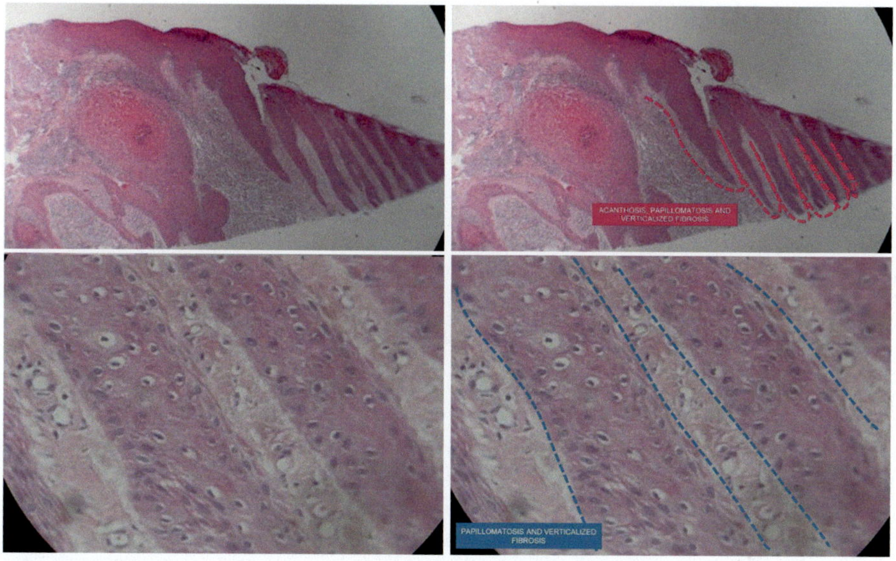

Fig. 18.11 Histological findings of a fibrokeratoma (H&E x4 and x10)

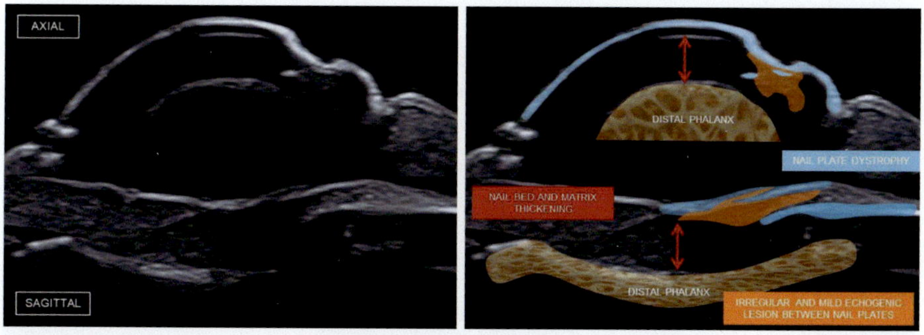

Fig. 18.12 Ultrasonographic findings of a fibrokeratoma with a 24 MHz probe (Aplio i800, Canon Medical Systems)

- Hypoechoic or slightly hyperechoic appearance.
- Usually located eccentrically in the nail fold and involving the nail matrix concurrently (dumbbell-shaped appearance).
- Hypovascularization on power Doppler imaging.
- Rare remodeling of the distal phalanx (only in large lesions).

18.2.7 MRI (Figs. 18.13 and 18.14)

- Round or fusiform mass presenting low signal intensity on T1 and T2 weighted images.
- Located eccentrically in the nail fold extending to nail matrix (dumbbell-shaped appearance).
- Absence of enhancement after gadolinium administration.

18.2.8 3D Images (Fig. 18.15, Video 18.2)

- Highly beneficial for treating for challenging recurrent cases, where anatomy is often distorted due to fibrosis and post-surgical changes.
- Facilitates visualization of the lesion's extent, aiding in the assessment of its relationship with adjacent structures, especially the nail matrix, which is often the site of origin. This detailed imaging is crucial, as preserving the nail matrix is essential for achieving better surgical outcomes and ensuring the regular growth of the nail plate.

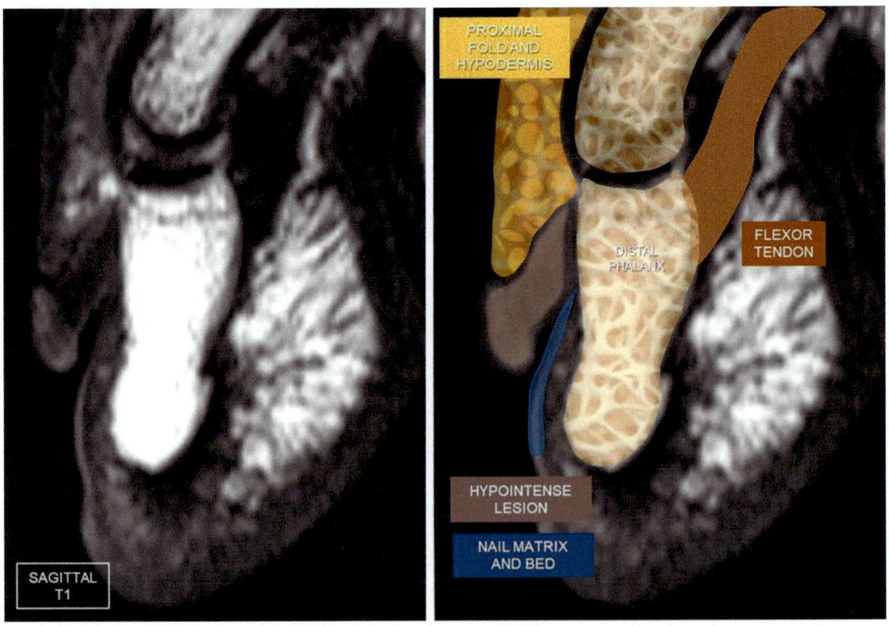

Fig. 18.13 MRI with surface coil findings of a fibrokeratoma in T1 weighted sequence (Magnetom Prisma 3T MRI, Siemens)

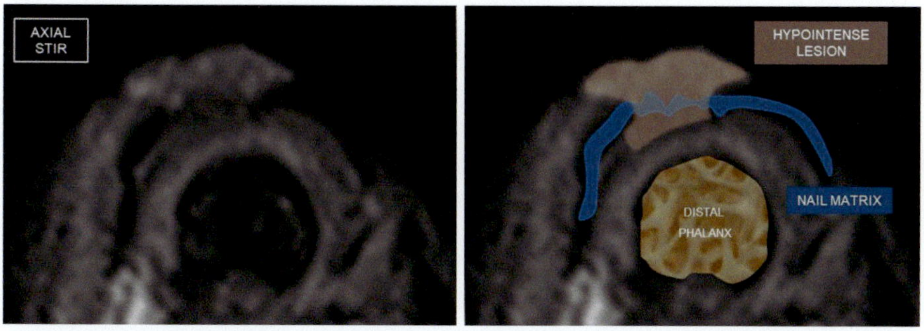

Fig. 18.14 MRI with surface coil findings of a fibrokeratoma in STIR sequence (Magnetom Prisma 3T MRI, Siemens)

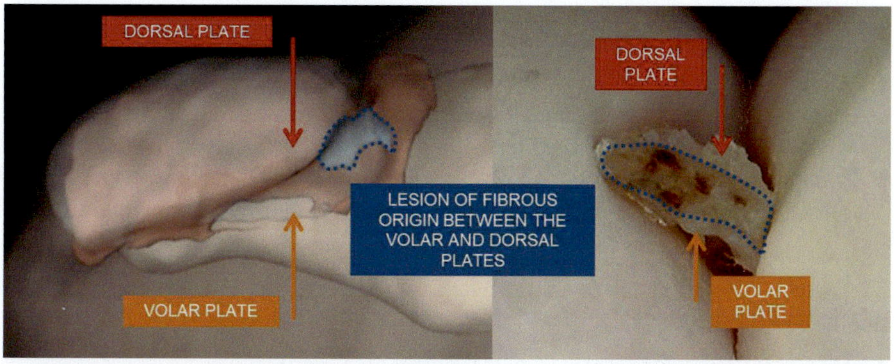

Fig. 18.15 3D virtual findings of a fibrokeratoma after image segmentation of MRI isotropic sequences for surgical planning

- Enhances precision in surgical interventions for complicate cases, where the fibroma grows between the nail plates, as precise imaging helps guide a more delicate surgical approach.
- Biomodels can be utilized to create physical replicas of the affected area, providing representations that support surgical planning and patient education.

18.3 Post-traumatic Subungual Hematoma

18.3.1 Definition [31, 32]

- Nail trauma involves injury to the fingernail or toenail and can affect the nail plate, nail bed, or surrounding structures. It often results from direct impact, crushing, or repetitive stress.

- In some cases, a subungual hematoma can present as a heterogeneous, expansile lesion on imaging, mimicking a true tumor and thus characterizing a pseudotumoral lesion.

18.3.2 Epidemiology [31]

- Nail trauma is a common occurrence, especially among individuals engaged in manual labor or sports.
- It accounts for a significant number of hand injuries seen in emergency departments and primary care settings.

18.3.3 Clinical Presentation (Fig. 18.16) [31]

- Patients with nail trauma typically present with pain, swelling, and visible damage to the nail or surrounding tissues.
- Common signs include subungual hematomas, nail plate detachment, and lacerations. The injury may limit the range of motion and cause throbbing pain.

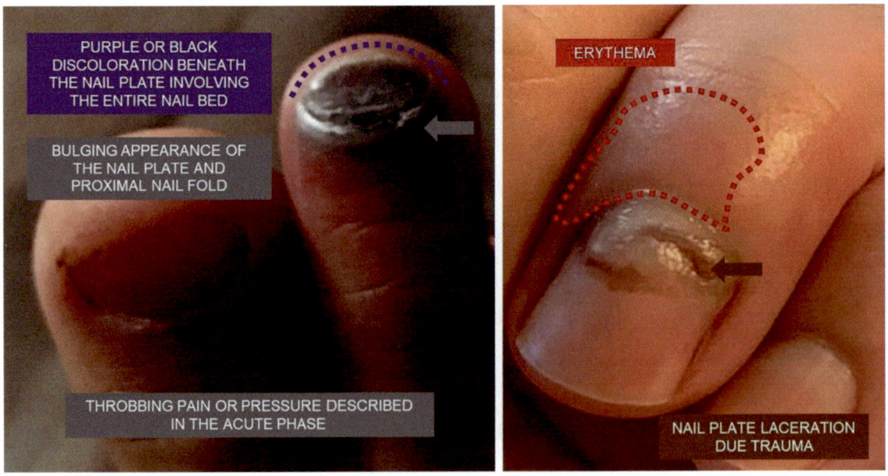

Fig. 18.16 Clinical photograph of a patient with a nail hematoma after a traumatic injury

18.3.4 Onychoscopy [31]

- Can be useful in evaluating nail trauma, providing detailed images of the nail plate and bed.
- It helps in assessing subungual hematomas, detecting hidden lacerations, and determining the extent of damage to the nail matrix.

18.3.5 Histopathology [31]

- Histological examination of nail trauma can reveal disrupted keratin layers, hematomas, and inflammatory responses.
- In severe cases, there may be damage to the nail matrix and surrounding tissues, leading to potential complications in nail regrowth.

18.3.6 Radiography and Computed Tomography (Fig. 18.17) [31]

- Radiographs are often used to assess for fractures of the distal phalanx and other bony structures.
- CT provides detailed images and is useful in complex cases to evaluate the extent of bone and soft tissue injuries.

18.3.7 Ultrasonography (Fig. 18.18) [32]

- Ultrasonographic examination of subungual trauma reveals several distinctive features. These include variations nail irregularity, distal phalanx fractures, nail bed and matrix lesions.
- A subungual hematoma typically appears as a hypoechoic to anechoic collection beneath the nail plate, depending on the age of the blood. In the acute phase, it may present as a more anechoic area, while in subacute or chronic stages, the hematoma can become more heterogeneous or hyperechoic, with internal echoes due to clot organization.
- These ultrasonographic changes may also suggest the presence of scarring and ongoing chronic inflammation.
- No internal vascular flow on power Doppler imaging, which helps distinguish it from vascularized tumors.

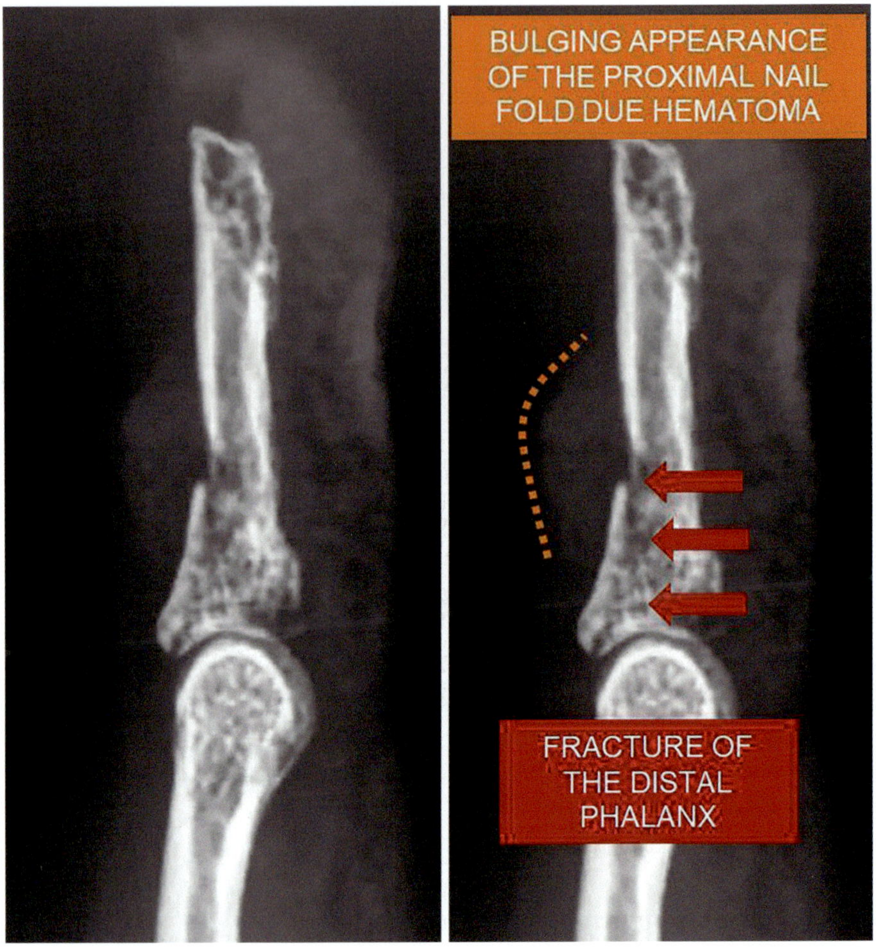

Fig. 18.17 Radiographic findings of a nail hematoma and bone fracture after a traumatic injury (Philips Duo Diagnost R&F Room Digital RF and Tomo System)

18.3.8 MRI (Fig. 18.19)

- Subungual hematomas often appear hyperintense on T2-weighted MRI images due to the presence of blood. On T1-weighted images, they may appear hypointense, depending on the age of the hematoma.
- Edema in the nail bed appears as increased signal intensity on T2-weighted images and may appear hyperintense on T1-weighted images with fat suppression techniques. This indicates fluid accumulation and inflammation.
- MRI can show displacement or separation of the nail plate from the nail bed. This may be visualized as a gap or altered alignment between the nail plate and underlying soft tissues.

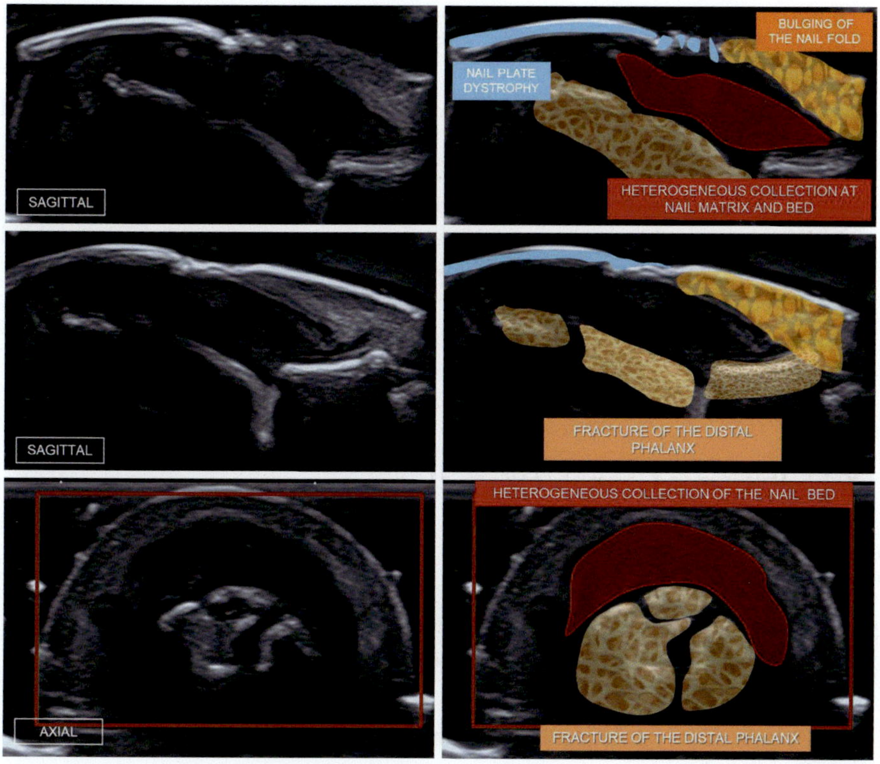

Fig. 18.18 Ultrasonographic findings of a nail hematoma after a traumatic injury with a 24 MHz probe (Aplio i800, Canon Medical Systems)

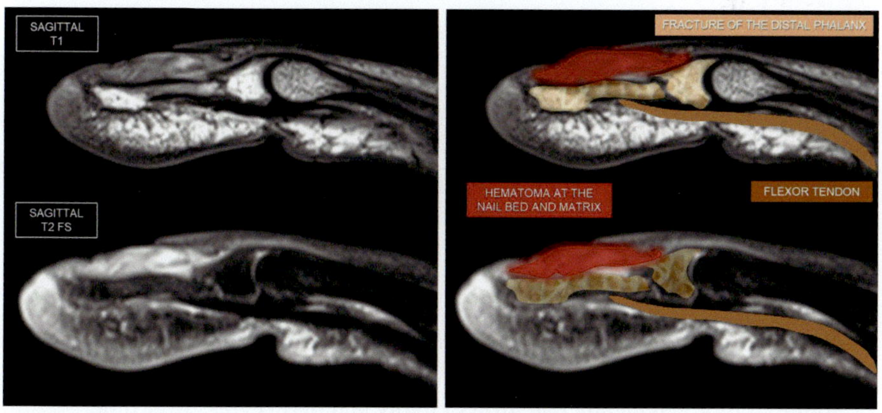

Fig. 18.19 MRI with surface coil findings of a nail hematoma after a traumatic injury in T1-weighted and STIR sequences (Magnetom Prisma 3T MRI, Siemens)

- Fluid collections under the nail plate appear as hyperintense areas on T2-weighted images. They are typically well-defined and may be surrounded by areas of edema.
- Soft tissue contusions or injuries around the nail bed show areas of increased signal intensity on T2-weighted MRI images. This may be due to bleeding or inflammation in the surrounding soft tissues.
- If there is associated trauma to the underlying bone (such as the distal phalanx), MRI may show bone marrow edema as hyperintense areas on T2-weighted images and hypointense areas on T1-weighted images.
- Chronic traumatic lesions may lead to fibrosis or scarring, which can appear as areas of hypointensity on T1-weighted images and may have varying signal characteristics on T2-weighted images.

18.4 Pyogenic Granuloma

18.4.1 Definition [33–35]

- Relatively common benign eruptive hemangioma.
- Factors that can induce this type of tumor include:
  - Penetrating skin injury.
  - Certain drugs (such as retinoids, antiretrovirals, and antineoplastic drugs).
  - Peripheral nerve injury.
  - Inflammatory systemic diseases (such as cutaneous sarcoidosis, psoriasis, and seronegative spondyloarthritis).

18.4.2 Epidemiology [25, 33, 34]

- More commonly found in young individuals.
- Pregnancy seems to be a contributing factor.
- The most frequent location is the proximal nail fold.

18.4.3 Clinical Presentation (Fig. 18.20) [33, 34]

- Solitary bright red papule that grows rapidly and may regress over time.
- Tends to be tender and prone to bleeding.
- Surface may become eroded, crusted, or ulcerated due to necrosis.
- Typically has a collarette surrounding the base of the lesion.
- Pain is almost always absent.

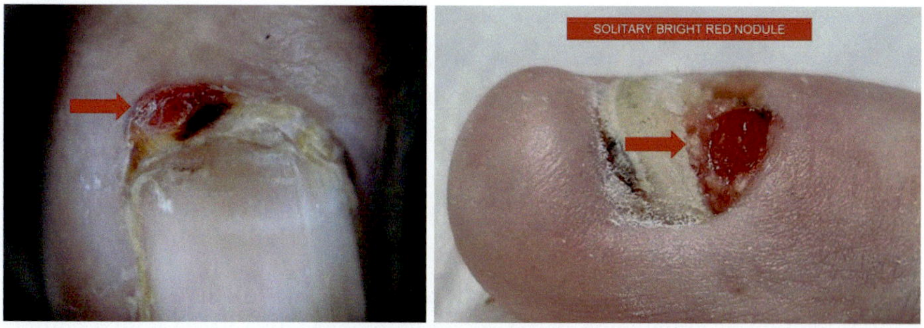

Fig. 18.20 Clinical photograph of a patient with a pyogenic granuloma

Fig. 18.21 Dermoscopy of a patient with a pyogenic granuloma (x20)

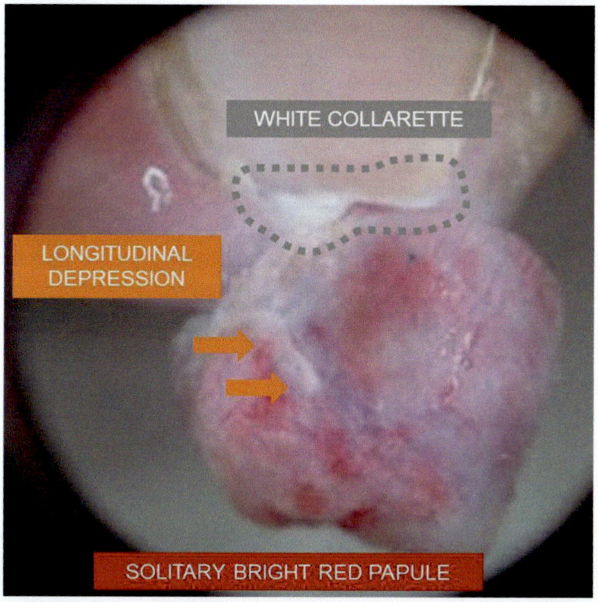

18.4.4 Onychoscopy (Fig. 18.21) [36–38]

- Reddish homogeneous area:
  - Homogeneous zone whose color varied from completely red to red with whitish zones.
- White collarette:
  - Ring-shaped or arcuate squamous structure located at the periphery of the lesion is the most specific structure for pyogenic granuloma.
- White rail lines represent whitish streaks or bands that intersect the lesion.

- Vascular structures:
  - Linear-irregular vessels are the most common.
  - The second most frequent was polymorphous or atypical vessels.

18.4.5 Histopathology (Fig. 18.22) [27]

- Also called capillary lobular hemangioma.
- Proliferation of granulation tissue, along with connective tissue with a chronic inflammatory process in distinct stages of organization.
- Often associated with erosion and ulceration.

18.4.6 Ultrasonography (Fig. 18.23) [28, 29, 34]

- Oval-shaped lesion.
- Appears hypoechoic and heterogeneous. The white collarette seen clinically around the lesion corresponds to a pedunculated structure, often appearing as a well-defined, echogenic tissue connected to the nail bed or matrix by a narrow stalk.
- Shows variable vascularity on power Doppler imaging.
- Typically located in the nail bed or proximal fold.
- When large and situated on the nail bed, can cause a "wavy shape" appearance of the nail plates.

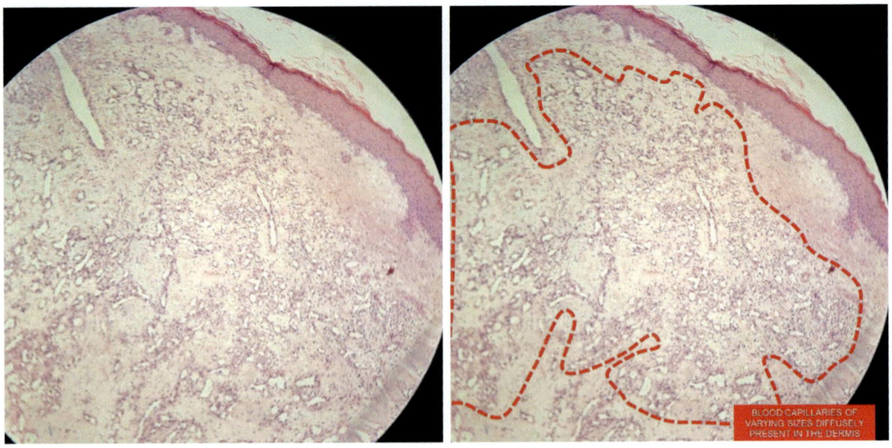

Fig. 18.22 Histological findings of a pyogenic granuloma (H&E x4)

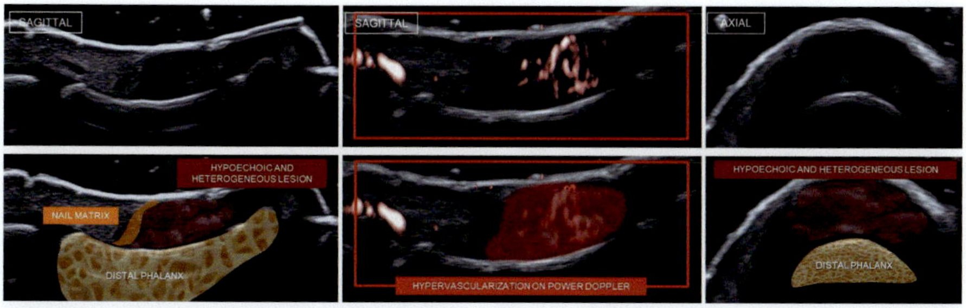

Fig. 18.23 Ultrasonographic findings of a pyogenic granuloma with a 24 MHz probe (Aplio i800, Canon Medical Systems)

18.4.7 MRI (Fig. 18.24) [21]

- Oval-shaped lesion with low signal intensity on T1-weighted images and high signal intensity on T2-weighted and STIR images. The white collarette can also be seen.
- Shows mild to moderate enhancement after gadolinium administration.
- Often presents with superficial erosions and ulceration.
- Typically located in the nail bed or proximal fold.

18.4.8 3D Images

- Extremely advantageous in managing difficult recurring cases.
- Improves the ability to see how far the lesion extends, helping to evaluate its connection with nearby structures, particularly the nail matrix. Sometimes, the white collarette seen clinically can also be visualized in 3D reconstructed images, providing additional detail that aids in surgical planning. Its identification helps delineate the base of pedunculated lesions and their precise point of attachment to the nail bed or surrounding tissue.
- Increases accuracy during complex surgical procedures.
- Biomodels can be used to produce physical models of the affected region, offering visual aids that aid in surgical preparation and patient education.

18.5 Keratoacanthoma

18.5.1 Definition [39]

- A rare, benign tumor with an appearance of aggressiveness.
- Shows a tendency for deep invasion and involvement of bone.

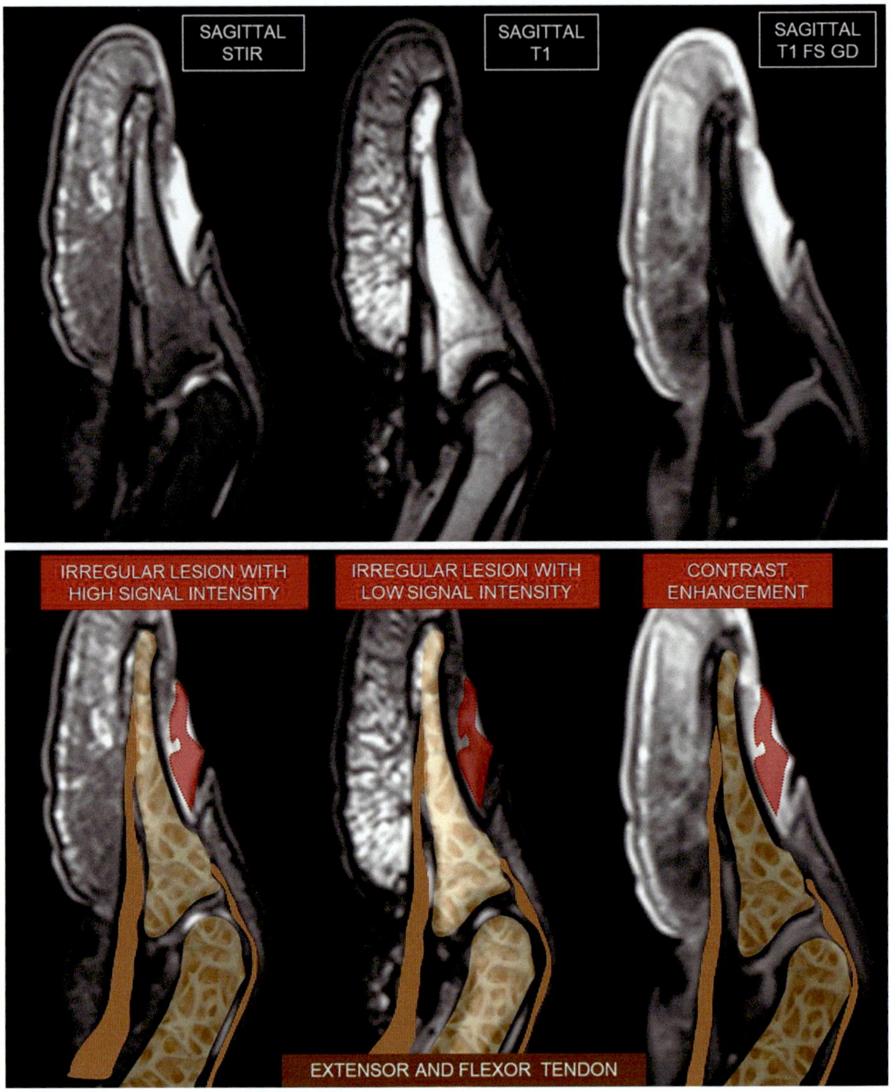

Fig. 18.24 MRI with surface coil findings of a pyogenic granuloma in T1, STIR e T1 FS GD weighted sequences after gadolinium administration (Magnetom Prisma 3T MRI, Siemens)

- The exact cause is still unclear, with suggestions of trauma and oncogenic HPV playing a role.
- Some researchers consider this tumor to be a well-differentiated variant of squamous cell carcinoma, possibly prone to spontaneous regression and having low potential for metastasis.

18.5.2 Epidemiology [39]

- More common in males.
- Typically occurs in the fifth decade of life.
- Predominantly affects the first three fingers, especially the thumb.
- In women, association with incontinentia pigmenti (genodermatosis with involvement of the skin, central nervous system, eyes, hair, nails, and teeth) should be ruled out.

18.5.3 Clinical Presentation (Fig. 18.25) [39]

- Can present as painful solitary or multiple tumors.
- Typically located below the free edge of the nail plate.
- Often tender to touch.
- Begins with partial onycholysis followed by the appearance of a keratotic-crusted nodule that grows rapidly into a dome-shaped structure with a central plug of horny material filling the crater.
- Applying pressure from the sides may cause the central keratotic plug to protrude from the crater.
- If situated more proximally under the nail fold, it may manifest as a painful chronic paronychia.

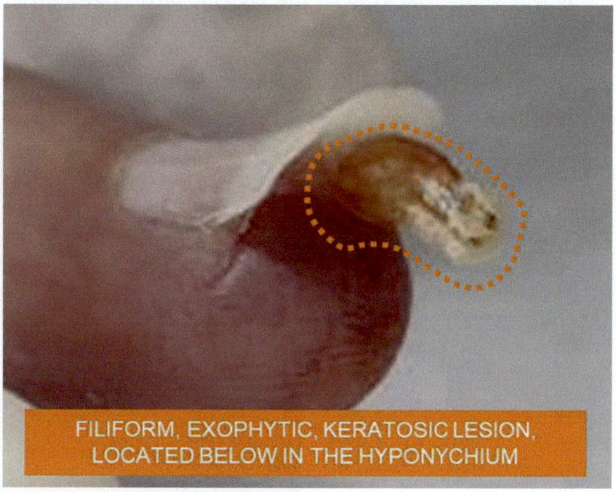

Fig. 18.25 Clinical photograph of a patient with a keratoacanthoma

18.5.4 Onychoscopy (Fig. 18.26) [13]

The nail plate exhibits:

- Irregular enlargement and deformation.
- Superficial fissuring and mild subungual hyperkeratosis [5].

18.5.5 Histopathology (Fig. 18.27) [40]

- Hematoxylin-eosin staining revealed epidermal hyperkeratosis, parakeratotic foci, and a central crater filled with amorphous keratin.
- Dyskeratotic cells, a small number of intraepithelial neutrophils and eosinophils, little nuclear atypia, patchy infiltrates of lymphocytes and plasma cells, and little or no fibrosis at the bases of the lesions.
- Staining for Ki-67 only revealed positivity in the stratum basale.

18.5.6 Radiography and Computed Tomography

- Underlying bony erosion characterized by well-defined margins and a cup-like appearance.
- The cup-like appearance of keratoacanthoma is an important diagnostic feature, as it is a specific sign of the lesion. This characteristic morphology is defined by

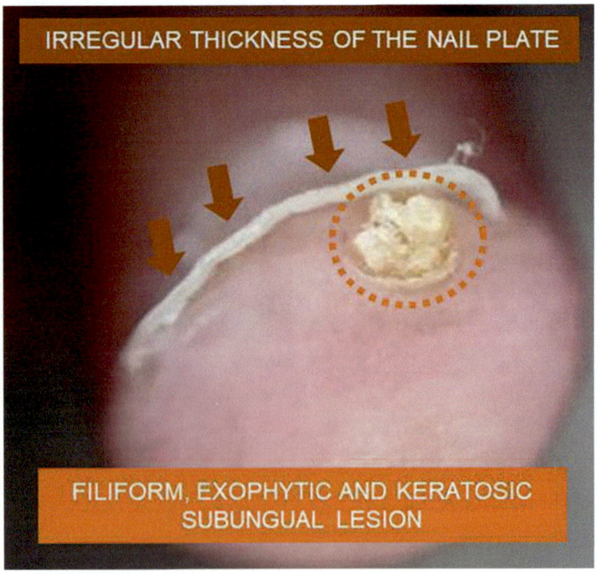

Fig. 18.26 Dermoscopy of a patient with a keratoacanthoma (x20)

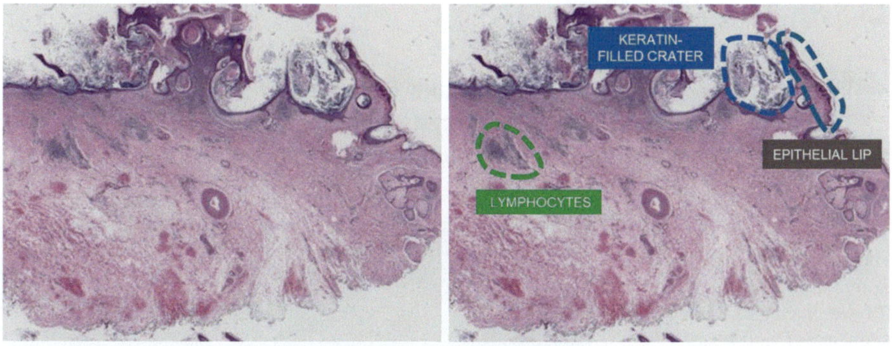

Fig. 18.27 Histological findings of a keratoacanthoma (H&E x4)

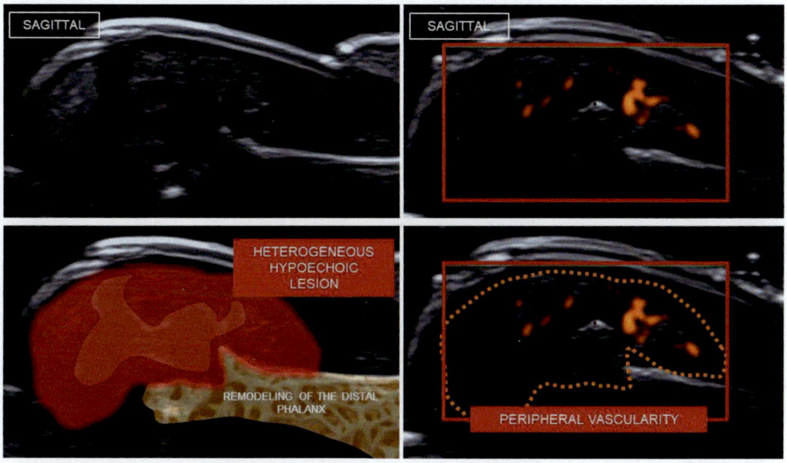

Fig. 18.28 Ultrasonographic findings of a keratoacanthoma with a 24 MHz probe (Aplio i800, Canon Medical Systems)

a central keratin-filled crater with regular, well-demarcated bone erosion, giving it a symmetrical, dome-shaped contour.

18.5.7 Ultrasonography (Fig. 18.28) [41]

- A heterogeneous hypoechoic lesion, sometimes with an anechoic center
- It features a thick hypoechoic wall surrounding an anechoic center, which represents the crater filled with keratin.
- Peripheral vascularity observed on power Doppler imaging.
- Remodeling or erosion of the distal phalanx with well-defined margins, characterizing the cup-like appearence

18.5.8 MRI (Fig. 18.29) [41]

- The lesion appears heterogeneous with a thick wall of low signal intensity on T1-weighted imaging and a centrally cystic appearance.
- Shows areas of hypointense calcification on all sequences.

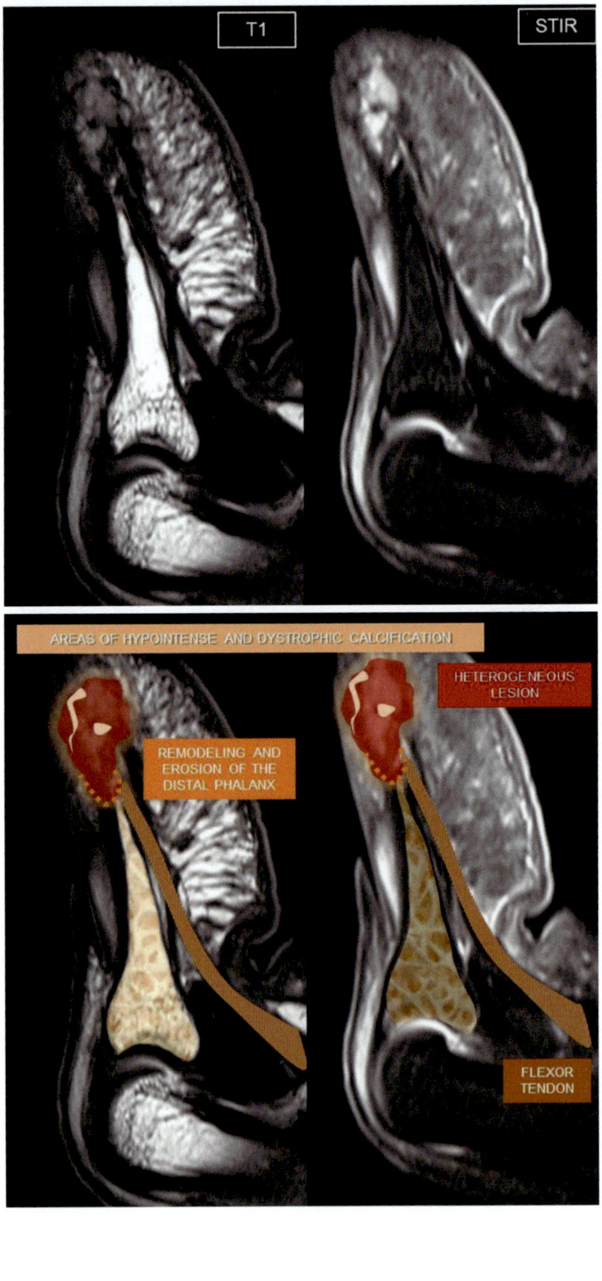

Fig. 18.29 MRI with surface coil findings of a keratoacanthoma in T1-weighted and STIR sequences (Magnetom Prisma 3T MRI, Siemens)

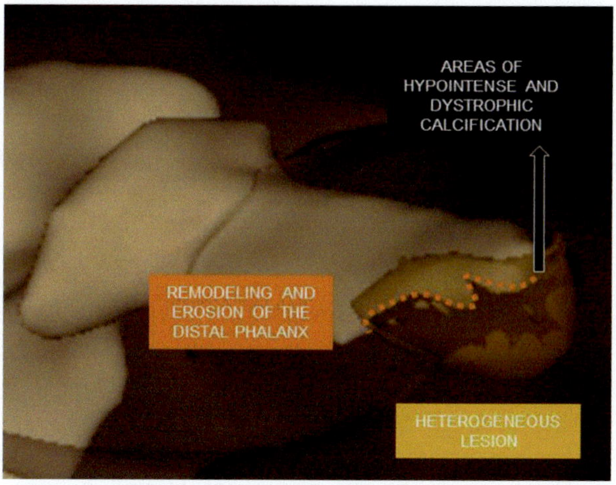

Fig. 18.30 3D virtual findings of a keratoacanthoma after image segmentation of MRI isotropic sequences for surgical planning

- There is no enhancement observed after gadolinium administration.
- Presents a classic chalice-shaped image due to well-defined bone erosion.

18.5.9 3D Images (Fig. 18.30, Video 18.3)

- Highly beneficial for addressing challenging recurrent cases, especially when the cup-like erosion of the distal phalanx is not well demonstrated by X-ray or ultrasonography
- Enhances visualization of the lesion's extent and its relationship with adjacent structures, notably the nail matrix and the distal phalanx. Also, It allows for a more accurate diagnosis of keratoacanthoma when the cup-like appearance of the distal phalanx is not clearly demonstrated by other imaging methods.
- Boosts precision in complex surgical interventions.
- Biomodels can generate physical replicas of the affected area, providing visual aids that support surgical planning and educate patients.

18.6 Neuroma

18.6.1 Definition [42, 43]

- Traumatic subungual neuromas are rare benign tumors resulting from abnormal proliferation of damaged sensory nerves following trauma.
- They typically arise in areas with previous trauma or surgery.

18.6.2 Epidemiology [42, 43]

- These neuromas are uncommon and have been reported infrequently in the literature.
- Subungual neuromas are especially rare compared to traumatic neuromas in other body parts.

18.6.3 Clinical Presentation (Fig. 18.31) [42, 43]

- Patients often present with a non-painful subungual lesion or changes in the nail, such as onycholysis or nail plate elevation.
- The lesion might be accompanied by other symptoms like chronic nail changes.
- There is usually no significant trauma history, and the lesion might be asymptomatic.

18.6.4 Onychoscopy (Fig. 18.32) [42, 43]

- Dermatoscopic examination might show changes such as nail plate elevation and linear ridging.
- Specific vascular or color changes may not be distinctly visible, making dermoscopy less useful in diagnosing traumatic subungual neuromas.

18.6.5 Histopathology [27, 42, 43]

- Histological examination reveals a proliferation of spindle cells arranged around small blood vessels, with a minor chronic inflammatory infiltrate.
- These spindle cells are positive for S100 protein, indicating a neuroma. There is typically no nuclear atypia.

18.6.6 Radiography and Computed Tomography

- Radiographs generally do not show bony changes in cases of subungual neuromas.
- Computed tomography may also be used to exclude bone involvement or other underlying conditions, though it is not usually definitive for neuromas.

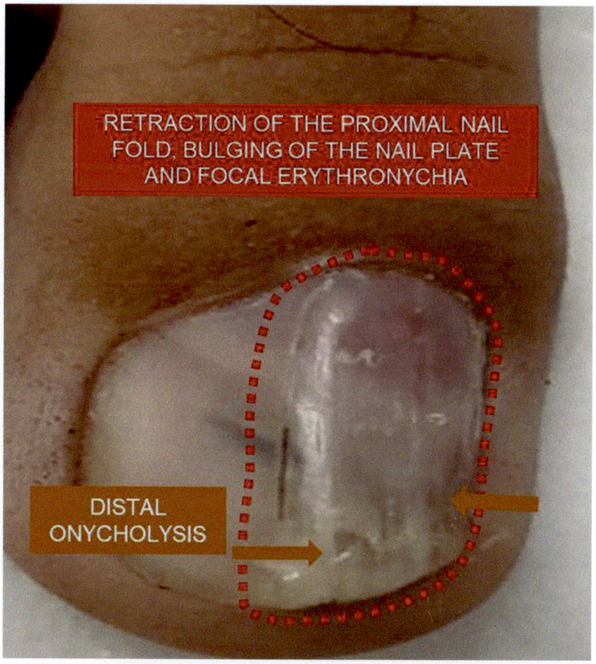

Fig. 18.31 Clinical photograph of a patient with a neuroma

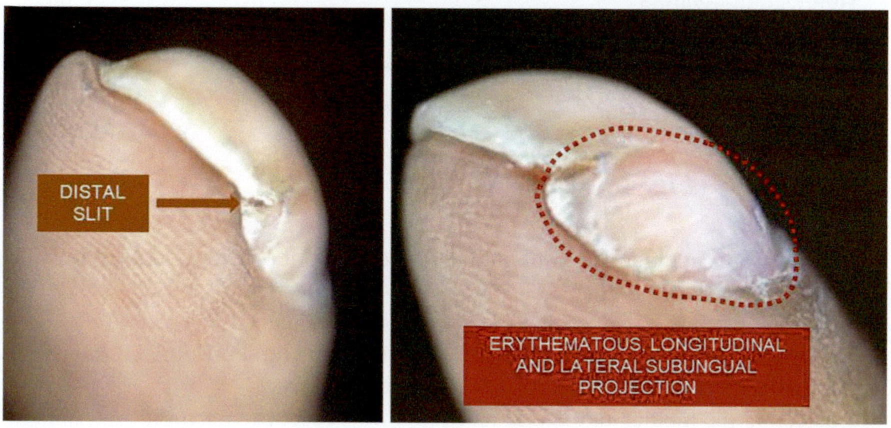

Fig. 18.32 Dermoscopy of a patient with a neuroma (x20)

18.6.7 Ultrasonography (Fig. 18.33) [44, 45]

- Oval and lobulated.
- Hypoechoic.
- Located in the medial and lateral nail folds with eccentric location.

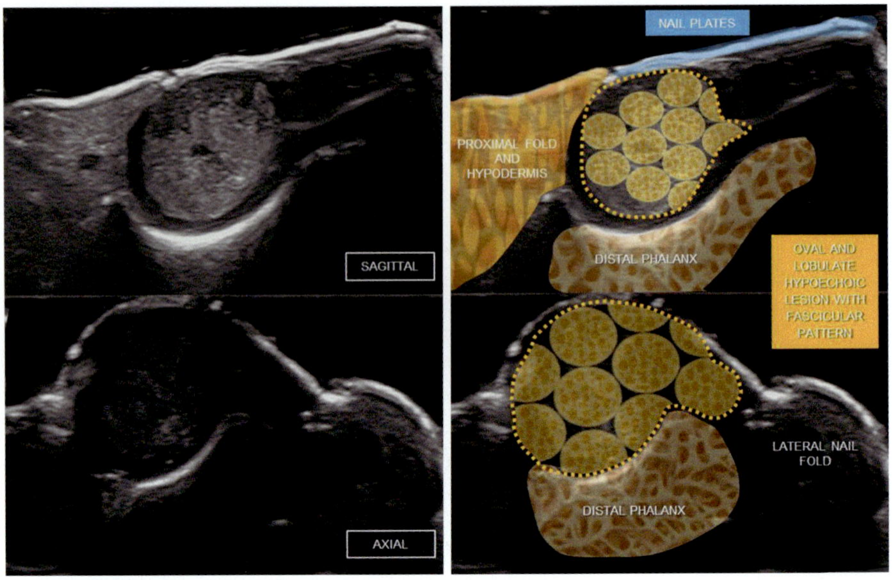

Fig. 18.33 Ultrasonographic findings of a neuroma with a 24 MHz probe (Aplio i800, Canon Medical Systems)

- Hypovascularization.
- Microcystic neural fascicular appearance in larger lesions.
- Absence of remodeling of the distal phalanx.

18.6.8 MRI (Fig. 18.34)

- MRI is useful in diagnosing subungual neuromas as it provides detailed imaging of soft tissue structures.
- Oval and lobulated, with fusiform pattern.
- Heterogeneous, predominantly hyperintense lesion on T2-weighted and STIR images, with microcystic neural fascicular appearance.
- Located in the medial and lateral nail folds with eccentric location.
- Mild enhancement after gadolinium administration.
- Absence of remodeling of the distal phalanx.

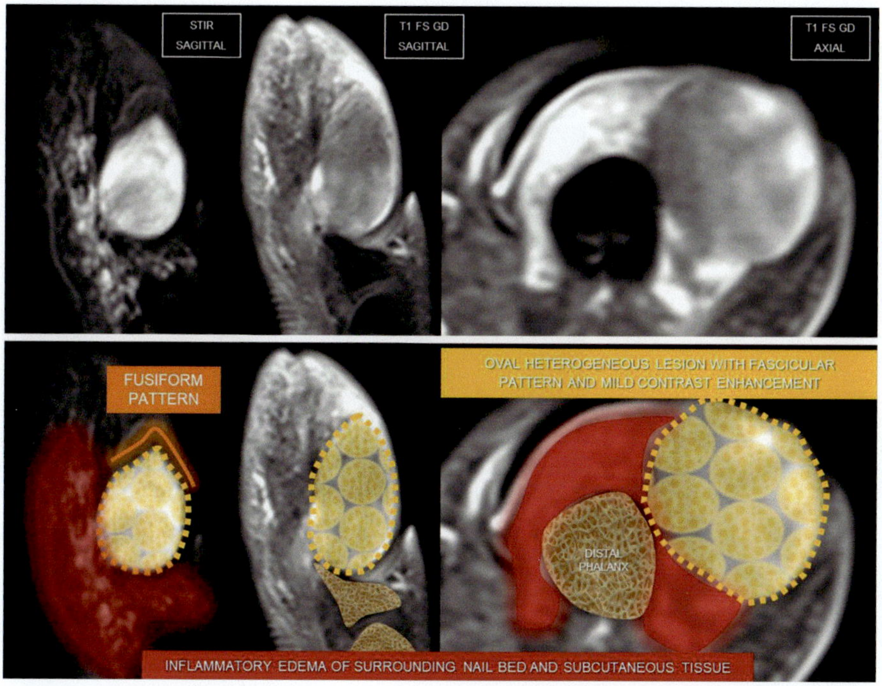

Fig. 18.34 MRI with surface coil findings of a neuroma in T1 FS weighted and STIR sequences after gadolinium administration (Magnetom Prisma 3T MRI, Siemens)

18.6.9 3D Images (Fig. 18.35, Video 18.4)

- Valuable for managing difficult recurring cases effectively.
- Improves the visualization of the lesion's extent and its connection to nearby structures, particularly the nail matrix.
- Increases surgical precision in complex procedures. The spatial information is particularly valuable when planning conservative excisions, as it allows the surgeon to better preserve critical structures like the nail matrix and surrounding skin, ultimately improving both functional and aesthetic outcomes.
- Biomodels can create physical replicas of the affected area, offering visual aids that assist in surgical planning and patient education.

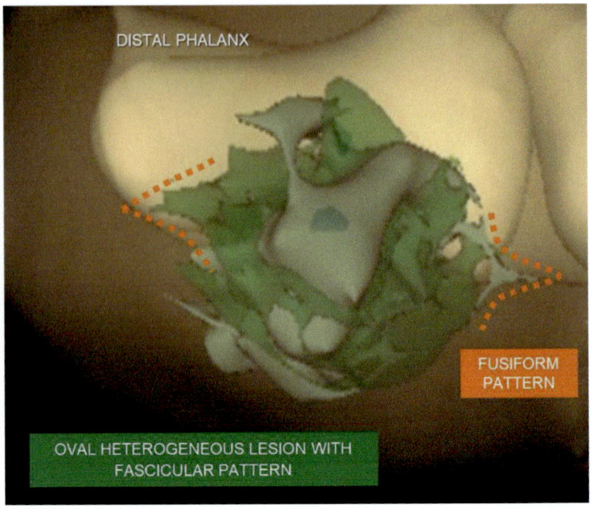

Fig. 18.35 3D virtual findings of a neuroma after image segmentation of MRI isotropic sequences for surgical planning

18.7 Onychopapilloma

18.7.1 Definition [46]

- Benign neoplasm affects the nail bed and distal matrix.
- Initially described in 1995 as "localized multinucleate distal subungual keratosis".
- Later renamed onychopapilloma in 2000.

18.7.2 Epidemiology [47, 48]

- Relatively common lesion, although it is predominantly described by a few specialized nail centers.
- It primarily affects middle-aged women.

18.7.3 Clinical Presentation [47–49]

- Most commonly a band of longitudinal erythronychia with thinning of the nail plate and distal subungual hyperkeratosis.
- However, presents heterogeneous morphological features:
  - Longitudinal leukonychia.
  - Melanonychia.

  - Yellow-brown chromonychia.
  - Splinter hemorrhages.
  - Nail plate fissuring with or without a v-shaped notch.
  - Onycholysis.
- The thumb is the most affected digit followed by the index, long, and ring finger.

18.7.4 Onychoscopy (Fig. 18.36) [47, 48, 50, 51]

- Band originates in the lunula area as a pale white-pink band with sharp margins or dome-shaped and convex morphology.
- Keratotic subungual papule in correspondence to the streak.
- Splinter hemorrhages are visualized as single or multiple thin purple to black interrupted irregular lines.

18.7.5 Histopathology [48, 50–52]

- Acanthopapilomatosis.
- In the area of distal papillomatosis, more superficially, spindle cells with eosinophilic cytoplasm form layers in a V-shaped pattern at the base, resembling the keratogenous zone of the nail matrix.
- Presence of thickened stromal vessels and, at the proximal border, there may be a cavity containing corneal material.
- There may also be long longitudinal or short splinter hemorrhages and distal fissures.

18.7.6 Ultrasonography (Figs. 18.37 and 18.38) [53, 54]

- The lesion appears as a hypoechoic oval or linear-shaped area in the nail bed, adjacent to the nail plates, and is best visualized on axial images.
- There is upward displacement and thickening of the nail plates.
- Focal hyperechoic spots are present on the nail plate, particularly on the distal portion, due to hyperkeratosis.
- Irregularities are noted on the ventral plate.
- No hypervascularity is seen on power Doppler imaging.

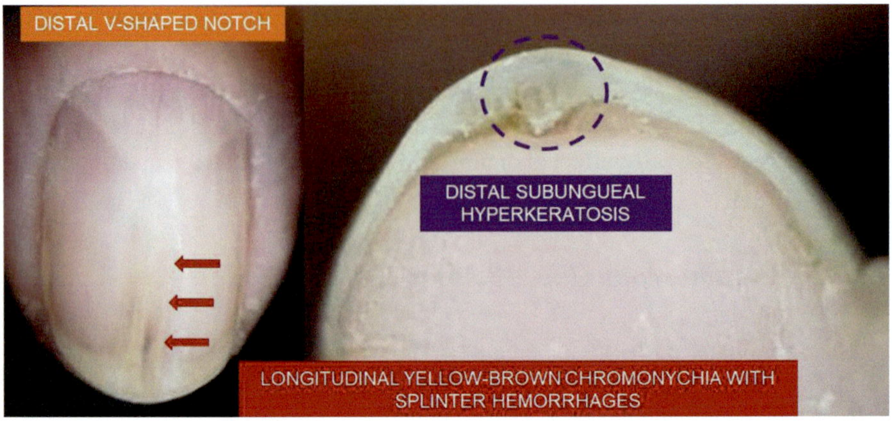

Fig. 18.36 Clinical photograph of a patient with an onychopapilloma (x20)

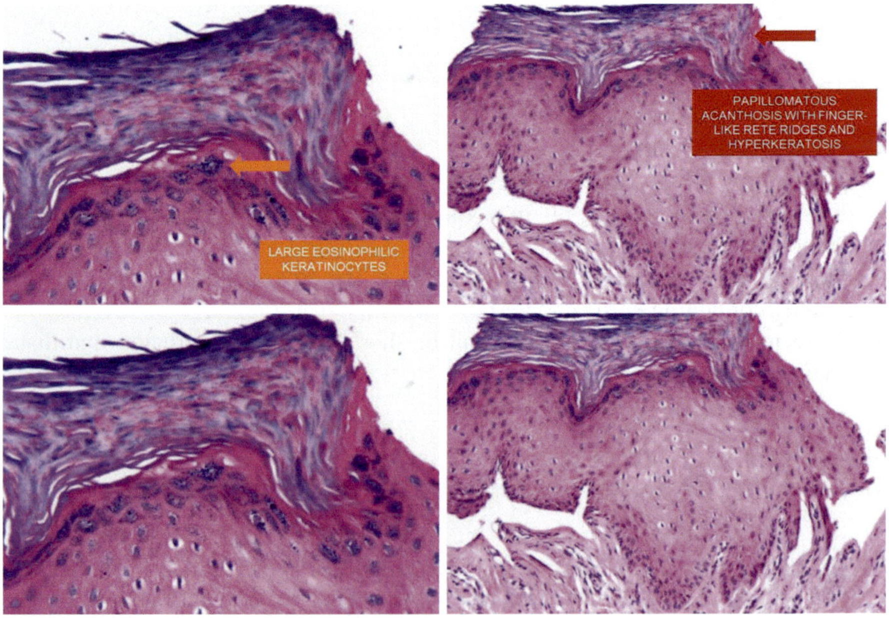

Fig. 18.37 Histological findings of an onychopapilloma (H&E x20)

18.7.7 MRI (Fig. 18.39)

- This lesion originates from the nail matrix and proximal nail bed, typically located within the nail plate.
- As a result, it is challenging to well observe the lesion on MRI, with the only observable signal being the indentation caused on the surface of the nail bed by the tumor.

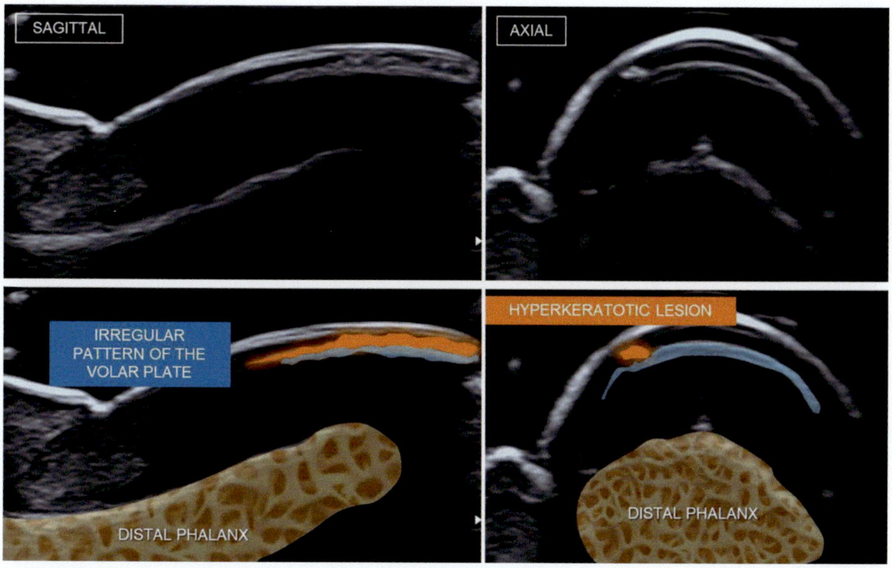

Fig. 18.38 Ultrasonographic findings of an onychopapilloma with a 24 MHz probe (Aplio i800, Canon Medical Systems)

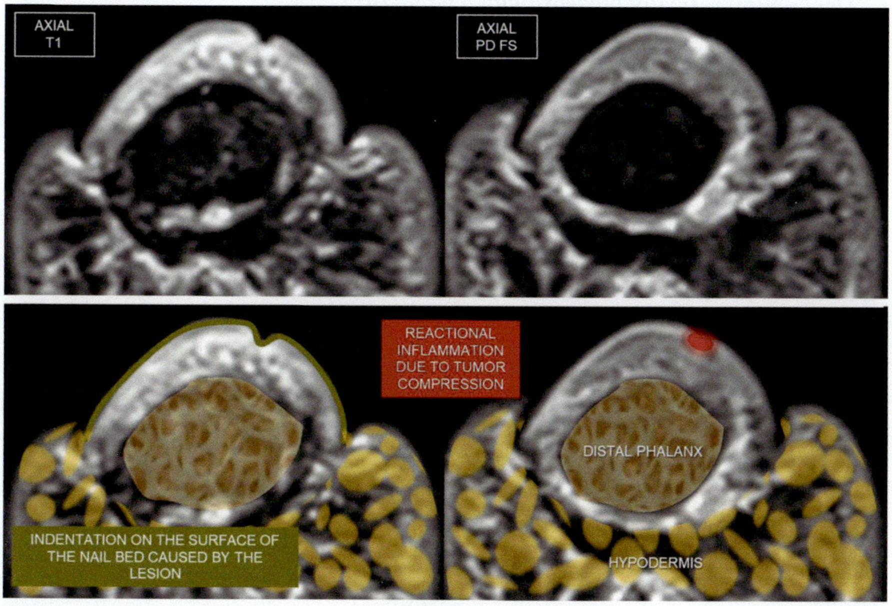

Fig. 18.39 MRI with surface coil findings of an onychopapilloma in PD FS weighted and STIR sequences (Magnetom Prisma 3T MRI, Siemens)

18.8 Onychomatricoma

18.8.1 Definition [55]

- First reported as a rare benign subungual tumor originating from the nail matrix.
- Recently, some authors have suggested that onychomatricoma may derive from the onychodermis, a specialized mesenchymal tissue containing onychofibroblasts located beneath the nail matrix and nail bed.

18.8.2 Epidemiology [56]

- It most commonly affects middle-aged individuals, with the highest incidence occurring around the fifth decade of life.
- There is no significant difference in prevalence between sexes.

18.8.3 Clinical Presentation (Fig. 18.40) [56–58]

- The tumor classically presents with a tetrad of:
  - Yellow discoloration with thickening of the nail plate.
  - Splinter hemorrhage.
  - Transverse nail plate overcurvature.
  - Worm-like cavitation of the nail plate.
- Other possible presentations are nail dystrophy, erythronychia, melanonychia, plate fracture, paronychia, and dorsal pterygium.
- Sections of the deep edge of the nail plate showed jigsaw-like variations, likely due to invasion by the finger-like projections of the tumor.
- More common on the fingers.

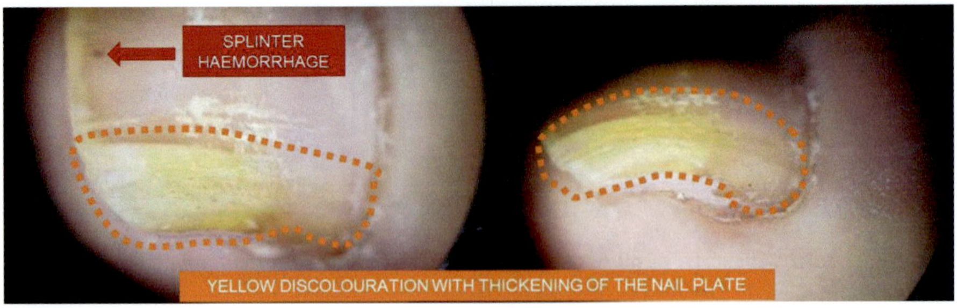

Fig. 18.40 Clinical photograph of a patient with a onychomatricoma

- Asymptomatic in most cases.
- Although no relevant relation has been found between the duration of the condition and the thickness of affected nail, longer than 5 years of evolution was more frequently associated with swelling and erythema.
- Some variants of onychomatricoma are described as follows:
  - Giant forms.
  - Pigmented forms are associated with a longitudinal melanonychia.
  - Associated with a dorsal pterygium.
  - Association with onychomycosis.
- Onychomatricoma may be complicated by fungal infection, and the tumor is often misdiagnosed as onychomycosis.

18.8.4 Onychoscopy [59–62]

- Perforations in the distal portion of the nail plate, hemorrhagic streaks, and white longitudinal grooves corresponding to channels in the nail plate.
- Parallel white lines and a distinct lateral demarcation of the lesion with parallel edges.
- Dark dots and pitting on the free edge of the nail plate.
- Architectural and vascular features include:
  - The "Sagrada Familia sign" (very regularly arranged hyperbolic crypts in the proximal part of the ventral aspect of the nail plate).
  - "Digitations" (finger-like extensions of the tumor above the lunula).
  - The "mirror" sign (symmetry of the components, such as crypts and digitations, across a perpendicular axis in the proximal nail fold).
  - Sagittal vessels.
  - Dotted vessels.
  - Irregular vessels.

18.8.5 Histopathology (Fig. 18.41) [57, 58, 62]

- This epithelial tumor originates from nail matrix cells and exhibits a vertical penetration pattern into the dermis.
- In its central region, it features longitudinally oriented parakeratotic cells expressing cytokeratin 14. The fibrous stroma is clearly separated from the tumor cells.
- If the nail plate is not sampled, this tumor may be misdiagnosed as a digital fibrokeratoma.

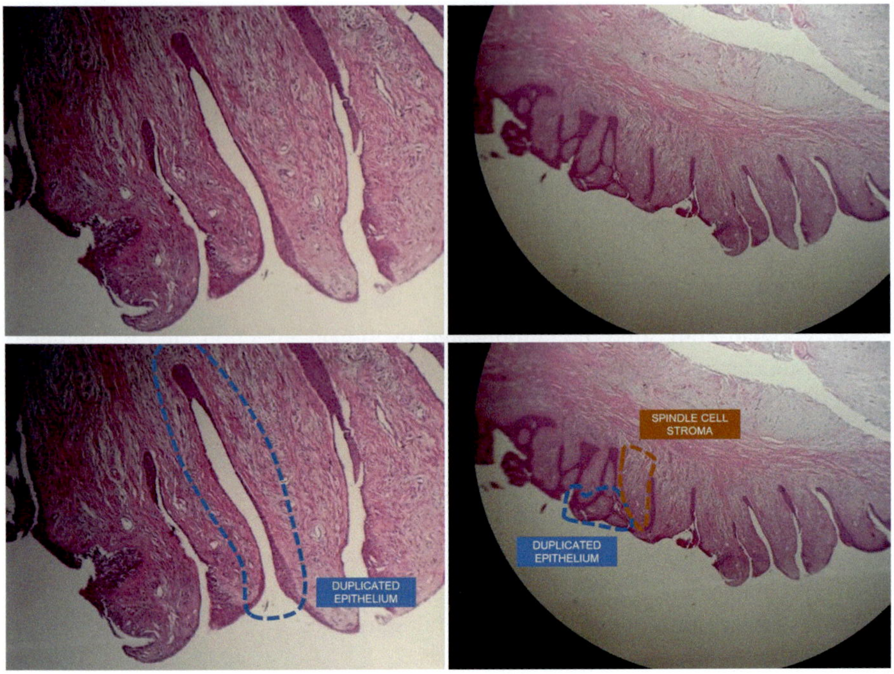

Fig. 18.41 Histological findings of a onychomatricoma (H&E x4)

- In longitudinal sections, it can be distinguished from fibrokeratoma by the presence of invaginations filled with corneal material, stroma organized in two layers, and absence of a distinct corneal layer.

18.8.6 Ultrasonography (Fig. 18.42) [29, 30]

- There is a heterogeneous and V-shaped thickening of the nail plates originating from the nail matrix.
- It appears as a hyperechoic linear band-like structure with hyperechoic lines within the nail plate.
- Shows hypovascularity on power Doppler imaging.
- There is no remodeling observed in the distal phalanx.

18.8.7 MRI (Fig. 18.43)

- This lesion originates from the nail matrix and proximal nail bed, typically located within the nail plate.

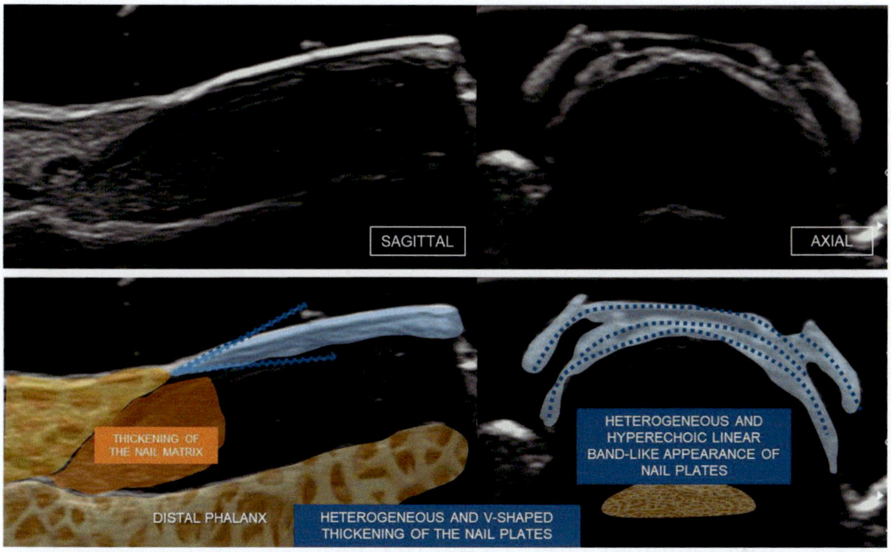

Fig. 18.42 Ultrasonographic findings of a onychomatricoma with a 24 MHz probe (Aplio i800, Canon Medical Systems)

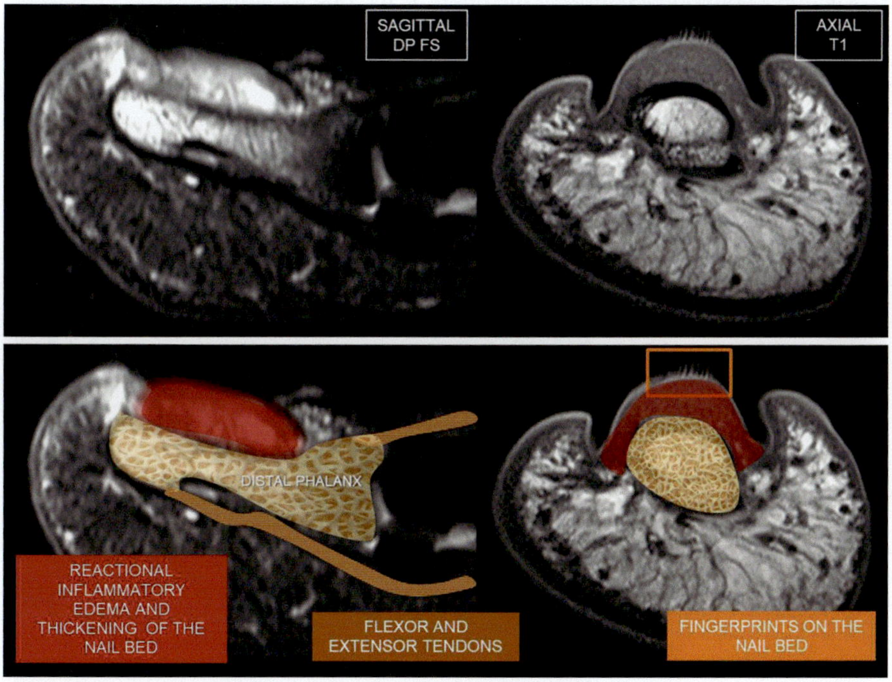

Fig. 18.43 MRI with surface coil findings of a onychomatricoma in PD FS weighted and STIR sequences (Magnetom Prisma 3T MRI, Siemens)

- As a result, it is challenging to well observe the lesion on MRI, with the only observable signal being the irregular and espiculated indentation caused on the surface of the nail bed by the tumor that is typical on T1 and T2-weighted images

18.9 Subungual Exostosis

18.9.1 Definition [63, 64]

- Isolated slow-growing benign outgrowths of normal bone or calcified cartilaginous remains. Trauma an etiologic factor despite history of trauma is only occasionally found.
- Finding of chromosomal translocation t(X;6)(q13-14;q22).

18.9.2 Epidemiology (Fig. 18.44) [63, 64]

- They are uncommon but may be underdiagnosed.
- Frequent in children and young adults.
- The most common location of the tumor is the first toenail.
- Female predisposition.

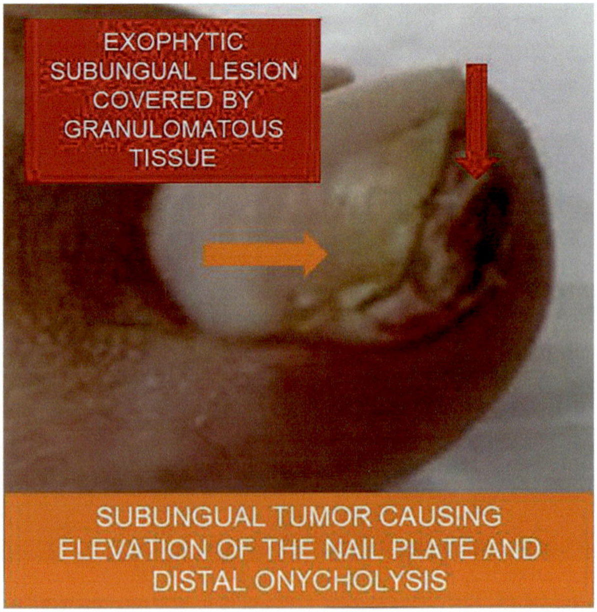

Fig. 18.44 Clinical photograph of a patient with an exostosis

18.9.3 Clinical Presentation (Fig. 18.44) [63–65]

- A solitary tumor causing elevation of the dorsal aspect of the distal phalanx with onycholysis or deformity.
- Firm and fixed to palpation, often hard.
- Initially presents with a shiny appearance and telangiectasia, later becoming hyperkeratotic over time.
- A peripheral collarette surrounds the tumor.
- The primary symptom is pain, although it can also be asymptomatic.

18.9.4 Onychoscopy (Fig. 18.45) [66, 67]

- Dermoscopic changes of the free nail edge:
  - Vascular ectasia (70%), an unusual vascular ectasia pattern like red coral: tortuous and dilated vessels were reminiscent of red coral with tentacle-like arms dancing in the sea.
  - Hyperkeratosis (60%).
  - Ulceration (30%).
- Dermoscopy of the nail plate reveled onycholysis (40%).

18.9.5 Histopathology [63, 68, 69]

- Peripheral fibrocartilaginous tissue with underlying peduncle composed of trabecular bone, which is attached to the underlying bone.

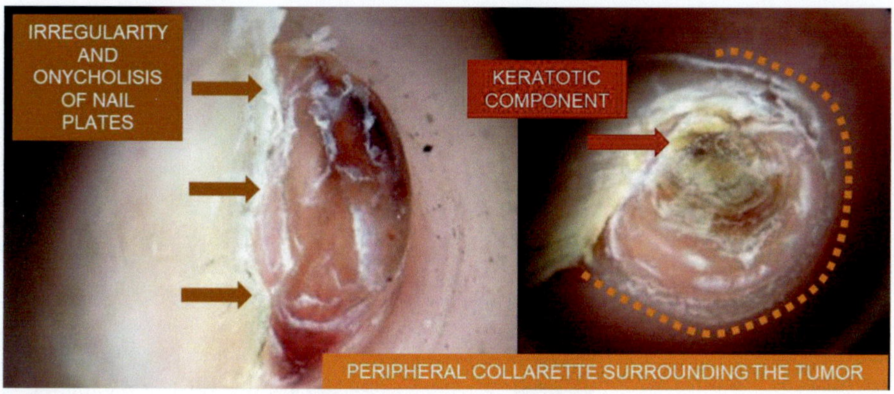

Fig. 18.45 Dermoscopy of a patient with an exostosis (x20)

- The amount of cartilaginous tissue is determined by the age of the lesion:
  - Early stage: cellular chondroid tissue with fibrous tissue proliferating from the background in the nail bed and may have no attachment to the underlying phalangeal bone. The cartilaginous layer may present hypercellularity and atypia of chondrocytes, with occasional mitosis. The cartilage matrix undergoes endochondral ossification over time.
  - Late stage: occasionally, the lesion is composed of irregular trabecular bone with an osteoblastic border with a thinned or even absent cartilaginous layer.

18.9.6 Radiography and Computed Tomography (Fig. 18.46) [70]

- In early stages, lesions may lack sufficient bone formation to be visible on radiographs.
- The tumor is a pedunculated bone projection originating from the dorsal aspect of the distal phalanx.
- On radiographic lateral views, smaller radiolucent lesions adjacent to the tumor typically represent the fibrocartilaginous cap.

18.9.7 Ultrasonography (Fig. 18.47) [71]

- The lesion appears as a heterogeneous linear structure with well-defined margins, resembling the adjacent cortical bone, which presents continuity with the bone, sometimes not clearly visualized by ultrasonography.

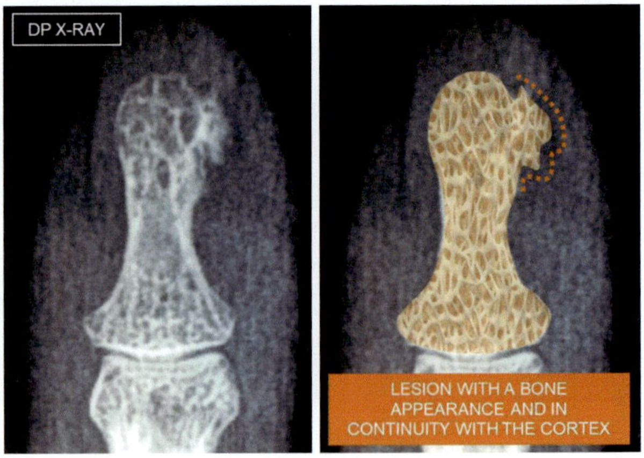

Fig. 18.46 Radiographic findings of an exostosis on dorso-palmar view (Philips Duo Diagnost R&F Room Digital RF and Tomo System)

- It exhibits calcifications with acoustic shadowing and a hypoechoic fibrocartilaginous cap.
- There is no detectable vascularity on power Doppler imaging.

18.9.8 MRI (Fig. 18.48) [21]

- The lesion presents as a heterogeneous oval structure with well-defined margins, extending into the cortical bone. The continuity with the cortical bone, is usually well observed on MRI, simulating a pedunculated lesion.
- Signal intensity is similar to that of the adjacent distal phalanx.
- The fibrocartilaginous cap appears hyperintense on T2-weighted and STIR images.
- There is only peripheral enhancement observed after gadolinium administration.

18.9.9 3D Images (Fig. 18.49, Video 18.5)

- Highly beneficial for effectively addressing challenging recurrent cases.
- Enhances visualization of the lesion's extent and its relationship with nearby structures, especially the cortical of the distal phalanx and the exact location and extension of the fibrocartilaginous cap.
- Enhances surgical precision during complex procedures, leading to a more conservative approach

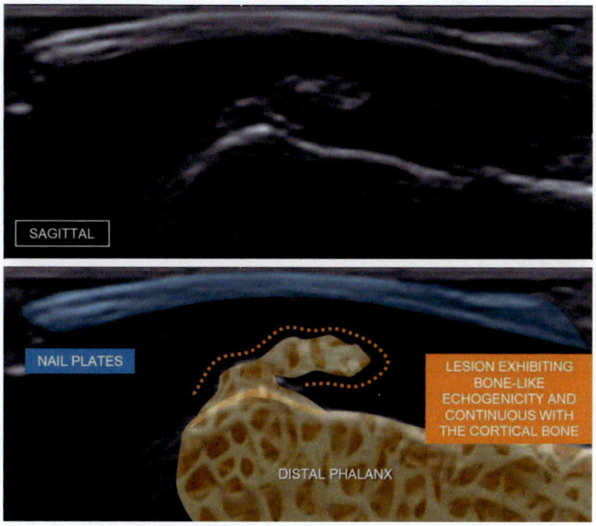

Fig. 18.47 Ultrasonographic findings of an exostosis with a 24 MHz probe (Aplio i800, Canon Medical Systems)

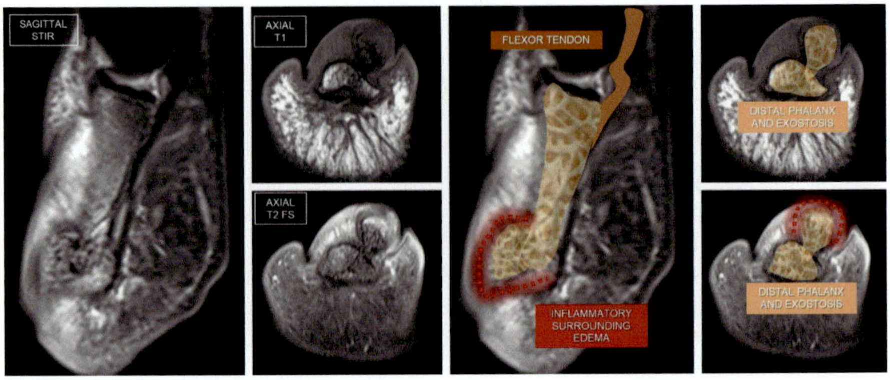

Fig. 18.48 MRI with surface coil findings of an exostosis in T1-weighted and STIR sequences (Magnetom Prisma 3T MRI, Siemens)

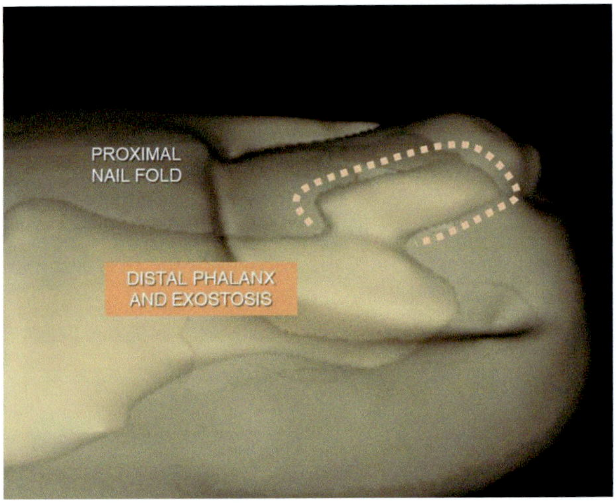

Fig. 18.49 3D virtual findings of an exostosis after image segmentation of MRI isotropic sequences for surgical planning

- Biomodels can generate physical replicas of the affected area, providing visual aids that support both surgical planning and patient education.

18.10 Lipoma

18.10.1 Definition [72–77]

- Lipomas are among the most common benign soft tissue tumors, typically found in areas such as the neck, trunk, and legs. They usually present as small subcutaneous nodules but can grow over time, potentially causing symptoms due to mechanical compression of surrounding organs, nerves, and tissues.

- The etiology and pathogenesis of lipomas are often unclear. Genetic, traumatic, and metabolic factors have been studied, but the conclusions are not always consistent.
- Periungual and subungual lipomas are extremely rare. Occasionally, lipomas may affect the phalanx and, when located near bones, can cause osteolysis and may infiltrate deeper structures like tendons and muscles.
- When lipomas involve the fingers, they should be considered in the differential diagnosis of benign soft tissue masses in unusual locations.

18.10.2 Epidemiology [74, 76]

- Lipomas are rarely found in the hand, accounting for 0.2–0.8% of benign tumors in this region. They infrequently affect the fingers, and involvement of the nail unit is extremely rare.
- They typically occur in adults, and those affecting the digits are notably rare.

18.10.3 Clinical Presentation (Fig. 18.50) [72–75]

- The clinical manifestation of a lipoma depends on its location and size.
- It presents as a solid tumor, and when located in the nail fold region, it is described as a palpable mass with a firm consistency and varying dimensions.
- If the nail matrix and nail bed are affected, onychodystrophy such as erythronychia, onycholysis, and longitudinal grooves may occur.
- The mass associated with the lipoma may not always be visible, depending on the size of the lesion. The spindle cell lipoma variant is rare and uncommon in subungual locations.

18.10.4 Onychoscopy [73, 74]

- The tumor usually appears as a volume increase with normal appearing overlying skin, reducing the initial value of dermoscopy.
- Dermoscopy becomes more useful when onychodystrophies are present, improving the detection of longitudinal grooves, erythronychia, and other related findings.
- Dermoscopic examination may reveal telangiectasias against a subtly yellowish background.
- The vascular pattern observed through dermoscopy can sometimes resemble other conditions, such as basal cell carcinoma. However, it aids in distinguishing the lipoma from other potential diagnoses.

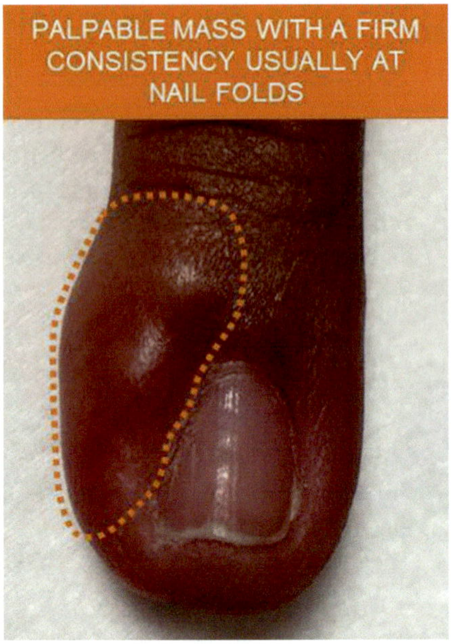

Fig. 18.50 Clinical photograph of a patient with a periungual lipoma

18.10.5 Histopathology (Fig. 18.51) [73]

- Lipomas occurring in the fingers, including in the subungual and periungual locations, are extremely rare, with few cases cited in the literature, usually presenting the classic form, circumscribed collection of mature adipose tissue with a thin capsule of connective tissue.
- Other variants include spindle cell lipoma and fibrolipoma.

18.10.6 Radiography and Computed Tomography (Fig. 18.52) [72, 78]

- Typically used to rule out bony abnormalities or erosions. For periungual lipomas, no significant osseous changes are observed.
- CT scan: Less commonly used but can help in visualizing the mass and its relationship with surrounding structures. It might show the lipoma as a well-defined, soft tissue mass.

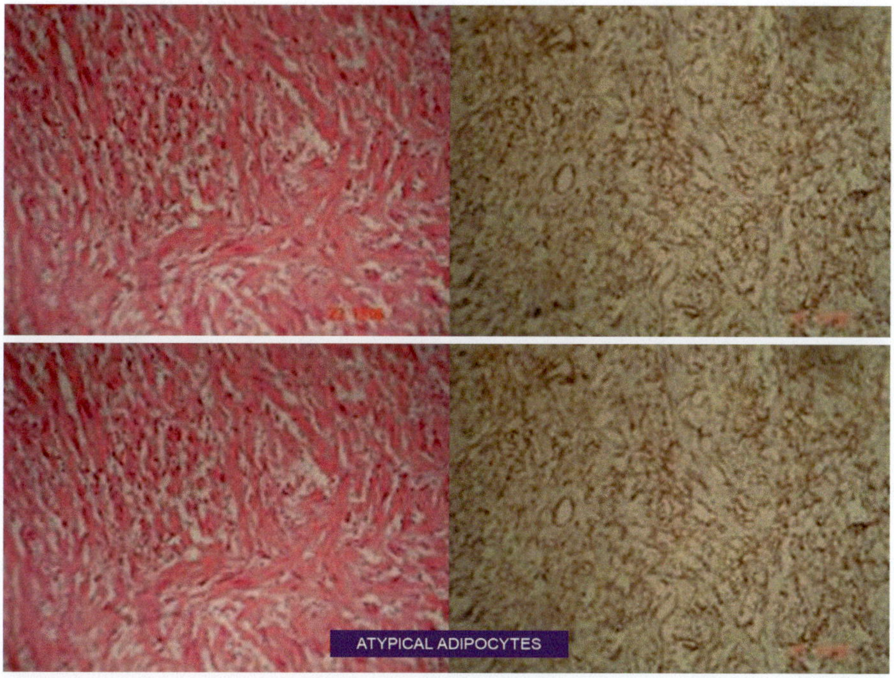

Fig. 18.51 Histology of a periungual lipoma (H&E x20 and Reticulin x20)

18.10.7 Ultrasonography (Fig. 18.53) [78]

- Usually shows a well-defined, hyperechoic mass with a thin capsule surrounding it.
- There is typically no internal blood flow detected, which helps in confirming the benign nature of the tumor.

18.10.8 MRI (Fig. 18.54) [79]

- MRI is the most effective imaging modality for diagnosing lipomas. It provides detailed images showing the lipoma as a homogeneous, high-signal-intensity mass on T1-weighted images.
- It helps in distinguishing the lipoma from other soft tissue tumors and in planning surgical excision.

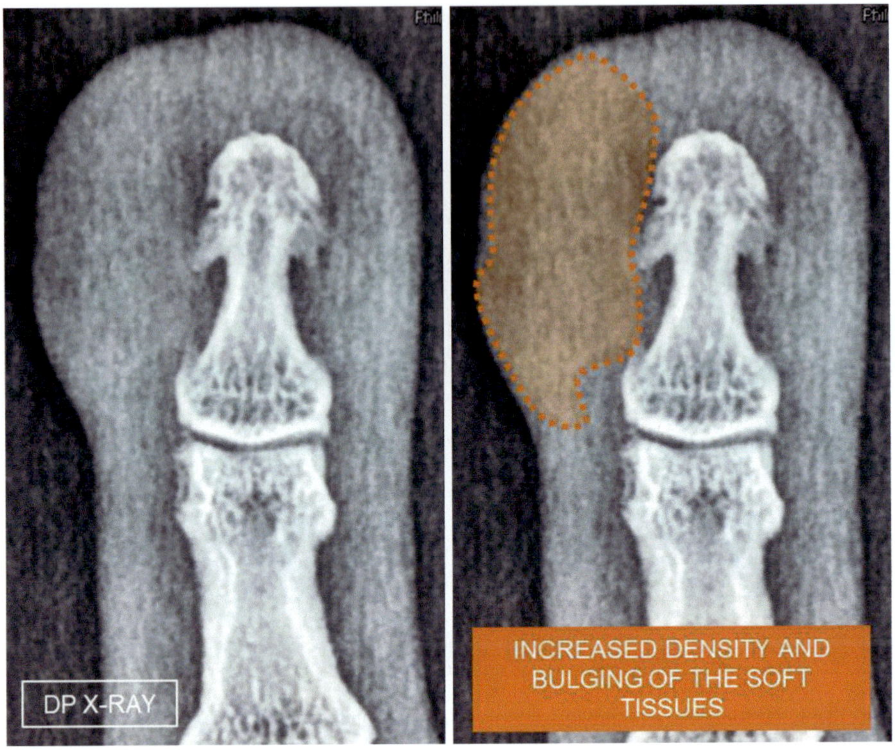

Fig. 18.52 Radiographic findings of a periungual lipoma (Philips Duo Diagnost R&F Room Digital RF and Tomo System)

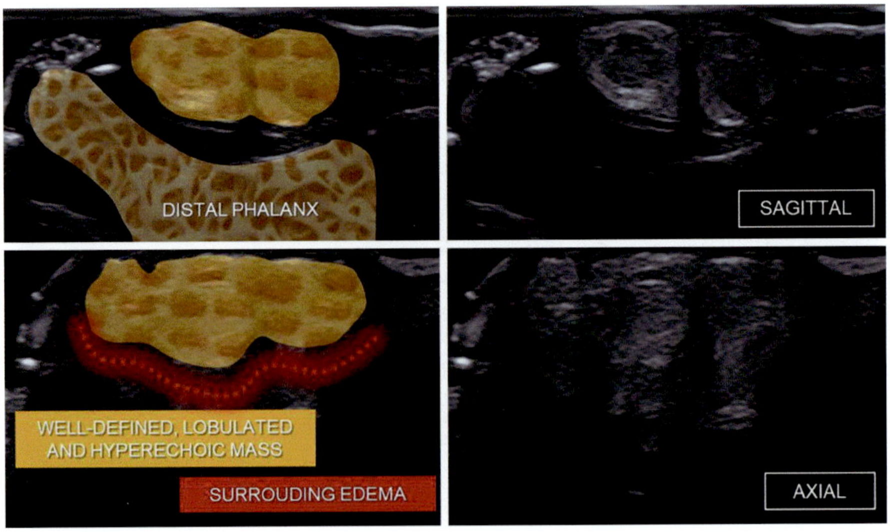

Fig. 18.53 Ultrasonographic findings of a periungual lipoma with a 24 MHz probe (Aplio i800, Canon Medical Systems)

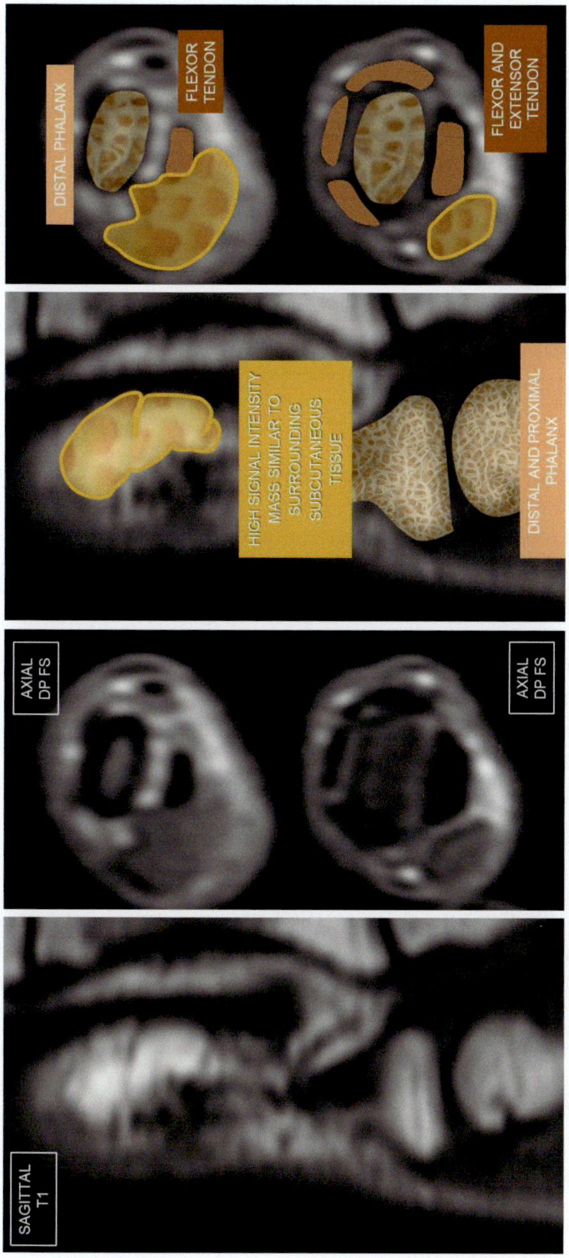

Fig. 18.54 MRI with surface coil findings of a periungual lipoma in T1 and DP FS weighted sequences (Magnetom Prisma 3T MRI, Siemens)

18.10.9 3D Images

- Highly advantageous for effectively managing challenging recurrent cases.
- Improves the visualization of the lesion's extent and its relationship with nearby structures, especially the nail matrix, adjacent tendons, and bone.
- Increases surgical precision during complex procedures.
- Biomodels can produce physical replicas of the affected area, offering visual aids that facilitate both surgical planning and patient education.

18.11 Cystic Lesions

18.11.1 Definition [80, 81]

- Mucous cysts.
  - Digital mucous cysts are lesions commonly associated with osteoarthritis of the distal interphalangeal (DIP) joint or thumb interphalangeal (IP) joint. These cysts result from the degeneration of collagen fibers.
- Myxoid cysts:
  - Benign tumors affecting the distal digits of fingers and toes.
  - Typically present as translucent nodules on the dorsum of the digit, between the distal interphalangeal joint crease and the proximal nail fold.
  - Less common variants may lie directly on the dorsal nail plate or beneath the proximal nail fold.
  - Can cause a longitudinal groove in the nail plate, varying in depth according to cyst volume.
- Onycholemal cyst.
  - Subungual onycholemmal cysts (SOCs) are uncommon cystic formations located beneath the nail. These cysts are characterized by their presence in the nail bed and are typically lined with stratified squamous epithelium.

18.11.2 Epidemiology [80–82]

- Mucous cysts.
  - Digital mucous cysts are ganglions that arise from the dorsum of the distal interphalangeal (DIP) joint.
  - Digital mucous cysts are frequently observed in individuals with osteoarthritis, particularly affecting the DIP or thumb IP joints.

- The condition equally affects men and women, with a mean age of onset around the seventh decade of life.

- Myxoid cysts:
  - More common in adults, with a slight female predominance.
  - Notable cases involving both thumbs and other fingers.
- Onycholemal cyst.
  - SOCs are rare and are often discovered incidentally during the evaluation of other nail abnormalities or suspected malignancies.
  - They most frequently occur in the great toenail or thumb and can be associated with past trauma to the nail.

18.11.3 Clinical Presentation (Fig. 18.55) [80–83]

- Mucous cysts.
  - Digital mucous cysts present as slow-growing masses over the dorsal aspect of the DIP joint, often located in the subcutaneous tissue. They are typically round, dome-shaped, firm, and can be transilluminated. Some cysts may cause deformities in the nail if they exert pressure on the germinal matrix, leading to longitudinal grooves. Skin overlying the cyst can be thin, ulcerated, or even infected.
- Myxoid cysts:
  - Presentation includes translucent nodules, often discharging a mucoid substance.

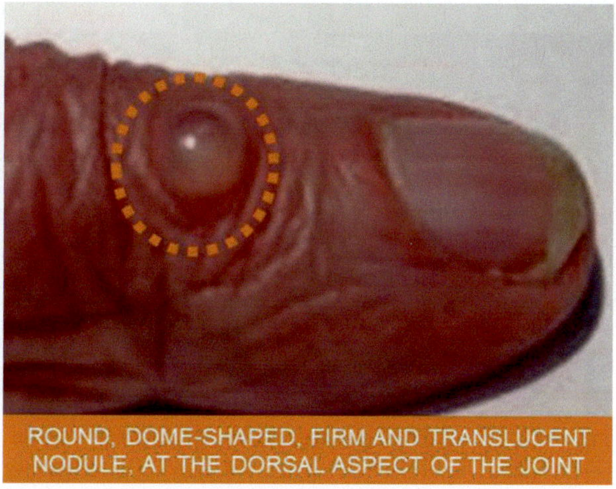

Fig. 18.55 Clinical photograph of a patient with a periungual synovial cyst

- Beneath the nail plate, cysts impact nail shape, integrity, and microvasculature.
- Clinical features such as color change in the lunula (red, blue, or longitudinal leukonychia), increased transverse nail curvature, and possible nail destruction.
- Symptomatic lateral ingrowing and secondary bacterial paronychia in some cases.

- Onycholemal cyst:
  - Also known as subungual epidermoid cysts or inclusions, these cysts are rarely diagnosed clinically as they typically do not cause any symptoms.
  - They consist of multiple small epidermal inclusion cysts occurring in the dermis of the nail bed, some with central solid keratinization. They are often related to trauma. Due to their potential for calcification, they can become visible on radiographs.

18.11.4 Onychoscopy (Fig. 18.56) [83]

- Mucous cyst.
  - Appearance without pressure:

    Predominantly shows a vascular pattern.
    Characterized by linear, branched, and serpentine vessels.

  - Appearance with pressure:

    Vascular pattern becomes less distinct.
    Lesion appears translucent with bright white areas.

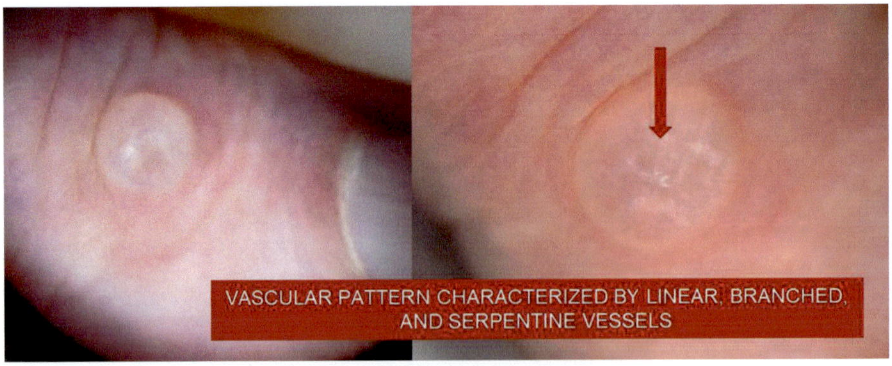

Fig. 18.56 Dermoscopy of a patient with a periungual synovial cyst (x10 and x20)

- Myxoid cysts.
  - Red lunula in most cases, with occasional blue hue or longitudinal leukonychia.
  - Increased transverse curvature and nail splitting.

18.11.5 Histopathology [80]

- Mucous cyst:
  - Digital mucous cysts lack an epithelial lining, making the term "cyst" somewhat misleading.
  - Myxomatous (superficial) type:

    Located near the proximal nail fold.
    Fluctuates and resembles focal mucinosis.
  - Ganglion (deep) type:

    Found on the dorsum of a finger near the distal interphalangeal (DIP) joint.
    Analogous to a ganglion cyst.
- Myxoid cysts:
  - Reveals a myxoid stroma bordered by compacted connective tissue without an epithelial lining.
  - Origin is often linked to the distal interphalangeal joint.
- Onycholemal cyst:
  - Histologically, SOCs are characterized by their lining of stratified squamous epithelium and the presence of onycholemmal keratin within the cysts.
  - The cysts do not show signs of cellular atypia or a granular layer. Immunohistochemical staining typically does not reveal melanocytic antigens, ruling out melanoma.

18.11.6 Radiography and Computed Tomography [80]

- CT scans are less frequently employed but can be useful in certain diagnostic contexts.
- Radiographic findings include joint arthritis and the absence of prominent arthritis in other cases.

18.11.7 Ultrasonography (Fig. 18.57) [29]

- Mucous cyst:
  - Round or oval, tortuous, anechoic (may contain echogenic areas when the content is more viscous), posterior acoustic enhancement, without vascularization, communication with the DIP joint, degenerative changes in the DIP joint, Heberden's nodes, and osteophytes.
- Mixoid cyst:
  - Appears as a round or oval structure, anechoic (without echoes) and may contain echogenic areas when the content is more viscous, with posterior acoustic enhancement. There is no vascularization present.
- Onycholemal cyst:
  - Poorly defined hyperechoic area in nail bed.

18.11.8 MRI (Fig. 18.58)

- Usuallt the T2-weighted MRI sequence is used to assess for bone and vascular involvement.
- The MRI showed a slight enlargement of the tumor involving the left thumbnail with an adjacent tissue reaction, but the cortical bone remains intact.

18.11.9 3D Images (Fig. 18.59, Video 18.6)

- Highly advantageous for effectively managing challenging recurrent cases.

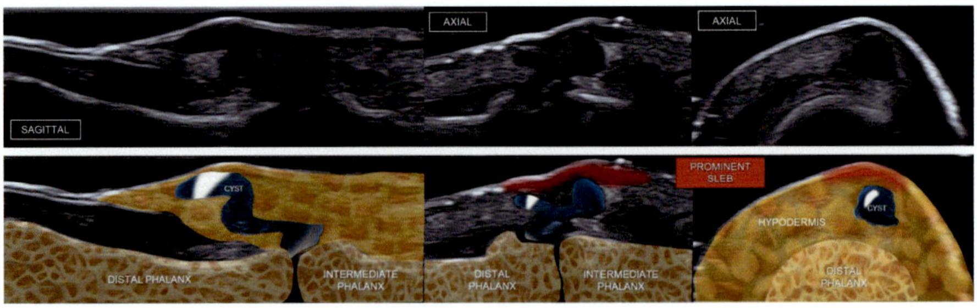

Fig. 18.57 Ultrasonographic findings of a periungual synovial cyst with a 24 MHz probe (Aplio i800, Canon Medical Systems)

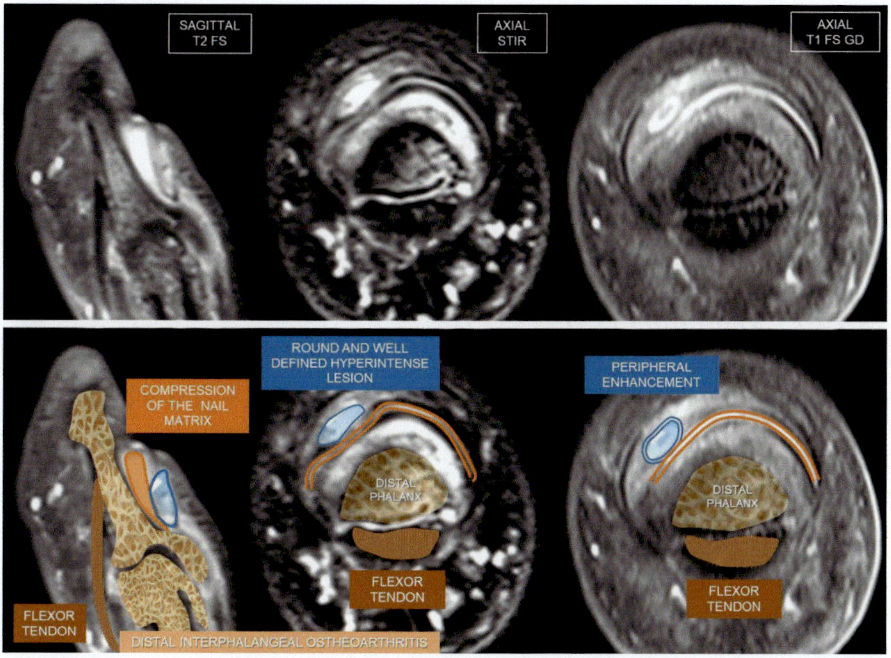

Fig. 18.58 MRI with surface coil findings of periungual synovial cyst in T1 FS, T2 FS weighted and STIR sequences after gadolinium administration (Magnetom Prisma 3T MRI, Siemens)

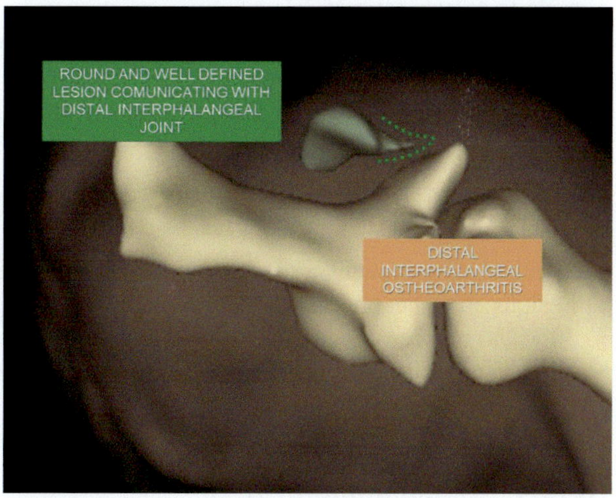

Fig. 18.59 3D virtual findings of periungual synovial cyst after image segmentation of MRI isotropic sequences for surgical planning

- Enhances visualization of the lesion's extent and its relationship with nearby structures, particularly the nail matrix and the communication with the pedicle that requires repair.
- Biomodels can create physical replicas of the affected area, providing visual aids that aid in both surgical planning and patient education.

18.12 Acral Fibromyxoma

18.12.1 Definition [84]

- Superficial acral fibromyxoma is a rare, benign, and slow-growing soft tissue tumor predominantly found in the periungual and subungual areas of adult fingers and toes.
- This neoplasm, first described in 2001, displays a distinct preference for these acral locations and often involves the nail apparatus.

18.12.2 Epidemiology [84]

- Fewer than 50 cases reported globally.
- Typically diagnosed in middle-aged adults, with a mean age of 43 years and a male-to-female ratio of 2:1.
- Cases are sporadically reported worldwide without any specific regional predilection.

18.12.3 Clinical Presentation (Fig. 18.60) [84]

- Painless, slow-growing masses located in the subungual or periungual regions.
- Lesions may be present for a prolonged period (ranging from 3 months to 30 years) before surgical intervention.
- Nodular growths disrupting the nail, with no clear history of trauma in most cases.

18.12.4 Histopathology [84]

- Moderately cellular, nonencapsulated tumor extending into the dermis and possibly the subcutis. It consists of stellate and spindle-shaped fibroblast-like cells within a myxocollagenous stroma.
- Presence of mast cells, occasional multinucleated stromal cells, and rare nuclear atypia and mitotic figures.

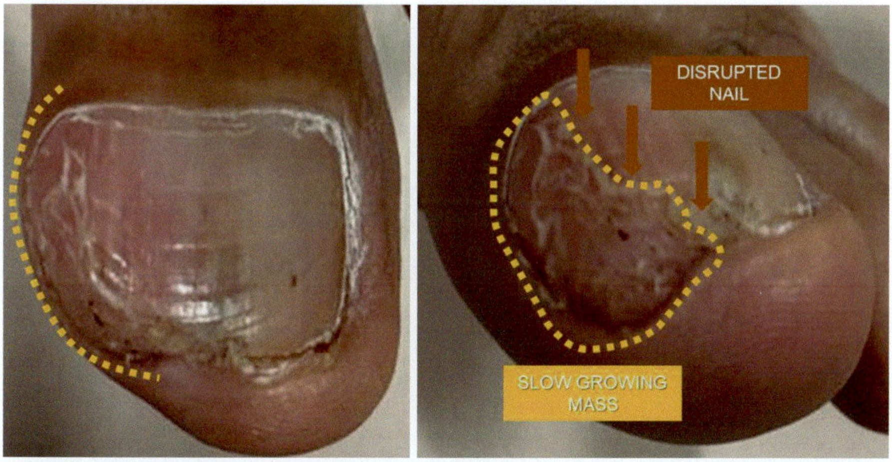

Fig. 18.60 Clinical photograph of a patient with an acral fibromyxoma

- Tumor cells show immunoreactivity for CD34, epithelial membrane antigen, CD99, and less frequently, CD10.

18.12.5 Radiography and Computed Tomography (Fig. 18.61)

- Smooth margin erosion or depression of the distal phalanx due to compression may be observed.

18.12.6 Ultrasonography [85]

- Ultrasonography can demonstrate the relationship between the fibromyxoma and the nail plate, though it has limited ability to differentiate fibromyxomas from glomus tumors.
- May demonstrate a well-circumscribed, hypoechoic mass within the soft tissues of the finger or toe, with eterogeneous appearence, aiding in preoperative planning and differential diagnosis.

18.12.7 MRI (Fig. 18.62) [86]

- Typically presents as a subungual or periungual mass, often displacing the nail plate.

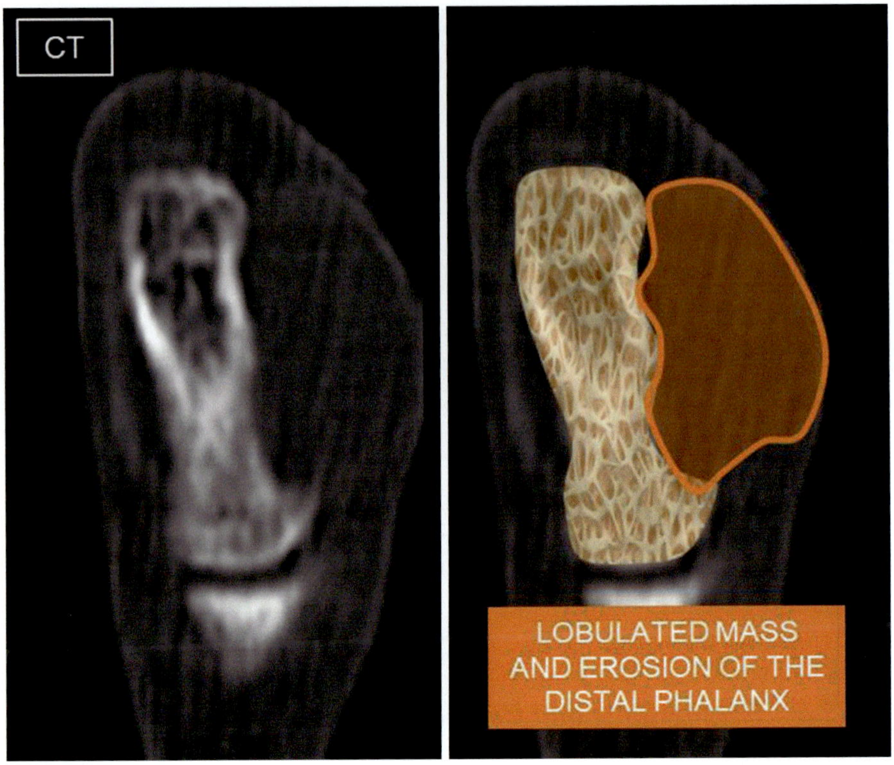

Fig. 18.61 Computed tomography findings of an acral fibromyxoma (Philips Brilliance CT 64-slice)

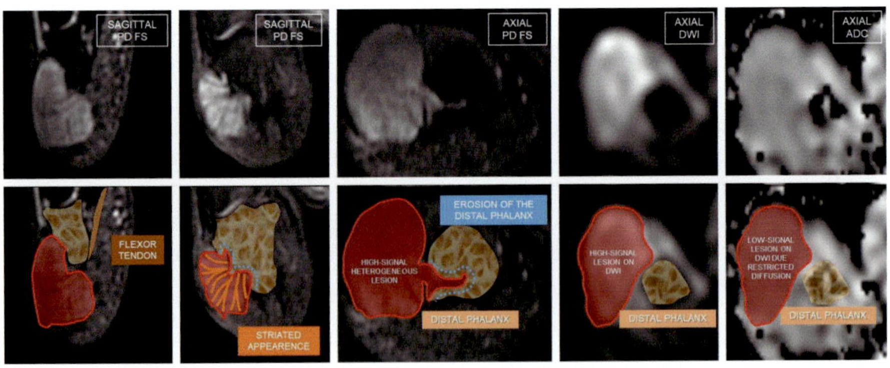

Fig. 18.62 MRI with surface coil findings of an acral fibromyxoma in PD FS weighted, DWI and ADC map sequences (Magnetom Prisma 3T MRI, Siemens)

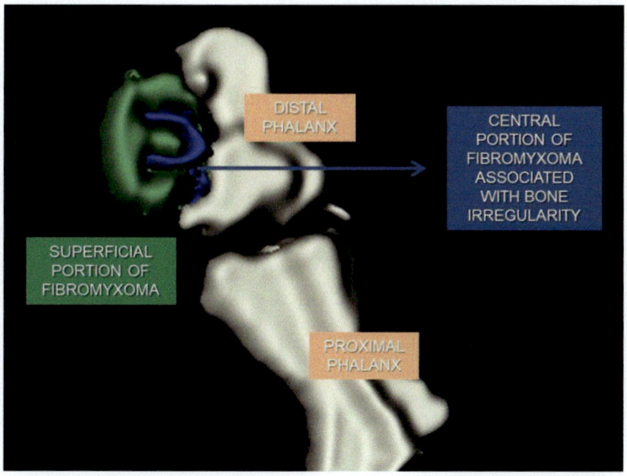

Fig. 18.63 3D virtual findings of an acral fibromyxoma after images segmentation of MRI isotropic sequences for surgical planning

- Appears as a high-signal lesion on T2-weighted MRI images, indicating a myxoid composition. Some lesions may display both fibrous (low signal on T2) and myxoid (high signal on T2) components.
- Post-contrast images show global enhancement of the lesion.
- Dynamic contrast-enhanced MRI reveals a type 5 enhancement curve, characterized by rapid initial enhancement followed by gradual slow enhancement, typical of tumors with large interstitial compartments, like myxoid tumors.

18.12.8 3D Images (Fig. 18.63, Video 18.7)

- 3D imaging is highly beneficial for managing complex recurrent cases, providing superior visualization of the lesion's extent and its relationship with nearby structures, such as the nail matrix and the pedicle requiring repair.
- It also reveals subtle findings like smooth margin erosion or distal phalanx depression due to chronic compression.
- Biomodels can generate physical replicas of the affected area, offering visual aids that facilitate both surgical planning and patient education.

18.13 Bowen's Disease

18.13.1 Definition [87, 88]

- Bowen's disease is an in situ squamous cell carcinoma of epidermis.
- Although very rare, it is the most common nail malignancy.

18.13.2 Epidemiology [89]

- Men between the ages of 35 and 60 are primarily affected.
- Bowen's disease is often misdiagnosed due to its resemblance to benign dermatoses and its slow, indolent progression.
- High-risk mucosal HPVs are reported to play a significant role in the development of lesions on the hand, including the periungual region.
- Predisposing factors may include radiation treatment, exposure to X-rays, ingestion of arsenic, chronic paronychia, or trauma.

18.13.3 Clinical Presentation (Fig. 18.64) [89]

- Classic patterns of periungual involvement include:
  - Hyperkeratotic, papillomatous, or warty proliferation.
  - Erosions or scaling of the nail fold.
  - Whitish cuticle.
  - Periungual swelling due to deep tumor proliferation.
- Fissure of the lateral nail groove, sometimes crusted with granulation-like tissue beneath the scab.
- Subungual involvement may present with onycholysis, sometimes associated with oozing erosion or ulceration of a crusty nail bed. Bleeding, nodularity, and ulceration indicate invasion.
- Other possible presentations include longitudinal melanonychia, subungual pseudofibrokeratoma, and longitudinal erythronychia.

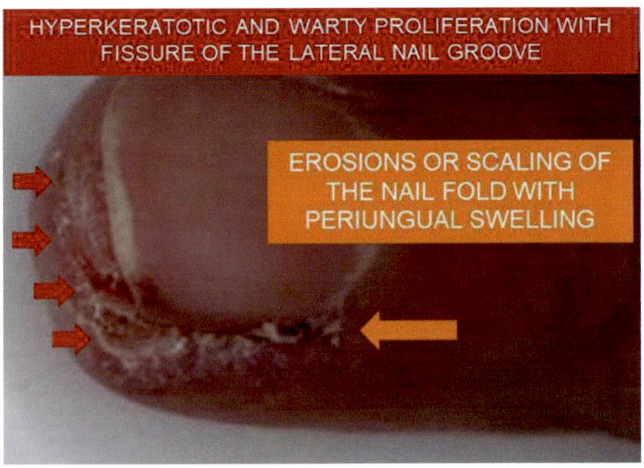

Fig. 18.64 Clinical photograph of a patient with a Bowen's disease

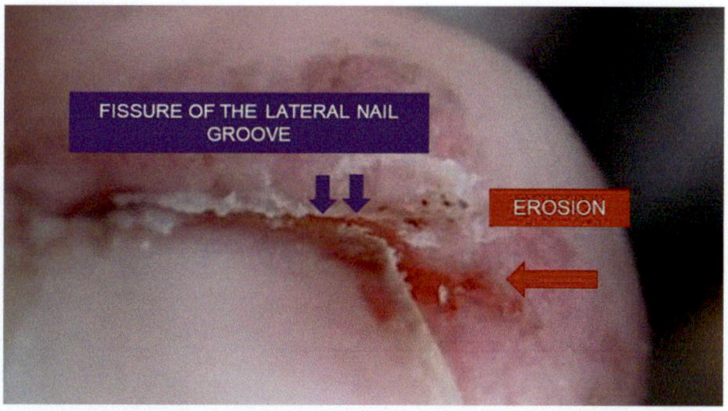

Fig. 18.65 Dermoscopy of a patient with a Bowen's disease (x20)

18.13.4 Onychoscopy (Fig. 18.65) [90, 91]

- In nonpigmented Bowen's disease:
  - Verrucous surface with brown-red streaky hemorrhages and clustering dot-like or glomerular vessel.
- In pigmented Bowen's disease:
  - Scaly surfaces, glomerular vessels, brownish dots along imaginary lines, or homogenous pigmentation.

18.13.5 Histopathology (Fig. 18.66) [92, 93]

- Histopathological findings are similar to those of Bowen's disease from other locations and may be associated with arsenical keratosis or HPV.
- It is an intraepithelial squamous cell carcinoma (in situ) without alternating parakeratosis, an important histopathological finding to differentiate from bowenoid actinic keratosis.

18.13.6 Ultrasonography (Fig. 18.67) [94]

- An irregular hypoechoic lesion with a solid component.
- Exhibits a superficial hyperechoic layer caused by keratinization, known as the "wave sign."
- Infiltration depth is limited to the epidermis.
- Power Doppler ultrasound reveals three types of blood flow:
  - Absence of internal blood flow signal.
  - Sparse punctiform blood flow signals within the lesion.
  - Profuse blood flow signals within the lesion.

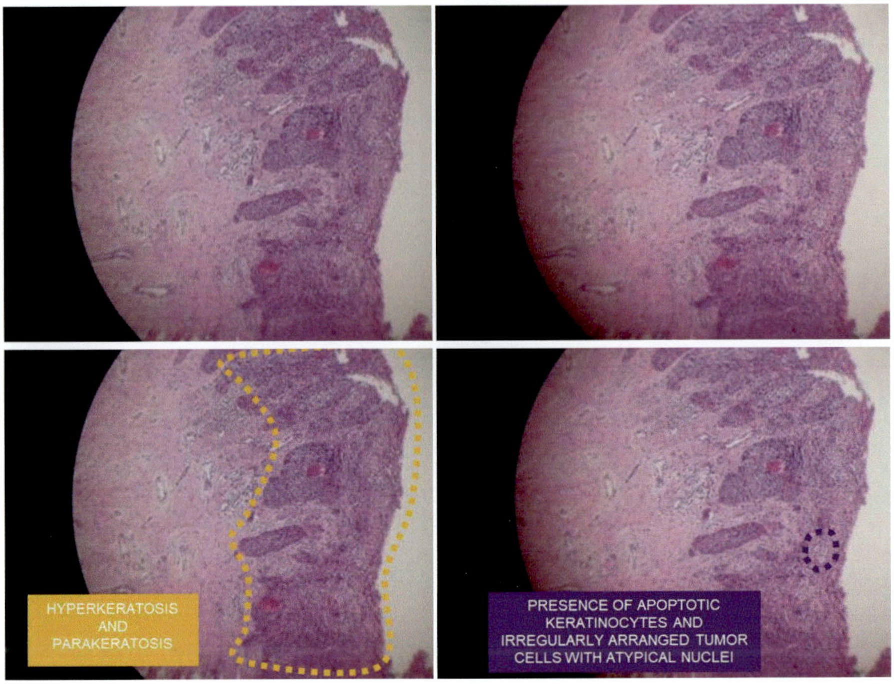

Fig. 18.66 Histological findings of a Bowen's disease (H&E x4)

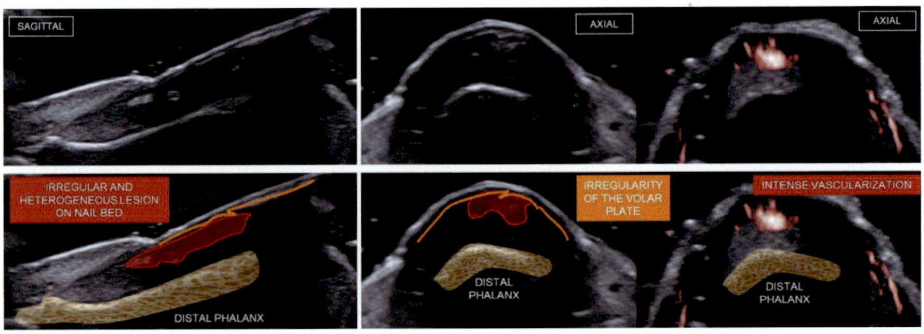

Fig. 18.67 Ultrasonographic findings of a Bowen's disease with a 24 MHz probe (Aplio i800, Canon Medical Systems)

18.14 Squamous Cell Carcinoma

18.14.1 Definition [95, 96]

- Rare malignant tumor that usually originates underneath the nail plate and grows slowly.
- Possible bone invasion.

18.14.2 Epidemiology [95, 96]

- Only 1–2% of primary tumors of the hand are malignant, and the most common hand malignancy is Squamous cell carcinoma.
- The majority originate from advanced Bowen's disease lesions.
- It is more common in fingernails of elderly men.
- Mainly in the thumb.
- Potential predisposing factors include trauma, chronic sun or arsenic exposure, radiation, burning, genodermatoses, tobacco or immunosuppression, and HPV infection.

18.14.3 Clinical Presentation (Fig. 18.68) [95–97]

- Most commonly arise from subungual region (57.4%), rarely from the proximal, lateral nail folds or hyponychium.
- Nonspecific features such as:
  - Onycholysis associated with yellow discoloration of the overlying nail and frequent oozing is considered a late symptom.
  - Destruction or discoloration of the nail plate.
  - Erosion of the nail bed associated or not with a nodule.
  - Hyperkeratosis.
  - Paronychia.
  - Longitudinal erythronychia.
- Pain, swelling, and inflammation may suggest bone involvement, nail Squamous Cell Carcinoma tend to become invasive more quickly.

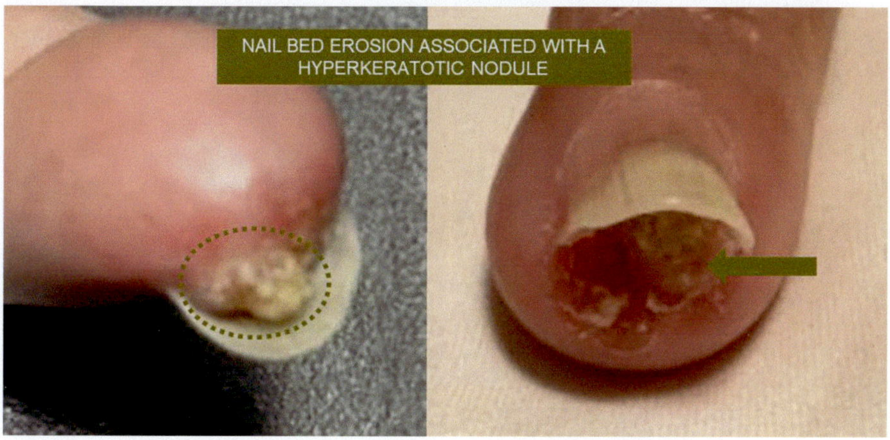

Fig. 18.68 Clinical photograph of a patient with an espinocelular carcinoma

18.14.4 Onychoscopy (Fig. 18.69) [97–100]

- The vascular polymorphism is the most important aspect.
- Onychoscopy criterion significantly associated with series of Squamous Cell Carcinoma was unparalleled lateral edges or fuzzy edges of the nail lesion.
- Common features are onycholysis, irregular vascularity, or hemorrhages with a rough-to-verrucous surface, white longitudinal lines, hyperkeratosis underneath the nail plate, and nail thickening.

18.14.5 Histopathology (Fig. 18.70) [96, 97]

- Histopathological findings are similar to those of squamous cell carcinoma from other locations, and may be associated with arsenical keratosis, Bowen's disease, or HPV.
- Extension inwards the dermis by irregular nests composed of atypical keratinocytes with an infiltrative aspect.
- Atypical, hyperchromatic, pleomorphic keratinocytes with nuclear aberrations, dyskeratosis, and increased number of mitoses, including atypical and off-basal mitosis.
- In 20% of cases, bone involvement occurs.

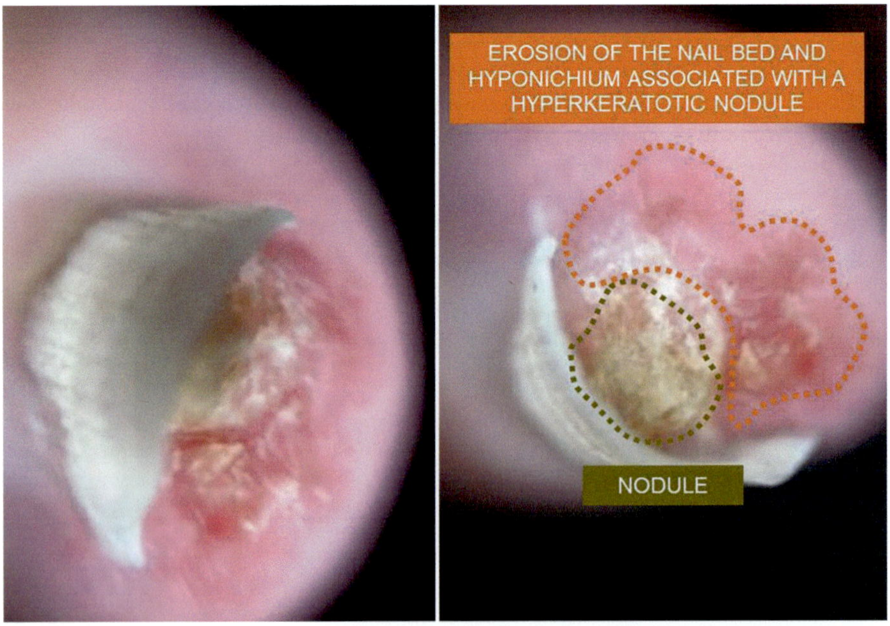

Fig. 18.69 Dermoscopy of a patient with an espinocelular carcinoma (x20)

18.14.6 Radiography and Computed Tomography

- Bone cortical irregularity, erosion, and periosteal reaction when distal phalanx is involved.

18.14.7 Ultrasonography (Fig. 18.71) [101, 102]

- Poorly defined heterogeneous and hypoechoic lesion that can demonstrates the "wave sign."
- Hypervascularization on power Doppler imaging.
- Eccentrically located in the nail bed.
- Deeper infiltration in dermis and epidermis with irregular and ill-defined appearence.
- Erosion of the nail plates and distal phalanx.

18.14.8 MRI (Fig. 18.72)

- Poorly defined heterogeneous lesion on nail bed with low signal intensity on T1-weighted images and high signal intensity on T2-weighted and STIR images.
- Intense contrast enhancement after gadolinium administration.
- Eccentrically located in the nail bed.
- Erosion of the nail plates and distal phalanx.

18.14.9 3D Images

- Highly advantageous for effectively managing challenging recurrent cases.
- Enhances visualization of the lesion's extent and its relationship with nearby structures, such as the irregular tumor margins, its depth of invasion, and its relationship with critical structures such as the nail matrix and underlying bone.
- It illustrates the extent of nail plate erosion and cortical disruption of the distal phalanx, aiding in preoperative planning and improving patient understanding of the surgical approach.
- Biomodels can create physical replicas of the affected area, providing visual aids that support both surgical planning and patient education.

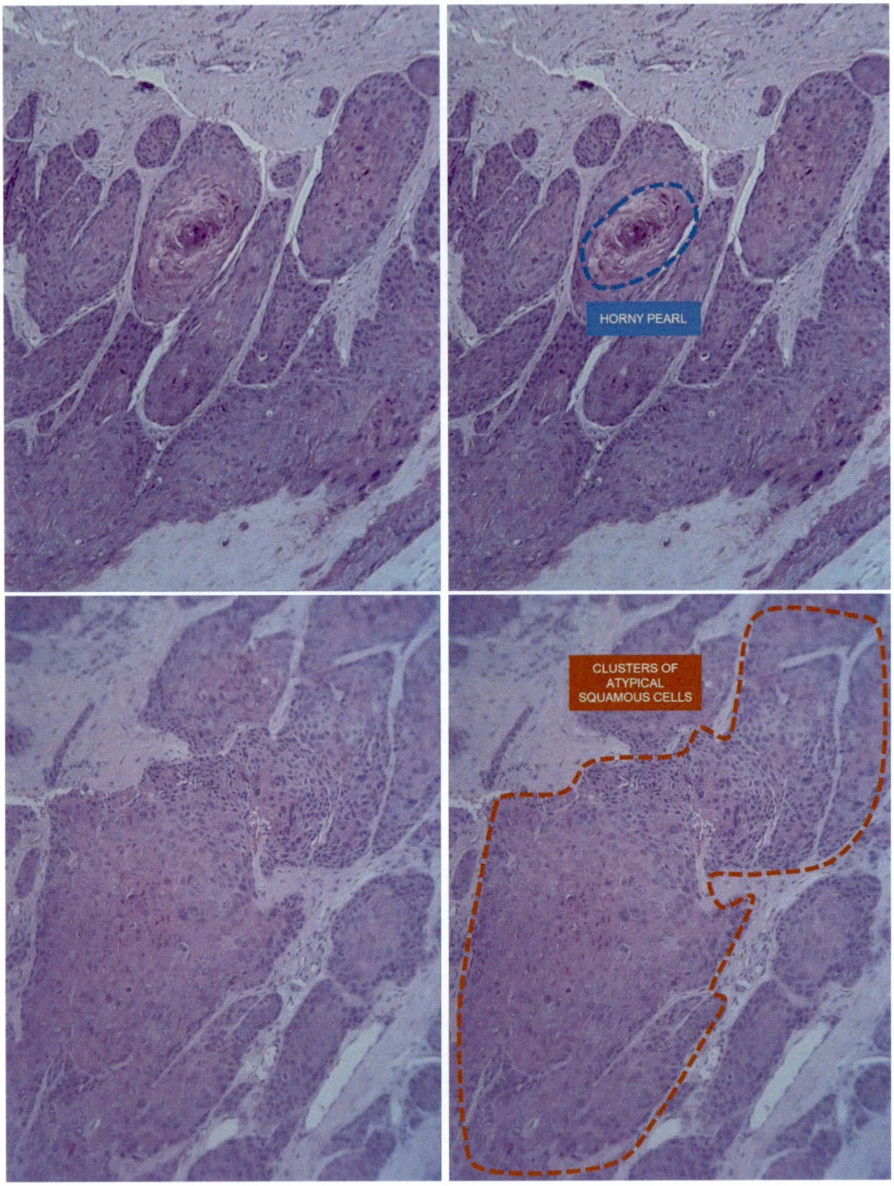

Fig. 18.70 Histological findings of an espinocelular carcinoma (H&E x10)

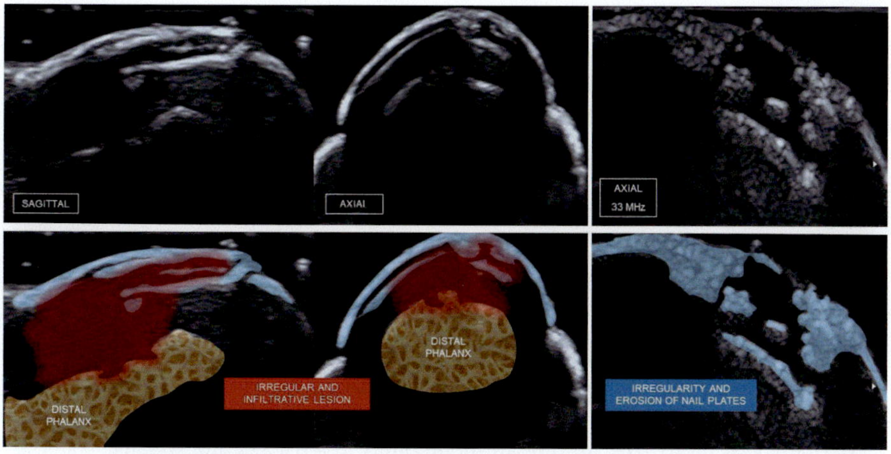

Fig. 18.71 Ultrasonographic findings of an espinocelular carcinoma with a 24 MHz probe (Aplio i800, Canon Medical Systems)

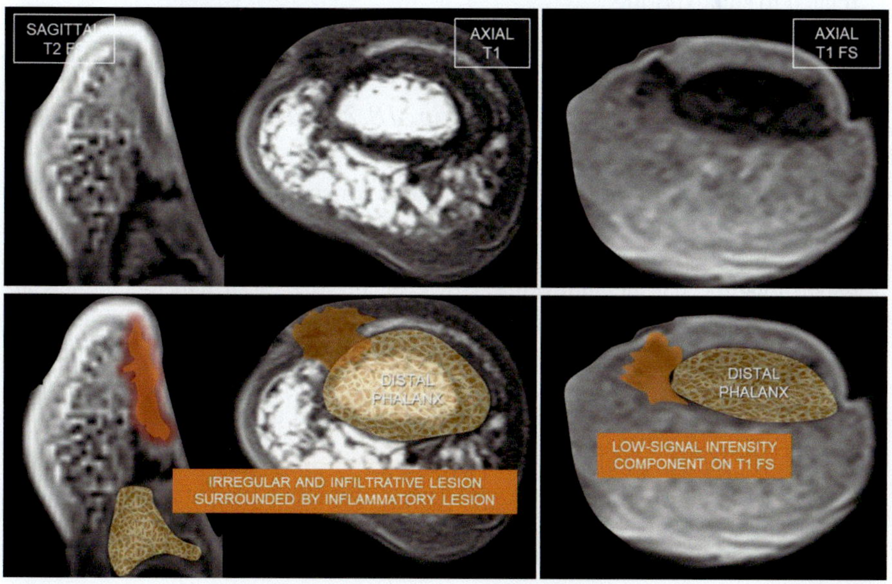

Fig. 18.72 MRI with surface coil findings of an espinocelular carcinoma in T1, T1 FS and T2 FS weighted sequences after gadolinium administration (Magnetom Prisma 3T MRI, Siemens)

18.15 Melanoma

18.15.1 Definition [103–105]

- Uncommon type of cutaneous melanoma with a poor prognosis.

18.15.2 Epidemiology [104–106]

- Between the ages of 50 and 70 years.
- Reported incidences between 0.7% and 3.5% of all melanoma.
- Incidence rates from 0.31% to 1.5% in Caucasian populations, with a relative frequency of up to 20% among all melanomas in Africans and Asians.
- Most nail melanomas appear to arise from abnormal nail matrix melanocytes. It has a predilection for the thumb and the hallux.
- Unlike cutaneous malignant melanoma, nail melanoma does not appear to be related to sun exposure.

18.15.3 Clinical Presentation (Fig. 18.73) [107, 108]

- Nail melanomas originate in the nail matrix, which houses the primary melanocytes in the nail unit.
- Approximately two-thirds of cases manifest clinically as a pigmented nail streak, called longitudinal melanonychia. However, up to 25% of nail melanomas are amelanotic, presenting as pink, red, or flesh-colored papules or longitudinal erythronychia. These may be accompanied by onycholysis, notching, splitting, bleeding, or ulceration.
- The ABCDEF rule of nail melanoma aids in clinical evaluation, although it has not been formally validated:
  - A: Age (peak incidence is 50–70 years), and ethnicity (African Americans, Asians, and Native Americans).
  - B: Bands with breadth >3 mm, Brown-black discoloration, and irregular Borders.
  - C: Change.
  - D: Digit most commonly involved (thumb > hallux > index finger).
  - E: Extension of pigment.
  - F: Family history of melanoma or dysplastic nevi.

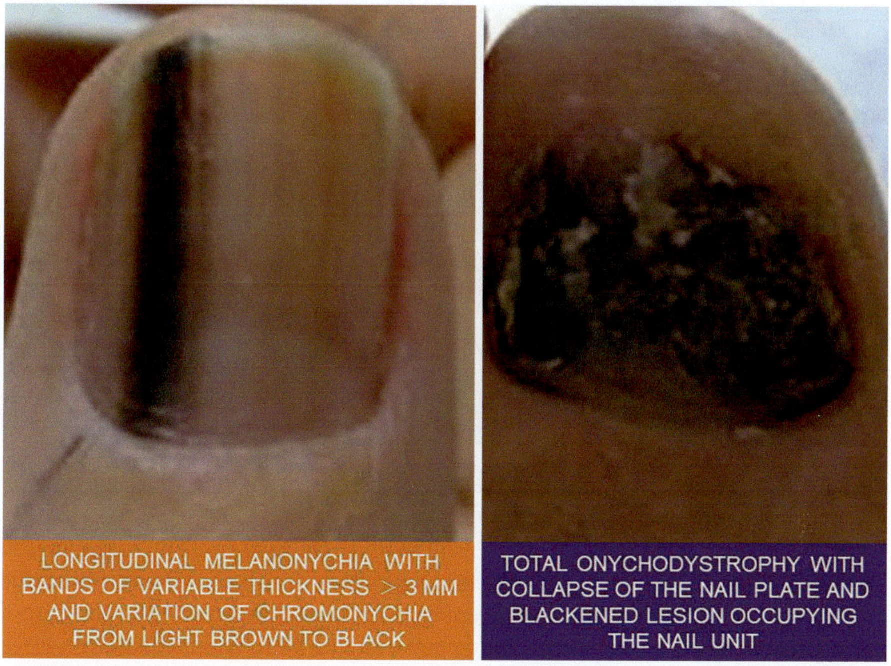

Fig. 18.73 Clinical photograph of a patient with a nail melanoma

- Additional concerning features include:
  - Color band heterogeneity.
  - Darkening or widening of bands.
  - Triangular band shape.
  - Purulence or bleeding.
  - Nail splitting.
  - Hutchinson's sign is characterized by pigment extension into the adjacent skin of the nail folds.

18.15.4 Onychoscopy (Fig. 18.74) [103, 106–108]

- Longitudinal melanonychia:
  - Width of the pigmented band covering more than two-thirds of the nail plate.
  - Gray and black coloration.
  - Irregularly pigmented lines.

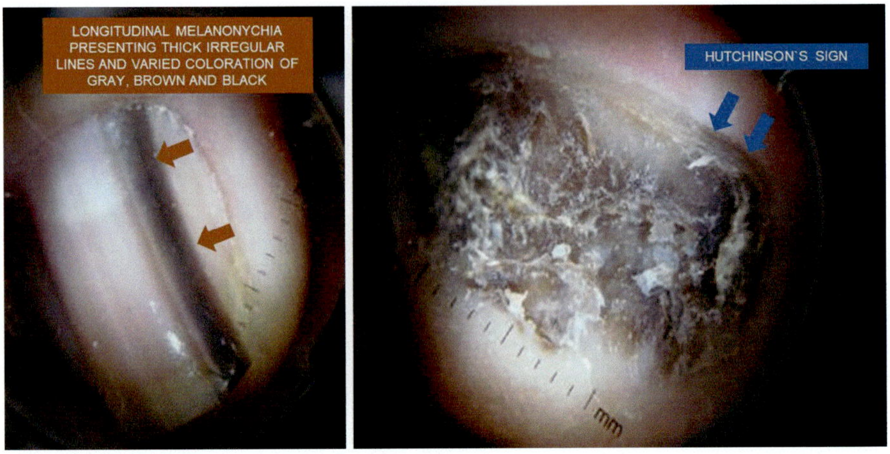

Fig. 18.74 Dermoscopy of a patient with a nail melanoma (x20)

- Hutchinson's and micro-Hutchinson's signs: In cases where pigmentation extends to the hyponychium, dermoscopy helps distinguish pigmentation due to melanocytic nevi (linear pigmentation in furrows or across skin lines) from Hutchinson's sign (disorderly pigmentation in a parallel ridge pattern).
- Nail dystrophy.
- Granular pigmentation.

- Free edge of the nail plate:
  - Pigmentation on the dorsum of the nail plate suggests a lesion originating from the proximal nail matrix.
  - Pigmentation on the lower part of the nail edge indicates a lesion of the distal matrix.
- Amelanotic nail melanoma:
  - Eroded nodules or granulated masses on the nail bed.
  - Whitish to milky-red veils or peripheral yellow-to-brown scaling and crusts.
  - Vascular polymorphisms with irregular vessels.

18.15.5 Histopathology (Fig. 18.75) [104, 109]

- In nail melanoma, the nail plate typically exhibits abundant diffuse melanin deposition. Histologically, sections from the matrix and nail bed reveal a melanocytic lesion characterized by:

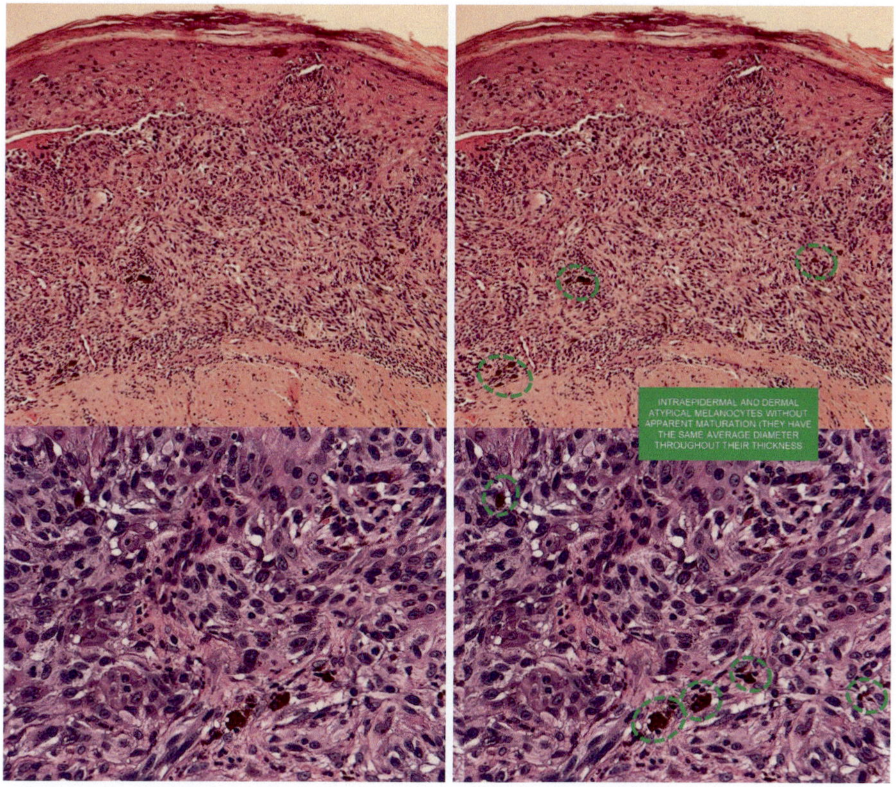

Fig. 18.75 Histological findings of a nail melanoma (H&E x4 and x10)

- Poor circumscription.
- Predominantly single-celled growth pattern.
- Pagetoid dispersion.
- Junctional nesting and confluence.
- Presence of epithelioid and dendritic cytomorphology in most cases.
- Nuclear atypia and conspicuous nucleoli, which may be subtle.

- Immunohistochemistry using markers such as Melan-A and SOX10 can be valuable in delineating the extent and pattern of the melanocytic lesion and confirming or ruling out dermal invasion. Proliferative markers like Ki-67 may also be utilized to highlight an increased proliferative index in the lesion.

18.15.6 Radiography and Computed Tomography

- Bone cortical irregularity, erosion, and periosteal reaction when distal phalanx is involved.

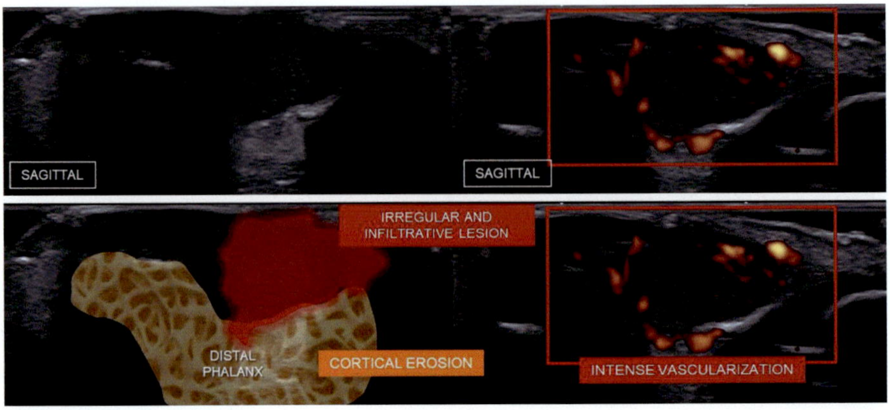

Fig. 18.76 Ultrasonographic findings of a nail melanoma with a 24 MHz probe (Aplio i800, Canon Medical Systems)

18.15.7 Ultrasonography (Fig. 18.76) [110, 111]

- In the early stages, it may present only as thickening and increased vascularity of the nail bed.
- Poorly defined heterogeneous and hypoechoic lesion with irregular appearence and infiltrative pattern
- Hypervascularization on power Doppler imaging.
- Erosion of the nail plates and distal phalanx.

18.15.8 MRI (Fig. 18.77) [112]

- The lesion on the nail bed appears poorly defined and heterogeneous.
- It shows mild high signal intensity on T1-weighted images, attributed to the melanocytic component, and high signal intensity on T2-weighted and STIR images.
- There is intense contrast enhancement observed after gadolinium administration.
- Erosion of the nail plates and distal phalanx is evident.

18.15.9 3D Images

- Highly beneficial for effectively managing challenging recurrent cases.
- A physical model can depict the lesion's asymmetric growth pattern, its relationship with the nail matrix and bed, and any associated bone changes.

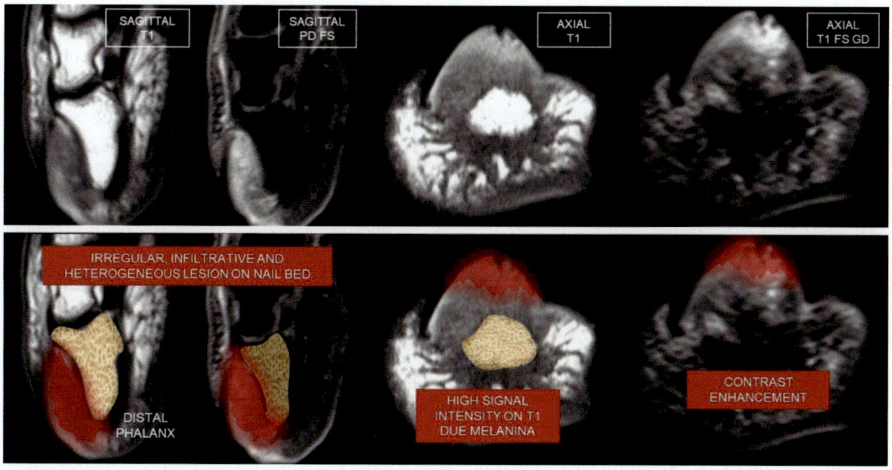

Fig. 18.77 MRI with surface coil findings of a nail melanoma in T1, PD FS and T1 FS weighted sequences after gadolinium administration (Magnetom Prisma 3T MRI, Siemens)

- Biomodels can produce physical replicas of the affected area, offering visual aids that aid in both surgical planning and patient education.

References

1. Gombos Z, Zhang PJ. Glomus tumor. Arch Pathol Lab Med. 2008;132:1448–52.
2. Sethu C, Sethu A. Glomus tumour. Ann R Coll Surg Engl. 2016;98:e1–2.
3. McDermott EM, Weiss A-PC. Glomus tumors. J Hand Surg Am. 2006;31A:1397–400. http://journals.sagepub.com/doi/10.1177/000331975000100601.
4. Netscher DT, Aburto J, Koepplinger M. Subungual glomus tumor. J Hand Surg. 2012;37:821–3. https://doi.org/10.1016/j.jhsa.2011.10.026.
5. Santoshi JA, Kori VK, Khurana U. Glomus tumor of the fingertips: a frequently missed diagnosis. J Family Med Prim Care. 2019;8:904–8. http://www.jfmpc.com/article.asp?issn=2249-4863;year=2017;volume=6;issue=1;spage=169;epage=170;aulast=Faizi.
6. Nazerani S, Motamedi MHK, Keramati MR. Diagnosis and management of glomus tumors of the hand. Tech Hand Up Extrem Surg. 2010;14:8–13.
7. Bhaskaranand K, Navadgi BC. Glomus tumour of the hand. J Hand Surg. 2002;27B:229–31.
8. Van Geertruyden J, Lorea P, Goldschimidt D, de Fontaine S, Schuind F, Kinnen L, et al. Glomus tumours of the hand. J Hand Surg. 1996;21:257–60.
9. Vieira FG, Nakamura R, Costa FM, Canella C, Marchiori E. Subungual glomus tumor. J Clin Rheumatol. 2016;22:331. http://journals.lww.com/00124743-201609000-00009.
10. Sprinkle RLB, Sangueza OP, Schwartz GA. Glomus tumor of the toe. J Am Podiatr Med Assoc. 2017;107:257–60. https://meridian.allenpress.com/japma/article/107/3/257/152324/Glomus-Tumor-of-the-ToeAn-Anatomical-Variant.
11. Baran R, Dawber RPR, de Berker DAR, Tosti A. Baran and Dawber's diseases of the nails and their management. New York: Wiley; 2008.
12. Maehara LDSN, Ohe EMD, Enokihara MY, Michalany NS, Yamada S, Hirata SH. Diagnóstico do tumor glômico pela dermatoscopia do leito e da matriz ungueal. An Bras Dermatol. 2010;85:236–8.

13. Starace M, Rubin AI, Di Chiacchio NG, Pampaloni F, Alessandrini A, Piraccini BM, et al. Diagnosis and surgical treatment of benign nail unit tumors. J Dtsch Dermatol Ges. 2023;21:116–29.
14. Alessandrini A, Starace M, Piraccini BM. Dermoscopy in the evaluation of nail disorders. Skin Appendage Disord. 2017;3:70–82.
15. Barnhill RL, Neil Crowson A, Magro CM, Piepkorn MW, Kutzner H, Desman GT. Barnhill's Dermatopathology. 4th ed. New York: McGraw Hill/Medical; 2019. [cited 2024 Aug 3]. https://dermatology.mhmedical.com/content.aspx?bookid=2802&sectionid=238125236.
16. Nakamura R, Baran R, da Unha D. Do Diagnostico ao Tratamento. 2a edição ed. Rio de Janeiro: Elsevier; 2018.
17. Glazebrook KN, Laundre BJ, Schiefer TK, Inwards CY. Imaging features of glomus tumors. Skeletal Radiol. 2011;40:855–62.
18. Gandhi J, Yang SS, Hurd J. The anatomic location of digital glomus tumor recurrences. J Hand Surg. 2010;35:986–9.
19. Ávila de Almeida C, Guarçoni S, Leverone A, Nakamura R, Marchiori E, Canella C. Characterization of a glomus tumor using 33-MHz ultrasound and superb microvascular imaging. Skin Res Technol. 2021;27(3):466–8.
20. de Almeida CÁ, Nakamura R, Leverone A, Marchiori E, Canella C. High-frequency ultrasonography for subungual glomus tumor evaluation—imaging findings. Skeletal Radiol. 2024;53:891–8.
21. Mundada P, Becker M, Lenoir V, Stefanelli S, Rougemont A-L, Beaulieu JY, et al. High resolution MRI of nail tumors and tumor-like conditions. Eur J Radiol. 2019;112:93–105. https://linkinghub.elsevier.com/retrieve/pii/S0720048X1930004X.
22. Kint A, Baran R, De KH. Acquired (digital) fibrokeratoma. J Am Acad Dermatol. 1985;12:816–21.
23. Navea OV, Navea MB, De la Fuente R. Acquired digital fibrokeratoma. Cureus. 2023.
24. Shih S, Khachemoune A. Acquired digital fibrokeratoma: review of its clinical and dermoscopic features and differential diagnosis. Int J Dermatol. 2019;58:151–8.
25. Rubin AI, Jellinek NJ, Ralph Daniel C, Scher RK. Scher and Daniel's nails: diagnosis, surgery, therapy. 4th ed. Berlin: Springer; 2018.
26. Rubegni P, Poggiali S, Lamberti A, Chiantini A, De Paola M, Peccianti C, et al. Dermoscopy of acquired digital fibrokeratoma. Australas J Dermatol. 2012;53:47–8.
27. Haneke E. Histopathology of the nail—onychopathology. Boca Raton, FL: CRC Press; 2017. https://www.taylorfrancis.com/books/9781351729840.
28. Singh R, Bryson D, Singh HP, Jeyapalan K, Dias JJ. High-resolution ultrasonography in assessment of nail-related disorders. Skeletal Radiol. 2012;41:1251–61.
29. Aluja Jaramillo F, Quiasúa Mejía DC, Martínez Ordúz HM, González Ardila C. Nail unit ultrasound: a complete guide of the nail diseases. J Ultrasound. 2017;20:181–92. http://link.springer.com/10.1007/s40477-017-0253-6.
30. Wortsman X, Jemec GBE. Ultrasound imaging of nails. Dermatol Clin. 2006;24:323–8. https://linkinghub.elsevier.com/retrieve/pii/S0733863506000283.
31. Lafreniere A-S, Misati G, Knox A. Approach to nail trauma for primary care physicians. Can Fam Physician. 2023;69:609–13.
32. Gungor F, Akyol KC, Eken C, Kesapli M, Beydilli I, Akcimen M. The value of point-of-care ultrasound for detecting nail bed injury in ED. Am J Emerg Med. 2016;34:1850–4. https://doi.org/10.1016/j.ajem.2016.06.067.
33. Piraccini BM, Bellavista S, Misciali C, Tosti A, De Berker D, Richert B. Periungual and subungual pyogenic granuloma. Br J Dermatol. 2010;163:941–53.
34. Lopez-Castillo D, Curto-Barredo L, Sánchez-Schmidt J, Pujol R. Multiple eruptive pyogenic granulomas on the proximal nail folds following cast immobilization: a case report with nail unit ultrasound findings. Acta Dermato Venereologica. 2020;100:adv00071-2. https://medicaljournalssweden.se/actadv/article/view/1914.
35. Hare AQ, Rich P. Nail tumors. Dermatol Clin. 2021;39:281–92.

36. Zychowska M. Dermoscopic rainbow pattern—now also in pyogenic granuloma. Int J Dermatol. 2020;59:369–70.
37. Zaballos P, Carulla M, Ozdemir F, Zalaudek I, Bañuls J, Llambrich Á, et al. Dermoscopy of pyogenic granuloma: a morphological study. Br J Dermatol. 2010;163:1229–37.
38. Zaballos P, Llambrich Á, Cuéllar F, Puig S, Malvehy J. Dermoscopic findings in pyogenic granuloma. Br J Dermatol. 2006;154:1108–11.
39. Baran G. Distal digital keratoacanthoma: a report of 12 cases and a review of the literature. Br J Dermatol. 1998;139:512–5.
40. González-Rodríguez AJ, Gutiérrez-Paredes EM, Montesinos-Villaescusa E, Burgués Gasión O, Jordá-Cuevas E. Queratoacantoma digital distal: importancia del diagnóstico diferencial con el carcinoma escamoso subungueal. Actas Dermosifiliogr. 2012;103:549–51.
41. Choi JH, Shin DH, Shin DS, Cho KH. Subungual keratoacanthoma: ultrasound and magnetic resonance imaging findings. Skeletal Radiol. 2007;36:769–72. http://link.springer.com/10.1007/s00256-007-0274-x.
42. Whitehouse HJ, Urwin R, Stables G. Traumatic subungual neuroma. Clin Exp Dermatol. 2018;43:65–6.
43. Choi R, Kim SR, Glusac EJ, Zubek A. Subungual neuroma masquerading as green nail syndrome. JAAD Case Rep. 2022;20:17–9.
44. Forte AJ, Boczar D, Oliver JD, Sisti A, Clendenen SR. Ultra-high-frequency ultrasound to assess nerve fascicles in median nerve traumatic neuroma. Cureus. 2019;11(6):e4871.
45. Wortsman X, Merino D, Catalan V, Morales C, Baran R. Perineurioma of the nail on sonography. J Ultrasound Med. 2010;29:1379–82.
46. Baran R, Perrin C. Localized multinucleate distal subungual keratosis. Br J Dermatol. 2006;133:77–82. https://academic.oup.com/bjd/article/133/1/77/6681911.
47. Starace M, Alessandrini A, Ferrari T, Wong V, Baraldi C, Piraccini BM. Clinical and onychoscopic features of histopathologically proven onychopapillomas and literature update. J Cutan Pathol. 2022;49:147–52.
48. Kim T, Bae K, Son J, Shin K, Kim H, Ko H, et al. Onychopapilloma: its clinical, dermoscopic, and pathologic features. J Eur Acad Dermatol Venereol. 2022;36(11):2235–40. https://onlinelibrary.wiley.com/doi/10.1111/jdv.18461.
49. Tambe S, Ansari SM, Nayak C, Chokkar R, Patil P. Surgical management of onychopapilloma, onychomatricoma, and subungual osteochondroma: case series. J Cutan Aesthet Surg. 2018;11:143.
50. Sarkissian L, Fattouh K, Kanitakis J, Villani A-P. DeRmpath clinic: onychopapilloma. Eur J Dermatol. 2017;27:336–7.
51. Delvaux C, Richert B, Lecerf P, André J. Onychopapillomas: a 68-case series to determine best surgical procedure and histologic sectioning. J Eur Acad Dermatol Venereol. 2018;32:2025–30.
52. Tosti A, Schneider SL, Ramirez-Quizon MN, Zaiac M, Miteva M. Clinical, dermoscopic, and pathologic features of onychopapilloma: a review of 47 cases. J Am Acad Dermatol. 2016;74:521–6.
53. Mattioli MA, Aromolo IF, Spigariolo CB, Marzano AV, Nazzaro G. Sonographic features of onychopapilloma: a single center retrospective observational study. J Clin Med. 2023;12:1795.
54. Canella C, Nakamura R, Leverone A, de Almeida CÁ, Iorizzo M, Yamada AF. Ultrasound imaging of onychopapilloma: evaluation of 43 cases. Eur J Radiol. 2024;170:111236.
55. Baran R, Kint A. Onychomatrixoma. Filamentous tufted tumour in the matrix of a funnel-shaped nail: a new entity (report of three cases). Br J Dermatol. 1992;126:510–5.
56. Lee D, Park J, Shin H, Yang J, Jang K, Kwon GY, et al. The presence and localization of onychodermis (specialized nail mesenchyme) containing onychofibroblasts in the nail unit: a morphological and immunohistochemical study. Histopathology. 2012;61:123–30.
57. Di Chiacchio N, Tavares GT, Padoveze EH, Bet DL, Gioia N, Chiacchio D. Onychomatricoma. Surg Cosmet Dermatol. 2013;5:10–4.

58. Fayol J, Baran R, Perrin C, Labrousse F. Onychomatricoma with misleading features. Acta Derm Venereol. 2000;80:370–2.
59. Lesort C, Debarbieux S, Duru G, Dalle S, Poulhalon N, Thomas L. Dermoscopic features of onychomatricoma: a study of 34 cases. Dermatology. 2015;231:177–83.
60. Ginoux E, Perier Muzet M, Poulalhon N, Debarbieux S, Dalle S, Thomas L. Intraoperative dermoscopic features of onychomatricoma: a review of 10 cases. Clin Exp Dermatol. 2017;42:395–9.
61. Di Chiacchio N, Tavares GT, Tosti A, Di Chiacchio NG, Di Santis E, Alvarenga L, et al. Onychomatricoma: epidemiological and clinical findings in a large series of 30 cases. Br J Dermatol. 2015;173:1305–7.
62. Okon LG, Saedi N, Schwartz L, Lee JB. A case of onychomatricoma: classic clinical, dermoscopic, and nail-clipping histologic findings. J Am Acad Dermatol. 2017;76:S19–21.
63. Chiheb S, Slimani Y, Karam R, Marnissi F, Hali F. Subungual exostosis: a case series of 48 patients. Skin Appendage Disord. 2021;7:475–9.
64. Perez-Palma L, Manzanares-Cespedes MC, de Veciana EG. Subungual exostosis systematic review and meta-analysis laura. J Am Podiatr Med Assoc. 2018;108:412. https://linkinghub.elsevier.com/retrieve/pii/S002234761400300X.
65. Zhang W, Gu L, Fan H, Shen X, Lu H. Subungual exostosis with an unusual dermoscopic feature. JAAD Case Rep. 2020;6:725–6.
66. Piccolo V, Argenziano G, Alessandrini AM, Russo T, Starace M, Piraccini BM. Dermoscopy of subungual exostosis: a retrospective study of 10 patients. Dermatology. 2017;233:80–5.
67. Piccolo V, Russo T, de Rezende LL, Argenziano G. Subungual exostosis in an 8-year-old child: clinical and dermoscopic description. An Bras Dermatol. 2019;94:233–5.
68. Sankar B, Ng BY, Hopgood P, Banks AJ. Subungual exostosis following toe nail removal—case report. Int J Clin Pract. 2005;59:132–3.
69. Singh R, Jain M, Goel R, Siwach R, Kalra R, Kaur K. Subungual exostosis of the great toe: a case report and tumor overview. Foot Ankle Spec. 2011;4:376–8.
70. Baek HJ, Lee SJ, Cho KH, Choo HJ, Lee SM, Lee YH, et al. Subungual tumors: clinicopathologic correlation with US and MR imaging findings. Radiographics. 2010;30:1621–36. http://pubs.rsna.org/doi/10.1148/rg.306105514.
71. Whittle C, Aguirre J, Catalán V, Fajre X, Vargas F. Subungual exostosis: high-resolution ultrasound findings. J Diagn Med Sonogr. 2019;35:387–90. http://journals.sagepub.com/doi/10.1177/8756479319836943.
72. Kolb L, Naga Yarrarapu SS, Atif Ameer M, Rosario-Collazo JA. Lipoma. In: StatPearls. Treasure Island, FL: StatPearls Publishing; 2023. https://www.ncbi.nlm.nih.gov/books/NBK507906/?report=printable.
73. Vélez NF, Telang GH, Robinson-Bostom L, Jellinek NJ. Subungual lipoma. Dermatologic Surg. 2014;40:1435–7.
74. Bardazzi F, Savoia F, Fanti PA. Subungual lipoma. Br J Dermatol. 2003;149:418. https://academic.oup.com/bjd/article/149/2/418/6635316.
75. Johnson CN, Ha AS, Chen E, Davidson D. Lipomatous soft-tissue tumors. J Am Acad Orthop Surg. 2018;26:779–88. https://journals.lww.com/00124635-201811150-00001.
76. Richert B, André J, Choffray A, Rahier S, De La Brassinne M. Periungual lipoma: about three cases. J Am Acad Dermatol. 2004;51:91–3.
77. Cunha N, De Sousa VC, Pinheiro R, Lencastre A. And next… adnexa: subungual lipoma. Eur J Dermatol. 2017;27:448–9.
78. Burt AM, Huang BK. Imaging review of lipomatous musculoskeletal lesions. SICOT J. 2017;3:34. http://www.sicot-j.org/10.1051/sicotj/2017015.
79. Le Nail L-R, Crenn V, Rosset P, Ropars M. Management of adipose tumors in the limbs. Orthop Traumatol Surg Res. 2022;108:103162.
80. Li K, Barankin B. Digital mucous cysts. J Cutan Med Surg. 2010;14(5):199–206.
81. De Berker D, Goettman S, Baran R. Subungual myxoid cysts: clinical manifestations and response to therapy. J Am Acad Dermatol. 2002;46:394–8.

82. Yamashita Y, Nagae H, Yamato R, Sedo H, Abe Y, Hashimoto I. Proximal nail fold flap for digital mucous cyst excision. J Med Investig. 2016;63:278–80. https://www.jstage.jst.go.jp/article/jmi/63/3.4/63_278/_article.
83. Salerni G, González R, Alonso C. Dermatoscopic pattern of digital mucous cyst: report of three cases. Dermatol Pract Concept. 2014;4:65.
84. Ashby-Richardson H, Rogers GS, Stadecker MJ. Superficial acral fibromyxoma: an overview. Arch Pathol Lab Med. 2011;135:1064–6.
85. Sechi A, Wortsman X. High-frequency ultrasound features of periungual superficial acral fibromyxomas. J Cutan Med Surg. 2023;27:536–8.
86. Lacroix M, Burns R, Campagna R, Larousserie F, Drapé JL. Acral fibromyxoma: findings on dynamic contrast-enhanced perfusion MRI. Diagn Interv Imaging. 2022;103:59–61.
87. Lee T, Jo G, Kim M, Lee S, Cho SI, Jo SJ, et al. Squamous cell carcinoma of the nail unit: a retrospective review of 19 cases in Asia and comparative review of Western literature. Int J Dermatol. 2019;58:428–32.
88. Cogrel O, Beylot-Barry M, Doutre M-S. Maladie de Bowen unguéale revelée par une érythronychie longitudinale. Ann Dermatol Venereol. 2008;135:883–5.
89. Haneke E. Important malignant and new nail tumors. J Dtsch Dermatol Ges. 2017;15:367–86.
90. Ghariani Fetoui N, Mokni S, Aounallah A, Ghariani N, Belajouza C, Boussofara L, et al. Bowen disease of the nailfold: dermoscopic diagnosis. Int J Dermatol. 2019;58:e252–3.
91. Baran R, Perrin C. Longitudinal erythronychia with distal subungual keratosis:onychopapilloma of the nail bed and Bowen's disease. Br J Dermatol. 2000;143(1):132–5.
92. Ishizuki S, Nakamura Y, Maruyama H, Okiyama N, Tanaka R, Oya K, et al. Pigmented Bowen's disease on the proximal nail fold with extensive, parallel pigmented lines in dermoscopy. J Dermatol. 2021;48:e88–9.
93. Perruchoud DL, Varonier C, Haneke E, Hunger RE, Beltraminelli H, Borradori L, et al. Bowen disease of the nail unit: a retrospective study of 12 cases and their association with human papillomaviruses. J Eur Acad Dermatol Venereol. 2016;30:1503–6.
94. Li M, Wang Q, Li X, Zhao C, Zhu R, Chen J, et al. Imaging findings of Bowen's disease: a comparison between ultrasound biomicroscopy and conventional high-frequency ultrasound. Skin Res Technol. 2020;26:654–63.
95. Starace M, Alessandrini A, Dika E, Piraccini BM. Squamous cell carcinoma of the nail unit. Dermatol Pract Concept. 2018;8:238–44.
96. de Sousa Padilha CB, de Almeida Balassiano LK, Pinto JC, de Souza FCS, Kac BK, Treu CM. Subungual squamous cell carcinoma. An Bras Dermatol. 2016;91:817–9.
97. Kok WL, Lee JSS, Chio MT. Subungual squamous cell carcinoma: the diagnostic challenge and clinical pearls. Case Rep Dermatol. 2016;8:272–7.
98. Haenssle H, Blum A, Hofmann-Wellenhof R, Kreusch J, Stolz W, Argenziano G, et al. When all you have is a dermatoscope—start looking at the nails. Dermatol Pract Concept. 2014;4:11–20.
99. Dijksterhuis A, Friedeman E, van der Heijden B. Squamous cell carcinoma of the nail unit: review of the literature. J Hand Surg Am. 2018;43:374–379.e2. https://doi.org/10.1016/j.jhsa.2018.01.010.
100. Teysseire S, Dalle S, Duru G, Phan A, Debarbieux S, Poulhalon N, et al. Dermoscopic features of subungual squamous cell carcinoma: a study of 44 cases. Dermatology. 2017;233:184–91.
101. Quintana-Codina M, Creus-Vila L, Iglesias-Plaza A, Iglesias-Sancho M, Melé-Ninot G, Lázaro-Simó AI, et al. Sonographic appearance of subungual squamous cell carcinoma in the hand. J Clin Ultrasound. 2018;46:212–4.
102. Sechi A, Alessandrini A, Patrizi A, Starace M, Caposiena Caro RD, Vara G, et al. Ultrasound features of the subungual glomus tumor and squamous cell carcinomas. Skin Res Technol. 2020;26:867–75. http://www.ncbi.nlm.nih.gov/pubmed/32585749.
103. Conway J, Bellet JS, Rubin AI, Lipner SR. Adult and pediatric nail unit melanoma: epidemiology, diagnosis, and treatment. Cells. 2023;12:964.

104. Carreño AM, Nakajima SR, Pennini SN, Candido Junior R, Schettini APM. Nail apparatus melanoma: a diagnostic opportunity. An Bras Dermatol. 2013;88:268–71.
105. Littleton TW, Murray PM, Baratz ME. Subungual melanoma. Orthop Clin N Am. 2019;50:357–66. https://doi.org/10.1016/j.ocl.2019.03.003.
106. Talavera-Belmonte A, Bonfill-Ortí M, Martínez-Molina L, Fornons-Servent R, Bauer-Alonso A, Ferreres-Riera JR, et al. Subungual melanoma: a descriptive study of 34 patients. Actas Dermosifiliogr. 2018;109:801–6. https://doi.org/10.1016/j.ad.2018.06.010.
107. Levit EK, Kagen MH, Scher RK, Grossman M, Altman E. The ABC rule for clinical detection of subungual melanoma. J Am Acad Dermatol. 2000;42:269–74.
108. Lieberherr S, Cazzaniga S, Haneke E, Hunger RE, Seyed Jafari SM. Melanoma of the nail apparatus: a systematic review and meta-analysis of current challenges and prognosis. J Eur Acad Dermatol Venereol. 2020;34:967–76.
109. Izumi M, Ohara K, Hoashi T, Nakayama H, Chiu C, Nagai T, et al. Subungual melanoma: histological examination of 50 cases from early stage to bone invasion. J Dermatol. 2008;35:695–703.
110. Guitera P, Li LX, Crotty K, Fitzgerald P, Mellenbergh R, Pellacani G, et al. Melanoma histological Breslow thickness predicted by 75-MHz ultrasonography. Br J Dermatol. 2008;159:364–9.
111. Hayashi K, Koga H, Uhara H, Saida T. High-frequency 30-MHz sonography in preoperative assessment of tumor thickness of primary melanoma: usefulness in determination of surgical margin and indication for sentinel lymph node biopsy. Int J Clin Oncol. 2009;14:426–30.
112. Seyed Jafari SM, Mazinani M, Beutler-Minth V, Lamos C, Heverhagen JT, Hunger RE, et al. Noncontrast-enhanced 3-Tesla MRI using surface coil as a complementary test for assessment of distribution and depth of locoregional cutaneous metastases of malignant melanoma. Melanoma Res. 2022;32:211–7. https://journals.lww.com/10.1097/CMR.0000000000000828.

Index

© The Editor(s) (if applicable) and The Author(s), under exclusive license to Springer Nature Switzerland AG 2025

C. Canella Moraes do Carmo (ed.), *Atlas of Diagnostic Imaging in Dermatology*,
https://doi.org/10.1007/978-3-031-77987-9

V

W

X